# Handbook of Plant and Animal Toxins in Food

# Handbook of Plant and Animal Toxins in Food

## Occurrence, Toxicity, and Prevention

Edited by

Gulzar Ahmad Nayik and Jasmeet Kour

CRC Press
Taylor & Francis Group
Boca Raton London New York

CRC Press is an imprint of the
Taylor & Francis Group, an **informa** business

First edition published 2022
by CRC Press
6000 Broken Sound Parkway NW, Suite 300, Boca Raton, FL 33487-2742

and by CRC Press
2 Park Square, Milton Park, Abingdon, Oxon, OX14 4RN

*CRC Press is an imprint of Taylor & Francis Group, LLC*



Library of Congress Cataloging-in-Publication Data
Names: Nayik, Gulzar Ahmad, editor. | Kour, Jasmeet, editor.
Title: Handbook of plant and animal toxins in food : occurrence, toxicity, and prevention / edited by Gulzar Ahmad Nayik & Jasmeet Kour.
Description: First edition. | Boca Raton : CRC Press, 2022. | Includes bibliographical references and index.
Identifiers: LCCN 2021048211 (print) | LCCN 2021048212 (ebook) | ISBN 9781032013954 (hardback) | ISBN 9781032013961 (paperback) | ISBN 9781003178446 (ebook)
Subjects: LCSH: Food--Toxicology. | Toxins.
Classification: LCC RA1258 .H365 2022 (print) | LCC RA1258 (ebook) | DDC 615.9/54--dc23/eng/20211220
LC record available at https://lccn.loc.gov/2021048211
LC ebook record available at https://lccn.loc.gov/2021048212

ISBN: 978-1-032-01395-4 (hbk)
ISBN: 978-1-032-01396-1 (pbk)
ISBN: 978-1-003-17844-6 (ebk)

DOI: 10.1201/9781003178446

Typeset in Times
by Deanta Global Publishing Services, Chennai, India

*Dedicated to our Beloved Family*

# Contents

# Preface

Food provides an ample amount of nutrients, and nutrients, in turn, provide energy for growth, activity, and to carry out pivotal functions of the body, including strengthening the immune system. Food has also been acknowledged as a reservoir of components concerning public health. It is a prerequisite for the survival of living organisms, followed by oxygen and water. Apart from this, the furtherance in science and technology has led to an impeccable improvement in the quality of food in various pivotal aspects. A significant amount of attention is drawn nowadays towards various scientific efforts aimed at designing functional food products embedded with health as well as nutrition. Nevertheless, while food is a storehouse of various natural chemicals such as carbohydrates, sugars, proteins, and vitamins, some foods possess potentially harmful natural toxins. A toxin may be identified according to its chemical structure, physiological expression induced in the animal body, and some kind of activity by which it can be recognized in the test-tube. These toxins, occurring naturally in food, act as defence mechanisms of several plants.

Owing to the ingress of modern and sophisticated analytical techniques, these toxicants in foods have become a hot-button issue. For a long time, the detection of toxins or poisons in foods was based on a trial-and-error method. Another noticeable feature is that these toxicants are also generated by natural origin apart from not highly industrialized society. Plants are credited with the production of a plethora of secondary metabolites with chemical structures varying from simpler ones, such as organic chemicals, to complex ones, such as proteins. These secondary plant metabolites have been reported for the outbreaks of deleterious health effects in humans and animals. They have been developed as an evolutionary response for self-protection. There is a dearth of human data available, although many inherent plant toxicants result in serious outbreaks or intoxication. The symptoms of ill health effects range from itching, nausea, and vomiting, to teratogenicity, arrhythmias, and psychosis. It is the chemical structure which defines the word toxicity, thereby making it highly substance-specific. The major mode of their action is by manipulation with enzymes, receptors, and even genetic material at particular cells and tissues.

In addition to plant toxins, animal toxins are an array of complex polypeptides, enzymes, and chemicals, leading to various physiological and pharmacological disturbances. These inherent animal toxins are highly toxic and have to be managed effectively to ensure food safety. This book elucidates various notable natural plant and animal toxicants which pose a special threat since their elimination is not readily acted upon by legislative action, which is not the case in chemicals intentionally incorporated in foods. One of the major highlighting features of this book is to accentuate the attention of food production and food safety personnel. The book has not only covered manifold naturally occurring toxic substances but has also tried to uncover hidden areas which require detailed evaluation. The entire material presented in this work is the collaboration of several experts in their distinguished fields. The expectations are that the entire information gathered will prove to be fulfilling in all the aspects with respect to uniqueness and usefulness for researchers, academicians, food toxicologists, and food scientists. This work will indeed be a boon in helping the general public to analyse efficiently the severity of prominent toxic constituents in plant- and animal-derived foods.

**Dr Gulzar Ahmad Nayik**
**Dr Jasmeet Kour**

# About the Editors

**Dr Gulzar Ahmad Nayik** completed his master's degree in food technology from Islamic University of Science & Technology, Awantipora, Jammu and Kashmir, India and PhD from Sant Longowal Institute of Engineering & Technology, Sangrur, Punjab, India. He has published more than 55 peer-reviewed research and review papers, 30 book chapters, edited 2 books with Springer Nature, published 1 book with Elsevier, and has delivered numerous presentations in various national and international conferences, seminars, workshops, and webinars. Dr Nayik was shortlisted twice for the prestigious Inspire-Faculty Award in 2017 and 2018 from Indian National Science Academy, New Delhi. He was nominated for India's prestigious National Award (Indian National Science Academy Medal for Young Scientists – 2019–2020). Dr Nayik also fills the roles of editor, associate editor, assistant editor, and reviewer for many food science and technology journals. He has received many awards, appreciations, and recognitions, and holds membership in various international societies and organizations. Dr Nayik is currently editing several book projects with Elsevier, Taylor & Francis, Springer, and Royal Society of Chemistry.

**Dr Jasmeet Kour** completed her master's degree in food science and technology from Government College for Women, Gandhi Nagar, Jammu, Jammu and Kashmir, India. She earned a doctoral degree at Sant Longowal Institute of Engineering and Technology, Longowal, Sangrur, Punjab, India from Department of Food Engineering and Technology in 2019. She has been serving as an assistant professor at the Department of Food Science and Technology, Government College for Women, Gandhi Nagar, Jammu, Jammu and Kashmir since 2009. She has conducted her vast research in various prominent nutraceuticals derived from plant origins and her work has been published in reputed journals with high-impact factors in eminent publishing houses in the field of food science. She has presented her research and reviewed paper presentations in various national and international conferences. She has authored as well as co-authored numerous book chapters and scientific articles published with international publishers Elsevier and Springer. She is also a part of various international projects. As a result of her impressive research work, she was cordially invited to share her newest research findings at Tokyo University of Agriculture, Japan, at the 6th International Conference on Agricultural and Biological Sciences (ABS 2020). She is currently working as editorial board member and peer reviewer of various journals of repute.

# Contributors

**Sheikh Firdous Ahmad**
ICAR-Indian Veterinary Research Institute
Izatnagar, Bareilly
UP, India

**Saghir Ahmad**
Department of Post-Harvest Engineering and Technology
Aligarh Muslim University
Aligarh, India

**Taslima Ahmed**
Department of Applied Food Science and Nutrition
Chattogram Veterinary and Animal Sciences University (CVASU)
Chattogram, Bangladesh

**Nadira Anjum**
Division of Food Science and Technology
Sher-e- Kashmir University of Agriculture Sciences and Technology Chatha
Jammu, India

**Aayeena Altaf**
Department of Food Technology
Jamia Hamdard, (Deemed to be University)
New Delhi India

**Zanoor ul Ashraf**
Department of Food Science and Technology
University of Kashmir Hazratbal
Srinagar, India

**Kanwate Balaji**
Department of Meat and Marine Science
CSIR-Central Food Technological Research Institute
Mysore, India

**Usma Bashir**
Department of Food Science and Technology
University of Kashmir Hazratbal
Srinagar, India

**Anju Bhat**
Division of Food Science and Technology
Sher-e- Kashmir University of Agriculture Sciences and Technology Chatha
Jammu, India

**Mohd.Munaff Bhat**
Department of Food Science and Technology
University of Kashmir Hazratbal
Srinagar, India

**Bharat Bhushan**
ICAR-Indian Veterinary Research Institute
Izatnagar, India

**Sunanda Biswas**
Department of Food and Nutrition
Acharya Prafulla Chandra College
Kolkata, India

**Hitesh Chopra**
Chitkara College of Pharmacy
Chitkara University
Punjab, India

**Aamir Hussain Dar**
Department of Food Technology
Islamic University of Science and Technology
Awantipora, India

**Subhamoy Dhua**
Department of Food Engineering and Technology
Tezpur University
Assam, India

**Triveni Dutt**
ICAR-Indian Veterinary Research Institute
Izatnagar, India

**Rakesh Gehlot**
Centre of Food Science and Technology
CCS Haryana Agricultural University
Hisar India

**Arun Kumar Gupta**
Department of Food Engineering and Technology
Tezpur University
Assam, India

**Younis Ahmad Hajam**
Department Of Biosciences, Division Zoology
Career Point University
Hamirpur, India

**Fozia Hameed**
Division of Food Science and Technology
Sher-e- Kashmir University of Agriculture Sciences and Technology Chatha
Jammu, India

**Monika Hans**
Govt PG College for Women Gandhi Nagar
Jammu, India

**Makhdoom Ibad Ullah Hashmi**
Department of Chemical Engineering
Khwaja Fareed University of Engineering & Information Technology
Rahim Yar Khan, Pakistan

**Muzzamal Hussain**
Institute of Home & Food Sciences
Government College University Faisalabad
Faisalabad, Pakistan

**Ali Ikram**
Institute of Home & Food Sciences
Government College University
Faisalabad, Pakistan

**Avinash Kumar Jha**
Department of Food Engineering and Technology
Tezpur University
Assam, India

**Ghulam Mustafa Kamal**
Department of Chemistry
Khwaja Fareed University of Engineering & Information Technology
Rahim Yar Khan, Pakistan

**Jaspreet Kaur**
Guru Nanak College
Mansa, India

**Ramandeep Kaur**
Department of Food Science and Technology
Punjab Agricultural University
Ludhiana,India

**Mandeep Kaur**
Department of Agriculture
Mata Gujri College
Punjab, India

**Naveet Kaushal**
Department of Agriculture
Mata Gujri College
Fatehgarh Sahib, India

**Muhammad Khalid**
Department of Chemistry
Khwaja Fareed University of Engineering & Information Technology
Rahim Yar Khan, Pakistan

**Waseem Khalid**
Institute of Home & Food Sciences
Government College University Faisalabad
Faisalabad, Pakistan

**Shafat Ahmad Khan**
Department of Post-Harvest Engineering and Technology
Faculty of Agricultural Sciences
Aligarh Muslim University
Aligarh, India

**Jasmeet Kour**
Department of Food Engineering and Technology
Sant Longowal Institute of Engineering and Technology Longowal
Punjab, India.

**Harish Kumar**
Amity Institute of Biotechnology
Amity University Rajasthan
Jaipur, India

**Parveen Kumar**
Academy of Scientific and Innovative Research (AcSIR),
CSIR-Indian Institute of Integrative Medicine
Jammu, India

**Rajesh Kumar**
Department of Biosciences
Himachal Pradesh University
Himachal Pradesh, India

**Varun Kumar**
Department of Home Science
R.J.M.College, Saharsa- B.N.Mandal University Madhepura
Bihar, India

**Javid Ahmad Malik**
Department of Zoology
Guru Ghasidas Vishwavidayalaya
Bilaspur, India

**Tanu Malik**
Food Technology & Nutrition
Lovely Professional University
Punjab, India

**Manimozhi E**
ICAR-Central Institute of Fisheries Education
Mumbai, India

**Arshied Manzoor**
Department of Post-Harvest Engineering and Technology
Faculty of Agricultural Sciences
Aligarh Muslim University
Aligarh, India

**F.A. Masoodi**
Department of Food Science and Technology
University of Kashmir Hazratbal
Srinagar, India

**Bharti Mittu**
National Institute Pharmaceutical Education and Research
Mohali, India

**Pal Murugan**
Defence Food Research Laboratory
Mysuru, India

**Zahoor Mushtaq**
ICAR-Central Institute of Fisheries Education
Mumbai, India

**Sabeera Muzzaffar**
Department of Food Science and Technology
University of Kashmir Hazratbal
Srinagar, India

**Aarifa Nabi**
Plant Physiology Section, Department of Botany
Aligarh Muslim University
Aligarh, India

**Sanusi Shamsudeen Nassarawa**
College of Biosystem Engineering and Food Science
Zhejiang University
Hangzhou, Peoples Republic of China

and

Department of Food Science and Technology
Bayero University Kano
Kano, Nigeria

**Gulzar Ahmad Nayik**
Department of Food Science and Technology
Govt. Degree College
Shopian, India

**Sadaf Nazir**
Department of Food Science and Technology
University of Kashmir Hazratbal
Srinagar, India

**Tuyiba Nazir**
Department of Food Science and Technology
University of Kashmir, Hazratbal
Srinagar, India

**Panchi Rani Neog**
Department of Molecular Biology and Biotechnology
Tezpur University
Assam, India

**Snehasmita Panda**
ICAR-Indian Veterinary Research Institute
Izatnagar, India

**Manjit Panigrahi**
ICAR-Indian Veterinary Research Institute
Izatnagar, India

**Suraj P Parihar**
International Centre for Genetic Engineering & Biotechnology
Institute of Infectious Diseases & Molecular Medicine
Cape Town, South Africa

**Nafia Qadir**
Department of Food Science and Technology
University of Kashmir, Hazratbal
Srinagar, India

**Ubaid Qayoom**
ICAR-Central Institute of Fisheries Education
Mumbai, India

**Shafiya Rafiq**
Department of Food Science and Technology
Sher-e-Kashmir University of Agricultural Sciences and Technology, Chatha
Jammu, India

**Summira Rafiq**
Division of Entomology
Sher-e-Kashmir University of Agricultural Sciences and Technology of Kashmir
Shalimar Campus
Srinagar, India.

**Reshu Rajput**
Department of Food Science and Technology
Punjab Agricultural University
Punjab, India

**Breetha Ramaiyan**
Athletebit Healthcare Pvt. Ltd.,
CSIR-CFTRI Campus
Mysore, India

**Payal Rani**
Maharaja Ranjit Singh Punjab Technical University
Bathinda, India

**Raksha Rani**
Department of Biosciences, Division Zoology
Career Point University
Hamirpur, India

**Rajeev Ranjan**
Department of Dairy Science and Food Technology
Banaras Hindu University
Varanasi, India

**Muzamil Ahmad Rather**
Department of Molecular Biology and Biotechnology
Tezpur University
Assam, India

**Farhan Saeed**
Institute of Home & Food Sciences
Government College University Faisalabad
Faisalabad, Pakistan

**Charanjiv Singh Saini**
Department of Food Engineering and Technology
Sant Longowal Institute of Engineering & Technology
Longowal, India

**Mukul Sains**
Dairy Engineering Division
ICAR-NDRI
Haryana India

**Sangeeta**
Guru Nanak College
Budhlada, India

**Nazmul Sarwar**
Department of Food Processing and Engineering, Faculty of Food Science and Technology
Chattogram Veterinary and Animal Sciences University (CVASU)
Chattogram, Bangladesh

**Gifty Sawhney**
Inflammation Pharmacology Division
CSIR-Indian Institute of Integrative Medicine
Jammu, India.

**Anil Dutt Semwal**
Defence Food Research Laboratory
Mysuru, India

**Asma Shabir**
Department of Chemistry
Khwaja Fareed University of Engineering & Information Technology
Rahim Pakistan

**Harish Kumar Sharma**
Department of Chemical Engineering
National Institute of Technology
Agartala, India

**Ram Kumar Sharma**
ICAR-IARI, PUSA
New Delhi. India

**Renu Sharma**
Department of Applied Sciences
Bhai Gurdas Degree College
Sangrur, India

**Sakshi Sharma**
Defence Food Research Laboratory,
Mysuru, Karnataka India

**Abhinay Shashank**
Department of Dairy Science and Food Technology
Banaras Hindu University
Varanasi, India

**Mohd Aaqib Sheikh**
Department of Food Engineering and Technology
Sant Longowal Institute of Engineering & Technology
Longowal, Punjab, India

**Rayees Ahmad Shiekh**
Department of Chemistry
Government Degree College Pulwama
Srinagar, India

**Mukesh S. Sikarwar**
Unit of Pharmaceutical Chemistry
Faculty of Pharmacy
AIMST University
Semeling, Malaysia

**Somya Singhal**
Department of Food Engineering and Technology
Tezpur University
Assam, India

**Ajay Singh**
Department of Food Technology
Mata Gujri College
Fatehgarh Sahib, India

**Ajay Singh**
Department of Food Technology
Mata Gujri College
Punjab, India

**Arashdeep Singh**
Department of Food Science and Technology
Punjab Agricultural University
Ludhiana, India

**Sukriti Singh**
Department of Food Technology
Uttaranchal University
Dehradun, India

**Talwinder Singh**
Department of Agriculture
Mata Gujri College
Fatehgarh Sahib, India

**Nitesh Sood**
Department of Agriculture
Mata Gujri College
Fatehgarh Sahib, India

**Salamatu Ahmad Sulaiman**
Department of Food Science and Technology
Faculty of Agriculture
Bayero University Kano
Kano, Nigeria

**Priyanka Suthar**
Department of Food Technology and Nutrition
Lovely Professional University
Phagwara, India

**Tabussam Tufail**
University Institute of Diet and Nutritional Sciences
The University of Lahore
Lahore, Pakistan.

**Jalal Uddin**
Department of Pharmaceutical Chemistry
College of Pharmacy
King Khalid University
Abha, Saudi Arabia

**Huma Bader Ul Ain**
University Institute of Diet and Nutritional Sciences
The University of Lahore
Lahore, Pakistan

**Zakiya Usmani**
Department of Pharmacy
Lingayas Vidayapeeth Nachauli
Faridabad, India

**D D Wadikar**
Defence Food Research Laboratory
Mysuru, India

**Idrees Ahmad Wani**
Department of Food Science and Technology
University of Kashmir Hazratbal
Srinagar, India

**Hauwa Ladi Yusuf**
Department of Food Science and Technology
Bayero University Kano
Kano, Nigeria

**Waliya Zubairi**
Department of Chemistry
Khwaja Fareed University of Engineering & Information Technology
Rahim Yar Khan, Pakistan

CHAPTER 1

# An Overview of Food Toxins

**Tabussam Tufail, Jasmeet Kour, Farhan Saeed, Huma Bader Ul Ain, Ali Ikram, Waseem Khalid, Muzzamal Hussain, and Hitesh Chopra**

## CONTENTS



DOI: 10.1201/9781003178446-1

## 1.1 INTRODUCTION

We have learned historically that everything is toxic; it is just the dose that differentiates the toxic and the non-toxic. If a large quantity (4–5 litres) is consumed in a relatively short time (2–3 hours), even water is toxic. Hyponatremia, followed by cerebral edema, seizures, and death, involves the pathogenesis of water intoxication (Villa et al., 2020). In the human environment, food, water, and air, as well as the soil are all inevitable components. The quality of human life is influenced by each of those elements, and each of them may be contaminated. Every year, almost two million deaths (including children) are linked to the utilization of hazardous food. More than 200 diseases are estimated to take place due to contaminated food by chemical substances, microbes, or harmful pathogens (Haque et al., 2020). Food is not only the primary source of nutrients but may also contain toxic natural chemical substances, e.g., cyanogenic glycosides (many plants), solanine (green potato parts). Akin to water, leading to hepatotoxicity, the acute poisonous effects may occur by excessive dosage levels, such as a pro-oxidant effect that may occur by the antioxidant vitamin A, or chronically elevated levels (Baker et al., 2016).

Some of the GRAS substances primarily salt and the trans fats present in hydrogenated vegetable based oils have been overlooked by The Food and Drug Administration (FDA) despite the fact that around 11 citizen petitions were filed by various consumer groups between 2004 and 2008. This is followed by lack of in-depth knowledge and its application by FDA in evaluating scientific information about their GRAS certified substances (Shames, 2010). The United States FDA's (FDA, 2001) labelling requirements provide consumers with useful information on the caloric value, potential allergens, proteins, carbohydrates, fat content, etc., however, on toxins it does not give information that is perhaps innate in or produced in the processing of food (Castro et al., 2019). Since foods cannot be separated from several food toxins as well as other food toxins that can be produced during processing or cooking, it is unavoidable to consume small amounts of food toxins. Food safety is vulnerable to new challenges, such as alteration in distribution procedures as well as production, increased contamination, emerging pathogens, and changes in food habits, among others, because of an increase in trade as well as travel (Heredia and Garcia, 2018). The WHO on World Health Day, 7 April 2015, decided to include food safety on its agenda. They have decided that, at all stages of food production, from harvesting, processing, storage, to preparation and transport, the execution of essential measures must comply with food safety (World Health Organization, 2015).

When consumed in large enough quantities, something as blameless as liquorice may be harmful. For instance, hypokalaemia, leading to cardiac arrest, was reported by Bannister in connection to the case of a 58-year-old woman who had eaten about 1.8 kg of liquorice per week (Afsah-Hejri et al., 2020). This intoxication with liquorice (liquorice's active component being glycyrrhizic, after glycyrrhizic acid) has effects similar to that of aldosterone, which holds back the renin-angiotensin-aldosterone axis, leading to potassium loss. Alkalosis hypokalemia, along with sodium retention muscle symptoms, oedema, severe hypertension, and cardiac arrhythmias are observed clinically at a rate of 100 g of liquorice/day may develop the syndrome, however withdrawal from using the liquorice reduces the impact slowly (Isbrucker & Burdock, 2006).

Regulators may, for their part, in food limit the quantities of potentially poisonous matters permitted and in situations where the surroundings of restrictions is ineffective, as well as where sufficient information given to the public provided by public health policymakers (for instance label information) can prevent plausibly foreseeable troubles to protect the consumer, wherever possible. Though, as for countries other than the US, regulatory information is included, legislation by the Food and Drug Administration is emphasized; as for other countries, readers are recommended to check with their precise region's regulations, as other countries' regulations and regulatory practices might be different from those of the US (Khaneghah et al., 2020).

Of the foods that are considered safe to eat, they cannot be toxic or unpalatable, and must contain nutritional value. Therefore, in the non-existence of contamination or spontaneous change, the conception of a poisonous food as such would seem to be an oxymoron. There are two main ways in which a foodstuff could then be poisonous: (1) a normally non-hazardous food has turned out to be poisonous for a small subpopulation; and (2) the over-eating of normally safe food. This move flanked by poisonous as well as safe or contaminated food for a chosen group has the prospective to create headaches for public health protection regulatory bureaus, but, as the reader will perceive on the subsequent pages, to achieve an acceptable risk balance and unavoidable circumstances, some realistic and thoughtful solutions have been developed by the Food and Drug Administration as well as other regulatory bureaus (Dolan et al., 2010).

## 1.2 TOXICITY

### 1.2.1 Environmental Contaminants

#### *1.2.1.1 Selenium in Grain*

Selenium (Se) joins the food chain by the transfer of inorganic selenium by plants and microorganisms to organically bound forms (Sors et al., 2005). Toxicity of selenium (that is selenosis) due to extreme intake of selenium happened to a wide degree in China in selenium areas owing to elevated selenium-retaining food consumption (an estimate on daily basis ingestion of 3–6.5 mg/day) (de Assis et al., 2020). Deformation, loss of nails, and loss of hair are the most common signs of selenosis. Increased levels of blood selenium, diarrhoea, weakness, garlic-like breath, and body odour, skin lesions, peripheral neuropathy, and irritability are other reported symptoms (Prakash et al., 1999). Intake levels of selenium that induce selenosis have not been well identified yet.

#### *1.2.1.2 Mercury in Seafoods*

The methyl derivative, methyl mercury, produced of anthropogenic as well as elemental mercury sources in a marine environment with bacterial activity is of concern to food toxicology. In marine settings, anthropogenic sources comprise coal combustion (which has mercury), the procedure of chloralkali, as well as other rudimentary mercury sources. A straight release of methyl mercury hooked on the atmosphere resulted in the Minamata Japan case. Neurological paresthesia, hearing defects, dysarthria, ataxia, as well as death may be caused by methyl mercury toxicity. Children born to mothers exposed to methyl mercury have been reported to suffer developmental delays (Caglayan et al., 2020). Rather than methyl mercury actual revelation, typically what happens is the introducing into the food chain of methyl mercury, going up as the weaker as well as fewer providential species are eaten by each predator. Methyl mercury is concentrated in fish near to the top of the food chain, counting Bluefin Tuna (*Thunnus spp.*), swordfish (*Xiphiasgladius*), shark (all species), marlin (*Makaira spp.*), mackerel (*Scomberomorus spp.*), halibut (*Hippoglossus spp.*), and bonito (*Sarda spp.*). The choice of these sorts was based on past data on the level of methyl mercury there was in fish eaten in the United States. The acceptable mercury amount, however, relies on whether the mercury was introduced; to be precise, as of an anthropogenic basis came the mercury attendance (that is the fish captured in a region recognized to have mercury discharged) or was not supplementary, as well as in the environment the effect was of course in attendance (Hutt et al., 2007).

### 1.2.2 Naturally Formed Substances

#### 1.2.2.1 *Thujone*

Thujone is attained as of several plants the chief element of essential oils, a monoterpene ketone, which comprises white cedar (*Thujaoccidentalis* L), wormwood (*Artemisia spp.*), tansy (*Tanacetumvulgare*), clary (*Salvia sclarea*), and salvia (*Salvia officinalis*) (Dolan et al., 2010). In herbal remedies, as of these plants, essential oils are second-hand across the world as flavourings in fragrances as well as alcoholic beverages (Food, 2006). Absinthe contains large amounts of thujone (made from wormwood) and is available in Spain, Denmark, and Portugal. Wormwood itself is a common vodka flavouring in Sweden, while all vermouth, chartreuse, and Benedictine contain small concentrations of thujone (Mahato et al., 2021). Sage oil is used in sausages, meats, condiments, and sauces to have the signature flavour and contains roughly 20–30% thujone (alpha- and beta-) (Lawrence, 2006; Ben, et al., 2000; Patocka & Plucar, 2003). Cedar essential oils as well as Sage, hyssop (Hyssopusofficinalis L.), and the entire restrain thujone as well are reported to contain induced symptoms on the CNS characterized by entirely clonic convulsions or tonic-colonic (Dietrich et al., 2021). The poisonous agent of absinthism, a condition created through the long-lasting utilization of absinthe, prepared as of the wormwood essence that is considered to be thujone. Addiction, hyperexcitability, and hallucinations characterize the condition (Bonkovsky et al., 1992; Adebo et al., 2021). In sub-chronic toxicity trials in female rats, the no-observed-effect-level (NOEL) for convulsions was 5 mg/kg bw/day (Hold, et al., 2001). Thujone detoxification is thought to occur through oxidation based on CYP450 and subsequent glucuronidation and excretion (Hold et al., 2001). When utilized, since it is a usual flavouring agent or usually matters when utilized in combination using flavours, the Food Drug Administration confines revelations of *Artemisia spp.* to al-thujone (Thakali and MacRae, 2021).

#### 1.2.2.2 *Prussic Acid (Plum, Apple and Peach Pits)*

Prussic acid (recognized as well as cyanide, hydrogen cyanide, or hydrocyanic acid) is produced when weakened cyanogenic glycosides inherit and get in touch with emulsion enzymes or beta-glycosidase present in apple, plum, leaves, oak moss, peach pits, as well as other plant tissues. As for the glycoside, the enzymes discharge the cyanide, and the cyanide inhibits oxygen from being utilized by the cells of the body, resultant in cellular necrosis as well as harm to the tissue. As they are oxygenated, the blood, as well as mucous membranes, is light red, but the oxygen cannot be used by the cells in the tissues. Rapid respirations, tremors, coordination, as well as, in severe circumstances, respiratory and/or heart arrest are clinical symptoms of prussic acid poisoning (Anandan

& Jankovic, 2021). A lot of trees of fruits have prussic acid glycosides in the seeds and leaves, but in the fleshy areas of the fruit, there are only marginal amounts (Kahn & Line, 2010). Since the dietary staple cassava is eaten in the western African tropics, and inadequate cassava handling before processing and ingestion will lead to cyanide poisoning, a chronic form that is called tropical ataxic neuropathy, resulting from the peripheral nerve tracts, auditory as well as optic demyelination (Panter, 2004).

In cherry pits (*Prunusavium* L.), peach leaves (*Prunuspersica* L.), elder tree leaves (*Sambucusnigra* L.) as well as cherry laurel leaves (*Prunuslaurocerasus* L.), prussic acid since establishing in the flavouring elements must be restricted to 25 ppm; although sour extract of almond (*Prunuspersica* L., *Prunusarmeniaca* L., or *Prunusamygdalus Batsch*) have to be prussic acid (21 CFR 182.20). There are no Food Drug Administration rules or recommendations regulating the presence of prussic acid in seeds of apple (*Malus spp.*), possibly for the reason that, as spice additives, extort of these seeds contain no mercantile advantage.

#### *1.2.2.3 Hypericin in St. John's Wort*

St. John's Wort is a herbal remedy thought to relieve depressive symptoms, and usually in tablet or pill form, St. John's Wort standardized extracts are eaten. Hypericin and hyperforin are believed to be the main active antidepressant ingredients in St. John's Wort (Wentworth et al., 2000; Karioti & Bilia, 2010). Hyperforin is also believed to stimulate CYP3A4 and CYP2C9 enzymes of cytochrome P450, which can lead to enhanced metabolism and the reduced therapeutic reaction of some drugs (Hammerness et al., 2003).

#### *1.2.2.4 Goitogens (Glucosinolates) in Brassica Species*

A few uncooked foods contain those matters, by interfering with the iodine uptake, in developing an important nutrient, hormonal equilibrium and cognitive function inhibit thyroid gland function. Cognitive deficits are considered to result from a lack of functional iodine (e.g., cretinism). The decline in the absorption of iodine contributes to an enlargement of the thyroid gland, creating a goitre. Pears, peaches, bananas, soybeans, sweet potatoes, cassava, peanuts, spinach, and Brassica genus vegetables, including rapeseed, radishes, mustard greens, cabbage, cauliflower, canola, sprouts of Brussels, and broccoli, have been classified as goitrogenic (Friedman et al., 2013). The ingestion of significant numbers of uncooked kale or cabbage has often been attributed to goitre.

Goitrogenic compounds, collectively called glucosinolates, are inactivated by elevated temperatures (i.e., cooking). Cassava (*Manihotesculenta*) in the tropics is an important dietary source of sugar but contains elevated amounts of glucosinolates linamarin. To significantly minimize the content of linamarin (Oberleas, 1973), the cassava has to be adequately processed: dried, fried, or immersed in water. Glucosinolates are compounds containing sulfur that are metabolized to figure nitriles, isothiocyanate, thiocyanates, as well as sulfur in the body by thioglucosidase. The isothiocyanates undergo cyclization under some conditions to figure goitrogens, elevating their powerful activity of goitrogenic (Brassica napus). Rapeseed oils should be analysed on behalf of possible gitorin to avoid the possible activity of goitrogenic oils. (Ven Etten et al., 1973). No FDA regulations have been established for acceptable glucosinolate concentrations in human foods.

#### *1.2.2.5 Erucic Acid in Rape*

A yearly mustard herb relative local to Europe, rape (*Brassica campestris* L. or *Brassica napus* L.) is cultivated in the US because it carries oil-wealthy seeds for cooking oil (Dolan et al., 2010). For hundreds of years, rapeseed oil has been used as oil for lamps and, further recently, as pc oil lubricant. Early research, however, confirmed that feeding to rats the elevated stages of rapeseed oil substantially improved adrenal gland cholesterol and cardiac tissue lipidosis levels (Carroll, 1953; Chien et al., 1983). This impact has additionally been observed in turkeys, ducks, and chickens that were fed with extended quantities of rapeseed oil, ensuing in epicardial increase retardation, thickening, and mortality and amplified fibrous tissue in various myocardial regions. Erucic acid has been defined because the contributory agent of those effects is rapeseed oil. EA is a fatty acid long-chain containing one C-C unsaturated bond (C22:1). While in humans, lipidosis of myocardial has not been reported due to the erucic acid intake, animal feeding experiments have confirmed the dose-dependent development of lipidosis of myocardial in several species of animal, by government agencies which have been the normative evaluation of the possible unfavourable belongings on humans. As of the rapeseed variety canola (low acid, Canadian oil) canola oil is derived, which was conventionally developed in Canada in the late 1970s to produce decreased amounts of erucic acid and glucosinolates (Dolan et al., 2010; Wagstaff, 1991). The amount of erucic acid in Canola oil is restricted by the FDA to no more than 2% of the portion of fatty acid (21 CFR 184.1555).

#### *1.2.2.6 Furocoumarins*

Furocoumarins constitute a class of constituents of natural foods with properties of photomutagenic and phototoxic. In plants that fit into the families, Umbelliferae (for instance carrots, parsnip, parsley, celery) and Rutaceae (for instance citrus fruits) are primarily present. They are developed to help plants protect themselves from animals, insects, fungi, bacteria, and viruses in response to stress and are called natural pesticides (Marzulli, 1970). After revelation to ultraviolet radiation, extended storage, increases temperature, treatment with copper sulphate or hypochlorite, concentrations can also increase (Wagstaff, 1991; Ashwood et al., 1986).

8-methoxypsoralen (8-MOP, xanthotoxin or methoxsalen), 5-methoxypsoralen (5-MOP, bergapten) and Psoralen are the three most important furocoumarins in the development of photodermatitis (NTP, 2006). In the presence of near ultraviolet light (320–380 nm) with DNA-crosslinks and DNA able to form adducts by these three linear furocoumarins. Cell death, defects, as well as gene aberrations are the results of these photo-additions to cells (Ashwood et al., 1986). In the presence of UVA radiation in laboratory animals are developed skin tumours by 8-MOP and 5-MOP. 8-MOP causes Zymbal gland carcinomas, kidney adenocarcinomas, adenomas, as well as elevated incidences of tubular cell hyperplasia in rats at a chronic rate of 37.5 mg/kg bw/day dietary dosage (NTP, 2006; Dolan et al., 2010; Stern et al., 1997; Dolan et al., 2010).

In their peels, citrus fruits, particularly grapefruit, generate a number of elements which might include adverse interactions of the drug. Using the entire fruit, including the peel, citrus fruit juice is usually made. The bergamottin (also recognized as bergamot), a usual furanocoumarin which is recognized to hold back certain cytochrome isoforms P450 enzyme (CYP) 3A4 (Girennavar et al., 2006), is one chemical present in the peel. Slowing down this enzyme inhibits the metabolism of oxidation of such pharmaceutical products, resultant in a high bloodstream drug concentration (Bailey et al., 1998). Other citrus elements, as well as bergamot (e.g., lemon, orange, grapefruit, and lime) oils (Duke, 1992), are also phototoxic and, when exposed to sunlight, induce severe skin toxicity (Placzek et al., 2007). The mainly phototoxic element of bergamot oil, methoxypsoralen, demonstrated activity of mutagenic bacterial clastogenic and assays consequences in cultured cells of mammalians as revelation to ultraviolet light (Marzulli, 1970).

Celery allegedly restrains 100 ppb of psoralene (100 mg/kg) as well as 40 ppm (40 mg/kg) of parsnip (Coulombe, 2001). On behalf of people consuming foods with furocoumarin-restraining (est. 80% of the populace), the average dietary consumption of furocoumarins is 1.31 mg/day (Wagstaff, 1991), on behalf of a 60 kg human that is roughly 0.022 mg/kg bw/day. This is nearly 1,000 times inferior for liver toxicity in rats than the 13-week dietary (NOAEL)

(25 mg 8-MOP/kg bw/day) as well as 1,700 times inferior to the nutritional dosage seen in rats to cause cancer (37.5 mg/kg).

The ingestion of celery roots, as well as other traditional vegetables under usual dietary habits, does not meet this phototoxic threshold dose, resulting in ingestion of about 2–8 mg of furocoumarin for each individual (Schlatter et al., 1991). FDA rules or recommendations in food-related advice to the furocoumarins being there are not available.

#### *1.2.2.7 Amylase Inhibitors*

In aqueous extort of kidney beans, rye, and maize, alpha-amylase naturally occurring inhibitors are found. In plant alpha-amylase inhibitors the physiological role is not well recognized, however, they can be shielded from infestation by insects. In mammals, a few inhibitors of amylase have been revealed in blood glucose to soothe the natural spike that occurs during starch intake. But, because pancreatic proteinases, pepsin, or gastric acid are inactivated by alpha-amylase inhibitors, their ability as 'starch blockers' is limited (Deshpande, 2002). For the reason of weight reduction to reduce the absorption of carbohydrate, inhibitors of alpha-amylase were formerly applied as 'starch blockers' to foods, but, the Food Drug Administration subsequently concluded that as a minimum this utilization of inhibitors of alpha-amylase was a drug and was subsequently occupied off the market (Dolan et al., 2010). A big allergen (referred to as Asp o 2) recognized as 'baker's asthma' disease that has been involved in the production of toxicity of work-related activities (Fränken et al., 1994) is the alpha-amylase inhibitor enzyme. Although in flour of wheat protein inhibitor of alpha-amylase is, of course, present, in flour alpha-amylase inhibitor protein is found as well in which of Aspergillus oryzaealpha-amylase has been additionally improving fermentation of yeast of carbohydrates (Moreno, et al., 2004). Consequently, the protein of the alpha-amylase inhibitor can theoretically be present in baked goods originating from sources other than wheat. In people who eat bread restraining protein inhibitor alpha-amylase, cases of food allergies have been identified. Dyspnea, cough, hoarseness, oropharyngeal itching, rhinorrhea, and sneezing are allergic signs (Granum, 1979).

In flour of wheat (590 units/g), entire flour of wheat (351 units/g) as well as entire flour of rye (186 units/g), inhibitor activity of high alpha-amylase in opposition to alpha-amylase in the human salivary gland has been detected. Bread baking decreases the operation, based on form, by 80–100%. The operation of raw spaghetti (248 units/g) is decreased by 15 minutes of boiling by more than 98%; 1.5 hours of boiling of red beans lowers operation to undetectable levels (Deshpande, 2002). However, when heated to 200°C, to maintain a few activities of allergenic the alpha-amylase has been revealed (Dolan et al., 2010).

#### *1.2.2.8 Lectins*

In legumes there is a group of glycoproteins which are lectins (for instance, lentils, kidney beans, lima beans, soybeans, and black beans). Without altering their covalent composition, reversibly lectins can connect to carbohydrates (Shibamoto and Bjeldanes, 1993). The castor bean lectin ricin is known to cause childhood deaths and has been used as a bioterrorism tool. Phytohaemagglutinin is a lectin present in legumes, for instance fava beans, green beans, and white or red kidney beans in large amounts (as much as 2.4–5% of total protein). There are a variety of distinct properties of PHA, including the capacity to cause mitosis, influence the transport of membranes, and red blood cells to agglutinate and protein permeability. A 6% phytohaemagglutinin-containing diet fed to rats demonstrates loss of weight-related with malabsorption of vitamin $B_{12}$, nitrogen, and lipid (Banwell, et al., 1983; Dobbins, et al., 1986). Symptoms of PHA toxicity in humans arise within 3 hours of intake, such as nausea, vomiting, or diarrhoea. In general, regeneration takes place contained by 4–5 hours of beginning (FDA, 2009).

Readily available are no Food Drug Administration laws or recommendations limiting in food the presence of the lectin. However, before eating legumes, the FDA does have recommended cooking practices. Phytohaemagglutinins (as well as erstwhile lectin) amounts are elevated in raw beans than in safe-to-eat beans. The majority of lectins decrease in moist, but not dry, weather (Buhler, 2004).

#### *1.2.2.9 Compounds of Anti-Thiamine*

Substances operating on vitamin supply are usually referred to as anti-vitamins. At the methylene linkage, thiaminase cleaves thiamine (vitamin $B_1$), leaving it dormant biologically. The thiaminase operation involves a co-substrate, generally a protein containing sulfhydryl or amine, for instance, cysteine or proline. Thiaminase is present in some fruits as well as vegetables, for instance red cabbage, Brussels sprouts, red beets, blackcurrants, and blueberries, as well as in fish, crabs, clams (Deshpande, 2002).

In humans, thiamine deficiency can result in losing weight and weakness. Extreme deficiency of thiamine, a condition characterized by muscle fatigue foremost to ataxia, heart enlargement, and anorexia, causes beri-beri (Cornell University, 2010). Thiaminase is killed in fish as well as other sources by frying. Food Drug Administration rules or recommendations in food-related to thiaminase presence are not available.

#### *1.2.2.10 Alkaloids of Pyrrolizidine*

Any plants in the family of *Scrophulariaceae*, *Rannuculaceae*, *Leguminosae* (*Crotalaria*), *Fabaceae*, Compositae (*Senecionae* and *Eupatoriae*), *Boraginaceae*, *Asteraceae*, and *Apocyanacae* are found to possess pyrrolizidine alkaloids (PAs). There are usually high amounts of PAs in herbs, for instance (Symphytum spp.) leaf as well as comfrey root, (*Tussilagofarfara*) flower, as well as (*Boragoofficinale*) leaf of borage. The unintentional exposure of foodstuffs and the deliberate consumption of PA-containing herbal medicines as well as vegetables subject humans to PAs. Severe disease incidences have been described in individuals who eat grain cereal that is infected utilizing PA-containing plant kernels. PAs are also found in cow and goat milk and honey (Prakash et al., 1999).

In the US as well as Canada (Christensen et al., 1977), the selling of comfrey goods for internal consumption has been forbidden. Comfrey tea, however, is still broadly available. Comfrey tea users are reported to be able to consume PAs equal to 5 mg of comfrey a day (Deshpande, 2002; Cawood et al., 1983) or 0.083 mg/kg bw/day.

## 1.3 TOXICOLOGY

Toxicology is the study of the unfavourable impact on live species of chemical or physical substances. A toxicologist is qualified to analyse as well as explain the existence of these impacts on environmental health, livestock, and humans. The study of toxicology showed that that the modes of activity of cells, biochemicals, and molecules, as well as functional consequences such as immunological and neurobehavioral effects, and measures the risk of their incidence. Characterizing the relationship between exposure, dose, and reaction is central to this method. The integration of different elements has demonstrated toxicology's emerging ethical complexities (Gilbert, 2005).

Secondly, along with extensive mechanistic studies, their job is to comprehend the enduring hazards to society as well as people. Much public policy, administrative, and judicial proceedings decisions have been precipitated by this, not to talk about expensive as well as occasionally intensive litigation. Ethics is increasingly regarded as playing a key function in deciding for public health involving contradictions among social justice, company, as well as individual agendas (Callahan & Jennings, 2002; Kass, 2001; Lee, 2002).

However, these wide over simplifications are not adequate to exclude these foodstuff additives as of the criteria of a rigorous security review. In the last decade, consumers have been particularly involved in the health-enhancing food qualities and the ingredients they contain. Substances such as soy isoflavones, vegetable oil, and phytosterols have been extracted and applied at higher amounts to other foods to impart cholesterol decrease in expertise.

These products have raised legal concerns as to whether these compounds, such as iron and vitamin C, can act as medicines and should be treated as such, or whether they have to be considered as fresh nutrients allowable in foodstuffs. Science of nutrition experts concur with the nutrients notion, and say that they have to be extended to incorporate an increasing figure of beneficial foodstuff components producing quantifiable physical condition gains associated with prevention of illness (Sansalone, 1999). This segregation as well as enrichment of fresh ingredients of food would entail a detailed review of protection at the level of planned consumption as well as for the general public (Gold et al., 1992).

Any of these compounds, perhaps antinutrients (e.g. saponins metabolites, lectins, chymotrypsin, as well as trypsin in soybeans, anti-thiamine, and phytate binders, which are present in soybean) found in plants and fish are also harmful to humans, for example cycasin and tomatine. The catalogue of unpredictable multipart metabolites of food, in that about 5,500 unpredictable substances are confirmed to exist in 1 or more of the 246 foods provides an understanding of the vast number of substances found in food. This is only the tip of the iceberg, though, since the unknown usual substances in foodstuff greatly go beyond the known number (Miller, 1989).

Around 2,000 of these are flavouring additives found in foodstuffs that are also non-nutritious (Burdock, 2002). Approximately one-third of the 2,000 flavouring additives which might be applied to foodstuff are utilized at attention underneath 10 ppm (Hall & Oser, 1968), around identical attention since is of course present.

Some contaminants, including biphenyls, dioxins, and dibenzofurans, or heavy metals, such as polyhalogenated aromatic hydrocarbons (PHAHs), are inherent in food due to their pervasive utilization, being there in the crust of the earth that has resulted in their presence in the atmosphere as a permanent or pervasive contaminant, or being there as part of the usual processing of food merchandise. As a consequence, food, as well as animal feed, mostly of animal origin (for instance, because of the lipophilicity of these compounds, polyhalogenated aromatic hydrocarbons accumulate in meat or milk products) and marine origin, produces inevitable pollutants at a certain stage. To make sure that they are healthy beneath planned or anticipated utilization conditions, tolerances in favour of the remainder of inevitable pollutants are recognized for food as well as additives of food.

### 1.3.1 Heavy Metals

Readily available are 92 usual components, of which about 22 are considered to be vital mammalian cadaver nutrients and are referred to as micronutrients (Concon, 1988). There are copper, molybdenum, iodine, cobalt, selenium, manganese, iron, zinc, and even arsenic as well as aluminium in the micronutrients. But cadmium, lead, and mercury are classified as contaminants among the 92 components or have as a minimum further requirements and restrictions in additives of food, e.g., Food Chemicals Codex Sources of heavy metals and their toxic effects are shown in Table 1.1.

#### *1.3.1.1 Lead*

While lead toxicity is renowned, the essential trace mineral may be lead. A lead deficiency-induced over one or more generations of rats feeding $< 50$ ppb (vs. 1,000 ppb in controls), developed

**Table 1.1 Source of Heavy Metals and Their Toxic Effect**

| Heavy Metal | Sources | Toxic Effect | References |
|---|---|---|---|
| Mercury | Marlin (Fish) | Mood swings, irritability, and nervousness | (Rice et al., 2014) |
| Cadmium | Cereals, nuts, vegetables, oilseeds, and pulses | Skeletal, urinary, reproductive, cardiovascular, central and peripheral nervous and respiratory systems | (Bernard, 2008) |
| Arsenic | Seafood | Darker skin, abdominal pain, diarrhoea, heart disease, numbness, and cancer | (Raikwar et al., 2008) |
| Chromium | Vegetables, fruits, and meats | Lung cancer, nasal irritation, nasal ulcer, and hypersensitivity | (Achmad & Auerkari, 2017) |
| Thallium | Vegetables | Lung, heart, liver, and kidney | (Peter & Viraraghavan, 2005) |
| Lead | Fruits and root vegetables | Convulsions and even death | (Pirooty & Ghasemzadeh, 2013) |

symptoms of the hematopoietic system, reduced the iron stocks in the spleen and liver, and reduced development, but not owing to a consequence on the absorption of iron (Kirchgessner, 1978).

In the past, the foods might turn out to be infected using lead if they are processed in circumstances, handled, and cultivated that may result in higher levels of lead being added in foodstuff, for instance where in the soil a crop root is fully fledged that was then erstwhile polluted by the utilization of pesticides of lead. Subsequent pollution of foodstuff could, under such circumstances, mean that consumers face a health risk.

#### *1.3.1.2 Arsenic*

It is an environmentally omnipresent feature; it positions 20th amongst the components of the crust of the earth as well as in the human body 12th in relative abundance (Concon, 1988). However, arsenic is mentioned elsewhere in this text in-depth, the conversation here is not enough to its association with food. For arsenic selenium absorption there is a little competition that is believed to reduce the arsenic toxicity; arsenic is as well recognized to provoke iodine synthesis. Readily available are various sources including arsenic, drinking water, air, and chemicals, but arsenic is mainly proportional to the volume of fish eaten by food (Newberne, 1987).

#### *1.3.1.3 Cadmium*

Cadmium is also used in conjunction with utilizing zinc, minerals, as well as fossil fuels in smaller quantities. While unusual, owing to its manufacturing utilization in plating, plastics, textiles, and pigments of painting, it is an almost ubiquitous feature in American society. Removal at smelters as well as processing facilities, the vehicle tires breakdown (restraining cadmium-overloaded rubber), resulting penetration hooked on the groundwater as well as soil, as well as incineration of cadmium-restraining resources inhalation also contribute to contamination to humans by secondary paths. The estimated annual cadmium discharges of motor vehicle varies between 5.2 and 6.0 metric tonnes (Davis, 1979; Lagerwerff and Specht, 1971).

#### *1.3.1.4 Chlorinated Organics*

These have been with us on behalf of a few occasions, given their durability of water as well as susceptibility to decay, microbial deterioration, UV light, as well as erstwhile causes of usual obliteration, for some time to come, though in minute quantities, chlorinated organics will continue to exist in the ecosystem. However, in the 1930s, by the utilization of chlorinated hydrocarbons since pesticides, insect vector-related illness such as malaria was almost eliminated.

#### *1.3.1.5 Food-Borne Moulds and Mycotoxins*

For decades, in food processing mould shave doled out to humans (e.g. ripening cheese) and have produced major therapeutic applications for numerous fungal metabolites; they may also generate secondary metabolites utilizing the ability to create substantial unfavourable physical condition consequences, counting alteration in behaviour (Cousins et al., 2005).

#### *1.3.1.6 Aflatoxins*

Among the numerous mycotoxins, owing to the highly hepatocarcinogenicity active in rats aflatoxin B toxicity, aflatoxins have been the focus of the most extensive studies. Epidemiological research performed in Asia and Africa indicates that it is a human being hepatocarcinogen, as well as several other types of research, contained in human toxicity occurrence included aflatoxins (Peers et al., 1976) of kneejerk electrophilic epoxide that make up RNA, DNA adducts, and covalent protein (IARC, 2002). To aflatoxin disparity in the reaction of organisms can in part be attributable to differences in biotransformation and vulnerability to initial biochemical lesions (Monroe & Eaton, 1987).

## 1.4 IDENTIFICATION AND QUANTIFICATION OF TOXICOLOGY

### 1.4.1 Identification and Quantification in Natural and Processed Cheeses

The connection between cancer and diet risk is quite complicated (Doll & Peto, 1981). Under one area of experimental conditions, factors that come to provoke carcinogenesis may retard or possess no effects in other experimental conditions provided (Pariza, 1988). Many reports regarding meat and dietary fat show the opposite relation flanked by utilization and esophagus cancer risk, i.e. more consumption lowers the risks of esophageal cancer (Tuyns et al., 1987; Pottern et al., 1981) plus stomach cancer (Geboers et al., 1985; Hill, 1987). These vexing verdicts recommend that the determination of anticarcinogenic components from plants and animals is of great importance for the identification of many risks of cancer. An isomeric derivative of c-9, c-12-octadecadienoic acid (linoleic acid) containing a conjugated double-bond structure (designated CLA) (Ha et al., 1987) has recently been derived from grilled ground beef. Synthetically prepared CLA restricted the start of skin carcinogenesis in mice by 7, 12-dimethylbenz[a]anthracene (Ha et al., 1987). The process behind inhibition is unknown. Research in this field is of special importance as CLA is being separated from many serum, duodenal juices, and bile (Cawood et al., 1983).

The centre of conjugated linoleic acid production in many liquids is still unknown, however, meats processed by heat plus other foods containing fats should be worked on, possibly involving springs. Although CLA formation process in foods is ambiguous, treatment by heat (Ha et al., 1987), linoleic acid free-radical-type rust (Cawood et al., 1983), as well as reactions of microbial enzymatic comprising rumen linolenic or linoleic acids (Viviani, 1970) are doubted as being important factors. With the process of GLC or spectrophotometric methods, conjugated dioic acids were isolated from butterfat (Bartlet and Chapman, 1961; Scott, et al., 1959) as well as milk fat (Riel, 1963; Parodi, 1977). In shortenings for the determination of conjugated linoleic acid as well as the capillary GC method for soy oil, (Lanza & Slover, 1981), as well as by means of HPLC, a combination of ultraviolet spectrophotometry (Brown & Snyder, 1982) were utilized respectively. These methods are short in precision. Efforts were exerted to detach individual isomers of conjugated linoleic acid synthesized as of isomerized-alkali linoleic acid utilizing either a capillary column non-polar or polar (Scholfield, 1981; Scholfield & Dutton, 1971).

### 1.4.2 Identification and Quantification of Photoheating in Roots of Rice

A survey of the United States market reported elevated attention of inorganic arsenic was found in rice as compared to other commodities (Schoof et al., 1999). Further research revealed that accumulated ion is more present in rice grains as well as shoots than that of barley and wheat (Williams et al., 2007). Hence, rice use might pose a critical risk, because of the presence of As in inorganic form, arsenate (As) and arsenate (As I), and that these are group 1 non-threshold carcinogens (ATSDR, 2000; Meharg et al., 2009). Arsenic accumulation in plants of rice is dependent on many conditions. During flood environment cultivation (Xu et al., 2008), through water irrigation, plus naturally contaminated soil are all provoking elements to upgrade the levels of As in grains of rice (Saha & Ali, 2007; Lu et al., 2009; Meharg et al., 2009; Raab et al., 2007). Because most of these are taken by transporters of phosphate and silicate, correspondingly, this may be because of resemblance in molecular structure by means of phosphate and silica (Meharg et al., 1994; Ma et al., 2006; Zhao et al., 2011).

Preparing (PCs) photoheating ability is dependent on factors of genetic plus availability of the sulfate (Cobbett & Goldsbrough, 2002; Zhao et al., 2011; Duan et al., 2011). Glutathione is the source of PCs (GSH). Zhang et al. (2011) and Duan et al. (2011) noted that GSH/PC plus sulfur lack heightened the change of location in rice flanked by roots to shoots as well as from shoots to grains, correspondingly. Reported by Duan et al. (2011), complicated arrangement of As as well as in plants of rice PC precipitation as of dissimilar cultivars showed the specific role of PCs in translocation and accumulation of As in grains of rice, devoid of quantifying or identifying the contributing thiols.

### 1.4.3 Identification and Quantification of Oligomers as Potential Migrants in Plastic Food Packaging

The utilization of plastic has increased since the time of its discovery. Plastic application exposed Europe as the largest user of plastic in 2013. PVC, PS, PET, PP, and PE are the most used polymers for plastic. Today, alternative to previously used petrochemical starters, plastic monomer units are being discovered and searched for as of a renewable basis akin to plants. Also, because of biodegradability issues, the production of new polymeric packaging (mass beverage packaging) upgraded along with the advancement of (co)polymer updates and the latest plastics materials. An important matter is that oligomers that all the time exist in polymers gain more consideration as potent migrants both from the quantitative and qualitative aspects. As the number of new co-monomers increase, probable compositional oligomer structures automatically increase. Various requirements are taken into consideration for (FCM) polymeric food contact materials; for instance, corporal shielding of the foodstuff as of mechanical shock, compression, and temperature also protects from oxygen, water vapour, plus oil.

FCM must shield the product from bacteria, viruses, mould, and fungi, and ultimately guarantees long-lasting quality and safety. Secondly, contents of food and FCM come in contact, hence the transfer of molecules of FCM to food occurs, this migration should never exceed up to the threatening level that renders health risks to consumers. The European regulation on plastic materials used for foodstuff, rules made for articles, as well as plastic materials are followed for their protective utilization.

Those are called deliberately additional materials. The migration of generic or specific restrictions of these substances. Compounds that emerge by demolishing of the additives or polymeric material, as well as initiators impurities area, added unintentionally as well as in the authorization list not included as it is not feasible to recognize the entire impurities. Those compounds are normally called NIAS (non-intentionally added substances). Non-approved compounds ought not to cross the stage of 0.01 mg/kg foodstuff (Nerin et al., 2013).

But, non-intentionally added substances cannot be quantified owing to difficulty as present classes of chemical substances have various analytical perceive aptitude plus factors of response.

Nowadays, high-resolution mass spectrometry (HRMS) is being used to identify unknown compounds. This gives the precise substance mass equipped to four decimal places that are important in favour of the identification compound (Nerin et al., 2013).

The oligomers' biological and toxicological properties and their migration rate are not well known. Prehistorically, little testing on oligomers' toxicity has been done and safety assessment was on the behalf of monomeric unit toxicity data, for example assuming that oligomers are completely hydrolyzed (Nelson et al., 2011). But, in fact, in the GI system oligomer humiliation is not well known, and hence it may be essential to test the structures of oligomeric independently as individual substances or evaluate their hydrolysis process.

## 1.5 FOOD SAFETY REGULATION AND PRECAUTION

### 1.5.1 Adverse Reactions to Food or Food Ingredients

It is revealed in an American appraisal that 30% of people specified that either they or persons of their instant families are food sensitive to one or another type. Even though the number is very high, up to 7.5% of the population might be allergically sensitive to food components (that is, their immune system of the body's stimulated opening to food ingredients) like a peanut allergy. Lactose intolerance (lack of disaccharide enzyme, lactase) is greater in some people; for instance, the chances by age 6 may raise to 33% in black children of 2 years. Food additives intolerant varieties as of 0.03 to 0.23% to 1–2% in the young northern European children.

People who consume tetracycline also avoid milk intake with this antibiotic. Standardized, there is a large number of actual and assumed side effects to food.

### 1.5.2 Food Allergy

The collusion of basophils, immunoglobulins, or mast cells (the concluding life form a basis of arbitrating materials counting bradykinin as well as histamine on behalf of unexpected responses plusleukotrienes and prostaglandins for slow-embryonic responses) as well as a necessary, preceding opening to the cross-kneejerk allergen or allergen are the factors that differentiate food allergy from other reactions. An allergic reaction can be obvious by one or more symptoms. The foods known to evoke allergies are large in number, plus are probably limited only by people's choice of eating food type.

### 1.5.3 Food Idiosyncrasy

The abnormal responses to a food additive or substance in a quantitative manner are termed food idiosyncrasies. It may sound like hypersensitivity, but it has physiological differences as immune mechanisms are not involved. Food idiosyncratic reactions occur in distinct groups of persons who might be genetically inclined. Intolerance of lactose is almost certainly the main ordinary distinctive response, in which enzyme lactase is essential for the lactose metabolism in milk is insufficient. In northern Europe at 3–8% the intolerance of lactose is lower, in Turkey and southern Italy 70% as well as in south-east Asia is about100%.

### 1.5.4 Metabolic Food Reactions

As of erstwhile types of unfavourable responses, the metabolic food reactions are dissimilar as the foods are commonly eaten extra or fewer as well as exhibit poisonous effects merely on overeating or improperly manufactured food. 'Voluntary' intake of food because of lack of supply of food or for a distinct food an irregular longing (Bannister et al., 1977), reported such an abnormal type of craving, hypokalemia followed by the cardiac arrest of a 58-year-old woman who had been eating about 1.8 kg of liquorice in a single week. In liquorice intoxication, or 'glycyrrhizin', the active component is glycyrrhizic acid, along by means of consequences like aldosterone, that dominates over the renin-angiotensin-aldosterone axis, ultimately potassium loss. Clinically, alkalosis hypokalemia symptoms, muscular symptoms, cardiac arrhythmias alongside oedema and sodium retention, as well as fierce hypertension are noted. At a stage of 100 g liquorice/day might occur syndromes, however ahead liquorice extraction gradually reduced (Isbrucker and Burdock, 2006).

## 1.6 REGULATIONS

Work-related safety provides attention to allergenic possessions since it is well known that enzymes are powerful inhalation sensitizers as well as being able to lead to allergic responses like asthma. However, poisonous materials that are mycotoxins plus bacterial toxins may as well be there in enzyme isolates, hence posing a risk to a consumer's health. Safety evaluation procedures sound good because no incidents have been observed since that time, hence suggesting lesser test parcels. Monitoring measures, as well as safety precautions demonstrated through industry, manage to lessen but not completely remove work-related dangers. The deficiency of harmonization legislation plus safety evaluation and the question of enzymes being sensitized are challenging to regulators and industrialists. EU can solve its challenges by developing harmony in its legislation regarding food safety enzymes. Industrial enzymes with growing entrepreneurship are internationally worth approximately US$2,000,000,000 where food enzymes contribute half of this amount. As the available number of food enzymes as well as their yearly profits both have been increasing contentiously, the principal industry organization Association of Manufacturers and Formulators of Enzyme Products (AMFEP) has scheduled enzymes, about 160 of which intended for the industry of food, 36 manufactured by hereditarily customized microorganisms.

Moreover, a few EU member states have established national legislation on enzymes of food. This legislation is meant to assure enzyme safety for final food production and sometimes encompasses details for activity as well as purity. In some situations, work-related fitness matters which may come out as enzymes handling and manufacturing are also included in the overview of regulatory practices. Scientific literature has discussed in detail the allergic reaction associated with workers handling enzymes, which are not enzymes specific among industrialists and concerned stakeholders, plus even in the general press.

## 1.7 PRECAUTIONS

Currently, a 'new science' call has been made by advocates of the precautionary principle to assure the aim of health policy of precaution-based environment and occupation. While a great concentration to epidemiology is erstwhile given, toxicology is the appropriate knowledge linked to prevention or precaution. In the field chances in favour of improving the toxicology function in public policy have to get biased currently. Hence, despite a 'new science', advocates should consider modification of ongoing scientific methods that are appropriate plus carry accurate scientific data (McGinn, 2000).

At this point the application of precaution does not need a new science, notwithstanding that, backdated studies have insisted that plausible proof of their risks have to contain performances by several states in the 1970s. With the revocation of a lot of the Delaney Clause (of the Cosmetic Act, Drug and Food) by the progress of the FQPA (Food Quality Protection Act), all pertinent United States law currently needs ceremonial risk tests to support narrow verdicts (O'Brien, 2000).

## 1.8 THE ROLE OF THE NEW TOXICOLOGY

The International High Production Volume (HPV) substances program is the early first authentic opportunity to introduce modern technologies in toxicology. Firstly, developed by an OECD Environmental Program unity choice, a self-imposed devotion with the chemical industry to give a short data set to help out initial risk or assessments of safety (U.S. Environmental Protection Agency, 2002).

The usage of a unique set of fast and profitable tests becomes a cause of creating the idiomatic improvement in this analysis, accepted by the countries of OECD, as a 'yardstick' in favour of judging accessible information. The deadlock recognized by the initial assessment of chemicals in comprehension was removed by this improvement, where it was impossible to elaborate an adequate set of information (NRC, 1984). According to the NGO analysis, the same studies were collected through the EPA as well as the United Study industry of chemicals. While their searches decided and elongated the Environmental Defence work, the self-imposed substances 'right to know' aim was accepted in the United States. It was developed to create enough data on behalf of an earlier security test in 2006 on almost 3,000 substances. Initial responsibility was of producers to develop this information, from one of many systems: repayment of up till now data of proprietary, contemporary testing completion, or the receipt of narrative schemes. This achievement is formidable, in the way of demands of fiscal as well as scientific, and on animal testing an enlarged freight. In addition the program of HPV, now readily available are national and international aims for testing mainly present substances (the European Union chemicals policy) or to ordeal for enlisted end points (for instance, in the OECD the international program of endocrine disruptor testing, in the United States the inventiveness of children's health, bioaccumulative/the unrelenting/poisonous substance identification program in the Nordic countries, in Japan the fresh initiative on endpoints of ecotoxicology). To achieve these objectives, as well as to fulfil links of the community safety of animals, there is an authentic demand to recognize, corroborate, as well as act on behalf of analysis of chemical use in modern technologies, counting methods of substitutional as well as enhanced structure-actions scrutinizes chemical groups hooked on types, whereas data are merely needed on a number of substances contained by a sensibly definite group.

## 1.9 EFFECT ON PROCESSING

A special or unusual challenge to the food industry is naturally present toxicant foods contamination by mycotoxins which is a highly inescapable and erratic toxin. Aspergillus species are responsible for producing aflatoxins which are poisoned mould metabolites. Effects of processing on the formation of toxic compounds are shown in Table 1.2.

Initial commodities having aflatoxin pollution include cottonseed, peanuts, and corn, as well as animal-imitative foods, for instance milk, when the aflatoxin-contaminated feed is fed by animal. Challenges linked with aflatoxin-contaminated foods are able to be minimized with usage unique procedures as well as cleanliness methods. The effectiveness of specific processes like the chemical stability of the mycotoxin(s)is influenced by different factors including the process nature, with

**Table 1.2 Effect of Processing on the Formation of Toxic Compounds**

| Toxic Compound | Processing | Food | References |
|---|---|---|---|
| N-Nitrosamines | Deep-fat frying | Cooked vegetables and meat products | (Park et al., 2015) |
| Aromatic hydrocarbons | Maillard-browning | High sugar foods and grilled foods | (Larsson et al., 1983) |
| Lipid polymerization | Lipid oxidation | Fish, beef, and vegetables | (Falowo et al., 2014) |

the matrix of food interaction and type, and, if present, the interaction with manifold mycotoxins. Decontamination practical processes have to be the following:

- Eliminate, inactivate, or destroy toxins.
- Do not generate or depart in the food the poisonous remainder.
- Hold on to the food dietary value.
- Do not change the acceptance of the technological characteristics of the product.
- Demolish fungal spores.

Much different strategies of decontamination and/or processing have been triumphant in minimizing concentrations of aflatoxin to a satisfactory stage. Manual maintenance as well as segregation processes, where the mould-spoilt kernel/seed is eliminated as of the whole product, are able to consequence a reduction of 40–80% in levels of aflatoxins. Division of remainder of aflatoxin hooked on minimum use part of the assets can be resulted from the processes of dry and wet milling. Moreover, the best process decontamination is one to be exact, accepted by agencies of regulatory, cost-effectual, as well as vigilance minimises the concentration of mycotoxin to satisfactory levels. Naturally occurring secondary moulds are afla-toxin metabolites formed at first by *A. parasiticus* as well as *Aspergillus flavus*. The initial farming setups linked by dirtiness of aflatoxin include dairy products, cottonseed, tree nuts, peanuts, and corn. Initial health of public concerned toxins contain B, G, and BG aflatoxin as well as M aflatoxin, an animal metabolite, that take place in milk when lactating dairy cows are fed with feed having aflatoxin B. The aflatoxins are toxins and influential liver carcinogens. According to IARC (the International Agency for Research on Cancer), aflatoxins are listed as a factor of human carcinogen (Stoloff, 1982).

There is a proof of epidemiological that against the aflatoxicos is humans not contain an immune system, as accounted in Kenya and India (Park & Stoloff, 1989); as well as, where further factors are there for instance hepatitis B virus, the event of carcinogenic be able to take place (Henry et al., 1999). Factors all of these encompass mentioned for aflatoxins the significance of set up proper management of food security programs (Park & Stoloff, 1989; Park et al., 1999;).

## 1.10 CLEANING AND SEGREGATION

The physical parting of the damaged mould kernel/seed/nut as of the whole as well as apparently non-contaminated product is the early first option for reducing aflatoxins. The processes, for instance, of hand picking, sorting, and cleaning (Dickens & Whitaker, 1975) are invasive and do not protect from change effectively. Segregation of density as well as flotation have been mentioned and designated as beneficial for separating aflatoxin-contaminated peanuts as well as corn (Cole, 1989).

Anyhow, the entire elimination of aflatoxins cannot be ordinary with manual technologies of parting. There have to be elevated residual levels of contamination, other actions have to be used to get rid of concentrations of aflatoxin in the fully ready product to levels of admissible aflatoxin. A mixture of separation as well as former techniques should be used by peanut industries to eliminate the levels of aflatoxin in products of peanut, for instance peanut butter. A fine option for the industry of food is physical separation. An earlier asset to buy sufficient tackle is compulsory; though, preservation charges are short.

### 1.10.1 Wet Milling

For the preparation of corn products, wet milling is hugely utilized. But, it is needed to recognize the separation outline of the toxins in dispensation side effects while utilizing this procedure. The fractions contaminated are able to be unfocused to low-risk utilization or subjected to procedures of decontamination. In trials studying the aflatoxin's fate through outcome wet milling, BJ aflatoxin was originated to divide first and foremost hooked on the steep water (39–42%) as well as fractions of fibre (30–38%). The aflatoxin remainder was present in gluten (13–17%), germ (6–10%), as well as (1%) fractions of starch (Wood, et al., 1982;). Comparatively little aflatoxin was smashed by means of this procedure. It is essential to appreciate the importance of the levels aflatoxin when scrutinizing suitable uses for the fractions of containing aflatoxin.

### 1.10.2 Dry Milling

The dry milling will also contain aflatoxin fractionalized found in grain with contaminated, similar to wet milling. On behalf of corn, the BJ aflatoxins uppermost levels subsequent to the process of milling were originated in the fractions of hull and germ, low-fat flour, and low-fat meal grits, included merely 6–10% of the unique BJ aflatoxin. Studies by means of rice (Achroder et al., 1986) as well as wheat demonstrated similar outlines, including bran with the enormous attentiveness of the toxins. As of an industrial perspective, dry milling may be a cost-reductive method of reducing the levels of aflatoxin in early manufactured goods into flour. Toxic fractions management is able to be effectual through substituted lower-risk utilizations.

### 1.10.3 Thermal Inactivation

Aflatoxins are approximately heat-stable and aren't damaged while boiled. Quite a lot of studies have resulting in the finding that scorching is perhaps a fine means for minimizing levels of aflatoxin in certain products, that is oil and dry-roasted peanuts (Peers et al., 1976), microwave-roasted peanuts (Luter et al., 1982), corn, coffee (Conway et al., 1978), and so on. Numerous of these studies were executed on samples ready by spiking artificially; consequently, it's significant to confirm dispensation consequences on incurred contaminant as the matrix belongings might as well be dissimilar by means of being spiked against usual contamination (Wood et al., 1982).

### 1.10.4 Irradiation

(2.5 Mrad) the gamma irradiation didn't considerably mortify aflatoxin in tainted meal of peanut. Because of the value of the instrument, incomplete optimistic consequences, as well as being short of customer receipt of the process of irradiation, irradiation doesn't come into view in fact.

### 1.10.5 Commercial Method

The utilization of no biological resources to absorb aflatoxins that bind covalently might be a fine means for decontamination of aflatoxin. Many adsorbent resources, that is, stimulated carbon and clays, are exposed to attach aflatoxins as of aqueous solutions, as well as amino silicates were revealed effectual with feeds of animal and oil (Machen et al., 1988). Though exact clays have been accounted to be effectual in aflatoxin binding as of aqueous solutions, lessening uptake aflatoxin in animals, in farm animals stopping aflatoxicosis as well as in milk lessening MI aflatoxin levels, their utilization for elimination of aflatoxin as of the feed isn't legal by regulatory agencies, so the enduring belongings as well as security of those managers haven't been strong-minded (Phillips et al., 1994).

### 1.10.6 Biological Decontamination

Biological demonstrating methods and effectual possessions are generally the termination of precise compounds formed through microorganisms. It is as a rule more inexpensive to put in the dynamic agent directly. On behalf of the industry fermentation, though, biological procedures are a fine alternative. Throughout the process of beer brewing, there is about a 70–80% decrease of BI aflatoxin contained by the preliminary resources. Subsequent to fermentation and cooking of corn milo, wheat, and corn, BI aflatoxin was abridged through 47% (Dam et al., 1977). The aflatoxin does not divide hooked on the distillate alcoholic, but the toxin contemplation in the exhausted grain. There is a need to mend defectactions for exhausted grain utilized for animal feed.

### 1.10.7 Chemical Inactivation

On behalf of changing the carcinogenic and toxic effects of aflatoxin in meals, cottonseed, peanuts, and corn. Ammonia is well thought to be very effectual. Through Park and Price the consequences of these studies have been abridged (Park & Price 2001).

The process of ammoniation has been effectively utilized for more than 20 years contained by France and the US. The system has also been utilized in South Africa, Mexico, Brazil, Sudan, and Senegal. Though a number of ammonia-based events are developed as well as studied, the elevated pressure/elevated-temperature processes that use (0.5–2.0%) ammonia beneath controlled (12–16%) moisture conditions (45–55 psi) pressure as well as (80–100°C) temperature on behalf of 20–60 minutes is the most proficient and produces a secluded product.

Throughout ammoniation, the molecule of aflatoxin is chemically adapted to compounds possessing abridged or non-obvious poisonous or mutagenic potentials. Extraction exhaustive, separation, and arid purification studies have revealed the poisonous/mutagenic potentials as well as the destiny of aflatoxin/ammonia response commodities to be non-obvious or numerous orders of enormity inferior to the aflatoxin of parent. The identified presence aflatoxin/ammonia responses products, that is., DI aflatoxin as well as a compound through a 206 molecular weight, in feeds of animal comprise no significance of health. In studies concluding the allocation and configuration of aflatoxin/ammonia responses, products in corn and cottonseed, approximately 12–14% of the original aflatoxin defect was misplaced as unstable compounds, by organic solvents responses products about 20–24% were extractable, as well as by methanol 6–13% of responses products were extractable. Subsequent treatment of the corn by acid and base as well as proteolytic enzymes, added responses products of about 19–22% were noticed.

The residual corn matrix or cottonseed contained merely 37% of the original concentration of aflatoxin as ammonia/reaction products. Excretions as well as metabolic studies in laboratory and farm livestock have revealed that over 98% of the feed-bound ammonia/aflatoxin merchandise was excreted in the faeces and urine. In milk flanked by 0.25–1.6% of the innovative contaminant was excreted. Thorough animal feeding studies have revealed that aflatoxin-ammonia responses merchandise have at least some consequence on the animals' health receipt food containing ammonia-treated cottonseed meals, peanut, and corn. One more effectual ammoniation process, the ambient temperature process, generally needs a 3–6-week management of the contaminated substance. This procedure as well requires secure checks to confirm effectual consequence.

Research has been done to intricate on the protection of the ammoniated creation. Nixtamalization, a characteristic treatment of alkaline of corn use contained by the produce of tortillas, has been revealed to considerably decrease levels of aflatoxin in corn (Ulloa & Herrera, 1970; Ulloa & Shroeder, 1969). Consequent studies have revealed that BI aflatoxin is rehabilitated ahead of acidification. Certain food additives unaccompanied or in amalgamation with H202 throughout the nixtamalization procedure result in important reductions of aflatoxin in tainted corn (Trujillo, 1997; Lopez-Garcia, 1998; Hagler et al., 1982; Burgos, 1998) as well as corn co-tainted through BI fumonisin (Park et al., 1996).

## 1.11 CONCLUSION

Food contamination through chemicals is considered as a potential hazard against health. This contamination is mainly caused by naturally occurring toxins and environmental pollutants or during the processing, packaging, preparing, storage, and transportation of food. The detection of such contaminants has become easier with the advancement in technology. However, there are several contaminants that are still unknown and research continues in this regard. Although the government has taken adequate steps to minimize the individual exposure to food contaminants, there are still measures that need to be taken to reduce the health risks and diseases that come with the chemical food contamination. In this article, a regulatory as well as toxicological overview of a small number of the contaminants found in a number of widely consumed foods was taken followed by addressing the measures taken to minimize consumer exposure, some of which are made possible by the US food regulatory process. Conclusively, the consumption of small quantities of food toxins is unavoidable because all food toxins cannot be removed from foods, and others may be created during processing or cooking.

## REFERENCES

Achmad, R. T. and Auerkari, E. I. 2017. Effects of chromium on human body. *Annual Research & Review in Biology* 1–8.

Achroder, H. W., Boller, R. A. and H. Hein, Jr. 1986. Reduction in aflatoxin contamination of rice by milling procedures. *Cereal Chemistry* 45: 574–580.

Adebo, O. A., Molelekoa, T., Makhuvele, R., Adebiyi, J. A., Oyedeji, A. B., Gbashi, S., and Njobeh, P. B. 2021. A review on novel non-thermal food processing techniques for mycotoxin reduction. *International Journal of Food Science & Technology* 56(1):13–27.

Afsah-Hejri, L., Hajeb, P. and Ehsani, R. J. 2020. Application of ozone for degradation of mycotoxins in food: A review. *Comprehensive Reviews in Food Science and Food Safety* 19(4): 1777–1808.

Anandan, C. and Jankovic, J. 2021. Botulinum toxin in movement disorders: An update. *Toxins* 13(1): 42.

Ashwood-Smith, M. J., Ceska, O., Chaudhary, S. K., Warrington, P. J. and Woodcock, P. 1986. Detection of furocoumarins in plants and plant products with an ultrasensitive biological photoassay employing a DNA-repair-deficient bacterium. *Journal of Chemical Ecology* 12(4): 915–932.

ATSDR, T. 2000. ATSDR (Agency for toxic substances and disease registry). Prepared by clement international corp., under contract 205: 88–0608.

Bailey, D. G., Malcolm, J., Arnold, O. and David Spence, J. 1998. Grapefruit juice–drug interactions. *British Journal of Clinical Pharmacology* 46(2): 101–110.

Baker, C. A., Rubinelli, P. M., Park, S. H. and Ricke, S. C. 2016. Immuno-based detection of Shiga toxin-producing pathogenic Escherichia coli in food–A review on current approaches and potential strategies for optimization. *Critical Reviews in Microbiology* 42(4): 656–675.

Bannister, B., Ginsburg, R. and Shneerson, J. 1977. Cardiac arrest due to liquoriceinducedhypokalaemia. *British Medical Journal* 2(6089): 738–739.

Banwell, J. G., Boldt, D. H., Meyers, J. and Weber, F. L., Jr, 1983. Phytohemagglutinin derived from red kidney bean (Phaseolus vulgaris): A cause for intestinal malabsorption associated with bacterial overgrowth in the rat. *Gastroenterology* 84(3): 506–515.

Bartlet, J. C. and Chapman, D. G. 1961. Butter adulteration, detection of hydrogenated fats in butter fat by measurement of cis-trans conjugated unsaturation. *Journal of Agricultural and Food Chemistry* 9(1): 50–53.

Bernard, A. 2008. Cadmium & its adverse effects on human health. *Indian Journal of Medical Research* 128(4): 557–564.

Bonkovsky, H. L., Cable, E. E., Cable, J. W., Donohue, S. E., White, E. C., Greene, Y. J. and Arnold, W. N. 1992. Porphyrogenic properties of the terpenes camphor, pinene, and thujone:(with a note on historic implications for absinthe and the illness of vincent van gogh). *Biochemical Pharmacology* 43(11): 2359–2368.

Brown, H.G. and Snyder, H.E. 1982. Conjugated dienes of crude soy oil: Detection by UV spectrophotometry and separation by HPLC. *Journal of the American Oil Chemists' Society* 59(7): 280–283.

Buhler, R. 2004. Eating raw, undercooked beans can be unpleasant. High Plains/Midwest AG Journal. Available online: http://www.hpj.com/archives/2004/nov04/nov15/Eatingrawundercooke ddrybean.cfm (accessed on 21 July 2010).

Burdock, G. A. 2002. Regulation of flavor ingredients. In *Nutritional Toxicology*, edited by F. N. Kotsonis, and M. A. Mackey 2: 316–339.

Burgos-Hernandez, A. 1998. *Evaluation of Chemical Treatments and Intrinsic Factors That Affect the Mutagenic Potential of Aflatoxin B1-Contaminated Corn*. Louisiana State University and Agricultural & Mechanical College.

Caglayan, M. O., Şahin, S. and Ustundag, Z. 2020. Detection strategies of Zearalenone for food safety: A review. *Critical Reviews in Analytical Chemistry* 1–20.

Callahan, D. and Jennings, B. 2002. Ethics and public health: Forging a strong relationship. *American Journal of Public Health* 92(2): 169–176.

Carroll, K. K. 1953. Erucic acid as the factor in rape oil affecting adrenal cholesterol in the rat. *Journal of Biological Chemistry* 200: 287–292.

Castro, V. S., Figueiredo, E. E. D. S., Stanford, K., McAllister, T. and Conte-Junior, C. A. 2019. Shiga-toxin producing Escherichia coli in Brazil: A systematic review. *Microorganisms* 7(5): 137.

Cawood, P., Wickens, D. G., Iversen, S. A., Braganza, J. M. and Dormandy, T. L. 1983. The nature of diene conjugation in human serum, bile and duodenal juice. *FEBS Letters* 162(2): 239–243.

Chien, K. R., Bellary, A., Nicar, M., Mukherjee, A. and Buja, L. M. 1983. Induction of a reversible cardiac lipidosis by a dietary long-chain fatty acid (erucic acid). Relationship to lipid accumulation in border zones of myocardial infarcts. *The American Journal of Pathology* 112(1): 68–77.

Christensen, C.M., Mirocha, C.l. and Meronuck, R.A. 1977. Mold, mycotoxin and mycotoxicoses. In *Agricultural Experiment Station*, Report 142. St. Paul: University of Minnesota.

Cobbett, C. and Goldsbrough, P. 2002. Phytochelatins and metallothioneins: Roles in heavy metal detoxification and homeostasis. *Annual Review of Plant Biology* 53(1): 159–182.

Cole, R. J. 1989. Technology of aflatoxin decontamination. In '*Mycotoxins and Phycotoxins* 88', edited by S. Natori, K. Hashimoto, and Y. Ueno (pp. 177–184). Elsevier Science Publishers.

Concon, J. 1988. Food Toxicology. Part B: Contaminants and Additives. New York: Dekker.

Conway, H. F., Anderson, R. A., & Bagley, B. 1978. Detoxification of aflatoxin-contaminated corn by roasting. *Cereal Chemistry* 55(1): 115–117.

Cornell University 2010. Plants poisonous to livestock. Thiaminases. Available online: http://www.ansci.cornell.edu/plants/toxicagents/thiaminase.html (accessed on 21 July 2010).

Coulombe, R. A. 2001. *Natural Toxins and Chemopreventives in Plants*. Boca Raton, FL: CRC Press.

Cousin, M. A., Riley, R. T. and Pestka, J. J. 2005. Foodborne mycotoxins: Chemistry, biology, ecology, and toxicology. In *Foodborne Pathogens: Microbiology and Molecular Biology*, edited by P. M. Fratamico, A. K. Bhunia, and J. L. (pp. 163–226). Caister Academic Press.

Dam, R., Tam, S. W. and Satterlee, L. D. 1977. Destruction of aflatoxins during fermentation and by-product isolation from artificially contaminated grains [Corn, wheat, corn-milo]. Cereal Chemistry (USA).

Davis, W. E. 1979. National Inventory of Sources and Emissions of Cadmium, Nickel, and Asbestos. Cadmium, Section 1. Report PB 192250. Springfield, VA: National Technical Information Service.

de Assis, D. C. S., da Silva, T. M. L., Brito, R. F., da Silva, L. C. G., Lima, W. G. and Brito, J. C. M. 2020. Shiga toxin-producing Escherichia coli (STEC) in bovine meat and meat products over the last 15 years in Brazil: A systematic review and meta-analysis. *Meat Science*, 108394.

Deshpande, S. E. 2002. Fungal toxins. In *Handbook of Food Toxicology* (pp. 413–417). New York: Marcel Dekker, Academic Press.

Dickens, J. W. and Whitaker, T. B. 1975. Efficacy of electronic color sorting and hand picking to remove aflatoxin contaminated kernels from commercial lots of shelled peanuts. *Peanut Science* 2(2): 45–50.

Dietrich, R., Jessberger, N., Ehling-Schulz, M., Märtlbauer, E. and Granum, P. E. 2021. The food poisoning toxins of Bacillus cereus. *Toxins* 13(2): 98.

Dobbins, J. W., Laurenson, J. P., Gorelick, F. S. and Banwell, J. G. 1986. Phytohemagglutinin from red kidney bean (Phaseolus vulgaris) inhibits sodium and chloride absorption in the rabbit ileum. *Gastroenterology* 90(6): 1907–1913.

Dolan, L. C., Matulka, R. A. and Burdock, G. A. 2010. Naturally occurring food toxins. *Toxins* 2(9): 2289–2332.

Doll, R. and Peto, R. J. 1981. The causes of cancer: Quantitative estimates of avoidable risks in the United States today. *Journal of the National Cancer Institute* 66(6): 1191–1308.

Duan, G. L., Hu, Y., Liu, W. J., Kneer, R., Zhao, F. J. and Zhu, Y. G. 2011. Evidence for a role of phytochelatins in regulating arsenic accumulation in rice grain. *Environmental and Experimental Botany* 71(3): 416–421.

Duke, J. A. 1992. *Database of Phytochemical Constituents of GRAS Herbs and Other Economic Plants.* CRC Press.

El-Banna, A. A., Pitt, J. I. and Leistner, L. 1987. Production of mycotoxins by Penicillium species. *Systematic and Applied Microbiology* 10(1): 42–46.

Falowo, A. B., Fayemi, P. O. and Muchenje, V. 2014. Natural antioxidants against lipid–protein oxidative deterioration in meat and meat products: A review. *Food Research International* 64: 171–181.

Food, U. S. 2006. Drug Administration Code of Federal Regulations. Department of Health and Human Services, Title, 21.

Fränken, J., Stephan, U., Meyer, H. E. and Konig, W. 1994. Identification of alpha-amylase inhibitor as a major allergen of wheat flour. *International Archives of Allergy and Immunology* 104(2): 171–174.

Friedman, M. and Rasooly, R. 2013. Review of the inhibition of biological activities of food-related selected toxins by natural compounds. *Toxins* 5(4): 743–775.

Geboers, J., Joossens, J. V. and Kesteloot, H. 1985. Diet and human carcinogenesis. *Excerpta Medica Amsterdam* 277: 494–501.

Gilbert, S. G. 2005. Ethical, legal, and social issues: Our children's future. *Neurotoxicology* 26(4): 521–530.

Girennavar, B., Poulose, S. M., Jayaprakasha, G. K., Bhat, N. G. and Patil, B. S. 2006. Furocoumarins from grapefruit juice and their effect on human CYP 3A4 and CYP 1B1 isoenzymes. *Bioorganic & Medicinal Chemistry* 14(8): 2606–2612.

Gold, L. S., Slone, T. H., Stern, B. R., Manley, N. B. and Ames, B. N. 1992. Rodent carcinogens: setting priorities. *Science* 258(5080): 261–265.

Granum, P. E. 1979. Studies on α-amylase inhibitors in foods. *Food Chemistry* 4(3): 173–178.

Ha, Y. L., Grimm, N. K. and Pariza, M. W. 1987. Anticarcinogens from fried ground beef: heat-altered derivatives of linoleic acid. *Carcinogenesis* 8(12): 1881–1887.

Hagler, W.M., Jr, Hutchings, J.E. and Hamilton, P.B. 1982. Destruction of aflatoxin in corn with sodium bisulfate. *Journal of Food Protection* 45(14):1287–1291.

Hall, R. L. and Oser, B. L. 1968. The safety of flavoring substances. *Residue Reviews/Rückstands-Berichte* 24: 1–17.

Haque, M. A., Wang, Y., Shen, Z., Li, X., Saleemi, M. K. and He, C. 2020. Mycotoxin contamination and control strategy in human, domestic animal and poultry: A review. *Microbial Pathogenesis* 142: 104095.

Henry, S. H., Bosch, F. X., Troxell, T. C. and Bolger, P. M. 1999. Reducing liver cancer--global control of aflatoxin. *Science* 286(5449): 2453–2454.

Heredia, N. and García, S. 2018). Animals as sources of food-borne pathogens: A review. *Animal Nutrition* 4(3): 250–255.

Hill, M. J. 1987. Dietary fat and human cancer. *Anticancer Research* 7(3 Pt A): 281–292.

Hold, K. M., Sirisoma, N. S. and Casida, J. E. 2001. Detoxification of α-and β-Thujones (the active ingredients of absinthe): Site specificity and species differences in cytochrome P450 oxidation in vitro and in vivo. *Chemical Research in Toxicology* 14(5)5: 589–595.

Hutt, P. B., Merrill, R. A. and Grossman, L. W. 2007. *Food and Drug Law.* New York: Foundation Press.

IARC Working Group on the Evaluation of Carcinogenic Risks to Humans, & International Agency for Research on Cancer. 2002. *Some Traditional Herbal Medicines, Some Mycotoxins, Naphthalene and Styrene* (Vol. 82). World Health Organization.

Isbrucker, R. A. and Burdock, G. A. 2006. Risk and safety assessment on the consumption of Licorice root (Glycyrrhiza sp.), its extract and powder as a food ingredient, with emphasis on the pharmacology and toxicology of glycyrrhizin. *Regulatory Toxicology and Pharmacology* 46(3): 167–192

Karioti, A. and Bilia, A. R. 2010. Hypericins as potential leads for new therapeutics. *International Journal of Molecular Sciences* 11(2): 562–594.

Kass, N. E. 2001. An ethics framework for public health. *American Journal of Public Health* 91(11): 1776–1782.

Khaneghah, A. M., Farhadi, A., Nematollahi, A., Vasseghian, Y. and Fakhri, Y. 2020. A systematic review and meta-analysis to investigate the concentration and prevalence of trichothecenes in the cereal-based food. *Trends in Food Science & Technology* doi:10.1016/j.tifs.2020.05.026.

Lagerwerff, J. V. and Specht, A. W. 1971. Occurrence of environmental cadmium and zinc, and their uptake by plants. *Trace Substances in Environmental Health* 4.

Lanza, E. and Slover, H. T. 1981. The use of SP2340 glass capillary columns for the estimation of thetrans fatty acid content of foods. *Lipids* 16(4): 260–267.

Larsson, B. K., Sahlberg, G. P., Eriksson, A. T. and Busk, L. A. 1983. Polycyclic aromatic hydrocarbons in grilled food. *Journal of Agricultural and Food Chemistry* 31(4): 867–873.

Lawrence, B.M. 2006. Progress in essential oils. Sage oil. In *Essential Oils*: 2001–2004, 25–30. Carol Stream, IL: Allured Publishing.

Lee, C. 2002. Environmental justice: Building a unified vision of health and the environment. *Environmental Health Perspectives* 110(suppl 2): 141–144.

Linder, M. C. 2002. Biochemistry and molecular biology of copper in mammals. In *Handbook of Copper Pharmacology and Toxicology*, edited by E. J. Massaro (pp. 3–32). Totowa, NJ: Humana Press.

Lopez-Garcia, R. 1998. Aflatoxin B (1) and Fumonisin B (1) Co-Contamination: Interactive Effects, Possible Mechanisms of Toxicity, and Decontamination Procedures. Louisiana State University and Agricultural & Mechanical College.

Lu, Y., Adomako, E. E., Solaiman, A. R. M., Islam, M. R., Deacon, C., Williams, P. N. and Meharg, A. A. 2009. Baseline soil variation is a major factor in arsenic accumulation in Bengal delta paddy rice. *Environmental Science & Technology* 43(6): 1724–1729.

Luter, L., Wyslouzil, W. and Kashyap, S. C. 1982. The destruction of aflatoxins in peanuts by microwave roasting. *Canadian Institute of Food Science and Technology Journal* 15(3): 236–238.

Ma, J. F., Tamai, K., Yamaji, N., Mitani, N., Konishi, S., Katsuhara, M. and Yano, M. 2006. A silicon transporter in rice. *Nature* 440(7084): 688–691.

Machen, M.D., Clement, B.A., Shepherd, E.C., Sarr, A.B., Pettit, R.E. & Phillips, T.D. 1988. Sorption of aflatoxins from peanut oil by aluminosilicates. *Toxicologist* 8:265.

Mahato, D. K., Devi, S., Pandhi, S., Sharma, B., Maurya, K. K., Mishra, S. and Kumar, P. 2021. Occurrence, impact on agriculture, human health, and management strategies of zearalenone in food and feed: A Review. *Toxins* 13(2): 92.

Marzulli, F. N. 1970. Perfume phototoxicity. *Journal of Cosmetic Science* 21: 695–715.

McGinn, A. P. 2000. Worldwatch Paper 153: Why Poison Ourselves. A Precautionary Approach to Synthetic Chemicals.

Meharg, A. A., Naylor, J. and Macnair, M. R. 1994. *Phosphorus Nutrition of Arsenate-Tolerant and Nontolerant Phenotypes of Velvetgrass* (Vol. 23, No. 2, pp. 234–238). American Society of Agronomy, Crop Science Society of America, and Soil Science Society of America.

Meharg, A. A., Williams, P. N., Adomako, E., Lawgali, Y. Y., Deacon, C., Villada, A. and Yanai, J. 2009. Geographical variation in total and inorganic arsenic content of polished (white) rice. *Environmental Science & Technology* 43(5): 1612–1617.

Miller, C. D. 1989. *Selected Toxicological Studies of the Mycotoxincyclopiazonic Acid in Turkeys*. Iowa State University.

Monroe, D. H. and Eaton, D. L. 1987. Comparative effects of butylatedhydroxyanisole on hepatic in vivo DNA binding and in vitro biotransformation of aflatoxin B1 in the rat and mouse. *Toxicology and Applied Pharmacology* 90(3): 401–409.

Moreno-Ancillo, A., Dominguez-Noche, C., Gil-Adrados, A. C. and Cosmes, P. M. 2004. Bread eating induced oral angioedema due to alpha-amylase allergy. *Journal of Investigational Allergology and Clinical Immunology* 14(4): 346–347.

National Research Council. 1984. Toxicity testing: strategies to determine needs and priorities.

National Toxicology Program. 2006. NTP technical report on the toxicology and carcinogenesis studies of 2, 3, 7, 8-tetrachlorodibenzo-p-dioxin (TCDD)(CAS No. 1746-01–6) in female Harlan Sprague-Dawley rats (Gavage Studies). *National Toxicology Program Technical Report Series* (521): 4–232.

Nelson, C. P., Patton, G. W., Arvidson, K., Lee, H. and Twaroski, M. L. 2011. Assessing the toxicity of polymeric food-contact substances. *Food and Chemical Toxicology* 49(9): 1877–1897.

Nerin, C., Alfaro, P., Aznar, M. and Domeño, C. 2013. The challenge of identifying non-intentionally added substances from food packaging materials: A review. *Analytica Chimica Acta* 2 (775): 14–24.

Newberne, P. M. 1987. Mechanisms of interaction and modulation of response. In *Methods for Assessing the Effects of Mixtures of Chemicals*, edited by V. B. Vouk, G. C. Butler, A. C. Upton, D. V. Parke and S. C. Asher, 555. New York: Wiley.

Oberleas, D. 1973. *Toxicants Occurring Naturally in Foods*. National Academy of Sciences. USA, pp. 363–371.
O'brien, M. 2000. *Making Better Environmental Decisions: An Alternative to Risk Assessment*. MIT Press.
Panter, K. E. 2004. *Natural Toxins of Plant Origin*. Boca Raton, FL: CRC Press.
Pariza, M. W. 1988. Dietary fat and cancer risk: Evidence and research needs. *Annual Review of Nutrition* 8(1): 167–183.
Park, D. L., López-García, R., Trujillo-Preciado, S. and Price, R. L. 1996. Reduction of risks associated with fumonisin contamination in corn. In *Fumonisins in Food*, edited by L. S. Jackson, J. W. DeVries, and L. B. Bullerman (pp. 335–344). Boston, MA: Springer.
Park, D. L., Njapau, H. and Boutrif, E. 1999. Minimizing risks posed by mycotoxins utilizing the HACCP concept. *Food Nutrition and Agriculture* 49–54.
Park, D. L. and Price, W. D. 2001. Reduction of aflatoxin hazards using ammoniation. *Reviews of Environmental Contamination and Toxicology* 171: 139–176.
Park, D. L. and Stoloff, L. 1989. Aflatoxin control—How a regulatory agency managed risk from an unavoidable natural toxicant in food and feed. *Regulatory Toxicology and Pharmacology* 9(2): 109–130.
Park, J. E., Seo, J. E., Lee, J. Y. and Kwon, H. 2015. Distribution of seven N-nitrosamines in food. *Toxicological Research* 31(3): 279–288.
Parodi, P. W. 1977. Conjugated octadecadienoic acids of milk fat. *Journal of Dairy Science* 60(10): 1550–1553.
Patocka, J. and Plucar, B. 2003. Pharmacology and toxicology of absinthe. *Journal of Applied Biomedicine* 1(4): 199–205.
Peers, F. G., Gilman, G. A. and Linsell, C. A. 1976. Dietary aflatoxins and human liver cancer. A study in Swaziland. *International Journal of Cancer* 17(2): 167–176.
Peter, A. J. and Viraraghavan, T. 2005. Thallium: A review of public health and environmental concerns. *Environment International* 31(4): 493–501.
Phillips, T. D., Clement, B. A. and Park, D. L. 1994. *Approaches to Reduction. The Toxicology of Aflatoxins: Human Health, Veterinary, and Agricultural Significance*, pp. 383–399. Press, 2003.
Pirooty, S. and Ghasemzadeh, M. 2013. Toxic effects of Lead on different organs of the human body. *KAUMS Journal (Feyz)* 16(7): 761–762.
Placzek, M., Frömel, W., Eberlein, B., Gilbertz, K. P. and Przybilla, B. 2007. Evaluation of phototoxic properties of fragrances. *Actadermato-venereologica* 87(4): 312–316.
Pottern, L. M., Morris, L. E., Blot, W. J., Ziegler, R. G. and FraumeniJr, J. F. 1981. Esophageal cancer among black men in Washington, DCI Alcohol, tobacco, and other risk factors. *Journal of the National Cancer Institute* 67(4): 777–783.
Prakash, A. S., Pereira, T. N., Reilly, P. E. and Seawright, A. A. 1999. Pyrrolizidine alkaloids in human diet. *Mutation Research/Genetic Toxicology and Environmental Mutagenesis* 443(1–2): 53–67.
Raab, A., Williams, P. N., Meharg, A. and Feldmann, J. 2007. Uptake and translocation of inorganic and methylated arsenic species by plants. *Environmental Chemistry* 4(3): 197–203.
Raikwar, M. K., Kumar, P., Singh, M. and Singh, A. 2008. Toxic effect of heavy metals in livestock health. *Veterinary World* 1(1): 28–30.
Rice, K. M., Walker Jr, E. M., Wu, M., Gillette, C. and Blough, E. R. 2014. Environmental mercury and its toxic effects. *Journal of Preventive Medicine and Public Health* 47(2): 74–83.
Riel, R. R. 1963. Physico-chemical characteristics of Canadian milk fat. Unsaturated fatty acids. *Journal of Dairy Science* 46(2): 102–106.
Saha, G. C. and Ali, M. A. 2007. Dynamics of arsenic in agricultural soils irrigated with arsenic contaminated groundwater in Bangladesh. *Science of the Total Environment* 379(2–3): 180–189.
Sansalone W (ed.). 1999. What is a Nutrient: Defining the Food-Drug Continuum. Proceedings, Georgetown University, Center for Food and Nutritional Policy, Washington, DC, p. 82.
Schlatter, J., Zimmerli, B., Dick, R., Panizzon, R. and Schlatter, C. H. 1991. Dietary intake and risk assessment of phototoxic furocoumarins in humans. *Food and Chemical Toxicology* 29(8): 523–530.
Scholfield, C. R. 1981. Gas chromatographic equivalent chain lengths of fatty acid methyl esters on a Silar 10C glass capillary column. *Journal of the American Oil Chemists' Society* 58(6): 662–663.
Scholfield, C. R. and Dutton, H. J. 1971. Equivalent chain lengths of methyl octadecadienoates and octadecatrienoates. *Journal of the American Oil Chemists' Society* 48(5): 228–231.
Schoof, R. A., Yost, L. J., Eickhoff, J., Crecelius, E. A., Cragin, D. W., Meacher, D. M. and Menzel, D. B. 1999. A market basket survey of inorganic arsenic in food. *Food and Chemical Toxicology* 37(8): 839–846.

Scott, W. E., Herb, S. F., Magidman, P. and Riemenschneider, R. W. 1959. Composition of edible fats, unsaturated fatty acids of butterfat. *Journal of Agricultural and Food Chemistry* 7(2): 125–129.

Shames, L. 2010. *Food Safety: FDA Should Strengthen Its Oversight of Food Ingredients Determined to be Generally Recognized as Safe*. DIANE Publishing.

Shibamoto, T. and Bjeldanes, L. F. 1993. *Introduction to Food Toxicology*. Academic Press, Inc.

Sors, T. G., Ellis, D. R., & Salt, D. E. (2005). Selenium uptake, translocation, assimilation and metabolic fate in plants. *Photosynthesis Research* 86(3): 373–389.

Stern, R. S., Nichols, K. T. and Vakeva, L. H. 1997. Malignant melanoma in patients treated for psoriasis with methoxsalen (psoralen) and ultraviolet A radiation (PUVA). *New England Journal of Medicine* 336(15): 1041–1045.

Stoloff, L. 1982. Mycotoxins as potential environmental carcinogens. *Carcinogens and Mutagens in the Environment* 1: 97–120.

Thakali, A. and MacRae, J. D. 2021. A review of chemical and microbial contamination in food: What are the threats to a circular food system?. *Environmental Research* 194: 110635.

Trujillo, S. 1997. *Reduction and Management of Risks Associated With Aflatoxin and Fumonisin Contamination in Corn*. Louisiana State University.

Tuyns, A. J., Riboli, E., Doornbos, G. and Péquignot, G. 1987. Diet and esophageal cancer in Calvados (France).

U.S. Environmental Protection Agency. Chemical right-to-know initiative [cited Oct 2002]. Available from: http://www.epa.gov/chemrtk

Ulloa, S. M. and Herrea, T. 1970. Persistencia de lasaflatoxinasdurante la fermantacion del pozol. *Revista Latinoamericana de Microbiología* 12: 19.

Ulloa-Sosa, M. and Schroeder, H. W. 1969. Note on aflatoxin decomposition in the process of making tortillas from corn. *Cereal Chemistry* 46: 397–400.

United States Food and Drug Administration (FDA) 2001. Chapter 10: Methyl mercury. In *Fish and Fisheries Products Hazards and Controls Guidance*, 3rd edition, June, 2001. Available online: http://www.fda.gov/Food/GuidanceComplianceRegulatoryInformation/GuidanceDocuments/Seaf ood/ucm092041.htm (accessed on 21 July 2010).

United States Food and Drug Administration (FDA). 2009. Bad Bug Book. Foodborne Pathogenic Microorganisms and Natural Toxins Handbook. Phytohaemagglutinin. Available online: http://www.fda.gov/food/foodsafety/foodborneillness/foodborneillnessfoodbornepathogens naturaltoxins/badbugbook/ucm071092.htm (accessed on 21 July 2010)

United States National Toxicology Program (NTP). Alpha-Thujone, December 10, 1997. Available online: http://ntp.niehs.nih.gov/index.cfm?objectid=03DB8C36-E7A1-98893BDF8436F2A8C51F (accessed on 21 July 2010).

VenEtten, C. H . and Woff, I. A. 1973. Natural sulfur compounds. In *Toxicants Occurring Naturally in Foods*, 2nd edition (pp. 210–234). Washington, DC: Committee on Food Protection, Food and Nutrition Board, National Research Council, National Academy of Sciences.

Villa, C. C., Galus, S., Nowacka, M., Magri, A., Petriccione, M. and Gutiérrez, T. J. 2020. Molecular sieves for food applications: A review. *Trends in Food Science & Technology* 102: 102–122.

Viviani, R. 1970. Metabolism of long-chain fatty acids in the rumen. *Advances in Lipid Research* 8: 267–346.

Wagstaff, D. J. 1991. Dietary exposure to furocoumarins. *Regulatory Toxicology and Pharmacology* 14(3): 261–272.

Wentworth, J. M., Agostini, M., Love, J., Schwabe, J. W. and Chatterjee, V. K. K. 2000. St John's wort, a herbal antidepressant, activates the steroid X receptor. *Journal of Endocrinology* 166(3): R11.

Williams, P. N., Villada, A., Deacon, C., Raab, A., Figuerola, J., Green, A. J. and Meharg, A. A. 2007. Greatly enhanced arsenic shoot assimilation in rice leads to elevated grain levels compared to wheat and barley. *Environmental Science & Technology* 41(19): 6854–6859.

Wood, G. M., Cooper, S. J. and Chapman, W. B. 1982. Problems associated with laboratory simulation of effects of food processes on mycotoxins. In Proc. of V. Int. Symp. Mycotoxins, Vienna, Austria (Vol. 142).

World Health Organization. 2015. *World health statistics 2015*. World Health Organization.

Xu, X. Y., McGrath, S. P., Meharg, A. A. and Zhao, F. J. 2008. Growing rice aerobically markedly decreases arsenic accumulation. *Environmental Science & Technology* 42(15): 5574–5579.

Zhang, H., Hu, S.L., Zhang, Z.J., Hu, L.Y., Jiang, C.X., Wei, Z.J., Liu, J., Wang, H.L. and Jiang, S.T. 2011. Hydrogen sulfide acts as a regulator of flower senescence in plants. *Postharvest Biology and Technology*, 60(3): 251–257.

Zhao, K., Tung, C.W., Eizenga, G.C., Wright, M.H., Ali, M.L., Price, A.H., Norton, G.J., Islam, M.R., Reynolds, A., Mezey, J. and McClung, A.M., 2011 .Genome-wide association mapping reveals a rich genetic architecture of complex traits in Oryzasativa. *Nature Communications* 467: 1–10.

# CHAPTER 2

# Phytates

**Arshied Manzoor, Aarifa Nabi, Rayees Ahmad Shiekh, Aamir Hussain Dar, Zakiya Usmani, Aayeena Altaf, Shafat Ahmad Khan, and Saghir Ahmad**

## CONTENTS



## 2.1 INTRODUCTION

Phosphorus is available in a number of plant tissues, in particular seeds and bran in the storage form of phytate or phytic acid (Cosgrove, 1980). In addition to phosphorus, inositol in plants is mainly in the form of phytate (inositol hexaphosphate, $InsP_6$), which is also believed to be the source of some other trace elements. Oilseeds contain near to about 60–80% phytates, cereals, and legumes are present in the form of phytates, which is actually a combination of phosphorus and inositol (Loewus, 2002). However, fruits, berries, tubers, and roots contain lower phytate concentrations. Phytates constitute almost 60–90% of total phosphate in dormant seeds and its formation occurs during the stage of maturation in plant seeds (Loewus, 2002). Phytates are reported as anti-nutrient compounds in some foods such as oats because of their complex formation with metals/proteins, thereby limiting their bioavailability in the gastrointestinal tract. Phytates are reported to be the complex compounds occurring naturally, responsible for altering the characteristics of foods based on the nutritional and functional properties. These substances have been known for a long time; however, a complete understanding of their role is not yet depicted in its entirety. Concerning the

DOI: 10.1201/9781003178446-2

health and nutrition of human beings, phytic acid is the most important among all the anti-nutritional components. Based on vegetarian diets, humans in rural areas of developing countries are reported to consume 2,000–2,600 mg daily which is only 150–1,400 mg based on the mixed diets (Reddy, 2002). Studies have reported that cereal-based foods contain less phytates as compared to legume-based foods, however, their rich sources include sesame seeds, soy protein concentrate, rice, maize bread, and peanuts (Kumar, Sinha, Makkar, & Becker, 2010).

## 2.2 CHEMISTRY

Weaver & Kannan (2002) described phytate as a chelating agent helpful in causing a reduction in the divalent cation bioavailability. The reduction in phytate content is favoured by some of the biological/thermal treatments among which fermentation, appertization, and germination are worth mentioning. Molecular ratio of phytate to zinc predicts the inhibitory effect on zinc caused by phytate and in this concern, a ratio of 10–15 was reported to furnish potential zinc inhibition.

IP6 or phytic acid is the highly reactive compound (acidic) having the property of binding mineral cations with it to form a complex technically called phytin. Studies have reported that phytic acid consists of 12 protons that are replaceable or called reactive sites. Out of the 12 protons, 2 have weak acidic nature (pK = 6), 6 with strong acidic nature (pK = 1.5–2), and the remaining 4 with weak acidic nature (pK = 9–11). The normal pH as reported in feeds and digestive tract of animals, furnishes phytin a negative charge that makes it much more proficient to bind with the di- and trivalent cations ($Zn^{2+}$, $Cu^{2+}$, $Ni^{2+}$, $Co^{2+}$, $Mn^{2+}$, $Fe^{2+}$, and $Ca^{2+}$) thereby forming stable complexes and hence making these minerals unavailable for the animals. Not confined to these cations, phytates can also form stable complexes with the Mg, Ca, and K (Bohn et al., 2007). Among all the minerals, $Zn^{2+}$ makes the most stable complex which bestows it the highest potential for the phytate hydrolysis inhibition by the phytase enzyme. Moreover, phytate to mineral molar ratio coupled with the pH of the solution determines the complex stability formed by the minerals. Among all the mineral-IP6 complexes, the complex formed by Ca is highly unstable and should inhibit the phytase enzyme to the minimum, however, these complexes are reported for a significant enzyme inhibition (both exogenous and endogenous) that is credited to the dietary Ca present. The IP6-metal complex precipitation is enhanced by the simultaneous presence of two cations. Phytate, an insoluble solid is formed in the excess presence of metal ions; however, abundance of phytic acid favours the formation of complexes soluble in nature (Torres et al., 2005). In addition, IP6 undertake the complex formation with the proteins through electrostatic binding (favoured at low pH) and salt bridges (favoured at high pH) and starches through hydrogen bonding present in different seeds respectively, making these macromolecules unavailable for absorption from the diets. pH is one of the most influencing factors affecting the phytic acid solubility of its Zn, Ca, Cu, and Cd salts. For example, up to pH 7.5, Mg-phytate shows 100% solubility while its salt of Ca, Cd, Zn, and Cu is soluble at pH $< 4$.

## 2.3 DISTRIBUTION

Seeds of cereals and legumes consist of phosphorous majorly in the form of Phytic acid. Phytic acid acts as an anti-nutrient crediting to its role in complex formation with minerals and proteins. Phytate distribution in cereals and legumes is decided either by the amount of photoassimilates and phosphorus that is transported to the cereal grains or by the metabolic pathways governing the substrate partitioning among different pools. For example, the amount of phosphorous (inorganic) in leaves predicts the phytate content which is otherwise predicted by the phosphorous supplied to the plant which ultimately enhances the phosphorous translocation to the grain. However, the mechanism deciding the regulation of phytate levels in plants is unknown as the protein level is also correlated with the protein storage bodies present. In addition to the environmental factors, the genetic variability also affects the phosphorous distribution in cereals such as beans (Santos, 1998). Fe, Zn, Mn like divalent cations help in the chelation of phytic acid which constitutes about 85% of phosphorous in wheat kernel. In aleurone, a protein-rich globoid cage protects the phytates which are present in the form of globules (Schlemmer, Frolich, Prieto, & Grases, 2009). Humans are devoid of the intestinal phytase enzymes, hence not assimilated in the human body due to their poor absorption. The growth and development of plants is enhanced by an increase in the phytase activity during the process of germination (Platel, Eipeson, & Srinivasan, 2010).

## 2.4 MODE OF ACTION OF PHYTATES

The phytic acid or phytate is present in many seeds as the main storage form of phosphorus and its structure generates the possibilities of interacting with protein residues and metal cations (Sharma et al., 2020; Silva et al., 2021). Mineral phosphorus is present in it and is tightly bound to it, forming a structure like a snowflake-like molecule. Various researchers have reported that the phytic acid protonation depends on the pH and the anions formed to have a varying degree of protonation. Twelve dissociable hydrogens are present in a phytic acid molecule (Oatway et al., 2001; Coulibaly et al., 2011). Phytic acid also binds with Zn, ca, Fe, Mg, and proteins. In germinating seeds, the breakdown of phytic acid occurs by the involvement of endogenous phosphatases and phytases. This process releases the secondary messenger of plants, calcium (chelated $Ca^{2+}$), for plant growth and development (Nissar et al., 2017; Grases et al., 2017). The involvement of $CaCl_2$ has been reported to enhance the activity of phytase and acid phosphatase activity by improving the $Ca^{2+}$ accumulation and influx in cells and ameliorates the degradation of phytic acid (Zhou et al., 2018; Rousseau et al., 2020).

Furthermore, it reduces inositol phosphates and activates the deprivation of PA releasing extra (P) to the germinating sprouts. Thus, phytic acid degradation depends on $Ca^{2+}$ regulation, accumulation, and mobilization (Eder et al., 2017; Mihrete, 2019). The positive or negative effect of mineral bioavailability depends on the higher (IP6 and IP5-negative effect) or lower inositol-phosphates (IP4 and IP3). It is a complex with the iron (Fe) and zinc (Zn), forming the zinc-calcium-phytate (Ca aids in phytic acid inhibition) and iron-calcium-phytate complexes, and the binding is dependent on the binding strength of minerals, making them unavailable for absorption (Rousseau et al., 2020). The biosynthesis of PA involves two routes (lipid-dependent and lipid-independent). The one operating in various plant organs is lipid-dependent, and the other working in seeds is lipid-independent. However, it involves multiple steps and enzymes; the enzymes for lipid-independent pathways are not well documented. The enzymes involved in phytate degradation are present in mature seeds, pollen, and form the constitutive ones and are responsible for phytate breakdown during imbibition. The others are synthesized de novo, either from the synthesis of enzymes at the transcriptional or from pre-existing mRNA. These form the germination-inducible, phytate-degrading enzymes (Greiner et al., 2007).

In the first step of biosynthesis, the enzyme MIPS (myo-inositol 3-phosphate synthase) acts upon the D-glucose-6-phosphate (Figure 2.1). It converts it into Myo-inositol 3-monophosphate, the phosphorylation of particular inositol through the involvement of different inositol phosphate kinases yield $InsP_6$ and constitute the lipid-independent route. The first phosphorylation step is catalyzed by MIK (myo-inositol kinase), and it converts the Ins to $InsP_1$ and then $InsP_1$ is converted to $InsP_2$ by a homolog of 2-PGK (2-phosphoglycerate kinase). The gene responsible for it detected in rice is *OsPGK1*. For the generation of $InsP_{3,4,5,6}$, further phosphorylation steps and inositol kinases are involved IPK1 (inositol polyphosphate 2-kinase), IPK2/IPMK (inositol polyphosphate multikinase), ITPK (inositol 1,3,4-trisphosphate 5-6-kinase) (Oh et al., 2004; Sparvoli and Cominelli, 2015; Madsen et al., 2020). In *Arabidopsis thaliana,* two inositol-phosphate kinases

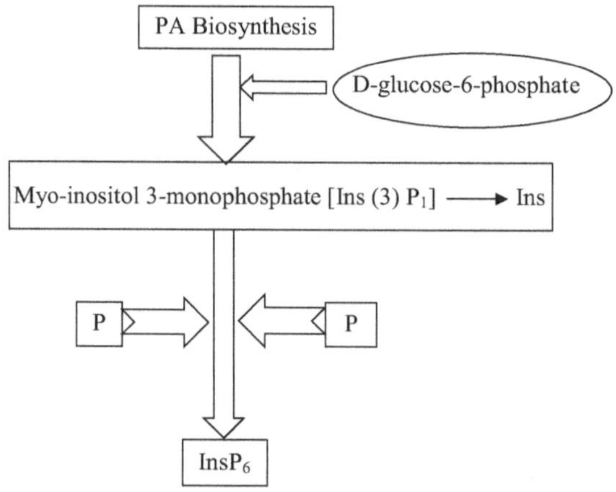


**Figure 2.1** Phytates: Mechanism of action.

(AtIpk2α and, AtIpk2β) encoded by various genes on chromosome 5 have been reported (Stevenson-Paulik et al., 2002).

For the hydrolysis of phytates, different classes of phytases (alkaline and HAPs) and phosphatases (protein phosphatases, high-molecular-weight HAPs [histidine acid phosphatases], high-molecular-weight HAPs [acid phytases], alkaline phosphatases, and purple acid phosphatases) act on it. This motif served as a nucleophile for the phosphomonoester hydrolysis and generated an intermediate, a covalent phosphohistidine. From the C-terminal conserved HD motif, the residue of aspartic acid donates oxygen atom to the phosphomonoester bond (scissile) (Wilson and Majerus, 1997; Qian et al., 2005; Sweetman et al., 2007; Cridland and Gillaspy, 2020). The phytate hydrolysis by alkaline phytase through catalytic mechanism occurs through a Ca-bound $H_2O$ molecule present in the active site. It attacks the phosphomonoester bond (calcium-phytate complex) of alkaline phytase. In this process, the first step is the substitution of Glu260, Glu211, and Asp314 (three calcium-binding residues), resulting in loss of catalytic activity. After that, the Ca-bound hydroxide ion replacement occurs at the enzyme active site cleft by fluoride, followed by nucleophilic attack by metal-bound hydroxide (Sacchi and Nocito, 2019; Laha et al., 2020). Besides these properties, substrate specificity is also an essential factor. It varies for HAPs (broad specificity), which prefer to hydrolyze metal-free phytates and alkaline phytases prefer to hydrolyze calcium-phytate complex (narrow specificity). A particular transporter for phytate (inositol hexakisphosphate) transport reported is AtABCC5. It helps in the storage of phytate in seeds and stomatal regulation in *Arabidopsis thaliana.* Its transport is AtABCC5-dependent (Nagy et al., 2009; Madsen and Pedersen, 2020). $H^+$/myo-inositol is a high-affinity plasma membrane-localized symporter that INOSITOL TRANSORTER4 encodes reported in *Arabidopsis* and is from the MPS protein family and is perhaps involved in sequestration of phytate (Haydon and Cobbett, 2007). Phytic acid plays a significant role in various plant processes besides acting as a signalling molecule (Gillaspy, 2013). It helps in various physiological and developmental processes, biosynthetic pathways involving the production of metabolites like pinitol, galactinol, pectic substances, and different polysaccharides (cell wall). It also plays an essential role in;

- Phosphorus homeostasis.
- Act as ligands for plant hormones.
- Cellular metabolism (mRNA nuclear export, chromatin remodelling, and modification).
- Signal transduction (energy sensing and metabolism, sugar signalling, downstream response to auxin, sugar, and ABA-mediated processes).

- Response to biotic and abiotic stress (anoxia, salt stress, heat stress, drought stress, exposure to elicitors and pathogens, resistance to herbivory and wounding).
- Maintaining the endomembrane structure and trafficking besides repressing the PCD (programmed cell death).

In yeast, the $InsP_4$ and $InsP_5$ have been reported to stimulate nucleosome mobilization by SWI/SNF complex. The InsPs have been reported to be structural cofactors of TIR1 and COI1, required for jasmonic acid and auxin signalling. Therefore, the Myo-inositol acts as a secondary messenger in signalling at the regulatory level and is involved in metabolism as it is also a precursor for themyo-inositol-polyphosphatases (Hitz et al., 2002, Secco et al., 2017). After the uptake of mineral nutrients like phosphorus from plants, they are stored in storage tissues. The phosphorus inside the plants is converted to phytate through the pathways operating in the cytoplasm. Specific transporter MRP-ABC is involved in its transport to PSV (protein storage vacuole). Some other nutrients like magnesium, potassium, and nitrogen also transport either through the same transporter or through antiporters and arrive at the storage tissue cell (Pfeiffer and Hager, 1993; Barragan et al., 2012). Gibberellic acid (GA) also plays a role in phytate degradation during seed development (acidification of PSV and events of hydrolysis, generation of the proton pump, germination, phosphate sensing, and biosynthesis (Ritchie et al., 2000; Jiang et al., 2001; Arcalis et al., 2014).

## 2.5 TOXICOLOGY OF PHYTATES

The ideal amount of phytate present in phytate-containing foods is 25 mg/100 g or less (0.035%). The phytate is an anti-nutrient and alters nutrient bioavailability (Ca, Mg, Zn, Fe) in various cereals and therefore deficient in particular nutrients and decreases protein digestibility in human and animal nutrition (Hamid and Kumar, 2017). Different anti-nutrients are present in the foods and lower the nutritive value of foods and include tannins, saponins, lectins, metal-binding ingredients, amylase and protease inhibitors, and metal-binding ingredients (Samtiya et al., 2020). If they are present in excess amounts, they become toxic and form complexes with the metal ions, hamper their absorption, and impart Zn deficiency in crop plants (Holmes et al, 2001; Gemede and Ratta, 2014). These problems are associated with the vegetarian diet and cause kidney stones and anaemia.

## 2.6 IDENTIFICATION AND QUANTIFICATION

Kolchev (1978) reported that it is water-based or acidic solvents which are employed for the extraction of PA in cereals and legumes. Apart from HCL, various other acids such as phosphoric, acetic, and sulfuric acids have also been reported to be employed at varied levels of concentrations for the extraction of PA. Nicolai Petry et al. (2014) evaluated the impact of PA on iron bioavailability from iron-biofortified beans. Sample preparation was done by milling the beans prior to freeze-drying. The concentration of phytic acid in bean slurries and bean seeds as well was done by the method of Makower (1970) with few modifications. Determination of the inorganic phosphate was done by following the method of Van Veldhoven and Mannaerts (1987). It was concluded from the study that in the biofortified bean seeds and meals, concentrations of native phytic acid were 35% higher than control samples. The dephytinization procedure followed led to a significant reduction in the concentration of phytic acid in the control sample and biofortified beans.

Mandizvo and Odindo (2020) analyzed the variation in four Bambara groundnut landraces with respect to concentration of phytic acid during crucial stages of seed development and maturation stage. Spectrophotometric determination of the phytates was done from 14–65 days after the flowering stage in terms of the total extractable phosphorus by measuring absorbance at wavelength of

720 nm. Determination of the pattern of phytate accumulation in Bambara groundnut landraces was targeted in this very significant work.

Ficco et al. (2009) adopted an HPLC technique by reporting linearity between phytic acid. In this work, the principle of phytic acid quantification in developing wheat seeds is that it is the storage compound of mineral phosphorus in seeds. Beer-Lambert's law was obeyed by the coloured complex over a range (0–75 ppm) of phosphorus working standards. A linear calibration curve was generated.

Mohamed et al. (1986) devised a direct spectrophotometric method for the analysis of phytate by precipitating phytates in the form of ferric phytate prior to its conversion into sodium phytate. Beer's Law was obeyed over a wide range of phytic acid and inorganic phosphate. Soybeans were reported to exhibit the highest concentration of phytic acid (23.35 mg/g of meal) and the lowest one was detected in black-eyed peas. The highlighting feature of this work was the advantage of new chromophore method over other ones in terms of the elimination of acid digestion of phytate to inorganic phosphate. The chromogenic reagent used in this method reacts directly with the phytic acid phosphorus leading to the formation of molybdenum blue colour complex. Darambazar (2018) reported a significant method for the determination of phytic acid in food, feed, and materials derived from plants based on the colorimetric method of Gao et al. (2007) with much modifications. Marolt and Kolar (2021) stated that the analysis of phytic acid and/or other inositol phosphates has been a daunting analytical task. Sample preparation involves the acidic extraction of inositol phosphates from dried and ground samples using HCl for 2–3 hours. One of the most successful and efficient techniques is high-performance ion-exchange chromatography for the separation of isomers of inositol phosphates, excluding the stereoisomers.

## 2.7 SAFETY, PRECAUTIONS, AND REGULATION

According to the study, phytate acts as an anti-nutrient since it can chelate iron, calcium, and zinc, influencing their absorption. A chelate's activity is, however, greatly influenced by its proportion of phytate to metal ions as well as pH. The World Health Organization (WHO) used phytate-to-zinc molar ratios of 5, 5–15, and > 15, as well as the amount and type of dietary protein, to characterize zinc absorption in diets as potentially comparatively high (50%), moderate (30%), or low (30%) (15%). Based on data from published isotopic studies on people focused primarily on single meals, individual foods, and certain whole-day diets, these absorption estimations were used to define three levels of dietary zinc requirements. The European Food Safety Authority has set adult nutritional zinc requirements for four tiers of phytate consumption, highlighting the urgent need for phytate food composition data.

## 2.8 EFFECT OF PROCESSING

### 2.8.1 Fermentation

When the sample of phytates was fermented at different temperatures it showed the reduction in phytate. As the temperature of the fermentation increased, the greater the amount of phytic acid was lost during fermentation. The lower the temperature, the greater the loss of phytate. According to some reports, phytase is hydrolyzed by several microorganisms during the fermentation of autoclaved flour and provides evidence for the low phytic acid content of the fermented autoclaved flour. Phytase from Pearl Millet was found to be highly beneficial to reducing phytate content fermented millet flour, which depended on fermentation pH and temperature, as Mahajan and Chauhan showed in their study of natural fermentation of raw Pearl Millet. Phytate reduction during fermentation has been reported in various foods, including corn meal (Chompreeda and Fields 1984), tempeh, rabadi, and Pearl Millet.

### 2.8.2 Cooking

Phytic acid and phytin phosphorous are significantly reduced when the phytates are cooked for three hours. The statistical data reveals that the loss of phytic acid content positively correlated with the cooking time.

### 2.8.3 Germination

The phytate or phytic acid present in many plant tissues is the phosphorous storage form, particularly in seeds and bran. Germination can result in an increase in phytase activity and phytate degradation. It was believed that phytase activity would increase as seed germination continued, causing oat seeds to have a lower phytate content during germination from 0.35% to 0.11%. It was reported by Larsson and Sandberg (1992) that temperatures of 37–40° and a pH of 4–4.5 were optimal germination conditions to reduce phytates in oat seeds by almost 79%.

### 2.8.4 Autoclaving

When the sample of phytate was autoclaved at 15 psi at 121°C with distilled water for 4 hours, it showed that the content of phytic acid reduced to 0.78%.

## 2.9 FUTURE SCOPE

Phytic acid was discovered in seeds in the late 19th century by chemists. Subsequently shown to be myoinositol (1,2,3,4,5,6) hexakisphosphate (InsP6 or "phytic acid"), this compound was originally thought to store phosphorus in seeds. It usually accounts for 75% of seed phosphorus and accounts for one to several percent of seed dry weight. Human health and animal nutrition are the two primary applications of seed InsP6 . This compound is a strong chelator of mineral cations, especially calcium, iron, and zinc (Sharply *et al.*, 1994). It forms mixed salts which are usually excreted by non-ruminants such as poultry, swine, and fish. Nutritional phytates might play both a positive and a negative role in human health. In the developing world, seed-derived dietary phytic acid may contribute to iron and zinc deficiency, a major public health concern. There is no doubt that the impact of dietary InsP6 must be analyzed on a case-by-case basis. The negative effects of dietary InsP6 acid seem to be most evident in the developing world, while the positive effects are more relevant in the developed world, dealing with inflammatory diseases and cancer management.

Since the early 1990s, our understanding of InsP6 and its role in cell biology have radically transformed. As one of the first results of the study, it was found that InsP6 is ubiquitous in eukaryotic species. In fact, the inositol phosphate that is most abundant in eukaryotic cells is phytic acid. An early move towards this development was the result of research focusing on inositol (1,4,5)-trisphosphate metabolism [Ins(1,4,5)P3] as a signal transduction pathway. Seed phytases may also increase phytase activity in the gut once a meal has been consumed by enhancing the level of seed phytases. The purpose of selecting a thermotolerant phytase was to ensure that it would retain activity after cooking. Researchers are still exploring the possibility of developing phytases that retain thermotolerance following expression and cooking.

## 2.10 CONCLUSION

The nutrient phytic acid is an example of a nutrient that can serve both good and bad purposes, depending on the situation. Plant compounds are generally healthy for humans. Aside from being an antioxidant, phytic acid may also have cancer-fighting properties. Phytates (phytic acid) can hinder iron, zinc, magnesium, and calcium absorption when consumed in whole grains, seeds, legumes, and some nuts. The presence of saponins in legumes and whole grains may interfere with the absorption of nutrients. There are many processes that help destroy phytates before they are consumed, such as cooking fermentation, germination autoclaving, heating, and soaking. Phytate is a highly reactive ligand capable of striking up interactions with various cations, small molecules, and polymers.

## REFERENCES


Arcalis, E., Ibl, V., Peters, J., Melnik, S. and Stoger, E. 2014. The dynamic behavior of storage organelles in developing cereal seeds and its impact on the production of recombinant proteins. *Frontiers in Plant Science* 5: 439.

Barragán, V., Leidi, E. O., Andrés, Z., Rubio, L., De Luca, A., Fernández, J. A. and Pardo, J. M. 2012. Ion exchangers NHX1 and NHX2 mediate active potassium uptake into vacuoles to regulate cell turgor and stomatal function in Arabidopsis. *The Plant Cell* 24(3): 1127–1142.

Bohn, L., Josefsen, L., Meyer, A. S. and Rasmussen, S. K. 2007. Quantitative analysis of phytate globoids isolated from wheat bran and characterization of their sequential dephosphorylation by wheat phytase. *Journal of Agricultural and Food Chemistry* 55(18): 7547–7552.

Cosgrove, D. J. 1980. Inositol Phosphates. Their Chemistry, Biochemistry and Physiology. Amsterdam, The Netherlands: Elsevier Scientific Publishing Co.

Coulibaly, A., Kouakou, B. and Chen, J. 2011. Phytic acid in cereal grains: Structure, healthy or harmful ways to reduce phytic acid in cereal grains and their effects on nutritional quality. *American Journal of Plant Nutrition and Fertilization Technology* 1(1): 1–22.

Cridland, C. and Gillaspy, G. 2020. Inositol Pyrophosphate Pathways and Mechanisms: What Can We Learn from Plants?. *Molecules* 25(12): 2789.

Darambazar, E. 2018. Method of phytic acid determination in food, feed, and plant materials. Assay protocol, University of Saskatchewan. Canada. Pp. 4. doi:10.13140/RG.2.2.14852.27520

Eder, K., Siebers, M., Most, E., Scheibe, S., Weissmann, N. and Gessner, D. K. 2017. An excess dietary vitamin E concentration does not influence Nrf2 signaling in the liver of rats fed either soybean oil or salmon oil. *Nutrition & Metabolism* 14(1): 1–15.

Ficco, D.B.M., Riefolo, C., Nicastro, G., De Simone, V., Di Gesu, A.M., Beleggia, R., Platani, C., Cattivelli, L. and De Vita, P., 2009. Phytate and mineral elements concentration in a collection of Italian durum wheat cultivars. *Field Crops Research* 111(3): 235–242.

Gao, Y, C. Shang, M. A. SaghaiMaroof, R. M. Biyashev, E. A. Grabau, P. Kwanyuen, J. W. Burton, and G. R. Buss. 2007. A Modified colorimetric method for phytic acid analysis in soybean. *Crop Science* 47:1797–1803

Gemede, H. F. and Ratta, N. 2014. Antinutritional factors in plant foods: Potential health benefits and adverse effects. *International Journal of Nutrition and Food Sciences* 3(4): 284–289.

Gillaspy, G. E. 2013. The role of phosphoinositides and inositol phosphates in plant cell signaling. *Lipid-Mediated Protein Signaling*: 141–157.

Grases, F., Prieto, R. M. and Costa-Bauza, A. 2017. Dietary phytate and interactions with mineral nutrients. In *Clinical Aspects of Natural and Added Phosphorus in Foods* (pp. 175–183). New York: Springer.

Greiner, R., Turner, B., Richardson, A. and Mullaney, E. 2007. Phytate-degrading enzymes: Regulation of synthesis in microorganisms and plants. *Inositol Phosphates: Linking Agriculture and the Environment*: 78–96.

Hamid, N. T. and Kumar, P. 2017. Anti-nutritional factors, their adverse effects and need for adequate processing to reduce them in food. *Agric International* 4: 56–60.

Haydon, M. J., & Cobbett, C. S. 2007. Transporters of ligands for essential metal ions in plants. *New Phytologist* 174(3): 499–506.

Hitz, W. D., Carlson, T. J., Kerr, P. S. and Sebastian, S. A. 2002. Biochemical and molecular characterization of a mutation that confers a decreased raffinosaccharide and phytic acid phenotype on soybean seeds. *Plant Physiology* 128(2): 650–660.

Holmes, R. P., Goodman, H. O. and Assimos, D. G. 2001. Contribution of dietary oxalate to urinary oxalate excretion. *Kidney International* 59(1): 270–276.

Jiang, L., Phillips, T. E., Hamm, C. A., Drozdowicz, Y. M., Rea, P. A., Maeshima, M. and Rogers, J. C. 2001. The protein storage vacuole: A unique compound organelle. *The Journal of Cell Biology* 155(6): 991–1002.

Kolchev, L.A., 1978. Method for producing phytin. United States Patent. N. 4070422.

Kumar, V., Sinha, A. K., Makkar, H. P. and Becker, K. 2010. Dietary roles of phytate and phytase in human nutrition: A review. *Food Chemistry* 120(4): 945–959.

Laha, D., Portela-Torres, P., Desfougères, Y. and Saiardi, A. 2020. Inositol phosphate kinases in the eukaryote landscape. *Advances in Biological Regulation*: 100782.

Loewus, F. 2002. Biosynthesis of phytate in food grains and seeds. In N. R. Reddy & S. K. Sathe (eds.), *Food Phytates* (pp. 53–61). Boca Raton, FL: CRC Press

Madsen, C. K. and Brinch-Pedersen, H. 2020. Globoids and phytase: The mineral storage and release system in seeds. *International Journal of Molecular Sciences* 21(20): 7519.

Makower, R.U., 1970. Extraction and determination of phytic acid in beans (Phaseolus vulgaris). *Cereal Chemistry* 47: 288–295.

Mandizvo, T. and Odindo, A.O., 2020. Spectrophotometric quantification of phytic acid during embryogenesis in bambara groundnut (Vigna subterranea L.) through phosphomolybdenum complex formation. *Emirates Journal of Food and Agriculture* 778–785.

Marolt, G. and Kolar, M., 2021. Analytical methods for determination of phytic acid and other inositol phosphates: A review. *Molecules* 26(1): 174.

Mihrete, Y. 2019. Review on mineral malabsorption and reducing technologies. *International Journal of Neurologic Physical Therapy* 5(1): 25–30.

Mohamed, A.I., Perera, P.A.J. and Hafez, Y.S., 1986. New chromophore for phytic acid determination. *Cereal Chemistry* 63(6): 475–478.

Nagy, R., Grob, H., Weder, B., Green, P., Klein, M., Frelet-Barrand, A. and Martinoia, E. 2009. The Arabidopsis ATP-binding cassette protein AtMRP5/AtABCC5 is a high affinity inositol hexakisphosphate transporter involved in guard cell signaling and phytate storage. *Journal of Biological Chemistry* 284(48): 33614–33622.

Nissar, J., Ahad, T., Naik, H. R. and Hussain, S. Z. 2017. A review phytic acid: As antinutrient or nutraceutical. *Journal of Pharmacognosy and Phytochemistry* 6(6): 1554–1560.

Oatway, L., Vasanthan, T. and Helm, J. H. 2001. Phytic acid. *Food Reviews International* 17(4): 419–431.

Oh, B. C., Choi, W. C., Park, S., Kim, Y. O. and Oh, T. K. 2004. Biochemical properties and substrate specificities of alkaline and histidine acid phytases. *Applied Microbiology and Biotechnology* 63(4): 362–372.

Petry, N., Egli, I., Gahutu, J.B., Tugirimana, P.L., Boy, E. and Hurrell, R., 2014. Phytic acid concentration influences iron bioavailability from biofortified beans in Rwandese women with low iron status. *The Journal of nutrition* 44(11): 1681–1687.

Pfeiffer, W. and Hager, A. 1993. A Ca 2+-ATPase and a Mg 2+/H+-antiporter are present on tonoplast membranes from roots of Zea mays L. *Planta* 191(3): 377–385.

Platel, K., Eipeson, S. W. and Srinivasan, K. 2010. Bioaccessible mineral content of malted finger millet (Eleusine coracana), wheat (Triticum aestivum), and barley (Hordeum vulgare). *Journal of Agricultural and Food Chemistry* 58: 8100–8103.

Qian, X., Mitchell, J., Wei, S. J., Williams, J., Petrovich, R. M. and Shears, S. B. 2005. The Ins (1, 3, 4) P 3 5/6-kinase/Ins (3, 4, 5, 6) P 4 1-kinase is not a protein kinase. *Biochemical Journal* 389(2): 389–395.

Reddy, N. R. 2002. Occurrence, distribution, content, and dietary intake of phytate. In N. R. Reddy & S. K. Sathe (eds.), *Food Phytates* (pp. 25–51). Boca Raton, FL: CRC Press.

Ritchie, S., Swanson, S. J. and Gilroy, S. 2000. Physiology of the aleurone layer and starchy endosperm during grain development and early seedling growth: New insights from cell and molecular biology. *Seed Science Research* 10(3): 193–212.

Rousseau, S., Kyomugasho, C., Celus, M., Hendrickx, M. E. and Grauwet, T. 2020. Barriers impairing mineral bioaccessibility and bioavailability in plant-based foods and the perspectives for food processing. *Critical Reviews in Food Science and Nutrition* 60(5): 826–843.

Sacchi, G. A. and Nocito, F. F. 2019. Plant sulfate transporters in the low phytic acid network: Some educated guesses. *Plants* 8(12): 616.

Samtiya, M., Aluko, R. E. and Dhewa, T. 2020. Plant food anti-nutritional factors and their reduction strategies: An overview. *Food Production, Processing and Nutrition* 2(1): 1–14.

Santos, JCP 1998. Nutritional status of common bean (Phaseolus vulgaris L.) and nutrient and phytate content in grains (Doctoral dissertation, Luiz de Queiroz College of Agriculture, University of São Paulo.).

Schlemmer, U., Frolich, W., Prieto, R. M. and Grases, F. 2009. Phytate in foods and significance for humans: Food sources, intake, processing, bioavailability, protective role and analysis. *Molecular Nutrition and Food Research* 53 Supplement 2: 330–375.

Secco, D., Bouain, N., Rouached, A., Prom-u-Thai, C., Hanin, M., Pandey, A. K. and Rouached, H. 2017. Phosphate, phytate and phytases in plants: From fundamental knowledge gained in Arabidopsis to potential biotechnological applications in wheat. *Critical Reviews in Biotechnology* 37(7): 898–910.

Sharma, N., Chaudhary, C. and Khurana, P. 2020. Wheat Myo-inositol phosphate synthase influences plant growth and stress responses via ethylene mediated signaling. *Scientific Reports* 10(1): 1–14.

Silva, V. M., Putti, F. F., White, P. J. and Dos Reis, A. R. (2021). Phytic acid accumulation in plants: Biosynthesis pathway regulation and role in human diet. *Plant Physiology and Biochemistry* 164:132–146.

Sparvoli, F. and Cominelli, E. 2015. Seed biofortification and phytic acid reduction: A conflict of interest for the plant?. *Plants* 4(4): 728–755.

Stevenson-Paulik, J., Odom, A. R., & York, J. D. (2002). Molecular and biochemical characterization of two plant inositol polyphosphate 6-/3-/5-kinases. *Journal of Biological Chemistry, 277*(45), 42711–42718.

Sweetman, D., Stavridou, I., Johnson, S., Green, P., Caddick, S. E. and Brearley, C. A. 2007. Arabidopsis thaliana inositol 1, 3, 4-trisphosphate 5/6-kinase 4 (AtITPK4) is an outlier to a family of ATP-grasp fold proteins from Arabidopsis. *FEBS Letters* 581(22): 4165–4171.

Torres, J., Domínguez, S., Cerdá, M. F., Obal, G., Mederos, A., Irvine, R. F. and Kremer, C. 2005. Solution behaviour of myo-inositol hexakisphosphate in the presence of multivalent cations. Prediction of a neutral pentamagnesium species under cytosolic/nuclear conditions. *Journal of Inorganic Biochemistry* 99(3): 828–840.

Van Veldhoven, P.P. and Mannaerts, G.P., 1987. Inorganic and organic phosphate measurements in the nanomolar range. *Analytical Biochemistry* 161(1): 45–48.

Weaver, C. M. and Kannan, S. 2002. Phytate and mineral bioavailability. In N. R. Reddy & S. K. Sathe (eds.), *Food Phytates* (pp. 211–224). Boca Raton, FL: CRC Press.

Wilson, M. P. and Majerus, P. W. 1997. Characterization of a cDNA EncodingArabidopsisthalianaInositol 1, 3, 4-trisphosphate 5/6-kinase. *Biochemical and Biophysical Research Communications* 232(3): 678–681.

Zhou, T., Wang, P., Yang, R., Wang, X. and Gu, Z. 2018. $Ca^{2+}$ influxes and transmembrane transport are essential for phytic acid degradation in mung bean sprouts. *Journal of the Science of Food and Agriculture* 98(5): 1968–1976.

# CHAPTER 3

# Tannins

**Nazmul Sarwar and Taslima Ahmed**

## CONTENTS



DOI: 10.1201/9781003178446-3

## 3.1 INTRODUCTION

The term "tannins" is derived from the primeval Celtic term for oak, and are either esters of galloyl or proanthocyanidins of a oligomeric and polymeric nature produced by the plant's secondary metabolism. They are water-soluble polyphenols with molecular masses ranging from 500 to 3,000 Da, but they can reach 20,000 Da when bound to proteins, saccharides, and alkaloids that exhibit phenol-specific reactions (Haslam 1989). Approximately 8,000 distinct tannins have been identified and chemically characterized till now, but their chemical composition is indistinguishable regardless of the species of plants that produce the substance. However, there are undoubtedly several other tannins whose chemical compositions have yet to be determined. The most abundant natural sources of tannins are fruits, vegetables, cereals, legumes, bark, seeds, roots, leaves, shrubs, and herbs (Hassanpour et al. 2011, Ghosh 2015). About 80% of the world population consumes tannins through the ingestion of common foods, including fruits, vegetables, grains, chocolate, and beverages, such as tea, coffee, and wine, and its intake is common among children due to its astringency that boosts the mood and attenuates fatigue (Morton 1992). It's also found in substantial quantities in kola nuts, which are regularly consumed in West African countries, and in Guarana seeds, which are used in the manufacturing process of soft drinks in Latin America (Kumar et al. 2018).

Tannins are bioactive compounds that have advantageous effects on the body when ingested in large amounts. They have a wide range of medicinal and therapeutic effects, as well as pharmacological properties such as anti-oxidant, anti-inflammatory, anti-diabetic, anti-microbial, anti-viral, anti-allergic, anti-toxic, anti-cancer, anthelmintic, dysentery remedial, and so on (Ghosh 2015).

Additionally, tannins have several negative effects, including anti-nutritional effects, increased indigestibility, carcinogenic and mutagenic activity, inducer and co-promoter of diverse illnesses, and inhibitory and hepatotoxic activity. Tannin is used in the tanning process to treat skins and hides of animals for producing leather. They protect the hide by binding and coating the collagen proteins, reducing water-solubility, increasing imperviousness to bacterial attack, and gradually making the hide more stable (Sharma et al. 2019).

## 3.2 CHEMISTRY

### 3.2.1 Biosynthesis

Because of the importance of plant polyphenols in human and animal life, as well as the scarcity of knowledge regarding tannin biosynthesis, several previous studies have focused on establishing understandable and rational biosynthetic routes. Two major routes of biosynthesis yielded tannins of varying basic complexity.

The first biosynthesis route (Figure 3.1) followed three consecutive steps, is originated from quinic acid, and ends with production of gallic acid. Herein, 1-galloyl-β-D-glucose is formed by the attachment of a galloyl unit, a fundamental intermediate and an important metabolite in the biosynthesis of hydrolyzable tannins (HT).

1. Initially, for the formation of di-, trigalloylglucoses, and pentagalloylglucoses, 1-galloyl—D-glucose acts as an acyl acceptor and acyl donor (the products are "simple" galloylglucose derivatives). Many plant families include the 2,3,4,6-tetra-O-galloyl-D-glucopyranose (TGG) and 1,2,3,4,6-penta-O-ga lloyl-D-glucopyranose (-PGG), which are essential mediators in the biosynthesis of almost all plant hydrolyzable tannins.
2. Galloylation of pentagalloylglucose produces hexa-, hepta-, octa-, and other galloylglucose derivatives, as well as an esteric interaction between two galloy moieties which are gallotannins or depsidic metabolites.
3. The final step is oxidation, which results in C-C linkages between well-oriented galloyl residues of glucogalloyl molecules and forming hexahydroxydiphenoyl (HHDP) units namely ellagitannins (Arapitsas 2012) (Figure 3.2).

During the second biosynthetic pathway, condensation of p-coumaroyl-CoA with malonyl-CoA produces chalcone that is a precursor of naringenin, and flavan-3-ols (He et al. 2008).

1. The glycosylation of a catechin unit to a gallotannin or ellagitannin unit starts the process.
2. The oligomerization of such catechin units resulted as a culmination of the linkage of one catechin unit's C-4 with the C-8 or C-6 of the next catechin unit and finally condensed tannins. (Khanbabaee and Van Ree 2001).

## 3.3 CLASSIFICATION

Condensed or polyflavonoid tannins and hydrolysable tannins are the two types of tannins that are commonly used. Condensed tannins are characterized by their oligomeric form, as opposed to the ostensibly nonpolymeric nature of hydrolysable tannins (Fengel and Wegener 1984, Tang et al. 1991, Haslam 1966, Roux 1992).

### 3.3.1 Hydrolysable Tannins

The central core of hydrolysable tannins (HTs) is a polyol (typically D-glucose) and carbohydrate's hydroxyl groups are partly or fully esterified with phenolic groups such as gallic acid

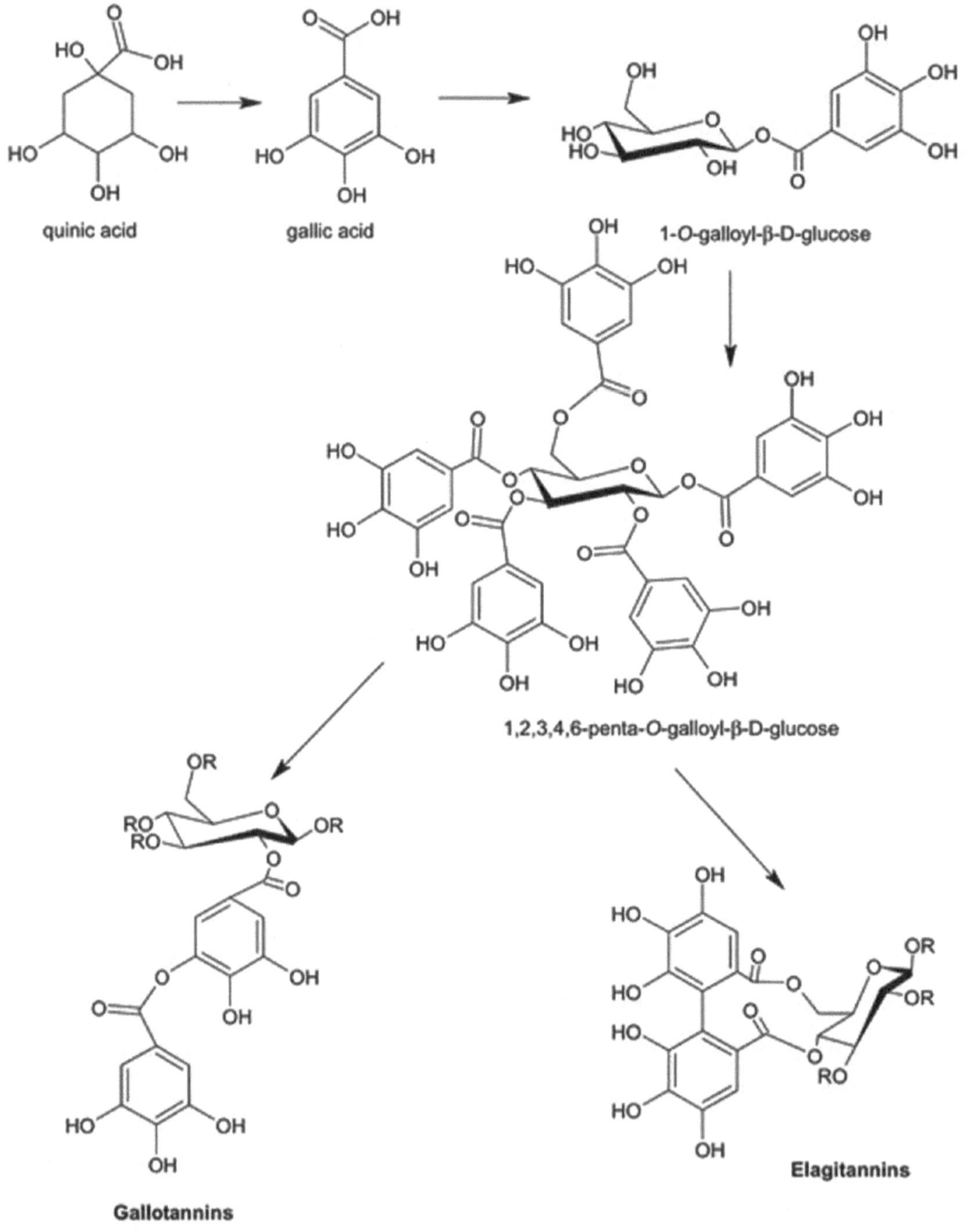


**Figure 3.1** Biosynthetic route of hydrolyzable tannins. (Source: Sieniawska and Baj 2017.)

(—>gallotannins) or ellagic acid (—>ellagitannins). Chestnut (*Castanea sativa*), divi-divi (*Caesalpina coraria*), myrabolans (*Phyllanthus emblica*), algarobilla (*Balsamocarpon brevifolium*), tara (*Tara spinosa*), valonea oak (*Quercus macrolepis*), as well as several other industrial tannin extracts are the most popular types of HTs. Numerous studies (Fengel and Wegener 1984; Tang, et al. 1991) identified the main elements of the commercial hydrolysable tannin. For instance, the positional isomers castalagin and vescalagin are observed in 14.2 and 16.2% respectively in chestnut

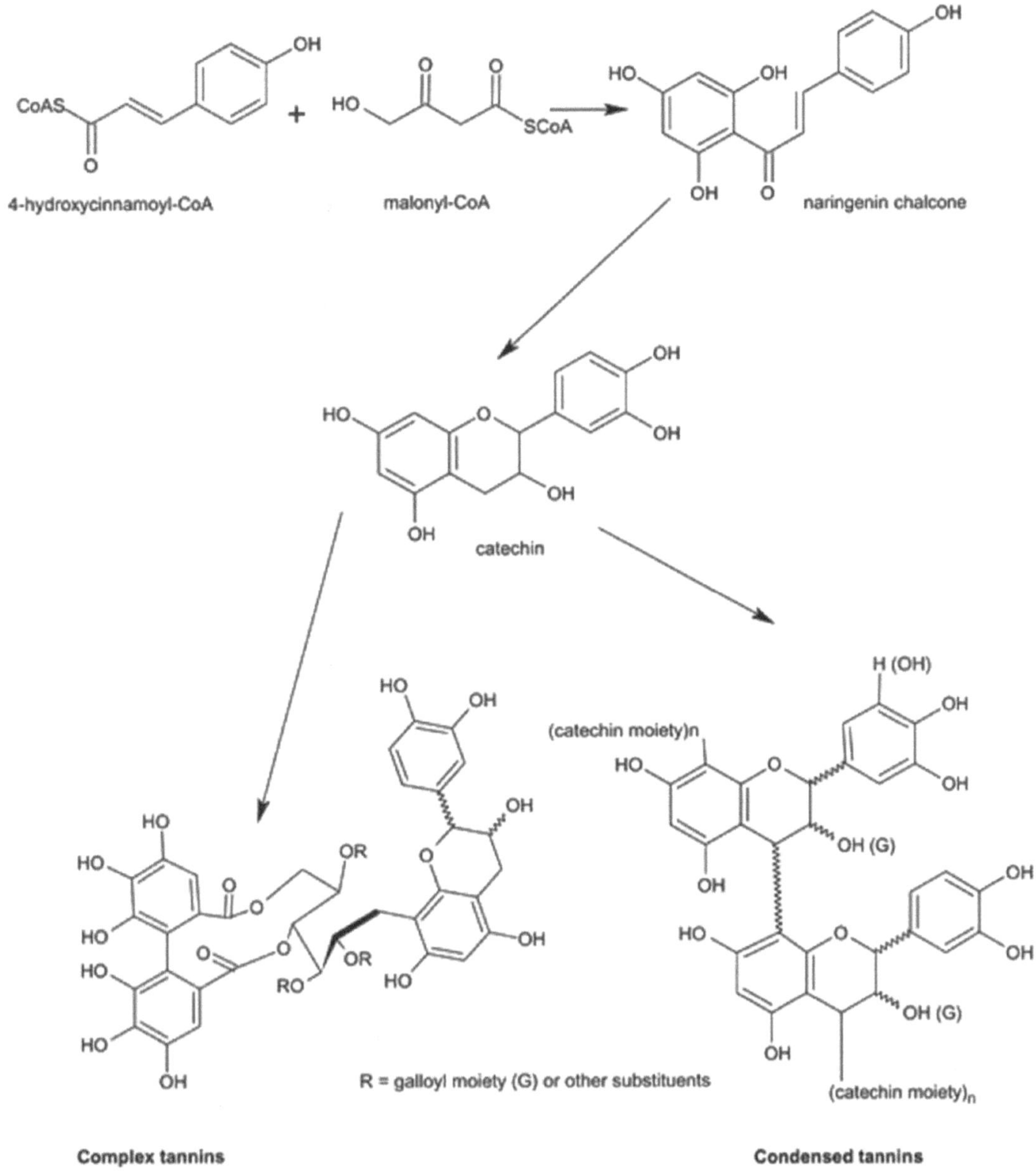


**Figure 3.2** Biosynthetic route of complex and condensed tannins. (Source: Sieniawska and Baj 2017.)

tannin extract as an ellagitannin. Among the rest of the tannins, the positional isomers castalin and vescalin contain 6.6%, gallic acid 6%, and pentagalloyl glucose monomer 3%.

In chestnut tannins, two groups of compounds have mass predominance: 28.8% of small molecules, whose formula is shown in Figure 3.3, and 25.4% of an unidentified and elusive fraction of a much high molecular mass (Tang et al. 1991) and a very low TLC Rf.

### 3.3.2 Condensed Tannins

Condensed tannins, also named proanthocyanidins (PAs), are the most abundant types of tannin, accounting for more than 90% of worldwide tannin production (Pizzi 1983). They are abundant in nature and can be present in high concentrations in the wood and bark of a variety of trees,

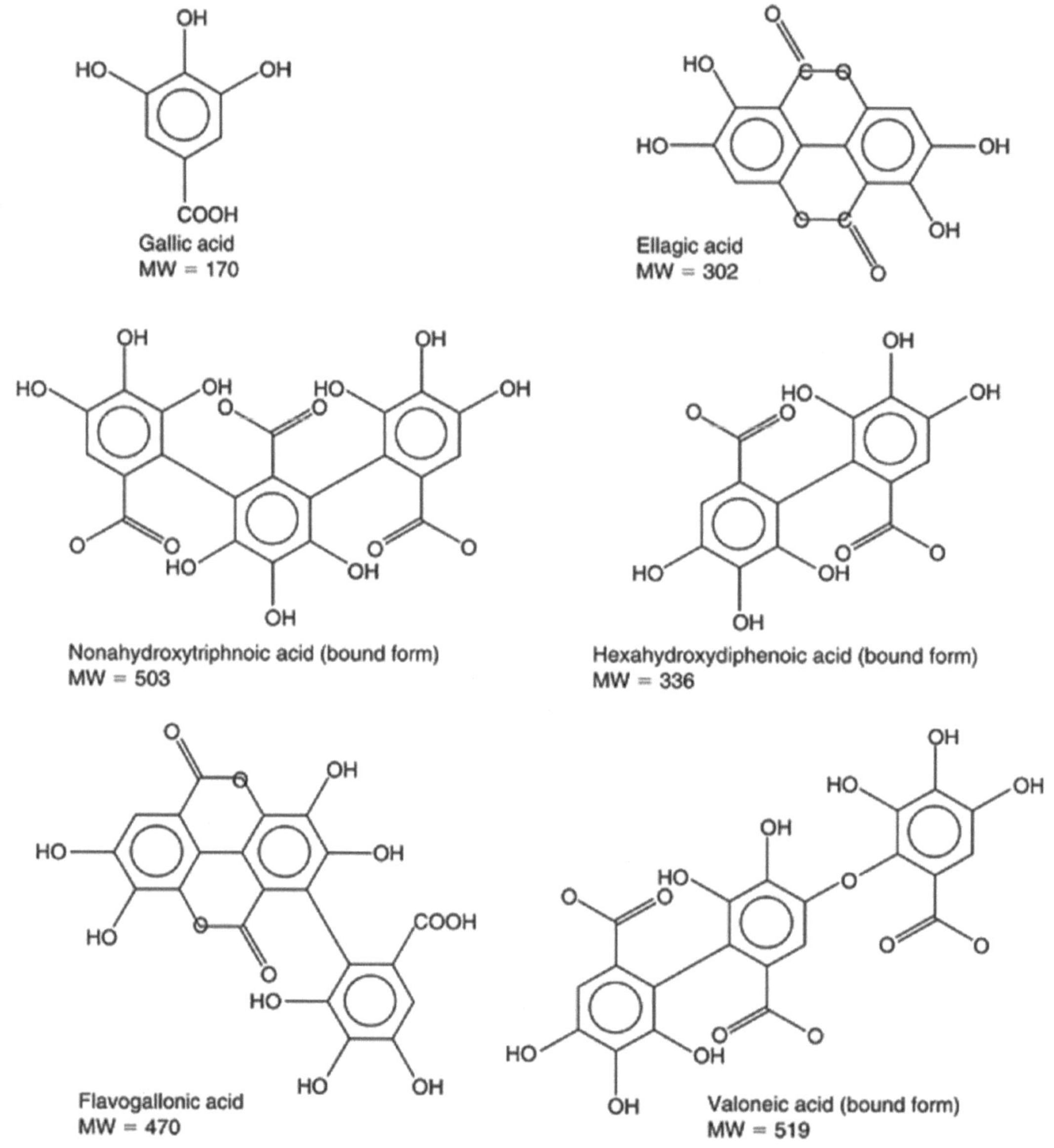


**Figure 3.3** Chemical species characteristic of the low molecular weight fraction of hydrolysable tannins. (Source: Pizzi 2008.)

including schinopsis, rhus, acacia, tsuga, and different pinus bark extract species. Flavonoid is the central monomer in the structure of condensed tannins. The flavonoid unit is echoed 2–11 times in mimosa and quebracho tannins, with an average degree of polymerization of 4–5, whereas it can be repeated up to 30 times in pine tannins, with an average degree of polymerization of 6–7 for their soluble extract component (Pizzi 1983, Pasch et al. 2001, Pizzi 1994). When the nucleophilic centres on a flavonoid unit's A-ring and B-ring are compared, the A-ring tends to be more reactive in aromatic substitution than the B-ring. The vicinal hydroxyl substituents are responsible for this since they cause general activation in the B-ring without any confined effects like those seen in the A-ring (Pizzi 1983).

Flavonoid analogues reflect the major polyphenolic pattern that is subjected to resorcinol A-rings and pyrogallol B-rings and comprises 70% of the tannins in mimosa bark's condensed tannins. The resorcinol A-rings and catechol B-rings form a secondary but parallel pattern. The secondary, parallel pattern is made up of resorcinol A-rings and catechol B-rings (Pizzi 1983, Roux 1965), and it accounts for around 25% of the overall mimosa bark tannin fraction. The remainder of the condensed tannin are the "nontannins" (Roux 1965) that are mainly comprise of carbohydrates, small amino and amino acid fractions, and hydrocolloid gums (Pizzi 1983; Roux 1965). Despite their low concentration, the hydrocolloid gums greatly contribute to the viscosity of the concentrate, ranging from 3 to 6% (Pizzi 1983, Roux 1965). Related flavonoid A- and B-ring patterns can be observed in wood extract of quebracho, but there is no phloroglucinol A-ring pattern, or just a small amount of it (Clark-Lewis and Roux 1959, King and White 1957, 1961; Roux and Paulus 1961, Roux et al. 1975). Hemlock and Douglas fir bark extract has features that are similar to wattle (mimosa) and quebracho. Pine tannins, on the other hand, exhibit two different patterns and relationships: one depicted by flavonoid analogues based on A-rings and B-rings of phloroglucinol and catechol respectively, and the other denoted by phloroglucinol A-rings and phenol B-rings, which is present in a much smaller proportion (Pizzi 2008, Porter 1974). Pine tannins' A-rings only contain the phloroglucinol type of structure, which is far more reactive to formaldehyde than its resorcinol-type equivalent, with widespread implications in the use of these tannins as adhesives.

## 3.4 DISTRIBUTION

Natural and synthetic tannins are the two primary categories of tannins that have a major effect on plant and human health in both positive and negative ways.

### 3.4.1 Natural Sources

Tea (*Camellia sinensis*), coffee (*Coffea spp.*), cocoa (*Theobroma cacao*), guarana (Paulliniacupana), kola nuts (*Cola vera*), are the main sources of tannins. Besides many cereals, legumes, fruits, vegetables, spices, herbs, and condiments also have plenty of tannins (Hassanpour et al. 2011). It is extensively dispersed in the kingdom *Plantae*, mainly among trees of higher plants, whereas lower plants contain trace amounts of tannins (Ashok and Upadhyaya 2012). Plants that adapted to heat and have broader leaves, such as Sericea lespedeza (*Lespedeza cuneata*), sorghum (*Sorghum bicolor*), etc., are reported to be the biorepository of tannins. Further other parts of some plants such as seed coat of Alfalfa (*Medicago sativa*) and leaves of White clover (*Trifolium repens*) are also reported to have a significant amount of tannins (MacAdam et al. 2013). Tannin can also be found in fruits, nuts, leaves, stems, roots, shells, and bark, among other places, depending on the crop (Table 3.1).

Tea, coffee, and cocoa are the predominant natural sources of tannins. Tea is used as a means of refreshment and is one of the most commonly consumed drinks following water (Kumar and Joshi 2016, Kumar et al. 2016, Joshi and Kumar 2017). Tea is grown all over the world, with India, Sri Lanka, Japan, Sumatra, Kenya, and Java supplying the most (Willson and Clifford 2012). Another source of tannins is coffee, a beverage made by percolating or infusing roasted seeds from trees referring to the botanical family Rubiaceae, genus Coffea, subgenus Eucoffea. It is grown all across the globe, with Brazil, Colombia, Ethiopia, Indonesia, and Vietnam being the top producers (Kumar et al. 2018). Two coffee plant species dominate world trade: the *Coffee Arabica*, or simply Arabica, which accounts for 75% of the total demand, and the *Coffee canephora*, which is more generally recognized by the fame of the most popular species: Robusta (Pohlan and Janssens 2010). Another decent source of tannins is cocoa, which is the main ingredient of chocolate production (Ghosh 2015). The Brazil, Cameroon, Ecuador Nigeria, Ghana, Ivory Coast, and Indonesia are the main producers, with Ghana being the second-largest producer and also known for providing

**Table 3.1 Presence of Tannins in Specific Parts of the Plant, as Well as Their Beneficial Effects**

| Sl. No. | Plant Part | Specific Location | Function |
|---|---|---|---|
| 1 | Non-woody items | Secondary xylem and phloem | Supports and controls tissue growth. |
| 2 | Heartwood | Coniferous heartwood | Exhibit anti-microbial activity, increasing the normal longevity of wood. |
| 3 | Bud | Buds outer layers | Provides anti-freezing security. |
| 4 | Leaf | Epidermis | Reduces the palatability of the food, making it less appealing to predators. |
| 5 | Root | Hypodermis | • Inhibits the colony development of Pathogen.<br>• Tannins, like other polyphenols, have an effect on plant growth and production.<br>• It also greatly influences plant reproduction by its interactivity with Gibberlic acid and auxin. |
| 6 | Seed | Layer within outer integument and aleurone | Aids in the upkeep of the plant's dormancy level. It also has allopathic and bactericidal effects. |
| 7 | Stem | Active growth region | Plays a key role in the development and control of these tissues. |

*Source:* Green & Corcoran (1975); Jacobson & Corcoran (1977); Ashok & Upadhyaya (2012).

premium quality cocoa beans (Kumar et al. 2018). Guarana is a soothing variety derived from the climbing shrub *Paullinia cupana*, which is native to Brazil, Bolivia, Venezuela, Uruguay, and Peru (Morton 1992).

Tannins are also found in a many of plant foods, including fruits and vegetables. Berries (blackberries, strawberries, blueberries, raspberries, and other berries), babul (*Acacia arabica*), amla (*Emblica officinalis*), majuphal (*Quercus infectoria*), munakka, dates (*Phoenix sylvestris*), red supari (*Areca catechu*), raisins (*Vitis vinifera*), peach (*Prunus persica*), plum (*Prunus domestica*), pomegranate (*Punica granatum*) (Kumari and Jain 2015). Vegetables aren't the ample sources of tannins but they are the most abundant ingredient after lignin, cellulose, and hemicellulose in most vegetables (Samanta et al. 2004).

Sorghum, the staple food of most Asian and African peoples, contains a high quantity of tannins. While cereals contain little tannins, barley, millets, and legumes including cowpeas, chickpeas, common beans, kidney beans, fava beans, and pinto beans are some of the most popular tannin-rich foods (Kumari and Jain 2012, Bennick 2002). Tannins can also be present in herbs such as Agrimoniapilosa, curry leaves (*Murraya koenigii*), Ephedeasinica, *Polygonum multiflorum*, *Prunella spica*, *Rheum palmatum*, and forages such as sainfoin, lespedeza, lotus, crown vetch, trefoil, and others (Ghosh 2015). Turmeric, chilies, coriander, tamarind, and other condiments and spices that are commonly used as flavouring agents in various dishes contain significant amounts of tannins. Table 3.2 gives a thorough explanation of the various tannin origins as well as their concentrations.

### 3.4.2 Synthetic Sources of Tannins

Cresols, naphthalenes, and other higher hydrocarbons are used as the primary ingredients in the artificial synthesis of tannins. E llagic acid, flavellagic acid, digallic acid, luteic acid, metellagic acid, Ordoval G, Neradol D, Neradol N, and tannic acids are commonly synthesized vegetable tannins that are used in a wide range of industrial applications in the food and leather industries. Both methyl and ethyl alcohols are soluble in digallic acid, but their solubility decreases in hot or cold water. It is hydrolyzed to produce gallic acid, which is then oxidized to produce luteic acid and ellagic acid. Ellagic acid is fully soluble in caustic potash, but partially soluble in ether, water, and alcohol. Because of its low cost and water solubility, Neradol D is more commercially important and

**Table 3.2 Different Sources of Tannins and Their Concentration**

| Sl. No. | Particulars | Name of Plant | Tannin (%) | References |
|---|---|---|---|---|
| 1 | Fruits | Amla (*Emblica officinalis*) | 4.15 | Kumari and Jain (2015), Del Bubba et al. (2009), Arogba (1997) |
| | | Babul (*Acacia arabica*) | 7.27 | |
| | | Badillayachi (*Amomum xanthiodes*) | 0.14 | |
| | | Dates (*Phoenix sylvestris*) | 0.23 | |
| | | Majuphal (*Quercus infectoria*) | 10.62 | |
| | | Mango kernel (*Ikanekpo variety*) | 4.48 | |
| | | Munakka (*Vitis vinifera*) | 0.23 | |
| | | Persimmon (*Kaki Tipo*) | 17–32 | |
| | | Persimmon (*Rojo Brillante*) | 9–27 | |
| | | Raisins (*Vitis vinifera*) | 0.11 | |
| | | Red Supari (*Areca catechu*) | 1.52 | |
| | | Ripened banana | 0.025–0.48 | |
| | | Sangiri (*Prosopis cineraria*) | 0.14 | |
| 2 | Leafy vegetables | Bathua (*Chenopodium album*) | 0.116 | Sriwichai et al. (2016), Gupta et al. (2013), Gupta et al. (2005), Goel et al. (2008), Lipsa et al. (2012) |
| | | Benghal dayflower (*Commelina benghalensis*) | 0.105 | |
| | | Broom creeper (*Cocculus hirsutus*) | 0.205 | |
| | | Buttercup (*Cucurbita maxima*) | 0.157 | |
| | | Canola (dehulled) | 3.91 | |
| | | Canola (whole) | 2.71 | |
| | | Desert horsepurslane (*Trianthema portulacastrum*) | 0.061 | |
| | | Drumstick (*moringa oleifera*) | 0.08 | |
| | | Edible Amaranth (*Amaranthus tricolor*) | 0.305 | |
| | | False amaranth (*Digera arvensis*) | 0.079 | |
| | | Fenugreek (*Trigonella foenum graecum*) | 0.163 | |
| | | Gotu kola (*Centella asiatica*) | 0.123 | |
| | | Joseph's coat (*Amaranthus gangeticus L.*) | 0.171 | |
| | | Mexican mint (*Coleus aromaticus*) | 0.015 | |
| | | Musk thistle (*Carduus leaves*) | 0.36 | |
| | | Plumed cockscomb (*Celosia argentea*) | 0.113 | |
| | | Punarnava (*Boerhaavia diffusa*) | 0.094 | |
| | | Shona cabbage (*Gynandropsis pentaphylla*) | 0.136 | |
| | | Snakeroots (*Polygala eriopter*) | 0.098 | |
| | | White Gulmohur (*Delonix elata*) | 1.330 | |

(*Continued*)

**Table 3.2 (Continued) Different Sources of Tannins and Their Concentration**

| Sl. No. | Particulars | Name of Plant | Tannin (%) | References |
|---|---|---|---|---|
| 3 | Cereals and millets | Bajra (*Pennisetum typhoideum*) | 0 | Rao and Prabhavathi (1982), Devi et al. (2014), Bennick 2002), Medugu et al. (2012), Balasubramanian et al. 2014) |
| | | Finger millets (Brown) | 0.12–3.47 | |
| | | Finger millets (White) | 0.04–0.06 | |
| | | Pearl millet | 0.152 | |
| | | Ragi (*Eleusine coracana*) | 0.36 | |
| | | Rice (*Oryza sativa*) | 0 | |
| | | Sorghum grain (red) | 1.54–7.44 | |
| | | Sorghum grain (white) | 0.55 | |
| | | Sorghum grain (yellow) | 0.2–2.0 | |
| | | Wheat (*Triticum aestivum*) | 0.041 | |
| 4 | Seeds/nutseeds | Almond | 0.07–0.09 | Murthy and Manonmani (2009), Kirubakaran et al. (2016), Bennick (2002), Kumari and Jain (2015), Venkatachalam and Sathe (2006) |
| | | Brazil nut | 0.01 | |
| | | Cashew nut | 0.03–0.04 | |
| | | Castor seeds | 0.7–3.8 | |
| | | Coffee (*Monsooned malabar*) | 0.08 | |
| | | Coffee (*Monsooned robusta*) | 0.15 | |
| | | Cumin seeds (*Cuminum cyminum*) | 0.23 | |
| | | Faba beans | 20 | |
| | | Fenugreek (on dry basis) | 0.01 | |
| | | Hazelnut | 0.04–0.23 | |
| | | Macadamia nut | 0.01 | |
| | | Mango seeds (*Mangifera indica*) | 0.35 | |
| | | Pecan | 0.84–0.88 | |
| | | Pine nut | 0.01 | |
| | | Pistachio | 0.02–0.22 | |
| | | Tamarind seeds | 0.07–0.29 | |
| | | Virginia peanut | 0.16–0.29 | |
| | | Walnut | 0.18–0.34 | |
| 5 | Legumes | Bengal gram | 0.33 | Medugu et al. (2012), Rao and Prabhavathi (1982) |
| | | Chickpea | 1.9–6.1 | |
| | | Cowpea (*Vigna catjang*) | 0.175 | |
| | | Green gram (*Phaseolus aureus*) | 0.437 | |
| | | Kidney bean (*Dolichos lablab*) | 1.024 | |
| | | Pigeon pea | 4.3–11.4 | |
| | | Red gram (*Cajanumcajan*) | 0.607 | |
| | | Soya bean (*Glycine max merr.*) | 0.045 | |

(*Continued*)

**Table 3.2 (Continued) Different Sources of Tannins and Their Concentration**

| Sl. No. | Particulars | Name of Plant | Tannin (%) | References |
|---|---|---|---|---|
| 6 | Condiments, spices, and herbs | Ajowan (*Carum copticum*) | 1.26 | Tur and Brenner (1998), Sriwichai et al. (2016), Rao and Prabhavathi (1982), Mansoori et al. (2006), Mamatha and Prakash (2016), Kumari and Jain (2015), Kirubakaran et al. (2016), Hoffmann et al. (2016) |
| | | Bisibele-bhat powder (formulated) | 0.216 | |
| | | Black pepper (*Piper nigrum*) | 0.94 | |
| | | Chilli powder (*Capsucum annuum*) | 0.98 | |
| | | Cinnamon (*Cinnamomum zeylanicum*) | 0.35 | |
| | | Coriander (*Coriandrum sativum*) | 0.311–0.82 | |
| | | Cumin seeds | 0.90 | |
| | | Dry ginger (*Zingiber officinale*) | 0.54 | |
| | | Garlic (*Allium sativum*) | 0.12 | |
| | | Kathaa (*Acacia catechu*) | 10.86 | |
| | | Mixed condiment powder | 0.611 | |
| | | Perilla leaves | 0.556 | |
| | | Potentilla officinalis | 15–25 | |
| | | Puliogare powder (formulated) | 0.206 | |
| | | Rasam powder (formulated) | 0.233 | |
| | | Sambhar powder (formulated) | 0.204 | |
| | | Tamarind (*Tamarindus indica*) | 0.6 | |
| | | Tamarind powder | 1.240 | |
| | | Turmeric (*Curcuma domestica*) | 3.350 | |
| | | Turmeric (*Curcuma longa*) | 0.11 | |
| 7 | Beverages | Apple juice | 0.005 | Bennick (2002), Khasnabis et al. (2015), Mousavinejad et al. (2009), Rao and Prabhavathi (1982) |
| | | Black tea | 13.36 | |
| | | Bordeaux | 0.15–0.49 | |
| | | Cranberry juice | 0.025 | |
| | | Dry red wines | 0.236 | |
| | | Dry white wines | 0.039 | |
| | | Green tea | 2.65 | |
| | | Madeira | 0.08 | |
| | | Oolong tea | 8.66 | |
| | | Pomegranate juice | 0.015–0.054 | |
| | | Red | 0.14–0.32 | |
| | | Red wine | 0.025–.031 | |
| | | Sparkling wines | 0.035 | |
| | | Sweet red wines | 0.096 | |
| | | Sweet white wines | 0.036 | |
| | | Tea (per cup) | 0.195 | |
| | | White | 0.025–0.031 | |

*(Continued)*

**Table 3.2 (Continued) Different Sources of Tannins and Their Concentration**

| Sl. No. | Particulars | Name of Plant | Tannin (%) | References |
|---|---|---|---|---|
| 8 | Masticatories/stimulants | Betel leaf (*Piper betle*) | 1.0–1.3 | Tur and Brenner (1998) |
| | | Betelnuts (*Areca catechu L*) | 8–15 | |
| | | Cassava leaves | 0.15–3.0 | |
| | | Coffee beans | 0.7 | |
| | | Dry tea leaves | 3.7 | |
| | | Guarana | 12 | |
| | | Katha (from catechu) | 11.7–14.2 | |
| | | Kola nuts (*Cola acuminata*, *Cola nitida*) | 3.9–4.4 | |
| | | Roasted coffee beans | 1.7 | |
| 9 | Gel | Aloe vera | 0.14 | Kumari and Jain (2015) |

*Source:* Sharma et al., (2019).

is used widely in the leather industry alongside natural tannins. Ordoval G, a synthetic tannin made by condensation of higher hydrocarbons with formaldehyde, is much more effective than natural tannins, as 40 kg of Ordoval G equals 100 kg of vegetable tannins (Grasser 2005). Synthetic tannins are generated using two distinct processes. The first is to synthesize tannic acid or similar tannins from hydroxybenzoic acids. In a second way, chemical compounds are produced that have little in common with the structure of natural tannins, but behave like true tannins when in contact with animal pelt, and are therefore of functional use since they can be manufactured on a commercial scale.

## 3.5 MECHANISM OF ACTION

Tannins are polymeric phenolic substances having astringent and hemostatic properties. They are soluble in water, alcohol, and acetone, and interact with carbohydrates, proteins, enzymes, polysaccharides, and bacterial cell membranes.

### 3.5.1 Reaction with Carbohydrates

Starch generates cavities where tannins and other hydrophobic complexes, such as lipid, are embedded. Tannins may directly react with cellulose especially with plant cell walls like lignin. But it's a matter of ambiguity whether there is a difference in the position of tannins and cell wall carbohydrates of living plants as well as in animals. Tannins are more susceptible to high molecular weight carbohydrates which are normally not very soluble and mobile in their structure.

### 3.5.2 Reaction with Proteins

The capability to assemble protein complexes is a distinguishing feature of tannins, which have been used to make leather from animal skins since ancient times. The interaction between tannins and proteins involves binding and gathering, resulting in the precipitate. The hydroxyl groups (OH) of tannins attach to the active collagen centres first, and then the tannins fill the interfibrillar gaps in leather. Tannins couple with the positively charged -NH3+ in collagen to draw out water. As a result, it prevents bacterial growth and protects leather, preventing odour (Heidemann 1993).

$$\mathrm{COO-.P.NH_3^+ + \left[Tannin\right]O^- + H^+ \rightarrow COOH.P.NH_3^+ + \left[Tannin\right]O^-}$$

$$\mathrm{COOH.P.NH_3^+ + \left[Tannin\right]O^- \rightarrow COOH.P.NH_3^+ + \left[Tannin\right]O}$$

$$\mathrm{COOH.P.NH_3\left[Tannin\right]O \rightarrow COOH.P.HN.\left[Tannin\right] + H_2O}$$

The development of tannin–protein networks is influenced by many conditions, including the chemistry of tannin and protein, solution concentration, the isoelectric point of protein, pH, and ionic strength, as well as the ubiquity of other compounds. Additionally, proline-rich proteins (PRPs), which are present in mammalian saliva, are highly susceptible to tannin reactions. These interactions are important in astringency, a sensation of lack of lubrication, and dryness, as well as protecting dietary nitrogen from polyphenols. Proteins can interfere with tannins when their level is greater than the tannins, but there is no precipitation, finding it challenging to know if the reaction took place. Only when the amount of tannins exceeds the amount of protein insoluble complexes and a hydrophobic outer layer form. Precipitation is critical, and caution should be exercised when combining herbs that contain tannins; a highly tanninized herb can bind beneficial constituents. One of the explanations why strong black tea is known to assist with diarrhoea is that it binds to the proteins in the gut wall, forming a membrane that prevents water loss (Elaine 2009).

### 3.5.3 Reaction with Iron

Tannic acid and tannins are major iron absorption inhibitors. They react with non-heme iron, which can be found in plant foods including beans, peas, leafy green vegetables, and nuts, as well as animal foods such as rice, chicken, and fish. Brune et al. (1989) found that 5 mg of tannic acid in a meal prevented absorption by 20% and 100 mg by 88%.

## 3.6 IDENTIFICATION AND QUANTIFICATION

Tannins are chemically complex polyphenolics with various biological functions, and their physiological and pharmacological effects are influenced by their polyphenolic skeleton properties (De Bruyne et al. 1999). Tannins are light yellow or white non-crystalline powders, free masses, nearly colourless, having an astringent taste and distinct smell. Tannins can bind with metal ions as well as macromolecules like proteins and polysaccharides to form complexes. Proteins and metal complexes precipitate in the solution following their extraction. Simple HT has a lower tendency to generate precipitates with enzymes than catechins with ester-binding properties. This results in the formulation of a cream (Sekiya et al. 1984), with tannin quantification dependent on the binding behaviour, explained earlier. The commercial hide powder process relies on binding with animal skin collagen, while the relative astringency and absolute preference to methylene blue are determined by applying methylene blue and blood under controlled pH. The structural configurations of tannins carrying two or three phenolic hydroxyl groups on a phenyl ring are responsible for such characteristics (Okuda and Ito 2011). Titrimetric method, colourimetric assays (Folin-Ciocalteu method, hide-powder method, vanillin-HCl method, butanol-HCl method, rhodanine assay, and Wilson and Hagerman assays), precipitation assays, and spectroscopic method are employed to determine the type or amount of tannins present in a sample.

### 3.6.1 Titrimetric Method

During the titrimetric method, $KMnO_4$ is used as a titrant that has been standardized with Oxalic acid (0.1N) before being used. The endpoint colour is produced by the formation of a complex between potassium permanganate and phenolic acids. Gallic acid, for example, combines with potassium permanganate to produce the reddish-brown compound $K_4[Mn(C_4H_4O_6)_2]5H_2O$. Other tannins also create complexes with potassium permanganate like gallic acid, resulting in the formation of a golden-yellow hue.

### 3.6.2 Colorimetric Assays

#### *3.6.2.1 Folin-Ciocalteu Method*

Folin-Ciocalteu (FC) reagent is prepared by mixing phosphomolybdic acid with phosphotungstic acid, which is reduced to a mixture of blue oxides of molybdenum blue tungsten following the oxidation with phenols. The absorption of the resulting blue coloration is measured at the wavelength of 750 nm at UV-Vis spectroscopy which is proportional to the sample's total phenolic compounds. Since the technique measures total free phenolic groups, it can also be used to determine soluble phenolics such as polyflavonoid tannins and hydrolysable tannins. Ascorbic acid, tyrosine, and potentially glucose are also measured by this method (Hemingway and Karchesy 2012).

#### *3.6.2.2 Hide-Powder Method*

The principle of this test relay on the precipitation of tannins in a mixture using hide powder as a binding agent. The amount of tannins in a sample is determined by the discrepancy between the overall polyphenols content determined with FC reagent and the quantity of polyphenols observed after the precipitation (Elgailani and Ishak 2014).

#### *3.6.2.3 Vanillin Assay*

The vanillin method is a specific test for condensed tannins analysis that relies on vanillin's reaction with condensed tannins and the formation of coloured complexes. A chromophore is formed when vanillin interacts with the metasubstituted flavanols A-ring. The amount of flavanols in a solution is proportional to its absorbance (Hemingway and Karchesy 2012). Figure 3.4 depicts the fundamental reaction.

The type of solvent used, the acid's structure and concentration, temperature, vanillin concentration, the type of reference parameters and reaction time used all play key roles in the assay's success (Dalzell and Kerven 1998, Makkar and Becker 1993, Sun et al. 1998, Scalbert 1992). At the same normality, sulfuric acid is a more powerful catalyst than hydrochloric acid in the vanillin assay, but increasing the normality of each acid results in a higher $A_{500}$ (Sun et al. 1998, Scalbert 1992).

#### *3.6.2.4 Butanol-HCl Assay*

Butanol-HCl assay detects condensed tannins in a sample by depolymerizing tannins in butanol with HCl to produce a red anthocyanidin that can be identified using spectrophotometry (Reaction is summarized in Figure 3.5). Undervalued tannins are those that have been cleaved into dimers or trimers. The degree of polymerization of the PAs can be estimated by combining the butanol-HCl and vanillin assays. The acid butanol assay determines the total amount of flavonoid residues present, while the vanillin assay determines the number of molecules. The butanol-HCl technique is also used to determine how much insoluble tannin is present in extraction residues (Hemingway and Karchesy 2012).

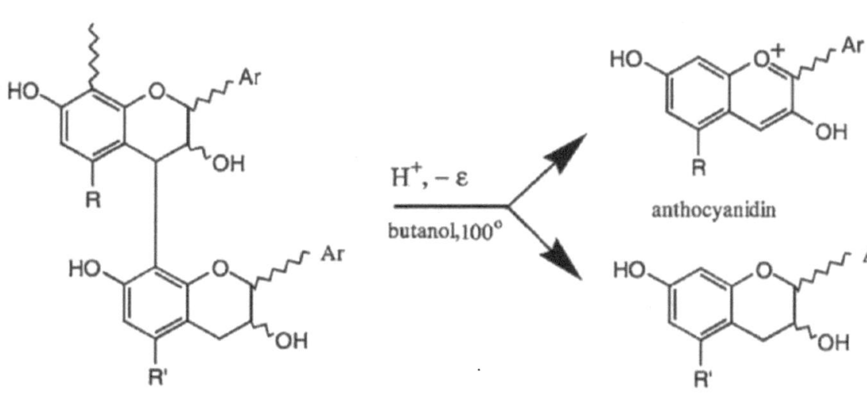


**Figure 3.4** Chemistry of Vanillin Assay. (Source: Schofield et al. 2001.)

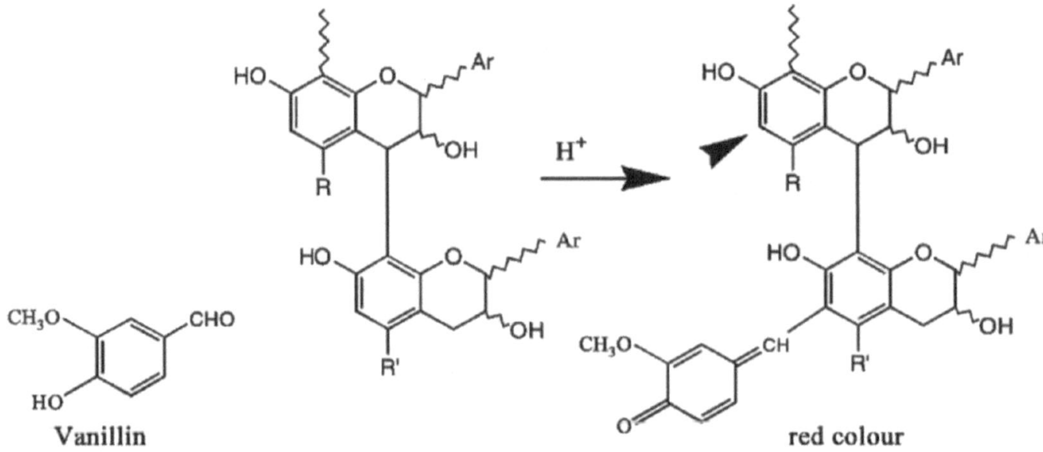


**Figure 3.5** Chemistry of Butanol-HCl Assay. (Source: Schofield et al. 2001.)

#### *3.6.2.5 Rhodanine Assay and Wilson and Hagerman Assay*

The former assay is designed to determine the existence of gallotannins, while the second is intended to evaluate the amount of ellagitannins. The sample is hydrolyzed to produce gallic acid or ellagic acid based on the results. Gallic acid reacts with the pigment rhodanine, and ellagic acid reacts with sodium nitrite to create a vigorous colour that can be analyzed spectrophotometrically (Hemingway and Karchesy 2012).

### 3.6.3 Precipitation Assay

This assay detects plant samples tannins having capacity to produce high tannin-protein complexes, further extraction yields low tannins. Having a higher affinity for tannins than proteins, polyethylene glycol 4,000 (PEG) binds to different types of tannins. The PEG-tannins compounds are insoluble in hot water, detergents (neutral and acidic), different organic solvents, and are stable over a pH range of 2 to 8.5 (Schofield et al. 2001).

### 3.6.4 Spectroscopic Determinations

The most of tannins are outside the spectrum of gas chromatography (GC) technique, so complex tannin extracts must be identified and estimated using the instrument named high-performance liquid chromatography (HPLC). When HPLC is combined with mass spectrometry (MS) and electron ionization (EI), researchers provide an effective instrument for analyzing tannins in crude and purified extracts. In LC/EI/MS, HPLC effluent is injected into an EI stream, resulting in standard EI spectra that can be screened for in a mass spectral library. Each approach produces various fragmentation patterns, but when used together, they provide structural elucidation with additional knowledge of a complementary nature (Barry et al. 2001). Hydrolyzable and complex tannins are normally easy to determine; however, condensed tannins must be acid depolymerized before HPLC and MS analyses (Zhang and Lin 2008).

## 3.7 HEALTH BENEFITS

While dietary tannins are often considered as hazardous due to their ability to impair protein digestibility or metal ion accessibility, tannins can sometimes be advantageous. Tannin-rich foods are becoming more prominent among persons of different ages, and these foods are helpful in certain way, providing us recovery from a variety of diseases, such as minimizing the risk of diabetes by increasing glucose uptake and thereby lowering blood sugar levels (Kumari and Jain 2015). When a diluted tannin solution is added to an open sore, the wound's collagen precipitates, developing a protective layer and stopping bleeding, causing the wound to heal faster (Ramakrishnan and Krishnan 1994). Allergic rhinitis, asthma, hypersensitive pneumonitis, mite allergens from carpet dust, and a range of many other allergies are all recovered by the application of condensed tannins (Chung et al. 1998). Tannins have biological properties include anti-inflammatory, anti-cancer, anti-allergic, anthelmintic, anti-microbial, and anti-viral properties against herpes simplex virus, poliovirus, and enteric virus (Athanasiadou et al. 2000, 2001, Ketzis et al. 2006, Muthukumar and Mahadevan 1981, Ghosh 2015). They are also used as anti-haemorrhoidal, anti-diarrheal, and hemostatic treatments in medicine. Tannin's propensity to create a protective coating and prevent infection in tissue makes it effective for curing skin ulcers, soaring throats, diarrhoea, dysentery, internal bleeding, and exhaustion (Ashok and Upadhyaya 2012). Furthermore, tannin serves as a precipitant in the liquor industry and has beneficial effects on vascular health (Ashok and Upadhyaya 2012). A comprehensive overview of the health effects of tannins are as follows.

### 3.7.1 Treatment of Diabetes Mellitus

Tannins inhibit human α-amylase and thereby delay starch digestion, are known to be effective antidiabetic functional foods. Tannins also reduce postprandial hyperglycemic secretion by suppressing carbohydrate digestion, glucose release, and absorption. Furthermore, they mingle with adipose tissue, inhibiting adipogenesis while increasing insulin production directly. Moreover, procyanidins have been shown to enhance the diabetic pathological oxidative condition (Sieniawska and Baj 2017, Kumari and Jain 2015).

### 3.7.2 Usage as Medicine

Tannin is used in Siddha and Ayurveda tooth powders as a gum-strengthening agent. Triphla churna is used to treat coughs in combination with honey and decoction is used to treat conjunctivitis. For treating ulcers and wounds, a diluted churna solution is used (Ramakrishnan and Krishnan 1994).

### 3.7.3 Healing of Wounds

When a diluted tannin solution is applied to an open wound, it aids in protein precipitation, the formation of a protective layer, and the prevention of bleeding, resulting in faster healing (Ramakrishnan and Krishnan 1994).

### 3.7.4 Cures Dysentery

In folk medicine, pomegranate rind decoction is said to treat various forms of dysentery (Ramakrishnan and Krishnan 1994).

### 3.7.5 Prevents Cardiovascular Diseases

Tannins' anti-oxidant properties protect the body from cardiovascular disease by preventing cholesterol oxidation, which is a precursor to plaque formation in vessels (Auger et al. 2002).

### 3.7.6 Anti-Carcinogenic

Green tea has been shown to suppress the growth of cancer cells. Peoples with frequent green tea were shown to have a diminished gastric cancer risk. Tannin, when consumed in adequate amounts, inhibits the production of carcinogens as well as tumour formation (Buzzini et al. 2008, Fujiki et al. 2002).

### 3.7.7 Anti-Mutagenic Activity

It has been documented that tannin extracted from grape seeds has anti-mutagenic activity against a variety of mutagens, including Benzo-(a)-pyrene, alfatoxinB, 2-aminofluorene, and others (Ghosh 2015, Yilmaz and Toledo 2004).

### 3.7.8 Anthelmintic Effect

The use of concentrated tannin resulted in a decrease in parasites. However, tannins were shown to have a direct effect in parasite cells at various stages of the life cycle, inducing reductions in invasive capability in the host, egg production in the third larval period, and egg excretion by an adult portion, as well as an indirect action, due to increased host resistance to invasion (Ketzis et al. 2006, Athanasiadou et al. 2000, 2001).

### 3.7.9 Anti-Oxidant Activity

Tannins have anti-oxidant activity due to their high molecular weight and a high degree of hydroxylation of aromatic rings, but tannin–protein complex formation limits this potential (Ketzis et al. 2006, Athanasiadou et al. 2000, 2001, Koleckar et al. 2008).

### 3.7.10 Anti-Microbial Activity

Tannins have anti-microbial properties due to the toxicity they trigger in bacteria, fungi, and yeasts. It also makes extracellular enzymes in different microorganisms inactive. Penicillium spp., HIV virus, *S. aureus*, *C. botulinum*, and other bacteria are all susceptible to it. Catechin, Epigallocatechin-3-gallate (EGCG), has a greater ability to disrupt membranes than hydrolyzable tannins, but has a lower anti-bacterial activity. By lowering the viability of H. pylori, hydrolyzable tannins (TG-I) have bactericidal effect (Chung et al. 1998, Muthukumar and Mahadevan 1981, Funatogawa et al. 2004, Khanbabaee and van Ree 2001).

### 3.7.11 Anti-Viral Activity

Tannins possess anti-viral effect because they suppress viral replication by inhibiting covalent closed circular DNA formation or causing protein aggregation by an inhibitory action based on their activity over certain proteases, integrases and transcriptases. Tannins also greatly reduce replication of P24 HIV-1. When tannins are incubated with red wines and high concentrated tannins, viruses such as enteric virus, herpes simplex virus, polio virus, and others are inactivated (Ashok and Upadhyaya 2012, Buzzini et al. 2008, Lu et al. 2004).

### 3.7.12 Anti-Inflammatory Activity

Individuals which are sensitive to selective cyclooxygenase-2 (COX-2) inhibitors or COX-nonselective nonsteroidal anti-inflammatory medications should use A-type and B-type procyanidins and derivatives for the treatment of inflammation and inflammation-related or associated diseases or disorders, as well as pain relief (Sieniawska and Baj 2017).

### 3.7.13 Effects on Vascular Health

Tannins in the proanthocyanidin group inhibit the formation of peptides that cause artery hardening (Ashok and Upadhyaya 2012).

## 3.8 TOXICOLOGY

While tannin is commonly used for its health benefits, it still has some negative side effects. Ingesting significant amounts of tannins may have negative health consequences. A miniscule fraction of the proper sort of tannins, on the other hand, can be useful to people's health (Chung et al. 1998). Tannin's tendency to impart astringency, which is desirable in the beverage sector, is a major downside in other food sectors because it reduces food palatability (Price and Butler 1980).

Tannin has anti-nutritional effects when it forms complexes with micro nutrients like vitamins and minerals, as well as macronutrients such as carbohydrates and proteins, making them inaccessible for the body to use (Hagerman et al. 1998, Waghorn et al. 1994). It also acts synergistically with enzymes involved in the metabolism of sugars, pectins, and proteins rendering them unable to function, resulting in nutritional content reduction of the product (Chung et al. 1998). Dietary tannins associate with proline-rich proteins, forming two groups of soluble and insoluble complexes that provide the astringent sensation (He et al. 2015). The tongue experiences astringency as a diffuse sensation that is accompanied by intense dryness and roughness in the mouth (Kaspchak et al. 2018). Tannins also limit the actions of intestinal microflora, resulting in less ingestion of organic matter and dietary fibre, which poses a threat to the digestive system's mucosal lining. Latest research suggests that the main consequence of tannins is a diminished efficiency in transforming ingested nutrients into new cell or tissue, rather than an inhibition on food intake or digestion.

Too much tannin in drinks like tea and coffee can lead to anaemia and osteoporosis, which can progress to cancer (Ricardo-da-Silva et al. 1991). Tannins have been linked to lower feed consumption, growth rate, feed production, and protein digestibility in laboratory animals (Aletor 2005). A comprehensive list of tannin's negative effects is as follows:

### 3.8.1 Anti-Nutritional Effects

Tannins act synergistically with minerals like phosphorus, calcium, and magnesium, rendering them inaccessible to monogastric species. Condensed tannins react with proteins in the diet and prevent nutrients from being digested. Tannin has a much greater affinity for protein than any other chemical for instances, 12 moles of protein can be bound with 1 mole of tannin. Tannin decreases the bioavailability of a variety of vitamins (vitamin A and vitamin B12) (Hagerman et al. 1998, Chung et al. 1998, Lacassagne et al. 1988, Waghorn et al. 1994, Longstaff and McNab 1991).

### 3.8.2 Enhance Indigestibility

Food consumption and digestibility are also diminished when condensed tannins are consumed (Acamovic and Brooker 2005, Dawson et al. 1999, Ketzis et al. 2006, Reed 1995).

### 3.8.3 Mutagenic and Carcinogenic

Tannins were graded as a class 1 carcinogen by the Occupational Safety and Health Administration (OSHA). Betel nuts are responsible for 11–26% of all oesophageal and cheek cancers. Due to mutagenesis, herbal tea along with a healthy diet induces stomach cancer (Chung et al. 1998).

### 3.8.4 Inducers or Co-Promoters

Tannins, when combined with other carcinogenic molecules, can serve as inducers and facilitate cancer (Mather 1997).

### 3.8.5 Relation with Migraines

The severity of migraine is increased when serotonin levels are reduced. This is due to the lack of starch, which is a precursor of serotonin and is bound by tannin (Chung et al. 1998).

### 3.8.6 Hepatotoxic Activity

Tannic acid is responsible for the onset of hepatic cell necrosis in both humans and livestock (Medugu et al. 2012).

### 3.8.7 Inhibitory Action

Endogenous enzyme activities are inhibited by condensed tannins, which form indigestible complexes. Enzymatic oxidation of tannins increases toxicity and has an inhibitory effect on enzymes (Awad et al. 2001).

Furthermore, many studies have examined the safety and effectiveness of gallic acid, ellagic acid, catechin, epicatechin, and proanthocynidin. Table 3.3 lists toxicity study details for these compounds as well as certain tannin-containing species.

## 3.9 APPLICATIONS OF TANNINS

Tannins play important role in the manufacturing industry, animal farming, refining, chemical industry, and tanning industry, in addition to biological roles. Condensed tannins are usually practiced in a variety of applications. Because of its complex relationship with protein, they have a lot of scope for use in animal nourishment and manufacturing processes (Cadahia et al. 1996). Table 3.4 summarizes the origins of concentrated tannins as well as their uses.

Tannins that can be hydrolyzed are often found in a variety of applications. These tannins interact with the protein in a variety of ways. As a result, it can be employed in numerous commercial applications and animal feed production(Cadahia et al. 1996). Table 3.5 summarizes the applications of hydrolyzable tannins.

## 3.10 SAFETY, PRECAUTIONS, AND REGULATION

Tannins are consumed from diverse food sources and it plays a vital role in ameliorating an individual's mood, cognitive function, and efficiency (Morton 1992). Daily tannin intake in the range of safe limit consumption for a healthy individual of 1.5–2.5 g and does not induce any adverse effects, although consumption exceeding this limit causes low iron absorption from the diet (Rao and Prabhavathi 1982). According to Kumari and Jain (2012), the amount of tannins consumed by children is lower than those consumed by adults. Tannins can be used in permissible and appropriate amounts for medicinal purposes, according to regulatory standards. Due to their low to a marginal risk factor and extended protective impact, natural sources of tannins such as tea, vegetables, herbs, chocolates, and wines can be eaten for a salubrious life (Ghosh 2015).

Average daily intake of added tannic acid by age groups of 0–5 Months, 6–11 Months, 12–23 Months and 2–65 + Years are 0.06 mg/kg, 0.36 mg/kg, 0.46 mg/kg and 0.21 mg/kg respectively. Calculations based upon the average body weight of 60 kg for an adult, and subsequently calculated weights of infants by age groups are 0–5 Months, 5 kg; 6–11 Months, 8 kg; 12–23 Months, 11 kg (Subcommittee on Review of the GRAS List 1972). While the literature defining the safe limits of

**Table 3.3 Tannins and Tannin-Containing Plants Toxicity Study**

| | | | Study Details | | |
|---|---|---|---|---|---|
| **Sl. No.** | **Compound** | **Reference** | **Study Type** | **Animal Used and study duration** | **No-Observed-Adverse-Effect Level (NOAEL)** |
| **Tannins** | | | | | |
| 1 | Gallic acid | Rajalakshmi et al. (2001) | Acute oral toxicity | Swiss Albino mice | 5,000 mg/kg |
| | | Sravan et al (2016) | Sub-acute toxicity | Swiss Albino mice (14 days) | 1,000 mg/kg/day |
| | | Niho et al. (2001) | Sub-chronic toxicity | F344 rat (13 week) | 115–128 mg/kg/day |
| 2 | Ellagic acid | Bhandary et al. (2013) | Sub-acute toxicity | Swiss Albino mice | 2,000 mg/kg/day |
| | | Takami et al. (2008) | Sub-chronic toxicity | F344 rats (13 weeks) | For male 3,011 and female 3,254 mg/kg BW/day |
| 3 | Catechin | Chengelis et al. (2008) | Repeated dose toxicity | Rats (28 days) | 2,000 mg/kg/day |
| | | Takami et al. (2008) | Sub-chronic toxicity | F344 rat (13 week) | For male 764 and female 820 mg/kg/day |
| | | Ogura et al. (2008) | Genotoxicity Study | SD rats | 2,000 mg/kg |
| 4 | Epigallocatechin-3-gallate (EGGG) | Isbrucker et al. (2006) | Acute oral toxicity | Rats | 200 mg/kg |
| | | | Sub-chronic toxicity | Rats (13 week) | 500 mg/kg/day |
| | | | Teratogenicity and reproductive toxicity | Rats | 200 mg/kg/day |
| 5 | Procyanidins | Yamakoshi et al. (2002) | Acute oral toxicity | F344 rats | 2 and 4 g/kg |
| | | | Sub-chronic toxicity | Rats (13 week) | For male 1,410 and female 1,501 mg/kg/day |
| | | Takahashi et al. (1999) | Dermal toxicity | Rats | 2,000 mg/kg |
| **Tannin-containing plants** | | | | | |
| 6 | Green tea (*Camellia sinensis*) | Sur et al. (2015) | Acute oral toxicity | Swiss albino mice | 2 g/kg |
| | | | Sub-chronic toxicity | ICR mice (13 week) | 250 mg/kg/day |
| | | Hua et al. (2011) | Repeat dose toxicity | Wistar rats (28 days) | 2,500 mg/kg /day |

*(Continued)*

**Table 3.3 (Continued) Tannins and Tannin-Containing Plants Toxicity Study**

| Sl. No. | Compound | Reference | Study Details | | No-Observed-Adverse-Effect Level (NOAEL) |
|---|---|---|---|---|---|
| | | | Study Type | Animal Used and study duration | |
| 7 | Grape seed (*Vitis Vinifera*) | Fiume et al. (2014) | Acute oral toxicity | F344/DuCrj rats | 4 g/kg |
| | | | Repeated dose toxicity | Sprague-Dawley rats (28 days) | For male 2,150 and female 1,780 mg/kg/day |
| | | Bentivegna and Whitney (2002) | Sub-chronic toxicity | IGS BR Sprague– Dawley rats (13 week) | For male 1.78 and female 2.15 g/kg/day |
| 8 | Pomegranate (*Punica granatum*) | Letizia et al. (2000) | Acute oral toxicity | Swiss Albino mice | 5 g/kg |
| | | | Sub-chronic toxicity | Wistar rats (13 week) | 600 mg/kg/day |
| | | Bhandary et al. (2013) | Repeated dose toxicity | Swiss Albino mice (28 days) | 2,000 mg/kg/day |
| 9 | Amla (*Emblica officinalis Gaertn*) | Jaijoy et al. (2010) | Acute oral toxicity | Sprague Dawley rats | 5 g/kg |
| | | | Chronic toxicity | Sprague Dawley rats (270 days) | 1,200 mg/kg/day |

*Source:* Laddha and Kulkarni (2019).

**Table 3.4 Applications of Condensed Tannins**

| Sl. No. | Types of Application | Main Features |
|---|---|---|
| 1 | Production of leather | Condensed tannins are widely used in tanneries for tanning leather. It is ideal for the tannery industry due to its higher shrinkage temperature and tolerance to detannage (Gustavson 1947, Mahdi et al. 2009, Hathway 1962, Lipsitz et al. 1949). |
| 2 | Animal food | Condensed tannins benefit animal health by using protein in the animal body and suppressing parasites in the gastrointestinal tract (Aguerre et al. 2020, Dentinho et al. 2020, Costes-Thire et al. 2019a, b, Lima et al. 2019, Aguerre et al. 2016). |
| 3 | Adhesive for plastic and wood | Condensed tannins having more excellent strength of wood composites, choicer of adhesiveness, and better water resistance characteristics react with formaldehyde and produce adhesives and plastics (Yang et al. 2020,Plomley et al. 1957, Pizzi 2008, Ping et al. 2012, Ping et al. 2011b, Ping et al. 2011a, Nico 1950, MacLean and Gardner 1952, Liu et al. 2020, Li et al. 2019a, Lei et al. 2008, Knowles and White 1954, Janceva et al. 2011, Hathway 1962, Hafiz et al. 2020, El Hage et al. 2011, Dalton 1950, Cui et al. 2015). |
| 4 | Wood preservation | Condensed tannins aid in the protection of wood from fungus and termite. It also lowers the leaching of boron to work as a fungicide and prevents photodegradation of wood by relieving $^1O2$ and suppressing phenoxyl radicals protection against preservative (Tomak and Gonultas 2018, Tascioglu et al. 2012, Thevenon et al. 2010, Tascioglu et al. 2013). |
| 5 | Wood properties improvement | Condensed tannins strengthen the mechanical properties, revamp the toughness properties, enhance the bending, compression, and hardness properties, and improve the dimensional stability of wood (Bariska and Pizzi 1986, Yalcin and Ceylan 2017). |
| 6 | Ceramics and oil industries | Condensed tannins are also widely employed in the oil and ceramic industries to minimize bentonite viscosity and promote better flow. They're often used to regulate mud viscosity and enhance the casting slip's suspending power (Hathway 1962, O'Flaherty et al. 1956). |
| 7 | Preservation of fishing nets | The use of different condensed tannins to preserve fishing nets is widespread because it prevents bacterial and fungal cellulases from degrading cellulose (Hathway 1962). |
| 8 | Fire-resistance of wood | To increase the fire-resistance properties of wood, tannin is combined with sodium hydroxide, phosphoric acid, hexamethylentetramine, and boric acid (Tondi et al. 2012). |
| 9 | Water and waste water treatment plant | Tannin is used in purifying water and effluent treatment plants because of its higher coagulation capacity and ability to absorb methylene blue and heavy metals. (Bello et al. 2020; Combs 2016; Grenda et al. 2020, Wang et al. 2019, Grenda et al. 2020). |
| 10 | Packaging | Tannins being biohybrid film with high tensile strength, thermal resilience, UV shielding capacity, and anti-oxidant properties are applied to the manufacture of food packaging and other materials (Li et al. 2019b). |
| 11 | Anti-corrosive for metal | Flavan-3-ol of condensed tannin structure possesses oxygen atoms in its functional assortments as well as aromatic rings, which can scavenge oxygen and prevent corrosion. In acidic media, oxygen's free electrons are protonated, the protonated molecules are adsorbed on the metal surface due to electrostatic interaction, and thus preventing metal corrosion (Shah et al. 2011, O'Flaherty et al. 1956,Nardeli et al. 2019, Byrne et al. 2020, Byrne et al. 2019). |
| 12 | 3D printing | Condensed tannins are used in 3D printing because they have a higher tensile property and have improved printing accuracy (Liao et al. 2020). |

tannins for human consumption is sparse, the safe limit for tannin is provided for only a few food items. According to the Joint FAO/WHO Food Standards Program (1995), whole sorghum's tannin content must not surpass 0.5% based on a dry weight basis and the tannin content of decorticated sorghum grains should be less than 0.3% based on the dry weight. As stated in the Food Safety and Standards Regulation (2009), Carob powder tannin content should be in the range 0.1 to 0.15%.

**Table 3.5 Applications of Hydrolyzable Tannins**

| Sl. No. | Types of Application | Main Features |
|---|---|---|
| 1 | Leather processing | Hydrolyzable tannins are also extensively utilized in tannery due to their capability of cross-links with the hide's collagen chains during the tanning process (Guo et al. 2020). |
| 3 | Preservation of wood | Hydrolyzable tannins, especially the gallic acid of hydrolyzable tannins can be used in the preservation of wood and thus, improve the durability of wood by hindering fungal attack (Tomak and Gonultas 2018). |
| 2 | Manufacturing of plastic resin and adhesives | Having better water defiance properties and tendency to form cross-linking with formaldehyde make hydrolysable tannins ideal for manufacturing of plastic resins and adhesives (Spina et al. 2013, Vazquez et al. 2013, Ghahri and Pizzi 2018, Vazquez et al. 2012). |
| 5 | Metal anti-corrosion agents | The hydrolyzable tannins' hydroxyl aromatic ring scavenges oxygen and prevents corrosion by blocking the metal surface by adsorption, and thus the tannins can be used as anti-corrosive (Byrne et al. 2019). |
| 4 | Improvement of wine quality | Wine quality is affected by polyphenols and anti-oxidants present in hydrolyzable tannins. In the wine industry, tannin derived from oak heartwood is widely used to enhance wine flavor, and ellagitannins play an important role in controlling the colour and quality of wine during ageing (Viriot et al. 1993, Vivas and Glories 1996; Vivas et al. 1996, Puech et al. 1999, Jordão et al. 2005). |
| 6 | Medication | Hydrolyzable tannins confer the advantageous impact on human well-being as it possesses anti-oxidant, anti-cancer, anti-mutagenic effects, and can reduce serum cholesterol, triglycerides, and insulin (Smeriglio et al. 2017,Ong et al. 1995, Yugarani et al. 1993). |

**Table 3.6 Maximum Level of Use of Tannic Acid in Various Foods**

| Sl. No. | Food | Maximum Level of Use (%) |
|---|---|---|
| 1 | Alcoholic beverages | 0.015 |
| 2 | Bakery items | 0.01 |
| 3 | Dairy desserts (frozen) and confectionery like soft candy | 0.04 |
| 4 | Fillings, gelatins, and puddings | 0.005 |
| 5 | Hard candy and throat lozenges | 0.013 |
| 6 | Meat and meat products | 0.001 |
| 7 | Non-alcoholic beverages and raw ingredients | 0.005 |

*Source:* Sharma et al. 2019.

The Food and Drug Administration (FDA) of the United States has estimated that the level of tannic acid in foods does not surpass 100 mg/kg, although there is no similar guideline exist for the European population. Tannic acid can be applied as a feed supplement in amounts to 15 mg/kg for whole animal species. Tannins, when used in permissible amounts (adult ruminants: 15,000 mg/kg, rabbits and laying hens: 10,000 mg/kg, pigs: 1,500 mg/kg, chickens: 1,000 mg/kg), seem to have no negative effects on babies, teenagers, adults, or pregnant women, according to numerous published studies (Aquilina et al. 2014, Jamroz et al. 2009, Anonymous 2006). According to the FEEDAP commission (The Panel on Additives and Products or Substances Used in Animal Feed), tannic acid could be employed as a feed additive, but only below the proposed circumstances, which would not pose any health risk to consumers (Anonymous 2006) (Table 3.6).

## 3.11 EFFECT OF PROCESSING ON TANNIN

Processing reduces or eliminates tannins in food and feedstuffs using appropriate techniques. Different processing techniques, such as application of heat and enzymes, washing, sprouting, irradiation, fermentation, dehulling and milling, microwave processing, high pressure processing, and extrusion can conveniently modify or mitigate the harmful effects of tannin as anti-nutritional factors prior to considering it as human and animal food or feed (Krupa 2008).

### 3.11.1 Dehulling

Dehulling is the act of removing a seed's outer coat/hull. Phenolic compounds, tannins, and fibres are often found in the grain's outer layers and seed coats, while phytate presents both in the external layers and the germ. As a result, dehulling has a significant effect on fibre, tannin, and other phenolic compounds elimination (Lestienne et al. 2007). Kaur et al. (2011) investigated the tannin content of various cereals bran and reported that wheat bran has 2.89 mg/g of tannins while barley bran contains 3.40 mg/g. When tannins are extracted from feedstuffs, protein content and its digestibility in legume seed meal increase significantly.

### 3.11.2 Fermentation

Fine wheat bran's tannin content was found to be slightly higher than the other two varieties, i.e., coarse and medium. This disparity is probably explained by the fact that the fine bran is predominantly composed of the seed coat. Hassan et al. (2008) have described a reduction in the tannin content of wheat bran after 4 h of fermentation.

### 3.11.3 Germination

The germination procedure, which is one of the cheapest processes, has been shown to minimize tannin content. Using response surface methodology, Hussain et al. (2011) controlled the time and temperature of germination in wheat and mung bean to minimize the content of tannins and phytic acid. The amount of raw wheat seeds tannin was 353 mg/100 g where the optimum time and temperature were 33.5°C and 60.3 h, and the minimum optimal value from multiple response optimizations was 295.7.

### 3.11.4 Enzyme Supplementation

Enzyme supplementation to lower tannin content is a useful process, but it may not be the most cost-effective. It has been shown to degrade tannins more effectively than other methods of processing like soaking, dehulling, and so on. Enzyme supplementation is beneficial in lowering tannins in protein feedstuffs in many trials (Avilés-Gaxiola et al. 2018, Towo et al. 2006). When sorghum is treated with polyphenoloxidase and phytase enzymes resulted in diminished hydrolysable and condensed tannins by 72.3% and 81.3% (Avilés-Gaxiola et al. 2018). Furthermore, Towo et al. (2006) found that treating sorghum grains with the three enzymes phytase, tannase, and paecilomyces variotii lowered all hydrolysable and condensed tannins by 40.6%, 38.92%, and 58.00%, respectively.

### 3.11.5 Soaking

Soaking is a low-cost conventional technique that has been used by animal nutritionists for decades. Adding sodium bicarbonate, soaking for very long time, or soaking at a higher temperature were found to be beneficial during the soaking phase in a sample (Schons, et al. 2012). According to Kyarisiima et al. (2004), sorghum soaked in wood ash extract lowered tannin levels without reducing nutritional content of sorghum grains. Leaching into the soaking water may be the cause of the drop in tannins while soaking (Tapiwa 2019). In addition, Iji et al. (2017) found a 73–82% decline in velvet beans.

### 3.11.6 Cooking

Cooking is thought to be beneficial in lowering the anti-nutrient activities of tannins. Cooking lowers the anti-nutrients found in tuber crops like cocoyam, according to Abeke and Otu (2008).

### 3.11.7 Autoclaving

Autoclaving has been shown to be one of the most efficient methods for removing anti-nutrients, but it is not cheap due to its dependence on electric energy (Manach et al. 2004).

### 3.11.8 Grinding

Since grinding increases the surface area, it decreases the interaction between the phenolic oxidase and tannins in the plant, making it an efficient tool for reducing tannin content (Vitti et al. 2005, Elizondo et al. 2010).

### 3.11.9 Extrusion

Anti-nutritional components have been found to be inactivated by extrusion (Navale et al. 2015, Kaur et al. 2015, Rathod and Annapure 2016). Extrusion cooking is a high-temperature, fast process that uses a combination of moisture, pressure, temperature, and mechanical shear to plasticize and cook starchy food materials (Alonso et al. 2000). Extrusion resulted in a substantial reduction in tannins and minimal oil loss in flaxseed meal (Imran et al. 2014). Since treatment with extrusion methods, lentil splits showed a drop in tannins, according to TV et al. (2018). In addition, Singh et al. (2017) found a decline in sorghum from 34.52% to 57.41%.

### 3.11.10 Combined Effects

A mingle of distinctive processing methods can help reduce anti-nutritional factors to a greater degree than a single process alone. Gunashree et al. (2014) investigated the effects of a range of conventional processing methods, including fermentation, germination, pressure cooking, soaking, blanching, milling, and kilning on the levels of various nutrients and anti-nutritional factors. Tannin concentration in all refined wheat was lower than in raw wheat, but fermentation had the maximum reduction of 85.1%, followed by germinated wheat. The tannin content of germinated seeds is mostly reduced due to the development of hydrophobic tannin interactions with seed enzymes and proteins rather than direct tannin depletion or degradation (Butler et al. 1984). The influence of germination and soaking on the level of anti-nutritional factors in wheat and other two grains were investigated by Patel and Dutta (2018). Wheat kernels were submerged in water (1:3) at room temperature for 10 h and then permitted to germinate at different temperatures of 36, 48, and 72 h at 30, 34, and 37°C and 85% relative humidity respectively. Tannin levels in soaked and germinated wheat reduced by 19.26 and 50.78%, respectively. The increased polyphenol oxidase and other catabolic enzyme activity may be accountable for the decrease in tannin during germination. These enzymes are triggered during germination, resulting in the hydrolysis of a variety of compounds such as glucose, protein, fibre, and lipid, as well as phenolic compounds.

## 3.12 FUTURE SCOPE

The impact of tannins in food on human health is a bone of contention among scientists. Tannins seem to be a two-edged blade. On the one side, tannin has health-preventive properties (anti-carcinogenic and anti-mutagenic), but on the other hand, it can also have anti-nutritional properties. Several trials have been accomplished to combat the negative impacts of tannins in foods such as fruits and vegetables. In a big development, fermentation with lactic acid bacteria was used in Xuan Mugua fruits, resulting in a reduction of up to 70% tannin content and a significant reduction in astringency, allowing the process to be used in the food industry (Shang, et al. 2019). Its benefits, on the other hand, may be reaped for the good of humanity if used under reasonable limits.

Since tannins are the raw material for sustainable green chemistry, it is now feasible to further utilize them as a result of current scientific investigation. Several enzymes such as tannase or tannin acyl hydrolase have recently been isolated, characterized, and categorized from microorganisms and fungi and the toxic influence of tannins is reduced by hydrolysis and oxidation (de Las et al. 2019, Prigione et al. 2018). In the leather tanning industry, tannase from several filamentous fungi is utilized for bioremediation. Tannins' chemical properties have proven them to be a possible replacement for metals or other chemical compounds used as coagulants or tannin inhibitors, which are harmful to human health and the environment. Tannins also have the potential to be used as coagulants, adhesives, superplasticizers, and floatation agents in the manufacture of modern environmentally safe products.

## 3.13 CONCLUSION

Tannins are essential natural bioactive compounds that belong to a variety of foods. They have enormous potentials in the manufacturing and nutraceuticals industries, but depending on their dosage they may exert both negative and positive effects on the human body. When consumed with food, tannins decrease the digestibility of the nutrient, even though different processing methods, either alone or in combination, are effective in modification or mitigation of its harmful effects. Tannins, on the other hand, can be isolated and purified to produce medicinal formulations that could be used to treat a wide variety of allergic reactions, inflammatory disorders, parasites, tumours, and other ailments. Further, tannins applications are not restricted to leather processing but also in the wood industry, oil and ceramics industry, water and waste treatment plants, animal food, metal anti-corrosive production, wine manufacturing, and the production of advanced materials.

## REFERENCES

Abeke, F.O. and Otu, M. 2008. Antinutrients in poultry feeds: concerns and options. In Proceedings of the 13th Annual Conference of the Animal Science Association of Nigeria (ASAN), 15$^{th}$ – 19$^{th}$ September 2008, A.B.U Zaria, Nigeria, pp. 396–398.

Acamovic, T. and Brooker, J.D. 2005. Biochemistry of plant secondary metabolites and their effects in animals. *Proceedings of the Nutrition Society* 64(3):403–412.

Aguerre, M.J., Capozzolo, M.C., Lencioni, P., Cabral, C. and Wattiaux, M.A. 2016. Effect of quebracho-chestnut tannin extracts at 2 dietary crude protein levels on performance, rumen fermentation, and nitrogen partitioning in dairy cows. *Journal of Dairy Science* 99(6):4476–4486.

Aguerre, M.J., Duval, B., Powell, J.M., Vadas, P.A. and Wattiaux, M.A. 2020. Effects of feeding a quebracho–chestnut tannin extract on lactating cow performance and nitrogen utilization efficiency. *Journal of Dairy Science* 103(3):2264–2271.

Aletor, V.A. 2005. Anti-nutritional factors as nature's paradox in food and nutrition securities. Inaugural lecture series 15, delivered at The Federal University of Technology, Akure, Nigeria (FUTA).

Alonso, R., Aguirre, A. and Marzo, F. 2000. Effects of extrusion and traditional processing methods on antinutrients and in vitro digestibility of protein and starch in faba and kidney beans. *Food Chemistry* 68(2):159–165.

Anonymous. 2006. Reassessment of one exemption from the requirement of a tolerance for tannin (CAS Reg. No. 1401-55-4). https://www.epa.gov/sites/production/files/2015-04/documents/tannin.pdf [Accessed 20 August 2019].

Aquilina, G., et al. 2014. Scientific opinion on the safety and efficacy of tannic acid when used as feed flavouring for all animal species. *EFSA Journal* 12(10):3828.

Arapitsas, P. 2012. Hydrolyzable tannin analysis in food. *Food Chemistry* 135(3):1708–1717.

Arogba, S.S. 1997. Physical, chemical and functional properties of Nigerian mango (Mangifera indica) kernel and its processed flour. *Journal of the Science of Food and Agriculture* 73(3):321–328.

Ashok, P.K. and Upadhyaya, K. 2012. Tannins are astringent. *Journal of Pharmacognosy and Phytochemistry* 1(3):45–50.

Athanasiadou, S., et al. 2000. Effects of short-term exposure to condensed tannins on adult Trichostrongylus colubriformis. *Veterinary Record* 146 (25):728–732.

Athanasiadou, S., Kyriazakis, I., Jackson, F., and Coop, R.L. 2001. Direct anthelmintic effects of condensed tannins towards different gastrointestinal nematodes of sheep: in vitro and in vivo studies. *Veterinary Parasitology*, 99(3):205–219.

Auger, C., Caporiccio, B., Landrault, N., et al. 2002. Red wine phenolic compounds reduce plasma lipids and apolipoprotein B and prevent early aortic atherosclerosis in hypercholesterolemic golden Syrian hamsters (Mesocricetus auratus). *The Journal of Nutrition* 132(6):1207–1213.

Avilés-Gaxiola, S., Chuck-Hernández, C. and Serna Saldivar, S.O. 2018. Inactivation methods of trypsin inhibitor in legumes: a review. *Journal of Food Science* 83(1):17–29.

Awad, H.M., Boersma, M.G., Boeren, S., van Bladeren, P.J., Vervoort, J. and Rietjens, I.M. 2001. Structure–activity study on the quinone/quinone methide chemistry of flavonoids. *Chemical Research in Toxicology* 14(4):398–408.

Balasubramanian, S., Yadav, D.N., Kaur, J. and Anand, T. 2014. Development and shelf-life evaluation of pearl millet based upma dry mix. *Journal of Food Science and Technology* 51(6):1110–1117.

Bariska, M. and Pizzi, A. 1986. The interaction of polyflavonoid tannins with wood cell-walls.*Holzforschung* 40(5):299–302.

Barry, K.M., Davies, N.W. and Mohammed, C.L. 2001. Identification of hydrolysable tannins in the reaction zone of Eucalyptus nitens wood by high performance liquid chromatography–electrospray ionisation mass spectrometry. *Phytochemical Analysis: An International Journal of Plant Chemical and Biochemical Techniques* 12(2):120–127.

Bello, A., Virtanen, V., Salminen, J.P. and Leiviskä, T. 2020. Aminomethylation of spruce tannins and their application as coagulants for water clarification. *Separation and Purification Technology* 242:116765.

Bennick, A. 2002. Interaction of plant polyphenols with salivary proteins. *Critical Reviews in Oral Biology and Medicine* 13(2):184–196.

Bentivegna, S.S. and Whitney, K.M. 2002. Subchronic 3-month oral toxicity study of grape seed and grape skin extracts. *Food and Chemical Toxicology* 40(12):1731–1743.

Bhandary, B.S.K., Sharmila, K.P., Kumari, N.S. and Bhat, S.V. 2013. Acute and subacute toxicity study of the ethanol extracts of Punica granatum (Linn). Whole fruit and seeds and synthetic ellagic acid in swiss albino mice. *Asian Journal of Pharmaceutical and Clinical Research* 6(4):192–198.

Bolobajev, J., Trapido, M. and Goi, A. 2016. Interaction of tannic acid with ferric iron to assist 2, 4, 6-trichlorophenol catalytic decomposition and reuse of ferric sludge as a source of iron catalyst in Fenton-based treatment. *Applied Catalysis B: Environmental* 187:75–82.

Brune, M., Rossander, L. and Hallberg, L. 1989. Iron absorption and phenolic compounds: importance of different phenolic structures. *European Journal of Clinical Nutrition* 43(8):547–557.

Butler, L.G., Riedl, D.J., Lebryk, D.G. and Blytt, H.J. 1984. Interactions of proteins with sorghum tannin: mechanism, specificity and significance. *Journal of the American Oil Chemists' Society* 61:916–920.

Buzzini, P., Arapitsas, P., Goretti, M., et al. 2008. Antimicrobial and antiviral activity of hydrolysable tannins. *Mini-Reviews in Medicinal Chemistry* 8(12):1179.

Byrne, C., D'Alessandro, O., Selmi, G.J., Romagnoli, R. and Deyá, C. 2019. Primers based on tara and quebracho tannins for poorly prepared steel surfaces. *Progress in Organic Coatings* 130:244–250.

Byrne, C., Selmi, G.J., D'Alessandro, O. and Deyá, C. 2020. Study of the anticorrosive properties of "quebracho colorado" extract and its use in a primer for aluminum1050. *Progress in Organic Coatings* 148:105827.

Cadahia, E., Conde, E., Garcia-Vallejo, M.C. and de Simón, B.F. 1996. Gel permeation chromatographic study of the molecular weight distribution of tannins in the wood, bark and leaves ofEucalyptus spp. *Chromatographia* 42(1–2):95–100.

Chengelis, C.P., Kirkpatrick, J.B., Regan, K.S., et al. 2008. 28-Day oral (gavage) toxicity studies of green tea catechins prepared for beverages in rats. *Food and Chemical Toxicology* 46(3):978–989.

Chung, K., Wong, T.Y., Wei, C., Huang, Y. and Lin, Y. 1998. Tannins and human health: a review. *Critical Reviews in Food Science and Nutrition* 38(6):421–464.

Clark-Lewis, J.W. and Roux, D.G. 1959. Natural occurrence of enantiomorphous leucoanthocyanidian:(+)-mollisacacidin (gleditsin) and quebracho (–)-leucofisetinidin. *Journal of the Chemical Society (Resumed)* 273:1402–1406.

Combs, C.A. 2016. *Tannins: Biochemistry, Food Sources and Nutritional Properties*. Nova Science Publishers, Inc., New York.

Costes-Thiré, M., Laurent, P., Ginane, C. and Villalba, J.J. 2019a. Diet selection and trade-offs between condensed tannins and nutrients in parasitized sheep. Veterinary Parasitology 271:14–21.

Costes-Thiré, M., Laurent, P., Ginane, C. and Villalba, J.J. 2019b. PSIII-42 Diet selection and trade-offs between condensed tannins and nutrients in parasitized sheep. *Journal of Animal Science* 97(3): 184–185.

Cui, J., Lu, X., Zhou, X., et al. 2015. Enhancement of mechanical strength of particleboard using environmentally friendly pine (*Pinus pinaster L.*) tannin adhesives with cellulose nanofibers. *Annals of Forest Science* 72(1):27–32.

Dalton, T.K. 1950. Tannin formaldehyde resins as adhesives for wood. *Australian Journal of Applied Science* 1:54–70.

Dalzell, S.A. and Kerven, G.L. 1998. A rapid method for the measurement of Leucaena spp proanthocyanidins by the proanthocyanidin (butanol/HCl) assay. *Journal of the Science of Food and Agriculture* 78(3), pp.405–416.

Das, A.K., Islam, M.N., Faruk, M.O., Ashaduzzaman, M. and Dungani, R. 2020. Review on tannins: extraction processes, applications and possibilities. *South African Journal of Botany* 135:58–70.

Dawson, J.M., Buttery, P.J., Jenkins, D., Wood, C.D. and Gill, M. 1999. Effects of dietary quebracho tannin on nutrient utilisation and tissue metabolism in sheep and rats. *Journal of the Science of Food and Agriculture* 79(11):1423–1430.

De Bruyne, T., Pieters, L., Deelstra, H. and Vlietinck, A. 1999. Condensed vegetable tannins: biodiversity in structure and biological activities. *Biochemical Systematics and Ecology* 27(4):445–459.

de Las Rivas, B., Rodríguez, H., Anguita, J. and Muñoz, R. 2019. Bacterial tannases: classification and biochemical properties. *Applied Microbiology and Biotechnology* 103(2):603–623.

Del Bubba, M., Giordani, E., Pippucci, L., Cincinelli, A., Checchini, L. and Galvan, P. 2009. Changes in tannins, ascorbic acid and sugar content in astringent persimmons during ontree growth and ripening and in response to different postharvest treatments. *Journal of Food Composition and Analysis* 22(7–8):668–677.

Dentinho, M.T.P., Paulos, K., Francisco, A., et al. 2020. Effect of soybean meal treatment with Cistus ladanifer condensed tannins in growth performance, carcass and meat quality of lambs. *Livestock Science* 236:104021.

Devi, P.B., Vijayabharathi, R., Sathyabama, S., Malleshi, N.G. and Priyadarisini, V.B. 2014. Health benefits of finger millet (*Eleusine coracana* L.) polyphenols and dietary fiber: a review. *Journal of Food Science and Technology* 51(6):1021–1040.

Elaine, M.A. 2009. Chapter 21 – *Phenols, A Handbook for Complementary Healthcare Professionals, Pharmacology* (pp. 149–166).

Elgailani, I.E.H. and Ishak, C.Y. 2014. Determination of tannins of three common Acacia species of Sudan. *Advances in Chemistry* 5, pp.45–53.

Elizondo, A.M., Mercado, E.C., Rabinovitz, B.C. and Fernandez-Miyakawa, M.E. 2010. Effect of tannins on the in vitro growth of Clostridium perfringens. *Veterinary Microbiology* 145(3–4):308–314.

Fengel, D. and Wegener, G. 1984. *Reactions in Alkaline Medium. Wood: Chemistry, Ultrastructure, Reaction* (pp. 296–318). Walter de Gruyter, Berlin and New York.

Fiume, M.M., Bergfeld, W.F., Belsito, D.V., et al. 2014. Safety assessment of Vitis vinifera (Grape)-derived ingredients as used in cosmetics. *International Journal of Toxicology* 33(3_suppl):48S–83S.

Fujiki, H., Suganuma, M., Imai, K. and Nakachi, K. 2002. Green tea: cancer preventive beverage and/or drug. *Cancer Letters* 188(1–2):9–13.

Ghahri, S. and Pizzi, A. 2018. Improving soy-based adhesives for wood particleboard by tannins addition. *Wood Science and Technology* 52(1):261–279.

Ghosh, D. 2015. Tannins from foods to combat diseases. *International Journal of Pharmaceutical Sciences Review and Research* 4(5):40–44.

Goel, G., Makkar, H.P., and Becker, K. 2008. Effects of Sesbania sesban and Carduus pycnocephalus leaves and Fenugreek (Trigonellafoenum graecum L.) seeds and their extracts on partitioning of nutrients from roughage-and concentrate-based feeds to methane. *Animal Feed Science and Technology* 147(1–3):72–89.

Grasser, G. 2005. Synthetic tannins. Project Gutenberg. Available from: http://www.gutenberg.org/files/7981/7981-8.txt [Accessed 20 August 2019].

Green, F.B. and Corcoran, M.R. 1975. Inhibitory action of five tannins on growth induced by several gibberellins. *Plant Physiology* 56(6):801–806.

Grenda, K., Arnold, J., Gamelas, J.A. and Rasteiro, M.G. 2020. Up-scaling of tannin-based coagulants for wastewater treatment: performance in a water treatment plant. *Environmental Science and Pollution Research* 27(2):1202–1213.

Gunashree, B.S., Kumar, R.S., Roobini, R. and Venkateswaran, G. 2014. Nutrients and antinutrients of ragi and wheat as influenced by traditional processes. *International Journal of Current Microbiology and Applied Sciences* 3 (7):720–736.

Guo, L., Qiang, T., Ma, Y., Wang, K. and Du, K. 2020. Optimisation of tannin extraction from Coriaria nepalensis bark as a renewable resource for use in tanning. *Industrial Crops and Products* 149:112360.

Gupta, S., Gowri, B.S., Lakshmi, A.J. and Prakash, J. 2013. Retention of nutrients in green leafy vegetables on dehydration. *Journal of Food Science and Technology* 50(5):918–925.

Gupta, S., Lakshmi, A.J., Manjunath, M.N. and Prakash, J. 2005. Analysis of nutrient and antinutrient content of underutilized green leafy vegetables. *LWT-Food Science and Technology* 38(4):339–345.

Gustavson, K.H. 1947. Reaction of tetra-oxalate-diol-chromiate with hide protein. *The Journal of the American Leather Chemists Association* 42:201.

Hafiz, N.L.M., Tahir, P.M., Lee, S.H., et al. 2020. Curing and thermal properties of co-polymerized tannin phenol–formaldehyde resin for bonding wood veneers. *Journal of Materials Research and Technology* 9(4):6994–7001.

Hage, R.E., Brosse, N., Navarrete, P. and Pizzi, A. 2011. Extraction, characterization and utilization of organosolv miscanthus lignin for the conception of environmentally friendly mixed tannin/lignin wood resins. *Journal of Adhesion Science and Technology* 25(13):1549–1560.

Hagerman, A.E., Riedl, K.M., Jones, G.A., et al. 1998. High molecular weight plant polyphenolics (tannins) as biological antioxidants. *Journal of Agricultural and Food Chemistry* 46(5):1887–1892.

Haslam, E. 1966. *Chemistry of Vegetable Tannins.* Academic Press, London.

Haslam, E. 1989. *Plant Polyphenols: Vegetable Tannins Revisited.* CUP Archive Oakleigh, Australia.

Hassan, E.G., Alkareem, A.M.A. and Mustafa, A.M.I. 2008. Effect of fermentation and particle size of wheat bran on the antinutritional factors and bread quality. *Pakistan Journal of Nutrition* 7(4):521–526.

Hassanpour, S., MaheriSis, N. and Eshratkhah, B. 2011. Plants and secondary metabolites (Tannins): a review. *International Journal of Forest, Soil and Erosion* 1(1):47–53.

Hathway, D.E. 1962. The condensed tannins. In *Wood Extractives and their Significance to the Pulp and Paper Industries* (191–228). Academic Press, London.

He, F., Pan, Q.H., Shi, Y. and Duan, C.Q. 2008. Biosynthesis and genetic regulation of proanthocyanidins in plants. *Molecules* 13(10):2674–2703.

He, M., Tian, H., Luo, X., Qi, X. and Chen, X. 2015. Molecular progress in research on fruit astringency. *Molecules* 20(1):1434–1451.

Heidemann, E. 1993. *Fundamentals of Leather Manufacture.* Eduard Roether KG, Darmstadt.

Hemingway, R.W. and Karchesy, J.J. 2012. *Chemistry and Significance of Condensed Tannins.* Springer Science & Business Media, New York.

Hua, C., Liao, Y., Lin, S., Tsai, T., Huang, C. and Chou, P. 2011. Does supplementation with green tea extract improve insulin resistance in obese type 2 diabetics? A randomized, double-blind, and placebocontrolled clinical trial. *Alternative Medicine Review* 16(2):157–163.

Hussain, I., Uddin, M.B. and Aziz, M.G. 2011. Optimization of antinutritional factors from germinated wheat and mungbean by response surface methodology. *International Food Research Journal* 18(3):957–963.

Iji, P.A., Toghyani, M., Ahiwe, E.U. and Omede, A.A. 2017. Alternative sources of protein for poultry nutrition. *Achieving Sustainable Production of Poultry Meat* 2:237–269.

Imran, M., Anjum, F.M., Butt, M.S. and Sheikh, M.A. 2014. Influence of extrusion processing on tannin reduction and oil loss in flaxseed (L inum usitatissimum L.) meal. *Journal of Food Processing and Preservation* 38(1):622–629.

Isbrucker, R.A., Edwards, J.A., Wolz, E., Davidovich, A. and Bausch, J. 2006. Safety studies on epigallocatechin gallate (EGCG) preparations. Part 2: dermal, acute and short-term toxicity studies. *Food Chemistry Toxicology* 44:636–650.

Jacobson, A. and Corcoran, M.R. 1977. Tannins as gibberellin antagonists in the synthesis of a-amylase and acid phosphatase by barley seeds. *Plant Physiology* 59(2):129–133.

Jaijoy, K., Soonthornchareonnon, N., Lertprasertsuke, N., Panthong, A. and Sireeratawong, S. 2010. Acute and chronic oral toxicity of standardized water extract from the fruit of Phyllanthus emblica Linn. *International Journal of Applied Research in Natural Products* 3(1):48–58.

Jamroz, D., Wiliczkiewicz, A., Skorupińska, J., Orda, J., Kuryszko, J. and Tschirch, H. 2009. Effect of sweet chestnut tannin (SCT) on the performance, microbial status of intestine and histological characteristics of intestine wall in chickens. *British Poultry Science* 50(6):687–699.

Janceva, S., Dizhbite, T., Telisheva, G., Spulle, U., Klavinsh, L. and Dzenis, M. 2011. Tannins of deciduous trees bark as a potential source for obtaining ecologically safe wood adhesives. In Environment. Technologies. Resources. Proceedings of the International Scientific and Practical Conference, Rēzekne, Latvia (Vol. 1, pp. 265–270).

Joint FAO and World Health Organization. 1995. Report of the twenty-first session of the Joint FAO/WHO, Codex Alimentarius Commission, Rome, 3–8 July 1995.

Jordão, A.M., Ricardo-da-Silva, J.M. and Laureano, O. 2005. Extraction of some ellagic tannins and ellagic acid from oak wood chips (Quercus pyrenaica L.) in model wine solutions. *South African Journal for Enology and Viticulture* 26(2):83.

Joshi, V.K. and Kumar, V. 2017. Influence of different sugar sources, nitrogen sources and inocula on the quality characteristics of apple tea wine. *Journal of the Institute of Brewing* 123(2):268–276.

Kaspchak, E., Mafra, L.I. and Mafra, M.R. 2018. Effect of heating and ionic strength on the interaction of bovine serum albumin and the antinutrients tannic and phytic acids, and its influence on in vitro protein digestibility. *Food Chemistry* 252:1–8.

Kaur, S., Sharma, S. and Nagi, H.P.S. 2011. Functional properties and anti-nutritional factors in cereal bran. *Asian Journal of Food & Agro-industry* 4(2):122–131.

Kaur, S., Sharma, S., Singh, B. and Dar, B.N. 2015. Effect of extrusion variables (temperature, moisture) on the antinutrient components of cereal brans. *Journal of Food Science and Technology* 52(3):1670–1676.

Ketzis, J.K., Vercruysse, J., Stromberg, B.E., Larsen, M., Athanasiadou, S. and Houdijk, J.G. 2006. Evaluation of efficacy expectations for novel and non-chemical helminth control strategies in ruminants. *Veterinary Parasitology* 139(4):321–335.

Khanbabaee, K. and van Ree, T. 2001. Tannins, classification and definition. *Natural Product Reports* 18(6):641–649.

Khasnabis, J., Rai, C., and Roy, A. 2015. Determination of tannin content by titrimetric method from different types of tea. *Journal of Chemical and Pharmaceutical Research* 7(6):238–241.

King, H.G.C. and White, T. 1957. Tannins and polyphenols Schinopsis (Quebracho) spp. Their genesis and interrelationship. *Journal- Society of Leather Technologists and Chemists* 41:368–383.

King, H.G.C. and White, T. 1961. Colouring matter of rhus cotinus wood (young fustic). *Journal of the Chemical Society* 3538–3539

Kirubakaran, A., Moorthy, M., Chitra, R. and Prabakar, G. 2016. Influence of combinations of fenugreek, garlic, and black pepper powder on production traits of the broilers. *Veterinary World* 9(5):470.

Knowles, E. and White, T. 1954. Tannin extracts as raw materials for the adhesives and resin industries. *Adhesives and Resin* 10:226–228.

Koleckar, V., Kubikova, K., Rehakova, Z., Kuca, K., Jun, D., Jahodar, L. and Opletal, L. 2008. Condensed and hydrolysable tannins as antioxidants influencing the health. *Mini Reviews in Medicinal Chemistry* 8(5):436–447.

Krupa, U. 2008. Main nutritional and antinutritional compounds of bean seeds-a review. *Polish Journal of Food and Nutrition Sciences* 58(2):149–155.

Krzyzowska, M., Tomaszewska, E., Ranoszek-Soliwoda, K., Bien, K., Orlowski, P., Celichowski, G. and Grobelny, J. 2017. Tannic acid modification of metal nanoparticles: possibility for new antiviral applications. In *Nanostructures for Oral Medicine* (pp. 335–363). Elsevier, Amsterdam.

Kumar, V. and Joshi, V.K. 2016. Kombucha, technology, microbiology, production, composition and therapeutic value. *International Journal of Food and Fermentation Technology* 6(1):13–24.

Kumar, V., Joshi, V.K., Vyas, G., Thakur, N.S. and Sharma, N. 2016. Process optimization for the preparation of apple tea wine with analysis of its sensory and physico-chemical characteristics and antimicrobial activity against food-borne pathogens. *Nutrafoods* 15:111–121.

Kumar, V., Kaur, J., Panghal, A., Kaur, S. and Handa, V. 2018. Caffeine: a boon or bane. *Nutrition & Food Science* 48(1):61–75.

Kumari, M. and Jain, S. 2012. Tannins, an antinutrient with positive effect to manage diabetes. *Research Journal of Recent Sciences* 1(12):70–73.

Kumari, M. and Jain, S. 2015. Screening of potential sources of tannin and its therapeutic application. *International Journal of Nutrition and Food Sciences* 4(2):26–29.

Kyarisiima, C.C., Okot, M.W. and Svihus, B. 2004. Use of wood ash in the treatment of high tannin sorghum for poultry feeding. *South African Journal of Animal Science* 34(2):110–115.

Lacassagne, L., Francesch, M., Carré, B. and Melcion, J.P. 1988. Utilization of tannin-containing and tannin-free faba beans (Vicia faba) by young chicks: effects of pelleting feeds on energy, protein and starch digestibility. *Animal Feed Science and Technology* 20(1):59–68.

Laddha, A.P. and Kulkarni, Y.A. 2019. Tannins and vascular complications of diabetes: an update. *Phytomedicine* 56:229–245.

Lei, H., Pizzi, A. and Du, G. 2008. Environmentally friendly mixed tannin/lignin wood resins. *Journal of Applied Polymer Science* 107(1):203–209.

Lestienne, I., Buisson, M., Lullien-Pellerin, V., Picq, C. and Trèche, S. 2007. Losses of nutrients and anti-nutritional factors during abrasive decortication of two pearl millet cultivars (*Pennisetum glaucum*). *Food Chemistry* 100 (4):1316–1323.

Letizia, C.S., Cocchiara, J., Wellington, G. A, Funk, C. and Api, A.M. 2000. Valencene. *Food and Chemical Toxicology* 8(S3):s235–s236.

Li, J., Zhu, W., Zhang, S., Gao, Q., Xia, C., Zhang, W. and Li, J. 2019a. Depolymerization and characterization of Acacia mangium tannin for the preparation of mussel-inspired fast-curing tannin-based phenolic resins. *Chemical Engineering Journal* 370:420–431.

Li, P., Sirviö, J.A., Haapala, A., Khakalo, A. and Liimatainen, H. 2019b. Anti-oxidative and UV-absorbing biohybrid film of cellulose nanofibrils and tannin extract. *Food Hydrocolloids* 92:208–217.

Liao, J., Brosse, N., Pizzi, A., Hoppe, S., Zhou, X. and Du, G. 2020. Characterization and 3D printability of poly (lactic acid)/acetylated tannin composites. *Industrial Crops and Products* 149:112320.

Lima, P.R., Apdini, T., Freire, A.S., et al. 2019. Dietary supplementation with tannin and soybean oil on intake, digestibility, feeding behavior, ruminal protozoa and methane emission in sheep. *Animal Feed Science and Technology* 249:10–17.

Lipsa, F.D., Snowdon, R., and Friedt, W. 2012. Quantitative genetic analysis of condensed tannins in oilseed rape meal. *Euphytica* 184(2):195–205.

Lipsitz, P., Kremen, S.S. and Lollar, R.M. 1949. Untersuchung uber vegetabilische Gerbung. VII. Das Gerbungspotential gereinigter Ligninsufonate und wirklicher Gerbstoffe. *The Journal of the American Leather Chemists Association* 44:194.

Liu, J., Wang, L., Li, J., Li, C., Zhang, S., Gao, Q., Zhang, W. and Li, J. 2020. Degradation mechanism of Acacia mangium tannin in NaOH/urea aqueous solution and application of degradation products in phenolic adhesives. *International Journal of Adhesion and Adhesives* 98:102556.

Longstaff, M. and McNab, J.M. 1991. The inhibitory effects of hull polysaccharides and tannins of field beans (Vicia faba L.) on the digestion of amino acids, starch and lipid and on digestive enzyme activities in young chicks. *British Journal of Nutrition* 65(2):199–216.

Lu, L., Liu, S.W., Jiang, S.B. and Wu, S.G. 2004. Tannin inhibits HIV-1 entry by targeting gp41. *Acta Pharmacologica Sinica* 25(2):213–218.

MacAdam, J.W., Brummer, J., Islam, A. and Shewmaker, G. 2013. *The Benefits of TanninContaining Forages.* Utah State University Plants, Soils, and Climate. AG/Forages/2013-03pr.

MacLean, H. and Gardner, J.A.F. 1952. Bark extract in adhesives. *Pulp and Paper Magazine of Canada* 53:111.
Mahdi, H.A.R.O.U.N., Palmina, K., Gurshi, A. and Covington, D. 2009. Potential of vegetable tanning materials and basic aluminum sulphate in Sudanese leather industry. *Journal of Engineering Science and Technology* 4(1):20–31.
Makkar, H.P. and Becker, K. 1993. Vanillin-HCl method for condensed tannins: effect of organic solvents used for extraction of tannins. *Journal of Chemical Ecology* 19(4):613–621.
Mamatha, C. and Prakash, J., 2016. Formulation of iron fortified masala powders and assessment of nutritional and sensory qualities. *The Indian journal of nutrition and dietetics*, 53(3):330–342.
Manach, C., Scalbert, A., Morand, C., Rémésy, C. and Jiménez, L. 2004. Polyphenols: food sources and bioavailability. *The American journal of clinical nutrition* 79(5):727–747.
Mansoori, B., Modirsanei, M., and Kiaei, S.M.M. 2006. Cumin seed meal with enzyme and polyethylene glycol as an alternative to wheat bran in broiler diets. *Journal of the Science of Food and Agriculture* 86 (15):2621–2627.
Mather, M. 1997. Migraines and tannins-any relationship? *Headache* 37(8):529–529.
Medugu, C.I., Saleh, B., Igwebuike, J.U. and Ndirmbita, R.L. 2012. Strategies to improve the utilization of tannin-rich feed materials by poultry. *International Journal of Poultry Science* 11(6):417.
Morton, J.F. 1992. Widespread tannin intake via stimulants and masticatories, especially guarana, kola nut, betel vine, and accessories. In *Plant Polyphenols* (pp. 739–765). Springer, Boston, MA.
Mousavinejad, G., Emam-Djomeh, Z., Rezaei, K. and Khodaparast, M.H.H. 2009. Identification and quantification of phenolic compounds and their effects on antioxidant activity in pomegranate juices of eight Iranian cultivars. *Food Chemistry* 115(4):1274–1278.
Murthy, P.S. and Manonmani, H.K. 2009. Physico-chemical, antioxidant and antimicrobial properties of Indian monsooned coffee. *European Food Research and Technology*, 229(4):645–650.
Muthukumar, G. and Mahadevan, A. 1981. Effect of tannins on soil microorganisms. *Indian Journal of Experimental Biology* 19:1083–1085.
Nardeli, J.V., Fugivara, C.S., Taryba, M., Pinto, E.R., Montemor, M.F. and Benedetti, A.V. 2019. Tannin: a natural corrosion inhibitor for aluminum alloys. *Progress in Organic Coatings* 135:368–381.
Navale, S.A., Swami, S.B. and Thakor, N.J. 2015. Extrusion cooking technology for foods: a review. *Journal of Ready to Eat Food* 2(3):66–80.
Nico, R. 1950. Lab. ensayo materiales e invest, tecnol. Prov. Buenos Aires (La Plata, Rep. Arg.) Ser. II, (38), p.5.
Niho, N., Shibutani, M., Tamura, T., Toyoda, K., Uneyama, C., Takahashi, N. and Hirose, M. 2001. Subchronic toxicity study of gallic acid by oral administration in F344 rats. *Food and Chemical Toxicology* 39(11):1063–1070.
O'Flaherty, F., Roddy, W.T. and Lollar, R.M. 1956. *Chemistry and Technology of Leather.*
Ogura, R., Ikeda, N., Yuki, K., Morita, O., Saigo, K., Blackstock, C., Nishiyama, N. and Kasamatsu, T. 2008. Genotoxicity studies on green tea catechin. *Food and Chemical Toxicology* 46(6):2190–2200.
Okuda, T. and Ito, H. 2011. Tannins of constant structure in medicinal and food plants—hydrolyzable tannins and polyphenols related to tannins. *Molecules* 16(3):2191–2217.
Ong, K.C., Khoo, H.E. and Das, N.P. 1995. Tannic acid inhibits insulin-stimulated lipogenesis in rat adipose tissue and insulin receptor function in vitro. *Experientia* 51(6):577–584.
Pasch, H., Pizzi, A. and Rode, K. 2001. MALDI–TOF mass spectrometry of polyflavonoid tannins. *Polymer* 42(18):7531–7539.
Patel, S., Dutta, S. 2018. Effect of soaking and germination on anti-nutritional factors of garden cress, wheat and finger millet. *International Journal of Pure and Applied Bioscience* 6 (5):1076–1081.
Ping, L., Brosse, N., Chrusciel, L., Navarrete, P. and Pizzi, A. 2011a. Extraction of condensed tannins from grape pomace for use as wood adhesives. *Industrial Crops and Products* 33(1):253–257.
Ping, L., Pizzi, A., Guo, Z.D. and Brosse, N. 2011b. Condensed tannins extraction from grape pomace: characterization and utilization as wood adhesives for wood particleboard. *Industrial Crops and Products* 34(1):907–914.
Ping, L., Pizzi, A., Guo, Z.D. and Brosse, N. 2012. Condensed tannins from grape pomace: characterization by FTIR and MALDI TOF and production of environment friendly wood adhesive. *Industrial Crops and Products* 40:13–20.
Pizzi, A. 1980. Wood adhesives: chemistry and technology, Volume I, Ed. Pizzi A. 1983. Marcel Dekker, New York. Chapter 4. *Journal of Macromolecular Science C* 18(2):247.

Pizzi, A. 1994. *Advanced Wood Adhesives Technology.* CRC Press, Dekker, New York.

Pizzi, A. 2008. Tannins: major sources, properties and applications. In *Monomers, Polymers and Composites from Renewable Resources* (pp. 179–199). Elsevier, Amsterdam.

Plomley, K.F., Gottstein, J.W. and Hillis, W.E. 1957. Australia Commonwealth Sei. Ind. Research Organ. Forest Prod. Newsletter No. 234. Forest Products. Newsletter No. 234.

Pohlan, H.A.J. and Janssens, M.J. 2010. Growth and production of coffee. *Plant Growth and Crop Production* 3:101.

Porter, L.J. 1974. Extractives of Pinus radiata bark. II. Procyanidin constituents (3rd ed.). *New Zealand Journal of Crop and Horticultural Science* 17:213–218.

Price, M.L. and Butler, L.G. 1980. Tannins and nutrition. Agric Expt Stn Bull 272, Purdue University, W. Lafayette, Indiana.

Prigione, V., Spina, F., Tigini, V., Giovando, S. and Varese, G.C. 2018. Biotransformation of industrial tannins by filamentous fungi. *Applied Microbiology and Biotechnology* 102(24):10361–10375.

Puech, J.L., Feuillat, F. and Mosedale, J.R. 1999. The tannins of oak heartwood: structure, properties, and their influence on wine flavor. *American Journal of Enology and Viticulture* 50(4):469–478.

Rajalakshmi, K., Devaraj, H. and Niranjali Devaraj, S. 2001. Assessment of the no-observedadverse-effect level (NOAEL) of gallic acid in mice. *Food Chemistry Toxicology* 39:919–922.

Ramakrishnan, K. and Krishnan, M.R.V. 1994. Tannin–classification, analysis and applications. *Ancient science of life* 13(3–4):232.

Rao, B.S. and Prabhavathi, T. 1982. Tannin content of foods commonly consumed in India and its influence on ionisable iron. *Journal of the Science of Food and Agriculture* 33(1):89–96.

Rathod, R.P. and Annapure, U.S. 2016. Effect of extrusion process on antinutritional factors and protein and starch digestibility of lentil splits. *LWT-Food Science and Technology* 66:114–123.

Reed, J.D. 1995. Nutritional toxicology of tannins and related polyphenols in forage legumes. *Journal of Animal Science* 73(5):1516–1528.

Ricardo-da-Silva, J.M., Cheynier, V., Souquet, J.M., Moutounet, M., Cabanis, J.C. and Bourzeix, M. 1991. Interaction of grape seed procyanidins with various proteins in relation to wine fining. *Journal of the Science of Food and Agriculture* 57(1):111–125.

Roux, D.G. 1965. *Modern Applications of Mimosa Extract* (pp. 34–41). Leather Industries Research Institute, Grahamstown, South Africa.

Roux, D.G. 1992. Reflections on the chemistry and affinities of the major commercial condensed tannins in the context of their industrial use. In *Plant Polyphenols* (pp. 7–39). Springer, Boston, MA.

Roux, D.G. and Paulus, E. 1961. Condensed tannins. 8. The isolation and distribution of interrelated heartwood components of Schinopsis spp. *Biochemical Journal* 78(4):785–789.

Roux, D.G., Ferreira, D., Hundt, H.K. and Malan, E. 1975. Structure, stereochemistry, and reactivity of natural condensed tannins as basis for their extended industrial application. *Applied Polymer Symposia* 28:335–353.

Samanta, S., Giri, S., Parua, S., Nandi, D.K., Pati, B.R. and Mondal, K.C. 2004. Impact of tannic acid on the gastrointestinal microflora. *Microbial Ecology in Health and Disease* 16(1):32–34.

Scalbert, A. 1992. Quantitative methods for the estimation of tannins in plant tissues. In *Plant Polyphenols* (pp. 259–280). Springer, Boston, MA.

Schofield, P., Mbugua, D.M. and Pell, A.N. 2001. Analysis of condensed tannins: a review. *Animal Feed Science and Technology* 91(1–2):21–40.

Schons, P.F., Battestin, V. and Macedo, G.A. 2012. Fermentation and enzyme treatments for sorghum. *Brazilian Journal of Microbiology* 43(1):89–97.

Sekiya, J., Kajiwara, T., Monma, T. and Hatanaka, A. 1984. Interaction of tea catechins with proteins: formation of protein precipitate. *Agricultural and Biological Chemistry* 48(8):1963–1967.

Shah, A.M., Rahim, A.A., Yahya, S., Raja, P.B. and Hamid, S.A. 2011. Acid corrosion inhibition of copper by mangrove tannin. *Pigment & Resin Technology* 40(2): 118–122

Shang, Y.F., Cao, H., Ma, Y.L., et al. 2019. Effect of lactic acid bacteria fermentation on tannins removal in Xuan Mugua fruits. *Food Chemistry* 274:118–122.

Sharma, K., Kumar, V., Kaur, J., et al. 2019. Health effects, sources, utilization and safety of tannins: a critical review. *Toxin Reviews.* DOI: 10.1080/15569543.2019.1662813

Sieniawska, E. and Baj, T. 2017. Chapter 10-Tannins. In *Pharmacognosy*, Elsevier, pp.199–232.

Singh, A., Gupta, S., Kaur, R. and Gupta, H.R. 2017. Process optimization for anti-nutrient minimization of millets. *Asian Journal of Dairy & Food Research* 36(4):1–5.

Singh, B., Bhat, T.K., and Sharma, O.P. 2001. Biodegradation of tannic acid in an in vitro ruminal system. *Livestock Production Science* 68 (2–3):259–262.

Smeriglio, A., Barreca, D., Bellocco, E. and Trombetta, D. 2017. Proanthocyanidins and hydrolysable tannins: occurrence, dietary intake and pharmacological effects. *British Journal of Pharmacology* 174(11):1244–1262.

Spina, S., Zhou, X., Segovia, C., Pizzi, A., Romagnoli, M., Giovando, S., Pasch, H., Rode, K. and Delmotte, L. 2013. Phenolic resin adhesives based on chestnut (Castanea sativa) hydrolysable tannins. *Journal of Adhesion Science and Technology* 27(18–19):2103–2111.

Sravan, K.R.T., Nagaraj, M.K., Ramakrishna, C., Vaikunta, R., Pranesha, S., Rathanakar, R.K. and MallikarjunaRao, D. 2016. Subacute toxicity of Gallic acid, isolated form Terminalia chebulain Swiss Albino Mice. *International Journal of Chemistry and Pharmaceutical Sciences* 4(10):439–443.

Sriwichai, W., Berger, J., Picq, C. and Avallone, S. 2016. Determining factors of lipophilic micronutrient bioaccessibility in several leafy vegetables. *Journal of Agricultural and Food Chemistry* 64(8): 1695–1701.

Subcommittee on Review of the GRAS List (Phase II). 1972. A Comprehensive Survey of industry on the Use of Food Chemicals Generally Recognized as Safe (GRAS). Committee on Food Protection, Division of Biology and Agriculture, National Research Council. National Academy of Sciences, Washington, DC for Department of Health, Education and Welfare (DHEW contract no. FDA 70-22)

Sun, B., Ricardo-da-Silva, J.M. and Spranger, I. 1998. Critical factors of vanillin assay for catechins and proanthocyanidins. *Journal of Agricultural and Food Chemistry* 46(10):4267–4274.

Sur, T.K., Chatterjee, S., Hazra, A.K., Pradhan, R. and Chowdhury, S. 2015. Acute and sub-chronic oral toxicity study of black tea in rodents. *Indian Journal of Pharmacology* 47(2):167.

Takahashi, T., Yokoo, Y., Inoue, T. and Ishii, A. 1999. Toxicological studies on procyanidin B-2 for external application as a hair growing agent. *Food and Chemical Toxicology* 37(5):545–552.

Takami, S., Imai, T., Hasumura, M., Cho, Y.M., Onose, J. and Hirose, M. 2008. Evaluation of toxicity of green tea catechins with 90-day dietary administration to F344 rats. *Food and Chemical Toxicology* 46(6):2224–2229.

Tang, H.R., Hancock, R.A. and Covington, A.D. 1991. Studies on commercial tannin extracts. In Proceedings of the XXI IULTCS (International Union of Leather Trades Chemists), *Proceedings*, Barcelona, Spain, (pp. 1503–1527d).

Tapiwa, K.A. 2019. Polyphenols in sorghum, their effects on broilers and methods of reducing their effects: a review. *Biomedical Journal of Scientific & Technical Research* 19:14058–14061.

Tascioglu, C., Yalcin, M., de Troya, T. and Sivrikaya, H. 2012. Termiticidal properties of some wood and bark extracts used as wood preservatives. *BioResources* 7(3):2960–2969.

Tascioglu, C., Yalcin, M., Sen, S. and Akcay, C. 2013. Antifungal properties of some plant extracts used as wood preservatives. *International Biodeterioration & Biodegradation* 85:23–28.

Thévenon, M.F., Tondi, G. and Pizzi, A. 2010. Friendly wood preservative system based on polymerized tannin resin-boric acid for outdoor applications. *Maderas. Ciencia y tecnología* 12(3):253–257.

Tomak, E.D. and Gonultas, O. 2018. The wood preservative potentials of valonia, chestnut, tara and sulphited oak tannins. *Journal of Wood Chemistry and Technology* 38(3):183–197.

Tondi, G., Wieland, S., Wimmer, T., Thévenon, M.F., Pizzi, A. and Petutschnigg, A. 2012. Tannin-boron preservatives for wood buildings: mechanical and fire properties. *European Journal of Wood and Wood Products* 70(5):689–696.

Towo, E., Matuschek, E. and Svanberg, U. 2006. Fermentation and enzyme treatment of tannin sorghum gruels: effects on phenolic compounds, phytate and in vitro accessible iron. *Food Chemistry* 94(3): 369–376.

Tur, E. and Brenner, S. 1998. Diet and pemphigus. In pursuit of exogenous factors in pemphigus and fogo selvagem. *Archives of Dermatology* 134(11):1406–1410.

TV, A.K., Mani, I., Pramod, A. et al. 2018. Effect of extrusion technique on antinutritional factors of sorghum-soya blends. *Indian Journal of Agricultural Sciences* 88(3):81–89.

Vázquez, G., Pizzi, A., Freire, M.S., Santos, J., Antorrena, G. and González-Álvarez, J. 2013. MALDI-TOF, HPLC-ESI-TOF and 13C-NMR characterization of chestnut (Castanea sativa) shell tannins for wood adhesives. *Wood Science and Technology* 47(3):523–535.

Vázquez, G., Santos, J., Freire, M.S., Antorrena, G. and González-Álvarez, J. 2012. DSC and DMA study of chestnut shell tannins for their application as wood adhesives without formaldehyde emission. *Journal of Thermal Analysis and Calorimetry* 108(2):605–611.

Venkatachalam, M., and Sathe, S.K. 2006. Chemical composition of selected edible nut seeds. *Journal of agricultural and food chemistry*, 54(13):4705–4714.

Viriot, C., Scalbert, A., Lapierre, C. and Moutounet, M. 1993. Ellagitannins and lignins in aging of spirits in oak barrels. *Journal of Agricultural and Food Chemistry* 41(11):1872–1879.

Vitti, D.M.S.S., Nozella, E.F., Abdalla, A.L., et al. 2005. The effect of drying and urea treatment on nutritional and anti-nutritional components of browses collected during wet and dry seasons. *Animal Feed Science and Technology* 122(1–2):123–133.

Vivas, N. and Glories, Y. 1996. Role of oak wood ellagitannins in the oxidation process of red wines during aging. *American Journal of Enology and Viticulture* 47(1):103–107.

Vivas, N., Glories, Y., Bourgeois, G. and Vitry, C. 1996. The heartwood ellagitannins of different oaks (*Quercus Sp.)* and chestnut species (*Castanea Sativa* Mill.). Quantity analysis of red wines aging in barrels. *Journal des Sciences et Techniques de la Tonnelerie* 2: 51–75.

Wang, G., Chen, Y., Xu, G. and Pei, Y. 2019. Effective removing of methylene blue from aqueous solution by tannins immobilized on cellulose microfibers. *International Journal of Biological Macromolecules* 129:198–206.

Willson, K.C. and Clifford, M.N. 2012. *Tea, cultivation to consumption.* Springer Science and Business Media, Amsterdam.

Yalcin, M. and Ceylan, H. 2017. The effects of tannins on adhesion strength and surface roughness of varnished wood after accelerated weathering. *Journal of Coatings Technology and Research* 14(1):185–193.

Yamakoshi, J., Saito, M., Kataoka, S. and Kikuchi, M. 2002. Safety evaluation of proanthocyanidin-rich extract from grape seeds. *Food and Chemical Toxicology* 40(5):599–607.

Yang, T., Dong, M., Cui, J., Gan, L. and Han, S. 2020. Exploring the formaldehyde reactivity of tannins with different molecular weight distributions: bayberry tannins and larch tannins. *Holzforschung* 74(7):673–682.

Yilmaz, Y. and Toledo, R.T., 2004. Major flavonoids in grape seeds and skins, antioxidant capacity of catechin, epicatechin, and gallic acid. *Journal of Agricultural and Food Chemistry*, 52(2):255–260.

Yugarani, T., Tan, B.K.H. and Das, N.P. 1993. The effects of tannic acid on serum lipid parameters and tissue lipid peroxides in the spontaneously hypertensive and Wistar Kyoto rats. *Planta Medica* 59(01):28–31.

Zhang, L.L. and Lin, Y.M. 2008. HPLC, NMR and MALDI-TOF MS analysis of condensed tannins from Lithocarpus glaber leaves with potent free radical scavenging activity. *Molecules* 13(12):2986–2997.

CHAPTER 4

# Solanine and Chaconine

**Sangeeta, Jaspreet Kaur, and Payal Rani**

## CONTENTS



DOI: 10.1201/9781003178446-4

## 4.1 INTRODUCTION

Solanine and chaconine are the major secondary metabolites of plants known as glycoalkaloids (Benkeblia, 2020; Omayio, Abong, and Okoth, 2016; Percival and Dixon, 1997). These glycoalkaloids occur naturally in plants and are toxic in nature. The main sources of these toxicants are the plants from family Solanaceae/nightshade including potatoes, tomatoes, eggplants, and the infamous deadly belladonna or nightshade. These glycoalkaloids are synthesized naturally in the tubers, leaves, roots, flowers, and other parts of the plant in varying amounts depending on the metabolic rate of that part (the higher the metabolic rate, the higher the glycoalkaloids level) (Omayio, Abong, and Okoth, 2016). Sprouts, in case of potato tuber, contain a high amount of glycoalkaloids (Friedman and Dao, 1992). Among all other sources, solanine and chaconine, present mainly in potato, and α-solanine and α-chaconineare, the prime glycoalkaloids of potato, comprise about 95% of total glycoalkaloids present (TGA) (Dale, Griffiths, and Bain, 1998; Sotelo and Serrano, 2000). As compared to other parts of the plant, dispersal of glycoalkaloids in potato tuber is less and not symmetrical as the periderm and cortex have a higher glycoalkaloid content which decreases markedly towards the pith (Dale, Griffiths, and Bain, 1998). The amount of glycoalkaloids in normal potato tubers varies from 12–20 mg/kg while the level increases to a great extent in green skin (1,500–2,200 mg/kg) and green tubers (250–280 mg/kg) (Omayio, Abong, and Okoth, 2016).

The function of glycoalkaloids in plants is their chemical defence mechanism as repellents or non-specific protectors against predators and potential pests (Omayio, Abong, and Okoth, 2016; Roddick, 1989). This is the reason that the plants having these components are unappealing and deadly to animals which might attempt to eat them. The important factor which protects the plants from fungi, insects, and predators is the presence of glycoalkaloid content in foliage. In spite of their defence mechanism in plants, solanine and chaconine are associated with food poisoning because of their toxicity. Solanine and chaconine are natural, bitter-tasting steroidal toxicants found in plants of Solanaceae family (Smith, Roddick, and Jones, 1996). So, these are considered as plant toxins and are mainly present in different parts of the potato plant and tuber. Millions of people consume potatoes (Solanaceae family) every day in a high amount. The main forms of these glycoalkaloids are α-solanine and α-chaconine alkaloids, which have a similar aglycone solanidine compound and different carbohydrates (sugars) in the side chain. The compound α-solanine has a glycosidic chain as the side chain comprising glucose, galactose, and rhamnose, whereas glucose and two rhamnose molecules are present in that of α-chaconine (Friedman and McDonald, 1999). The variation in cytotoxic effects of α-solanine and α-chaconine has been considered to be due to this slight compositional difference of the glycosidic chain, i.e., sugars of the triose (Friedman, 2006). The accumulation of solanine and chaconine is higher in damaged, greened, and stored potatoes, but the accumulation level is very low in the majority of current commercial varieties. These glycoalkaloids, if consumed in a higher concentration, may cause acute poisoning, including neurological and gastro-intestinal disturbances in man. The upper non-toxic limit of glycoalkaloids, which is recognized as safe was reported and the normal level in potatoes was reported to be 20–100 mg/kg, which is not of toxicological concern as per the WHO (Badowski and Urbanek-Karłowska, 1999). In this chapter, different aspects of solanine and chaconine, such as their chemistry, distribution, toxicology, effect of processing, and their mechanism of action, etc., are discussed.

## 4.2 CHEMISTRY

Solanine and chaconine are the vital glycoalkaloids of potato tubers and their alpha form is about 95% of total glycoalkaloids present in it (Friedman, McDonald, and Filadelfi-Keszi, 1997; Smith, Roddick, and Jones, 1996; Kuiper-Goodman and Nawrot, 1993). Solanine and chaconine as shown in Figure 4.1 are nitrogen-containing steroidal alkaloids, bearing the same alkaloid solanidine

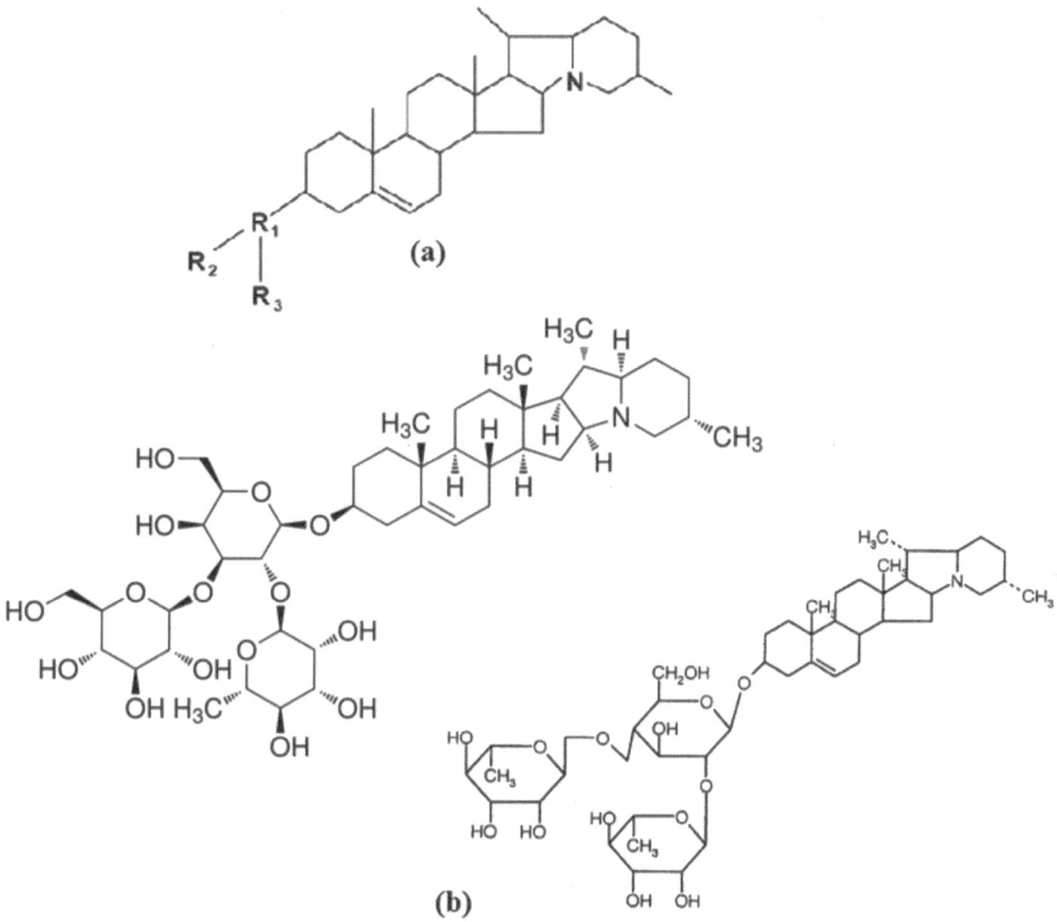


**Figure 4.1** (A) The basic structure of glycoalkaloids (α-solanine and α-chaconine): same aglycone solanidine; side chain having different trisaccharides (R1; R2; R3) in α-solanine and α-chaconine (R1 = β-D-galactose, R2 = β-D-glucose, R3 = α-L-rhamnose for α-solanine and R1 = β-D-glucose, R2 = R3 = α-L– rhamnose for α-chaconine). (B): Structure of solanine and chaconine. (Source: Modified from Uluwaduge 2018; Sucha and Tomsik 2016.)

(aglycone), but the trisaccharide side chain differs slightly in them (Ostry, Ruprich, and Skarkova, 2010; Widmann et al., 2008). The side chain sugars in α-solanine are galactose, glucose, and rhamnose, and the trisaccharide present in α-chaconine is a glucose molecule and two rhamnose residues (Uluwaduge, 2018; Widmann et al., 2008). A minor percentage of glycoalkaloids (5%) present are β-chaconine, γ-chaconine, β-solanine, and γ-solanine (Uluwaduge, 2018; Widmann et al., 2008).

Solanine alkaloids were first isolated in 1820 (Friedman, McDonald, and Filadelfi-Keszi, 1997), and later in 1861, the presence of a side chain of glycoside was reported (Zwenger and Kind, 1861). In 1954, it was observed that glycoalkaloid solanine was a mixture of α-solanine and α-chaconine, two prime glycoalkaloids (GAs) bearing the same compound, solanidine (non-sugar). Since then more than 90 different glycoalkaloids have been reported to be isolated and elucidated on the basis of a structure from different species of the Solanaceae family (Al-Sinani and Eltayeb, 2017). Diversification in glycoalkaloids is mainly due to the compositional difference in side chain (glycosides in nature). The carbohydrate present in glycoalkaloids is either a tri-saccharide (chacotriose or solatriose) or a tetra-saccharide (lycotetraose) (Friedman, McDonald, and Filadelfi-Keszi, 1997).

**Table 4.1 Different Glycoalkaloids Present in *S. Tuberosum* (Aglycone Solanidine and Sugar Moeity)**

| Glycoalkaloids (S. tuberosum) | Aglycone (non-sugar) | Sugars (glycoside side chain) |
|---|---|---|
| α-solanine | Solanidine | galactose + glucose + rhamnose |
| β-solanine | Solanidine | galactose + (glucose or rhamnose) |
| γ-solanine | Solanidine | galactose |
| α-chaconine | Solanidine | glucose + rhamnose + rhamnose |
| β-chaconine | Solanidine | glucose + rhamnose |
| γ-chaconine | Solanidine | glucose |

(*Source:* Modified from Lachman et al., 2001; Sinden, Sanford and Osman 1980)

In commercial potato cultivars (Solanum tuberosum), the main glycoalkaloids present are α-solanine and α-chaconine, having the similar non-sugar compound solanidine and the different side chain carbohydrates solatriose and chacotriose, respectively, which are presented in Table 4.1. The intact glycoside is referred to by the prefix alpha (α-), whereas beta (β-), gamma (γ-), and delta (δ-) are the corresponding glycoalkaloids with progressively different carbohydrates (truncated) in their side chains (glycosidic) composed due to acidic or enzymatic hydrolysis (Milner et al., 2011; Friedman, 2006). The difference in sugars (type and number) present in the side chain of the non-sugar component (solinidine) influence the biological activity of these compounds (Rayburn, Bantle, and Friedman, 1994). It has been reported that the sugar units, if removed stepwise from the side chain (chacotriose and solatriose) result in a general decrease of embryo toxicity (Benkeblia, 2020).

## 4.3 DISTRIBUTION

These compounds are distributed throughout the plant (mainly found in potato) and the concentrations vary significantly depending on the anatomical part or the genetic variety (Benkeblia, 2020; Uluwaduge, 2018; Nahar, 2011; Smith, Roddick, and Jones, 1996). The profile of glycoalkaloids in each part of the tuber was not revealed by most of the past records and only the total glycoalkaloid content was reported by many studies (Uluwaduge, 2018; Smith, Roddick, and Jones, 1996; Gelder, 1990). However, the content of α-chaconine is reported to be slightly higher than α-solanine in potato (Goodman and Nowrot, 1993). A broad range for total glycoalkaloids for a given part of the plant was reported by many studies owing to considerable variation of the compound among potato plants (Smith, Roddick, and Jones, 1996; Goodman and Nowrot, 1993). Synthesis of these glycoalkaloids has been reported in each part of the plant and higher concentrations are reported in parts with high metabolic rates (Peksa et al., 2002). Flowers (215–500 mg/100 g), sprouts (200–730 mg/100 g), and young leaves (23–100 mg/100 g) are comparatively rich in these glycoalkaloids (Gelder, 1990; Uluwaduge, 2018). Normally, the potato tubers contain glycoalkaloids in the range of 1–15 mg/100 g of potato tubers (fresh weight basis) (see Table 4.2). Most of the edible tubers contain a low amount of glycoalkaloids (less than 10 mg/100 g fresh weight) (Uluwaduge, 2018). Whereas in potato peels, higher levels of glycoalkaloids are usually observed but of less concern as the peel comprises only < 20% weight of the total tuber weight and is removed during processing in most of the cases (Sinden, Sanford, and Webb, 1984). The highest levels are confined to the skin and the peel, while lower amounts have been observed towards the pith (Goodman and Nowrot, 1993; Omayio, Abong, and Okoth, 2016). The pith had undetectable levels of glycoalkaloids, indicating that the tubers are safe to consume, though there had been few reported occasions with banned levels of glycoalkaloids in tubers (Nahar, 2011; Hellenas et al., 1995). These compounds are mainly concentrated in the "eye" regions of the tuber and consumption of potatoes rich in those parts may cause potential health risks (Goodman and Nowrat, 1993). Small tubers are reported to be rich in glycoalkaloids on

**Table 4.2 Distribution of Total Glycoalkaloid Content in Various Tissues of Potato Tuber and Potato Plant Parts**

| Part (tuber) | Total glycoalkaloid content (mg/100 g fresh weight) |
|---|---|
| Whole tuber | 1–15 |
| Skin of tuber (2–3% of tuber) | 15–107 |
| Peel of tuber (10–12% of tuber) | 30–64 |
| Flesh | 1.2–10 |
| Bitter-tasting tuber | 25–80 |
| Peel from bitter tuber | 150–220 |
| **Part (Plant)** | **Total glycoalkaloid content (mg/100 g fresh weight)** |
| Sprouts | 200–730 mg/100 g |
| Flowers | 215–500 mg/100 g |
| Young leaves | 23–100 mg/100 g |

(*Source:* Modified from Uluwaduge 2018; Omayio, Abong, and Okoth 2016; Gelder, 1990)

a weight for weight basis than larger ones (Smith, Roddick, and Jones, 1996). Green potatoes often show bitterness, and this off flavour is due to the accumulation of excess amounts of glycoalkaloids in the peel.

The glycoalkaloid levels in modern cultivars are much lower than in wild progenitors and this information is useful for commercial potato breeders (Smith, Roddick, and Jones, 1996). These compounds are not transported between various parts of the plant and therefore the amount present in each part is propionate to synthesis (Nahar, 2011). Genetic engineering approaches could be useful for the manipulation of the level of glycoalkaloids according to commercial needs, such as to reduce their levels in tubers to enhance the edibility and safety and to increase the content in leaves to ensure protection from diseases and predators (Ginzberg, Tokuhisa, and Veilleux, 2009).

Both genetic and environmental factors have been shown to affect the levels of glycoalkaloid in potato tubers. Environmental factors (external factors) during the pre-harvest period (composition of soil and climate), and post-harvest time (light, temperature, humidity, mechanical injury, sprouting, and storage time, etc.) may increase the glycoalkaloid content (Friedman, McDonald, and Filadelfi-Keszi, 1997). Exposure to light may stimulate chlorophyll synthesis leading to "greening" and those tubers are reported to be rich in glycoalkaloids (Percival, Dixon, and Sword, 1996). Extreme temperatures and dry or wet growing seasons may influence the synthesis of glycoalkaloids during the growth of the plant (Nahar, 2011; Percival and Dixon 1993). Water-logging and drought stress are other environmental factors which could enhance the production of glycoalkaloids in significant amounts in some cultivars (Bejarano et al., 2000; Papathanasiou, Mitchell, and Harvey, 1998). It has been reported that a double nitrogen rate during cultivation increased glycoalkaloid content by 10% in some varieties (Tajner-Czopek, Jarych-Szyszka, and Lisinska, 2008). A perusal of the literature indicates that early harvested tubers may show cultivar-specific impacts on glycoalkaloid accumulation than late harvested tubers (Peksa et al., 2002; Hellenas et al., 1995). The potato breeds grown in biodynamic conditions (use of natural environment) were rich in glycoalkaloids and solanidine compared to the breeds grown in classic conditions (use of fertilizers and other chemicals) (Widmann et al., 2008). Hence the need for natural phytorepellents such as glycoalkaloids is not as great in artificial conditions. Home Guard potato tubers had a higher glycoalkaloid content and showed a little increase in response to adverse environmental conditions (Papathanasiou, Mitchell, and Harvey, 1998).

Tubers subjected to post-harvest stress factors such as physical damage (cutting and bruising during harvest or transit), microbial or herbivore attack, improper handling, and inadequate storage conditions are known factors which may influence the content of these compounds in potato tubers (Dale, Griffiths, and Bain1998). Tubers which are exposed to the mentioned factors if used for skin-on or peel-based products have higher glycoalkaloid levels and therefore cause potential health risks. However, safe handling and monitoring of other storage conditions such as temperature and light are important to improve the quality of potatoes in commercial varieties (Uluwaduge, 2018).

Ability to produce glycoalkaloids is inherited to potato cultivars (Valkonen et al., 1996; Kozukue and Mizuno, 1990). This information regarding distribution of glycoalkaloids is useful for commercial production of edible cultivars of potato with low level through different breeding and biotechnological methods. However, genotypes with elevated glycoalkaloid content may be developed by various breeders for pharmaceutical purposes (Valkonen et al., 1996). It is recommended to grow potatoes with inherently low glycoalkaloid and to protect them from other inducers of glycoalkaloid synthesis to enhance the quality of the commercial potato destined for consumption. Development for new varieties via breeding to obtain characteristics such as resistance to disease and ability to withstand cold and other changes in agricultural practices should be accompanied by careful control of the glycoalkaloid levels (Uluwaduge, 2018; Nahar, 2011).

## 4.4 MECHANISM OF ACTION

Glycoalkaloids (GA) solanine and chaconine are compounds that are toxic in nature and biosynthesized naturally for the protection of the plants. In spite of the toxic properties of these compounds, many beneficial health properties have also been reported. These compounds are studied for various therapeutic and biological properties, such as anticancer, antifungal, antimicrobial, and insecticidal activity, etc. (Nielsen et al., 2020). However, the mechanism behind the action of these compounds related to these properties does not seem to be clear, but, as per available literature, different properties of these alkaloids and their mechanism of action are discussed in this section.

### 4.4.1 Toxicity of Glycoalkaloids (GA) (Solanine and Chaconine):

The toxic glycoalkaloids (solanine and chaconine) exhibit a natural defence mechanism within the plant and its parts (mainly present in potatoes) towards harmful/infectious agents, insects, and predators. Upon consumption of food with a high amount of these toxins (exceeding the safe limit) may result in GA toxicity having different adverse symptoms (Uluwaduge, 2018; Nielsen et al., 2020). General symptoms in humans because of glycoalkaloid poisoning are nausea, diarrhoea, vomiting, abdominal cramps, rapid and weak pulse, headache, fever, rapid breathing, and hallucination, etc. (Nahar, 2011). Even comas and deaths have resulted in serious cases (Nahar, 2011; Smith, Roddick, and Jones, 1996). There are two main biological mechanisms behind the glycoalkaloids poisoning. The major mechanism behind GA toxicity is the inhibitory action of glycoalkaloids on the enzymes acetylcholine esterase and butyrylcholin esterase. Both of these enzymes are involved in the hydrolysis of acetylcholine (the neurotransmitter) at the cholinergic synapses (McGehee et al., 2000; Nigg et al., 1996). Glycoalkaloids thus exhibit anti-acetylcholine esterase activity, which is manifested by various neurological symptoms such as weakness, confusion, and depression, etc. (McGehee et al., 2000).

Additionally, the disruption of the membrane has also been observed due to the interference of GA with the ion-transport mechanism in cell membranes (Friedman, 2006). The mechanism behind this is their ability to bind with the membrane sterols, which cause the membrane architecture's disruption, leading to the leakage of cellular contents. This in turn raises gastrointestinal disturbances, having various symptoms like abdominal cramps, vomiting, and diarrhoea (Friedman et al., 1997). Intoxication due to solanine (up to 2–5 mg/kg level) accelerates various gastrointestinal related problems such as abdominal pain, diarrhoea, vomiting, and neurological disturbance like headaches and hallucinations, etc. (Uluwaduge, 2018; Nielsen et al., 2020). Potato tubers exhibit a bitter taste if their glycoalkaloids levels exceed the limit of 14 mg/100 g, whereas a burning sensation in the throat and mouth was observed when the levels exceed 22 mg/100 g. Due to this toxicity, maximum safety level of glycoalkaloids in various raw and processed products have been decided by the European Commission and other leading authorities. Glycoalkaloid content of commercial varieties tends to be less than that of the accepted safety limit (20 mg/10 0g fresh weight) (Smith, Roddick, and Jones, 1996). The total GA content of potato protein powder used for various food applications must not exceed the limit of 150 μg/g, as prescribed by the European Commission (Nielsen et al., 2020).

However, differential diagnosis of glycoalkaloid poisoning is complicated because the symptoms of acute intoxication and other gastrointestinal disorders share common features (Benkeblia, 2020; Smith, Roddick, and Jones, 1996).

### 4.4.2 Anticancer Activity

α-solanine and α-chaconine from Solanum spp. are used traditionally for curing metastasis, as well as many other disorders. The ability of these compounds to disrupt cellular structure may be the possible reason for treating cancer cells, as examined by some researchers. Extracts containing these compounds have been used for centuries to treat cancer as they possess cytotoxic activity, as observed in many studies. These compounds possess an inhibiting action against proliferation and promoting effect for apoptosis on multiple cells of cancer, e.g., cancer cells of melanoma, clone, and liver, etc. (Lv et al., 2014). The whole range of molecular mechanism for apoptosis inducing the effect of glycoalkaloid α-solanine and α-chaconine is known. The release of Ca2 + from mitochondria caused by α-solanine increases the cytoplasmatic Ca2+concentration in HepG2 cells, and lowered the membrane potential of mitochondria which in turn promotes apoptosis (Gao, Wang, and Ji, 2006). The induction of apoptosis by these glycoalkaloids has been proved in HepG2 cells, and it is demonstrated that different doses of α-solanine show sub-G0 apoptosis peak and also a dose-dependent decrease in antiapoptotic protein Bcl-2 with α-solanine and α-chaconine (Ji et al., 2008). Within the mitochondrial pathway of apoptosis, cytochrome c is released if treated with an adequate dose of α-solanine as it stimulates p53 and Bax (proapoptotic protein) but suppresses Bcl-2 and helps in induction of apoptosis (Sun, Lv, and Yang et al., 2014; Mohsenikia, Alizadeh, and Khodayari et al., 2013).

Another mechanism for the effect of these compounds in cells of cancer is due to the inhibition action against cell migration and invasion. This may be caused due to inhibiting the phosphorylation process of PI3-K/Akt/JNK, and, thus, the hindrance of Matrix metalloproteinase-2 and −9 (MMP-2 and −9 expressions). Additionally, the cells treated with α-solanine demonstrate a down regulation of NF-κB (nuclear content) (Lu et al., 2010). This action of these glycoalkaloids accelerates the inhibition of metastasis cancer (Sun, Lv, and Yang et al., 2014). The glycoalkaloid α-chaconine as compared to α-solanine caused the more potential enhancement of apoptosis in the cell line of human colorectal adenocarcinoma (HT-29 cells). It persuades the activation of caspase-3 activity (apoptosis) without any change in the expression of protein Bax and Bcl-2 (apoptotic activator). The level of phosphorylated ERK has been decreased further by α-chaconine without any change in the expression of ERK, which leads to cell death (Yang et al., 2006; Lu et al., 2010).

The combination of gallic acid and chaconine has been reported to be potent in reducing the multiplication of cancer cell lines of prostate (LNCaP and PC-3). This amalgamation activates caspase-dependent apoptosis (in LNCaP cells). This apoptotic effect may be due to the activation of JNK produced by the combined effect of gallic acid and chaconine (Reddivari et al., 2010). Further, it has been reported that the type, number, and presence of sugars in the side chain of glycoalkaloids can affect their cytotoxicity. The glycoalkaloid γ-chaconine (hydrolysis product of α-chaconine glycoalkaloid) showed lower cytotoxicity against the cell of colon in comparison to their higher activity against the cells of liver. The cytotoxicity of glycoalkaloid γ-chaconine against the cells of liver has been reported to be greater than that of β1 and β2-chaconine and almost similar to that of α-chaconine. The inhibitory action of α-solanine (100 μg/mL level) was reported to be similar for both cell types (liver and colon) and the inhibitory action was lower than that of α-chaconine at reduced concentration. This difference in cytotoxic activity might be due to the difference in sugars of side chain in different glycoalkaloids (Lee et al., 2004)

### 4.4.3 Antifungal, Antimicrobial, and Insecticidal Activity

The antimicrobial, insecticidal, and fungicidal properties of these glycoalkaloids have been reported in literature. The protective activity of these compounds against several herbivores, insects, and pests may be due to these properties. The glycoalkaloids (Chaconine and Solanine), and their extracts exhibit toxic effect against the pests and insects of stored products (e.g., flour and seed), leaf-eating insects, mosquitoes, termites and cockroaches, and predatory species, etc. (Chowanski, Adamski, and Marciniak et al., 2016). It has been reported in some studies that α-solanine exhibits much higher toxicity than α-chaconine, whereas some studies reported contradictory results (Friedman, Huang, and Quiambao et al., 2018). This may be due to the difference in nature and/or number/type of the sugars in the side chain of the molecules which affects the activity of these compounds as reported in literature. Synergetic effect of two major glycoalkaloids is reported to be significantly greater as membrane-disruptive property as compared to their effect alone (Friedman, Huang, and Quiambao et al., 2018).

### 4.4.4 Other Biological Activities

Glycoalkaloids possess some other biological activities like antibiotic, antipyretic, antiallergenic, anti-inflammatory, and antihyperglycaemic etc., which are dose- and condition-dependent, reported in literature. The potato extract in solvent ethanol has been studied for the analgesic (pain-relieving) and anti-inflammatory attributes of these compounds and the antinociceptive effect of these compounds were observed (Choi and Koo 2005). This might be due to reduction in influx of Ca2 + at axon terminal of afferent nerve and in turn a reduction in adenylyl cyclase activity has been induced. This further resulted in the decrease of levels cyclic AMP and efflux of K + ions. Nerve hyperpolarisation as influenced due to the latter finally shows a clear cut antinociceptive effect (Yaksh, 1999). The glycoalkaloids α-chaconine and solanidine (sublethal concentrations) exhibit a significant reduction (22% reduction by α-chaconine and 35% reduction by solanidine) in both interleukin-2 and −8 cytokines (proinflammatory cytokines) production as reported in literature (Kenny, McCarthy, and Brunton et al., 2013). The potential therapeutic effect of α-solanine for treatment of inflammatory diseases has also been reported (Shin et al., 2016). This anti-inflammatory effect may be due to regulation of inflammatory cytokines in LPS-induced systemic inflammation mouse model and in RAW 264.7 macrophages (Shin et al., 2016).

## 4.5 TOXICOLOGY

Solanine and chaconin are toxic glycoalkaloids and accumulated mainly in different parts of the potato plant, sprouts, and tuber under certain conditions. It is a well-known fact for many years that, if these compounds exceed the safety limit level, they may cause poisoning in humans as well as animals. The toxicity of glycoalkaloids is more towards human beings in comparison to other animals. The toxic effects of glycoalkaloids has been studied and reviewed by various researchers (Uluwaduge, 2018; Sucha and Tomsik, 2016). The toxic effect of these compounds depends on various factors, mainly route of administration, dose, and species, etc. In comparison to oral administration, parenteral administration is much more toxic. The anticholinesterase activity of glycoalkaloids on the central nervous system may be the reason behind their toxicity. Additionally, the toxic effect of glycoalkaloids may be due cell membrane disruption, which affects various organs as well as the digestive system of the body (Sucha and Tomsik, 2016).

Different studies reported that a bitter taste occurs if the content of glycoalkaloid in potatoes exceeds up to 14 mg/100 g (on fresh weight basis) and a burning sensation in the mouth when the level exceeds from 22 mg/100 g (fresh weight basis). A strong bitter taste and the problem of a burning sensation are produced if the total glycoalkaloid content exceeds from 60 mg/100 g (on fresh weight basis). The total glycoalkaloid in commercial cultivars of potatoes should not exceed from 10 mg/100 g (fresh weight basis). The glycoalkaloid solanine in potatoes should not be more than 20 mg/100 g as limited by the US Food & Drug Administration (FDA). The toxicological effects, known toxic doses, and administration type of these compounds (solanine and chaconine) are summarized in Table 4.3. The main symptoms of poisoning caused by solanine include vomiting, stomach/abdominal cramps, diarrhoea, headache, fever, nausea, weak/rapid pulse, hallucinations, delirium, rapid breathing, and sometime coma in severe cases (Uluwaduge, 2018; Sucha and Tomsik, 2016). The absorption of glycoalkaloids is poor in the gastrointestinal tract and reported higher in the spleen (Sucha and Tomsik, 2016). The distribution of these glycoalkaloids is reported to be greatest after 5 h of ingestion in the blood and after about 21 h is their biological half-life (Barceloux, 2009; Mensinga et al., 2005). Thus, glycoalkaloids if consumed on a daily basis accumulate in the body and possess adverse health effects (Mensinga et al., 2005).

### 4.5.1 Toxicological Findings in Animals and Humans

Some of the data (as per availability in literature) related to toxicological effect of glycoalkaloids on animals and humans have been reviewed in this section. Intraperitoneal injection of α-solanine induces irritation for about one min in mice and the subjected animals seem to be sleepy, unresponsive, quiet, exhibit rapid breathing, dyspnoea (shortness of breath), and paralysis (hind leg), etc. (Sucha and Tomsik, 2016; Patil et al., 1972). However, oral administration of α-solanine and α-chaconine mixture (doses up to 33.3 mg/kg) did not cause any serious gastrointestinal toxicity in hamsters. But, problems such as distended gas, intestines/stomach filled with fluid have been observed (Langkilde et al., 2009). A dose of 20 mg/kg (α-solanine) if given to pregnant mice resulted in embryotoxicity, exhibited as abortion and is potentiated by aspirin (Sucha and Tomsik, 2016; Bell et al., 1976). The malformation and mortality of Xenopus embryos has been observed

**Table 4.3 Toxicity of Glycoalkaloids (α-solanine, α-chaconine)**

| Compound | Administration | Model organism | Toxicological effects | References |
|---|---|---|---|---|
| *α-solanine* | Oral (p.o.) | Mice | 1,000 mg/kg – not lethal | Sucha and Tomsik 2016;Chiu and Lin 2008 |
| | Intraperitoneal (i.p.) | Mice | LD50 = 30 mg/kg | Sucha and Tomsik 2016; Nishie, Norred and Swain 1975 |
| | | | dose up to 50 mg/kg – death within 1–3 h | Sucha and Tomsik 2016; Bell et al., 1976 |
| | | Rabbits | lowest lethal dose – 40 mg/kg | Sucha and Tomsik 2016; Nishie, Norred and Swain 1975 |
| | Intravenous (i.v.) | Rabbits | Lethal dose – 10 mg/kg | Sucha and Tomsik 2016; Chiu and Lin 2008 |
| *α-chaconine* | Intraperitoneal (i.p.) | Mice | LD50 = 27.5 mg/kg | Sucha and Tomsik 2016; Nishie, Norred and Swain 1975 |
| | | Rabbits | lowest lethal dose – 50 mg/kg | |

because of the synergic effect of compounds α-solanine and α-chaconine when given in combination (Sucha and Tomsik, 2016). Among different potato glycoalkaloids, the most toxic alkaloid is α-chaconine (Sucha and Tomsik, 2016; Korpan et al., 2004). The lowest lethal dose (LD) of α-chaconine in rabbits was 50 mg/kg (intraperitoneal injection), whereas in mice, LD50 was 27.5 mg/kg (Sucha and Tomsik, 2016; Nishie, Norred and Swain, 1975) (Table 4.3). As per the literature, the half-life of α-chaconine is about 44 h, longer than that of α-solanine (Sucha and Tomsik, 2016; Mensinga et al., 2005).

The toxic effect of these glycoalkaloids on human beings has also been reported in literature. Some of the findings as per available literature related to glycoalkaloids (solanine and chaconine) toxicity have been highlighted in this section. In the documented history of a hotel proprietor from Britain, it has been reported that steroidal glycoalkaloid poisoning (from potatoes) occurred until 1917 as a result from an outbreak of solanine poisoning (Uluwaduge, 2018; Wilson, 1959). The causative agent identified for this poisoning was baked potatoes having skin. The symptoms showed by victims were abdominal pain, vomiting, and diarrhoea (Wilson, 1959). Due to consumption of potatoes in diet, an outbreak of sickness among agricultural workers was recorded in a clinical observation in a village near Berlin (Unverricht, 1937). An incidence of poisoning among school boys has been reported due to consumption of potatoes having high glycoalkaloid content (α-solanine and α-chaconine). As per the literature available, toxicological data from cumulative assessment suggests that glycoalkaloids (solanine and chaconine) at a very lower dose are toxic to humans when compared with other animal models (Uluwaduge, 2018; Friedman, McDonald, and Filadelfi-Keszi, 1997).

## 4.6 IDENTIFICATION AND QUANTIFICATION

Over time, for the productive isolation of glycoalkaloids, different methodologies were formulated by various researchers and later the protocols were refined for pharmacological and other precise purposes. Common processes for glycoalkaloid extraction include maceration, Stas-Otto process, Soxhlet, Kippenberger's process, Manske's process, pressurized solvent extraction, negative pressure cavitation, ultrasonic-assisted extraction, steam distillation, and pulse electric field, etc. (Azmir, Zaidul, and Rahman et al., 2013, Jayakumar and Murugan, 2016). The glycoalkaloids extracted by these techniques as stated above were likely to have impurities. To remove these impurities extracted alkaloids have to be treated further. Different solvents, such as acid solution/precipitating alkaloids, suitable acids (organic/mineral), and/or different chromatographic techniques (partition, column, or ion-exchange techniques, etc.) are suggested to further remove or avoid these impurities (Yubin et al., 2014). X-ray crystallography or NMR spectroscopies are being used for identification of individual alkaloids fraction (Pan et al., 2016).

For the determination of total as well as individual glycoalkaloids, a number of analytical methods have been reported. The commonly used extraction processes employed in these analytical methods are bisolvent/aqueous/organic systems followed by glycoalkaloid precipitation with an aqueous base. For the quantification of glycoalkaloids, methods usually consist of three parts, similar to most analytical methods: extraction, clean-up, and quantification (Friedman, McDonald, and Filadelfi-Keszi, 1997; Coxon, 1984); or extraction, separation, and analysis (Jadhav, Sharma, and Salunkhe, 1981), described differently by different scientists. In spite of their different names, the aims behind these steps commonly involve (1) extraction of required compounds; (2) elimination of impurities, i.e., removing all unwanted compounds, which can create problems during analysis; and finally (3) determination of the quantity of glycoalkaloids present. Sometimes, as per the requirement of analysis, modifications such as derivatization or hydrolysis may also be included. The conversion of glycosidic compounds to non-sugar compounds (aglycones) is required before evaluation in several analytical techniques like gas chromatography (GC) and the colorimetric method, whereas derivatization of alkaloids is required in some other GC methods. Extraction and modification in combination is used in several methods of analysis. Extraction of glycoalkaloids with strong acid like sulfuric acid (3.5 *M*) allows extraction and hydrolysis simultaneously (Coxon, Price, and Jones, 1979). For the improvement in determination and quantification, new, modified, and improved methods are being proposed time to time, but sometimes it is hard to know the more responsible step for the improvement (Friedman, McDonald, and Filadelfi-Keszi, 1997; Coxon, 1984).

### 4.6.1 Extraction

The solvents used for the extraction of glycoalkaloids should be nonaqueous or acidic in nature or both because all the glycoalkaloids, excluding the leptines, are only sparingly soluble in aqueous solvents (pH $\geq$ 7). More than 20 different solvents are used for extracting glycoalkaloids as described in the literature. Extractions of glycoalkaloids have been carried out normally at room temperature, and combination of heat and acid is avoided due to hydrolysis caused by them. However, some methods of gas chromatography and colorimetric require hydrolysis prior to analysis (Friedman, McDonald, and Filadelfi-Keszi, 1997).

Extraction efficiency of different solvents was studied by various researchers. According to the literature available, ten solvent systems were evaluated in a preliminary study for their efficiency for extraction. The evaluation of the glycoalkaloids solanine and chaconine was done by using fresh, dried, and processed potato tubers and the extraction, clean-up, and determination processes (HPLC) used were the same for all the solvents studied (Friedman and McDonald, 1995). Different solvents studied by different researchers were ethanol; ethanol-based solution of acetic acid (3%); 2% solution of acetic acid; TCAA solution (5% trichloroacetic acid in 50% methanol and 75% methanol; 2:1 methanol-chloroform; 10:1:9 of chloroform-acetic acid-methanol solvent; acetic acid (5%); tetrahydrofuran-water-acetonitrile-acetic acid in ratio 5:3:2:0.1; sodium bisulfite (0.5%) in acetic acid (2%); 1-heptanesulfonic acid (0.4%) in acetic acid (1%); methanol-acetic acid-water in a ratio of 94:1:6; Na-1-heptanesulfonate (0.02 *M*) in acetic acid (0.17 *M*) (Friedman and McDonald, 1995). Variation in results was observed to be wide for α-solanine as compared to α-chaconine. The solvent reported best in case of dried sample is acetic acid (2%) (Friedman and McDonald, 1995; Birner, 1969). This reinforces other researchers' results that solvents of a nonaqueous nature do not show efficient results with dried samples (Speroni and Pell, 1980; Bushway, Bureau, and Stickney, 1985). Alcohol-based acetic acid solvent has been reported as a poor solvent for extraction of solanine (Jayakumar and Murugan, 2016; Friedman, McDonald, and Filadelfi-Keszi, 1997).

### 4.6.2 Clean-Up

Purification of glycoalkaloids is commonly done by any one of these methods: precipitation with ammonium hydroxide (Friedman and Dao, 1992); segregation (partitioning) using aqueous solutions of Na,SO or butanol (water-saturated) (Wang, Bedford, and Thompson, 1972; Crabbe and Fryer, 1980; Friedman, Levin, and McDonald, 1994); or by passing via Clg ion-pair chromatography a cartridge (Houben and Brunt, 1994). These techniques in combination may also be used if required. The basic nature solvent method like ammonia precipitation method (pH 10) has some disadvantages because of the insolubility of solanine in basic solutions, whereas it has partial solubility for chaconine. The loss due to this method should not matter for large samples, but could be significant on samples of a small-scale. The problems like their partial loss in rejected layer or by obstruction due to salts formed can be prevented with the use of a water-saturated solvent like n-butanol. The pure hydrolyzed systems and extracts of freeze-dried samples in acetic acid solvents worked well with this (Friedman and McDonald, 1995, Friedman and Dao, 1992). However, it is not successful with fresh samples or extract of nonaqueous solvents because of interfering compounds which may be present. Solid-phase extraction (SPE) is reported as the most popular method of clean-up used during glycoalkaloid determination by HPLC. The use of various cartridges has been reported and recommended for clean-up prior to glycoalkaloid determination like commercial "C cartridges"; SPE; SPECN cartridges; c 1g (low lipid samples) and NH (high lipid sample), cartridges depending on the type of sample and method of determination (Houben and Brunt, 1994; Jonker, Koops, and Hoogendoorn, 1992). The selection of method used for clean-up depends to a large extent on the nature of solvent used for extraction and analysis method. So, these cartridges as mentioned above may not prove to be best for all types of procedures (Friedman, McDonald, and Filadelfi-Keszi, 1997).

### 4.6.3 Analysis

Evaluation of glycoalkaloids is not an easy task, as optimization of one section may cause problems in another section of the procedure. This may be due to the reason that sometimes the most efficient solvent for extraction may extract interfering compounds also and create the requirement of extensive clean-up. These problems might be avoided by other solvents but then extraction might not be so much efficient. Different analytical methods as reported in literature are highlighted in this section. Determination of solanine was done by gravimetric method followed by alkaline precipitation for the first 100 years (Bomer and Mattis, 1924). However, precipitation is only being used as part of the clean-up process in recent times. The use of liquid (LC) and paper chromatography (PC) has been reported for qualitative and quantitative separation of glycoalkaloids (Paseshnichenko and Guseva, 1956). Later on, PC has been replaced by TLC, and LC is used as part of the purification process only. For the evaluation of glycoalkaloids and their related compounds, methods which are in use include: colorimetry; TLC; GC; HPLC; and immunoassays (ELISA). The most important methods include TLC, gas-liquid chromatography, HPLC and colorimetry or titrimetry, etc. (Friedman, McDonald, and Filadelfi-Keszi, 1997; Jayakumar and Murugan, 2016). As compared to other methods, the test kit ELISA has good efficiency, reproducibility, and sensitivity, and provides a very quick as well as simple screening method, even for samples of large numbers. Freeze-dried samples have been recommended in comparison to other samples because of several advantages: fewer compositional changes (moisture-dependent, enzyme-catalyzed, and wound-induced), as glycoalkaloid content is affected by these changes; analysis of sample at different periods of time and by different analysts is possible as transportation and storage of freeze-dried samples without change is possible; makes easy to relate nutrition and safety with composition; additionally, freeze-dried extracts are easy to clean up; no browning during handling (Friedman, McDonald, and Filadelfi-Keszi, 1997).

However, further studies are required to evaluate various analytical techniques on a variety of samples for efficient and precise results.

## 4.7 SAFETY, PRECAUTIONS, AND REGULATION

In human beings, toxic dose of glycoalkaloids is in range of 1–5 mg/kg (body weight) and lethality dose is 3–6 mg/kg (body weight) through the oral route (Uluwaduge, 2018; Smith, Roddick, and Jones, 1996). Therefore, the safe limit of glycoalkaloid level as defined by the USDA and other leading authorities is 20 mg/100 g (fresh weight) and 100 mg/100 g (dry weight) in edible tubers (Aziz et al., 2012; Nahar, 2011). Glycoalkaloid poisoning in human beings vary from individual to individual (Smith, Roddick, and Jones, 1996). Therefore, it is difficult to establish a safe level of intake from analysis of the toxicological data on human subjects and considerable efforts are required further (Goodman and Nawrot, 1993). It has been proposed that the safety limit of glycoalkaloids has to be brought down to a level less than that recommended because of the variations in glycoalkaloid level based on different factors like pre- and post-harvest factors and the individual-dependent variations of the toxic dose (Uluwaduge, 2018; Cantwell, 1996).

Glycoalkaloid content of commercial varieties tends to be less than that of the accepted safety limit (20 mg/100 g fresh weight) (Smith, Roddick, and Jones, 1996). Glycoalkaloid level of potato tubers exceeding that of 14 mg/100 g exhibit a bitter taste, while a sensation of burning in the throat and mouth was observed with levels in excess of 22 mg/100 g (Sinden, 1987). Therefore, the quality of tubers is directly affected by the quantity of glycoalkaloids present. Since the off flavours of tubers as caused by high glycoalkaloid content will reduce the value of tubers from a commercial point of view. So, routine testing of edible tubers and potato-based products for glycoalkaloid content is necessary to ensure the safety of the consumer (Uluwaduge, 2018; Sucha and Tomsik, 2016).

### 4.7.1 Regulatory Control of Glycoalkaloid Level

The glycoalkaloids solanine and chaconine are mainly found in potatoes and the current safe level set by several leading authorities is 20 mg/100 g (fresh weight basis). Any cultivar exceeding this value is not recommended for consumption by humans (Uluwaduge, 2018; Aziz et al., 2012). However, different varieties of potatoes with the acceptable glycoalkaloid content have been released for commercial production, but the safe level could be exceeded occasionally, maybe because of several factors like environmental, physical, and storage conditions, etc. An example of this is that two potato cultivars "*Lenape*" and "*Magnum Bonum*" were not accepted and withdrawn from United States and Swedish markets due to unacceptable levels of glycoalkaloid. The reported average values of these glycoalkaloids were 30 mg/100 g in "*Lenape*" and 25.4/100 g in that of "*Magnum Bonum*" cultivar (Nahar, 2011; Hellenas et al., 1995). Therefore, as a safety regulation, it is being advised to monitor glycoalkaloid content, especially of produce which faced adverse conditions (environmental and other) during the tuber bulking. The amount of these compounds in these types of batches should also be screened before market release as a safety precaution. Further, the glycoalkaloid levels of tubers generated from breeding programs should also be assessed. It is highly recommended to avoid the genetic transmission of glycoalkaloids from wild species to hybrid progeny at undesirable levels. Otherwise, it may result in wasted effort, time, and money (Uluwaduge, 2018; Gregory, 1984).

The post-harvest factors causing the stress in tubers such as damage due to physical factors like cutting and bruising during harvest or transit, herbivore or microbial attack, inadequate storage, and improper handling are known to influence the level of glycoalkaloid content in potato tubers (Uluwaduge, 2018; Dale, Griffiths, and Bain, 1998). Products prepared from these tubers, especially peel- or skin-based products, can cause potential health risks because of higher glycoalkaloid levels. However, proper monitoring, adequate storage condition, safe handling, and proper control on other responsible factors such as temperature and light may improve the quality of commercial varieties of tubers (potatoes) (Uluwaduge, 2018).

### 4.7.2 Safety Measures to Optimize Toxicity of Edible Tubers

As per the data available, the following strategies (Table 4.4) would be helpful for grower, farmer, commercial producers, retailers, and consumers for improving the quality of edible potatoes in terms of toxicity.

In spite of the toxic and bitter-tasting nature of the solanine and chaconine, major glycoalkaloids present in potatoes (staple food for humans) show that it is safe for consumption (as observed throughout the long history of consumption). This may be due to the reason that glycoalkaloid level in most of the commercial varieties of potato is less than the acceptable safety limit, i.e. $<20$ mg/100 g fresh weight of edible tubers (Uluwaduge, 2018). As precautionary measures and from a food safety perspective, precise review on cultural and marketing practices is important for

**Table 4.4 Recommended Strategies for the Control of Glycoalkaloid Formation or Accumulation in Potatoes and Potato-Based Products**

| Stages | Strategies |
|---|---|
| Farmers/grower/ commercial producers | 1. Selection of low glycoalkaloids containing cultivars<br>2. Manipulating environmental factors carefully (low temperature, desired soil nitrogen content)<br>3. Minimizing the level of tuber damage during post- harvest processing/handling<br>4. Careful screening and evaluation of glycoalkaloid content of newly developed varieties prior to release in market |
| Retailer | 1. Proper packaging (opaque plastic films or paper bags to protect from light)<br>2. Stock rotation in retail displays<br>3. Storage under shaded and cold environment |
| Consumers/final customer/processor | 1. Proper selection of tuber (intact tubers; moderate/large size)<br>2. Proper peeling any processing<br>3. Reject tubers having bitter taste and green colour |

(*Source:* Modified from Uluwaduge 2018)

farmers and retailers to ensure that the tubers and other products containing these glycoalkaloids contain a safe level of glycoalkaloids at each level from field through storage to retail market and finally to consumer (i.e. from the field to plate) (Uluwaduge, 2018).

Processed products have increased popularity and therefore, in addition to selection criteria, processing methods adopted are also important to ensure the safety of edible tubers because of processing methods like drying, baking, cooking, fermentation, heat treatment, freezing, etc., also affect the quality of product in terms of their glycoalkaloid content present in them (Uluwaduge, 2018).

## 4.8 EFFECT OF PROCESSING

Glycoalkaloids are naturally bitter-tasting, heat-stable toxicants present mainly in potatoes and other crops of the Solanaceae family. The majority of these compounds are confined to the peel in edible tuber. High content of glycoalkaloids impart an off flavour to the potatoes and exhibit toxicity to animals and humans. Due to the reason of a higher glycoalkaloid level, there have been many food safety issues associated with the regular intake of potato and its products. The glycoalkaloid content of edible potatoes, if it exceeds the safe limit, can be a major determinant in terms of quality and safety (Uluwaduge, 2018). Different processing methods affect these glycoalkaloid levels and the quality of products containing these compounds. Various researchers reported the effect of processing methods (like peeling, baking, microwave processing, drying, drying, etc.) on the level of glycoalkaloid and their effect on the quality of products containing these compounds (Tajner-Czopek et al., 2014; Lachman et al., 2013, Mulinacci et al., 2008). Preliminary processing, e.g., peeling, cooking, boiling, etc., have the potential to reduce these compounds (Rytel et al., 2005). Baking, frying, or microwave cooking and other processing methods have been reported for their capability in reducing the level of glycoalkaloids in snacks or other dried products of potato at a significant level (Pezksa et al., 2006; Friedman, McDonald, and Filadelfi-Keszi, 1997). Due to the toxicity of glycoalkaloids and their significant reduction by processing methods, a precise review on the changes in glycoalkaloid level, resulting from different processing technologies, is required. As reported in literature, some of the common processing methods and their effect on glycoalkaloid content are discussed in this section and summarized in Table 4.5.

### 4.8.1 Peeling

Peel or skin and the portion immediately beneath the skin contain a major portion of glycoalkaloids. Higher concentrations of these compounds are found in the potato eyes and area around it

**Table 4.5 Effect of Different Processing Methods on the Glycoalkaloids (α-solanine and α-chaconine)**

| | | Reduction in Glycoalkaloids | | | |
|---|---|---|---|---|---|
| **Method** | **Conditions** | **α-solanine** | **α-chaconine** | **α-solanine and α-chaconine** | **Reference** |
| *Peeling* | Steam peeling | 43.6% | 30.5% | – | Lachman et al., 2013 |
| | | – | – | 40–77% | Rytel et al., 2005; Mader, Rawel and Kroh 2009 |
| | Mechanical peeling | – | – | 25% | Pezksa et al., 2006 |
| | Manual peeling | – | – | 60% | Tajner-Czopek, Jarych-Szyszka and Lisinska, 2008 |
| *Microwave processing* | 750 W/10 min | – | – | 45%, | Lachman et al., 2013 |
| | 2000 W/8 min | – | – | 12.4–13.3 mg/100 g | Bushway and Ponnampalam 1981 |
| | – | – | – | 3–45% | Schrenk et al., 2020 |
| *Baking* | 425°F/1 h | 54% | 47% | – | Bushway and Ponnampalam 1981 |
| | 180°C/45 min | 47% | 54% | | Lachman et al., 2013 |
| | – | – | – | 20–50% | Schrenk et al., 2020 |
| *Frying* | 170–180°C/5–6 min | | | 39%–92%, | Tajner-Czopek et al., 2014 |
| | 170–180°C/1–5 min | | | 62–87% | Rytel et al., 2005 |
| | 170°C/5 min;<br>150°C/5 min;<br>210°C/10 min | | | 21%<br>3%<br>38% | Takagi et al., 1990 |
| | 177°C/4 min | | | 16–22% | Bushway and Ponnampalam 1981 |
| *Boiling* | 25 min | | | 26% | Lachman et al., 2013 |
| | – | – | – | > 3.5% | Friedman 2006 |
| | 25 min | 0.04–0.08 mg/100 g | 0.04–0.06 mg/100 g | – | Bushway and Ponnampalam 1981 |
| *Cooking* | – | 18% | 23% | – | Tajner-Czopek, Jarych-Szyszka and Lisinska, 2008 |
| | – | – | – | 27–42 mg/100 g | Smith, Roddick, and Jones 1996 |
| *Drying* | 120–160°C/1–2 h | – | – | 27–67% | Mader, Rawel, and Kroh 2009 |
| | 160°C/2 h | – | – | 25% | Elzbieta. 2012 |
| | Air drying/177°C | – | – | 11% | Elzbieta 2012 |
| | Fluidized | – | – | 3.11 mg/100 g | Elzbieta 2012 |
| *Freezing* | 4–8°C/6 week | – | – | 50% | Griffiths, Bain, and Dale 1997 |
| | 10°C/45 days | | | 30.4 mg/100 g | Griffiths, Bain, and Dale 1997 |
| *Blanching* | 80°C/15 min | – | – | 25% | Elzbieta 2012 |
| | 75°C/20 min | – | – | 19% | Rytel et al., 2018 |

(Peksa et al., 2002). Peeling reduced the glycoalkaloid level up to 50–95% (Frydecka-Mazurczyk and Zgorska, 1997). Peeling resulted in the significant reduction of these compounds in potatoes because α-chaconine and α-solanine present in higher ratio in peel in comparison to flesh of tuber (Elzbieta, 2012). The process of peeling on an average decreased the glycoalkaloid content up to 34.7% (α-solanine up to 43.6% and α-chaconine to up to 30.5%) in non-peeled tubers

(Lachman et al., 2013). Steam peeling of potato resulted in a decrease of 77% and 40% of glycoalkaloids during its processing for products like potato granules and French fries, respectively (Mader, Rawel, and Kroh, 2009; Rytel et al., 2005). During the process of chips manufacturing, manual peeling (25% reduction) was observed to be more effective as compared to mechanical peeling (60% reduction) (Pezksa et al., 2006; Tajner-Czopek, Jarych-Szyszka, and Lisinska, 2008). The process of peeling and cooking significantly reduced solanine to chaconine ratio in cooked potatoes (Tajner-Czopek, Jarych-Szyszka, and Lisinska, 2008). The process of peeling in combination with cooking reduces the level of glycoalkaloids in potatoes from 75%–80% depending on the type and cultivar. The reduction reported in the level of glycoalkaloids has been two times higher for peeling in comparison to the cooking process. As compared to chaconine, solanine losses were reported significantly higher in both processes, i.e., peeling and cooking. Potatoes with peel, if cooked, were found to be bitterer than potato cooked without peel due to their (glycoalkaloid) migration into the cortex during the process of cooking (even though the mobility is less) (Mondy and Gosellin, 1988). Most of the data in literature claimed that peeling in comparison to cooking removes higher amount of glycoalkaloids (approximately twice) (Tajner-Czopek et al., 2014).

### 4.8.2 Boiling

Boiling in combination with peeling reported to be more effective as compared to boiling alone because these compounds are heat stable in nature and found mainly within or beneath the peel. Boiling of peeled potato reduced the glycoalkaloid content up to 26% (Lachman et al., 2013). Lowest value of these glycoalkaloids has been reported in canned boiled potato products (25 min), i.e. 0.04–0.08 mg/100 g (α-chaconine) and 0.04–0.06 mg/100 g (α-solanine) may be due peel removal and moisture loss during canning (Bushway and Ponnampalam, 1981). Boiling reduced glycoalkaloid content in potatoes (up to 3.5%) as compared to peeling (50–95%) (Friedman, 2006).

### 4.8.3 Cooking

Cooking methods like boiling also have a similar effect on the glycoalkaloid as reported in literature. During the cooking process of unpeeled potato, glycoalkaloids migrate into the cortex which gives a bitter taste as compared to peeled potato (Mondy and Gosellin, 1988). Cooking does not cause a higher reduction in glycoalkaloids (average reduction – 22%) (Tajner-Czopek, Jarych-Szyszka, and Lisinska, 2008), but the losses reported were higher for α-chaconine (23%) than for α-solanine (18%). As explained above, cooking was not as effective as peeling as it removes a higher amount of glycoalkaloids (approximately twice) than cooking (Tajner-Czopek et al., 2014).

### 4.8.4 Blanching

Blanching of sliced potatoes in water (15 min/80°C) showed a significant decrease in the glycoalkaloid content (25%). Higher reduction in α-chaconine content (29%) has been reported than that of α-solanine (21%) (Elzbieta, 2012). Two-stage water blanching at 80°C reduced the glycoalkaloid level up to 40% in French fries (Rytel et al., 2005).

### 4.8.5 Microwave Processing

Microwave processing (750 W for 10 min) reduces the glycoalkaloid content up to 45% (267–146 mg/kg reduction on dry basis) (Lachman et al., 2013) whereas much lower reductions up to 15% have also been reported in some studies (Takagi et al., 1990). Non-significant effects of microwave processing on glycoalkaloids content of unpeeled potatoes as compared with fresh potatoes have been reported (Mulinacci et al., 2008). Microwave processing at (2,000 W) for 8 min showed the significant decrease in glycoalkaloid content, i.e. 12.4–13.3 mg/100 g (Bushway and Ponnampalam, 1981). Unpeeled potatoes during microwave processing have been reported for the reduction in the glycoalkaloid content, i.e. from 3–45% (Schrenk et al., 2020).

### 4.8.6 Baking

Baking process (425°F/1 h) resulted in the significant reduction of α-chaconine (47%) in comparison with α-solanine (54%) (Bushway and Ponnampalam, 1981). Baking significantly reduced the glycoalkaloid level of diced (small cubes) non-peeled tubers (i.e. from 267 to 134 mg/kg on dry basis) (Lachman et al., 2013). The reduction (20–50%) in the level of these glycoalkaloids has also been reported by oven baking of unpeeled potatoes (Schrenk et al., 2020).

### 4.8.7 Frying

The Frying process also affects the glycoalkaloid content of potato as reported in various studies. Reduction of 62–79% glycoalkaloids in blanched potato strips was observed after first-stage frying (1 min), whereas the reduction was 75–87% after second-stage frying (after more than 5 min) (Rytel et al., 2005). A maximum of 92% reduction was reported after frying (175°C/5–6 min) of blanched potato strips (Tajner-Czopek et al., 2014). Different fried products were reported for reduction in glycoalkaloids and the reduction was found higher in ready French fries products (94%), followed by first-stage fried French fries (92%) and in crisps (83%) (Lachman et al., 2013; Omayio, Abong, and Okoth, 2016). No significant reduction in glycoalkaloids has been reported at 150°C, whereas a 21% reduction was observed at frying temperature of 170°C and the reduction increased with increase in temperature (up to 38% at 210°C) (Takagi et al., 1990). The ratio of α-chaconine and α-solanine has been reported to be constant in some studies regardless of the difference in conditions of frying (e.g., time and temperature) (Pezksa et al., 2006; Rytel et al., 2018).

### 4.8.8 Drying

Drying does not affect the stability of α-solanine and α-chaconine as observed during dried powder production from potato at temperature up to 150°C for 2 h. However, the degradation of these compounds has been reported when processed above 150°C and reported stability is lesser for α-chaconine than α-solanine (Nie et al., 2018). Drying of potatoes (at temperature 120°C and 160°C/1–2 h) after peeling and slicing resulted in a higher reduction of these compounds in final products (flakes, dried dices, and powder), i.e., from 29%–67% (Mader, Rawel, and Kroh, 2009). At high temperature reduction of these compounds was found to be significant (25% when dried for 2 h at 160°C) (Elzbieta, 2012). Air drying (177°C) of potatoes reduced the glycoalkaloids by 11%, whereas fluidized drying resulted less of a decrease in these compounds (3.39 mg/100 g–3.11 mg/100 g) (Elzbieta, 2012).

### 4.8.9 Freezing and Low Temperature Storage

Freezing and low temperature storage increases the glycoalkaloid levels in potato tubers during the storage of the initial 3 months (10°C/45 days) (Love et al., 1994). Further decrease in storage temperature (up to 4.4°C) increased the total glycoalkaloid content but at a minor level (1 mg/100 g fresh weight) (Love et al., 1994). Almost twice an increase in the total glycoalkaloid content has been reported in potato tubers during storage of 6 weeks at temperature 4–8°C in comparison to tubers stored at 12–15°C (Maga and Fitzpatrick, 1980). Development of bitterness at low temperature storage due to higher total glycoalkaloid content has been reported (Griffiths, Bain, and Dale, 1997)

Most of the studies revealed that peeling was the most effective method for reducing glycoalkaloid content in comparison to other processes like cooking, frying, baking, roasting microwaving, and boiling, etc., because of the reason that these compounds are stable to heat unless the processing temperature was high (above 150°C in most cases) (Rytel et al., 2018; Bushway and Ponnampalam, 1981). A comparative study on different processes reported that the total glycoalkaloids content in tubers was induced by various heat processes such as frying, roasting, cooking, and only frying at higher temperatures resulted in a decrease in these compounds (Rytel et al., 2018). However, contradictory results were also reported in literature. Some studies reported that under normal home cooking conditions, potato glycoalkaloids are relatively stable and only little reduction was reported for microwave treatment and boiling (Lachman et al., 2013). Thus, on the basis of most of the studies, removal of peel of the tubers before any cooking and further processing is advisable to reduce the glycoalkaloid content and improve the quality of products.

## 4.9 FUTURE SCOPE

In spite of their toxic effect, these compounds have a huge scope in future as it shows some remedial effects on mankind. Solanine and chaconine are mainly present in different parts of the potato plant, and among the total glycoalkaloids found in potato, α-solanine and α-chaconine are the major glycoalkaloids (95%), which functions as a self-defensive compound against fungal, bacterial, and insect attacks (Hossain et al., 2015). Additionally, these compounds have also been reported for various health beneficial properties in human as well as animals as discussed in above sections. Glycoalkaloids and their hydrolysed/derivatized products may also have cholesterol-lowering benefits by disrupting cell membranes which contain cholesterol by forming strong complexes with cholesterol as well as other phytosterols in vitro. So, the glycoalkaloids have great scope in future for the researcher/scientist as well as at pharmacological scale. Additionally, there is a great scope for plant breeders for further research due to incomplete data regarding biology and plant physiology of these secondary metabolites. Requirement for the development of potato and other related plants strains with reduced toxic glycoalkaloids and their metabolites while maintaining their self-defensive properties should be there. Researchers and scientists related to the food and biomedical (microbiologists, pharmacologists, and nutritionists) industry have plenty of future scope because of further challenges to define the effective use of these glycoalkaloids for their self-defensive, beneficial health effects.

## 4.10 CONCLUSION

Solanine and chaconine are the naturally synthesized glycoalkaloids present in plants of the Solanaceae family and their toxic nature may be for the self-protection of the plant against various phytopathogens and other adverse environmental factors. In spite of their toxic effect, these glycoalkaloids are also reported for their beneficial health properties in animals as well as humans. The difference in the toxicity and properties of these glycoalkaloids has been reported due to a difference in their chemical composition, mainly the sugars in the glycosides side chain. Among all the processing methods, peeling and frying at higher temperatures (above 150°C) have been reported as the most efficient methods for the significant reduction in level of these glycoalkaloids. Requirement for the development of potato and other related plants strains with reduced toxic glycoalkaloids and their metabolites while maintaining their self-defensive properties should be there. Now a day's glycoalkaloid level found in commercial cultivars is usually below the safety level as decided by various regulatory bodies. Researchers and scientists related to the food and biomedical (microbiologists, pharmacologists, and nutritionists) industry have plenty of future scope because of further challenges to define the effective use of these glycoalkaloids for their self-defensive, beneficial health effects.

## REFERENCES


Al-Sinani, S.S.S. and Eltayeb, E.A. 2017.The steroidal glycoalkaloids solamargine and solasonine in Solanum plants. *South African Journal of Botany* 112:253–69.

Aziz, A., Randhawa, M.A., Butt, M.S. Asghar, A., Yasin, M. and Shibamoto, T. 2012. Glycoalkaloids (α-chaconine and α-solanine) contents of selected Pakistani potato cultivars and their dietary intake assessment. *Journal of Food Science* 77:58–61.

Azmir, J., Zaidul, I.S.M., Rahman, M.M., Sharif, K.M., Mohamed, A., Sahena, F., Jahurul, M.H.A., Ghafoor, K., Norulaini, N.A.N. and Omar, A.K.M. 2013. Techniques for extraction of bioactive compounds from plant materials: A Review. *Journal of Food Engineering* 117:426–36.

Badowski, P. and Urbanek-Karłowska, B. 1999. Solanine and Chaconine: Occurrence, properties, methods for determination. *Roczniki Panstwowego Zakladu Higieny* 50:69–75.

Barceloux, D.G. 2009.Potatoes, tomatoes, and solanine toxicity (Solanum tuberosum L., Solanum lycopersicum L.). *Disease-a-month* 55:391–402.

Bejarano, L., Mignolet, E., Devaux, A., Espinola, N., Carrasco, E. and Larondelle, Y. 2000. Glycoalkaloids in potato tubers: The effect of variety and drought stress on the α-solanine and α-chaconine contents of potatoes. *Journal of the Science of Food and Agriculture* 80:2096–2100.

Bell, D.P., Gibson, J.G., McCarroll, A.M. and McClean, G.A. 1976. Embryotoxicity of solanine and aspirin in mice. *Reproduction* 46:257–59.

Benkeblia, N. 2020. Potato glycoalkaloids: Occurrence, biological activities and extraction for biovalorisation–A review. *International Journal of Food Science and Technology* 55:2305–2313.

Birner, J. 1969. Determination of total steroid bases in Solanum species. *Journal of Pharmaceutical Sciences* 58:258–59.

Bomer, A. and Mattis, H. 1924. The solanine content of potatoes.*Z.Unters. Nuhr-u. Genussmittel* 47:97–127.

Bushway, R.J. and Ponnampalam, R. 1981. alpha.-Chaconine and. alpha.-solanine content of potato products and their stability during several modes of cooking. *Journal of Agricultural and Food Chemistry* 29:814–17.

Bushway, R.J., Bureau, J.L. and Stickney, M.R. 1985. A new efficient method for extracting glycoalkaloids from dehydrated potatoes. *Journal of Agricultural and Food Chemistry* 33:45–46.

Cantwell, M. 1996. A review of important facts about potato glycoalkaloids. *Perishables Handling Newsletter* 87:2–27.

Chiu, F.L. and Lin, J.K. 2008. Tomatidine inhibits iNOS and COX-2 through suppression of NF-κB and JNK pathways in LPS-stimulated mouse macrophages. *FEBS Letters* 582:2407–12.

Choi, E. and Koo, S. 2005. Anti-nociceptive and anti-inflammatory effects of the ethanolic extract of potato (Solanum tuberlosum). *Food and Agricultural Immunology* 16:29–39.

Chowanski, S., Adamski, Z., Marciniak, P., Rosinski, G., Buyukguzel, E., Buyukguzel, K., Falabella, P., Scrano, L., Ventrella, E., Lelario, F. and Bufo, S.A. 2016. A review of bioinsecticidal activity of Solanaceae alkaloids. *Toxins* 8:60.

Coxon, D.T. 1984. Methodology for glycoalkaloid analysis. *American Potato Journal* 61:169–83.

Coxon, D.T., Price, K.R. and Jones, P.G. 1979. A simplified method for the determination of total glycoalkaloids in potato tubers. *Journal of the Science of Food and Agriculture* 30:1043–49.

Crabbe, P.G. and Fryer, C. 1980. Rapid quantitative analysis of solasodine, solasodine glycosides and solasodiene by high-pressure liquid chromatography. *Journal of Chromatography* 187:87–100.

Dale, M.F.B., Griffiths, D.W. and Bain, H. 1998. Effect of bruising on the total glycoalkaloid and chlorogenic acid content of potato (*Solanum Tuberosum*) tubers of five cultivars. *Journal of the Science of Food and Agriculture* 77:499–505.

Elzbieta, R. 2012. The effect of industrial potato processing on the concentrations of glycoalkaloids and nitrates in potato granules. *Food Control* 28:380–84.

Friedman, M. and Dao, L. 1992.Distribution of glycoalkaloids in potato plants and commercial potato products. *Journal of Agricultural and Food Chemistry* 40:419–23.

Friedman, M. and McDonald, G.M. 1995.Extraction efficiency of various solvents for glycoalkaloid determination in potatoes and potato products. *American Potato Journal* 72:66A.

Friedman, M. and McDonald, G.M. 1999. Postharvest changes in glycoalkaloid content of potatoes. *Impact of Processing on Food Safety* 121–43.

Friedman, M. 2006. Potato glycoalkaloids and metabolites: Roles in the plant and in the diet. *Journal of Agricultural and Food Chemistry* 54:8655–81.

Friedman, M., Huang, V., Quiambao, Q., Noritake, S., Liu, J., Kwon, O., Chintalapati, S., Young, J., Levin, C.E., Tam, C. and Cheng, L.W. 2018. Potato peels and their bioactive glycoalkaloids and phenolic compounds inhibit the growth of pathogenic trichomonads. *Journal of Agricultural and Food Chemistry* 66:7942–47.

Friedman, M., Levin, C.E. and McDonald, G.M. 1994. Alpha.-tomatine determination in tomatoes by HPLC using pulsed amperometric detection. *Journal of Agricultural and Food Chemistry* 42:1959–64.

Friedman, M., McDonald, G.M. and Filadelfi-Keszi, M. 1997. Potato glycoalkaloids: Chemistry, analysis, safety, and plant physiology. *Critical Reviews in Plant Sciences* 16:55–132.

Frydecka-Mazurczyk, A. and Zgorska, K. 1997.The content of glycoalkaloids in potato tubers. *Ziemniak Polski* 4:10–12.

Gao, S.Y., Wang, Q.J. and Ji, Y.B. 2006. Effect of solanine on the membrane potential of mitochondria in HepG2 cells and [Ca2+] in the cells. *World Journal of Gastroenterology: WJG* 12:3359.

Gelder, W.M.J. 1990. Chemistry, toxicology, and occurrence of steroidal glycoalkaloids: Potential contaminants of the potato (*Solanum Tuberosum* L.). In *Poisonous Plant Contamination of Edible Plants*, edited by AF.M. Rizk (pp. 117–156). Boca Raton, FL: CRC Press.

Ginzberg, I., Tokuhisa, J.G. and Veilleux, R.E. 2009. Potato steroidal glycoalkaloids: Biosynthesis and genetic manipulation. *Journal of the European Association for Potato Research* 52:1–15.

Goodman, T. and Nawrot, P.S. 1993.Solanine and chaconine. *WHO Food Additive Series*, 30.

Gregory, P. 1984. Glycoalkaloid composition of potatoes: Diversity and biological implications. *American Potato Journal* 61:115–22.

Griffiths, D.W., Bain, H. and Dale, M.F.B. 1997. The effect of Low-temperature storage on the glycoalkaloid content of potato (*Solanum Tuberosum*) tubers. *Journal of the Science of Food and Agriculture* 74:301–7.

Hellenas, K.E., Branzell, C., Johnsson, H. and Slanina, P. 1995. High levels of glycoalkaloids in the established Swedish potato variety Magnum Bonum. *Journal of the Science of Food and Agriculture* 68:249–55.

Hossain, M.B., Aguiló-Aguayo, I., Lyng, J.G., Brunton, N.P. and Rai, D.K. 2015.Effect of pulsed electric field and pulsed light pre-treatment on the extraction of steroidal alkaloids from potato peels. *Innovative Food Science & Emerging Technologies* 29:9–14.

Houben, R.J. and Brunt, K. 1994. Determination of glycoalkaloids in potato tubers by reversed-phase high-performance liquid chromatography. *Journal of Chromatography* 661:169–74.

Jadhav, S.J., Sharma, R.P. and Salunkhe, D.K. 1981. Naturally occurring toxic alkaloids in foods. *CRC Critical Reviews in Toxicology* 9:21–104.

Jayakumar, K. and Murugan, K. 2016. Solanum alkaloids and their pharmaceutical roles: A review. *Journal of Analytical and Pharmaceutical Research* 3:00075.

Ji, Y.B., Gao, S.Y., Ji, C.F. and Zou, X. 2008. Induction of apoptosis in HepG2 cells by solanine and Bcl-2 protein. *Journal of Ethnopharmacology* 115:194–202.

Jonker, H.H., Koops, A.J. and Hoogendoorn, J.C. 1992. A rapid method for the quantification of steroidal glycoalkaloids by reversed phase HPLC. *Journal of the European Association for Potato Research* 35:451–55.

Kenny, O.M., McCarthy, C.M., Brunton, N.P., Hossain, M.B., Rai, D.K., Collins, S.G., Jones, P.W., Maguire, A.R. and Obrien, N.M. 2013. Anti-inflammatory properties of potato glycoalkaloids in stimulated Jurkat and Raw 264.7 mouse macrophages. *Life Sciences* 92:775–82.

Korpan, Y.I., Nazarenko, E.A., Skryshevskaya, I.V., Martelet, C., Jaffrezic-Renault, N. and Anna, V. 2004. Potato glycoalkaloids: True safety or false sense of security? *Trends in Biotechnology* 22:147–51.

Kozukue, N. and Mizuno, S. 1990. Effects of light exposure and storage temperature on greening and glycoalkaloid content in potato tubers. *Journal of the Japanese Society for Horticultural Science* 59:673–77.

Lachman, J., Hamouz, K., Musilova, J., Hejtmankova, K., Kotikova, Z., Pazderu, K., Domkarova, J., Pivec, V. and Cimr, J. 2013.Effect of peeling and three cooking methods on the content of selected phytochemicals in potato tubers with various colour of flesh. *Food Chemistry* 138:1189–97.

Lachman, J., Hamouz, K., Orsak, M. and Pivec, V. 2001. Potato glycoalkaloids and their significance in plant protection and human nutrition –*Review. Rostlinna Vyroba* - UZPI(Czech Republic) 47(4):181–19.

Langkilde, S., Mandimika, T., Schroder, M., Meyer, O., Slob, W., Peijnenburg, A. and Poulsen, M. 2009.A 28-day repeat dose toxicity study of steroidal glycoalkaloids, α-solanine and α-chaconine in the Syrian Golden hamster. *Food and Chemical Toxicology* 47:1099–1108.

Lee, K.R., Kozukue, N., Han, J.S., Park, J.H., Chang, E.Y., Baek, E.J., Chang, J.S. and Friedman, M. 2004. Glycoalkaloids and metabolites inhibit the growth of human colon (HT29) and liver (HepG2) cancer cells. *Journal of Agricultural and Food Chemistry* 52:2832–39.

Love, S.L., Herrman, T.J., Thompsonjohns, A. and Baker, T.P. 1994. Effect and interaction of crop management factors on the glycoalkaloid concentration of potato tubers. *Potato Research* 37:77–85.

Lu, M.K., Chen, P.H., Shih, Y.W., Chang, Y.T., Huang, E.T., Liu, C.R. and Chen, P.S. 2010. α-Chaconine inhibits angiogenesis in vitro by reducing matrix metalloproteinase-2. *Biological and Pharmaceutical Bulletin* 33:622–30.

Lv, C., Kong, H., Dong, G., Liu, L., Tong, K., Sun, H., Chen, B., Zhang, C. and Zhou, M. 2014. Antitumor efficacy of α-solanine against pancreatic cancer in vitro and in vivo. *PLoS One* 9(2):e87868.

Mader, J., Rawel, H. and Kroh, L.W. 2009. Composition of phenolic compounds and glycoalkaloids α-solanine and α-chaconine during commercial potato processing. *Journal of Agricultural and Food Chemistry* 57:6292–97.

Maga, J.A. and Fitzpatrick, T.J. 1980. Potato glycoalkaloids. *Critical Reviews in Food Science and Nutrition* 12:371–405.

McGehee, D.S., Krasowski, M.D., Fung, D.L., Wilson, B., Gronert, G.A. and Moss, J. 2000. Cholinesterase inhibition by potato glycoalkaloids slows mivacurium metabolism. *The Journal of the American Society of Anesthesiologists* 93:510–19.

Mensinga, T.T., Sips, A.J., Rompelberg, C.J., Twillert, K., Meulenbelt, J., van-den-Top, H.J. and van-Egmond, H.P. 2005. Potato glycoalkaloids and adverse effects in humans: An ascending dose study. *Regulatory Toxicology and Pharmacology* 41:66–72.

Milner, S.E., Brunton, N.P., Jones, P.W., OBrien, N.M., Collins, S.G. and Maguire, A.R. 2011. Bioactivities of glycoalkaloids and their aglycones from Solanum species. *Journal of Agricultural and Food Chemistry* 59:3454–84.

Mohsenikia, M., Alizadeh, A.M., Khodayari, S., Khodayari, H., Karimi, A., Zamani, M., Azizian, S. and Mohagheghi, M.A. 2013. The protective and therapeutic effects of alpha-solanine on mice breast cancer. *European Journal of Pharmacology* 718:1–9.

Mondy, N.I. and Gosellin, B. 1988. Effect of peeling on total phenols, total glycoalkaloids, discoloration and flavor of cooked potatoes. *Journal of Food Science* 53:756–59.

Mulinacci, N., Ieri, F., Giaccherini, C., Innocenti, M., Andrenelli, L., Canova, G., Saracchi, M. and Casiraghi, M.C. 2008.Effect of cooking on the anthocyanins, phenolic acids, glycoalkaloids, and resistant starch content in two pigmented cultivars of Solanum tuberosum L. *Journal of Agricultural and Food Chemistry* 56:11830–37.

Nahar, N. 2011. Regulation of sterol and glycoalkaloid biosynthesis in potato (*Solanum Tuberosum* L.): Identification of key genes and enzymatic steps. *Acta Universities Agriculture Sueciae* 2011(15): 1–66.

Nie, X., Zhang, G., Lv, S. and Guo, H. 2018.Steroidal glycoalkaloids in potato foods as affected by cooking methods. *International Journal of Food Properties* 21:1875–87.

Nielsen, S.D., Schmidt, J.M., Kristiansen, G.H., Dalsgaard, T.K. and Larsen, L.B. 2020. Liquid chromatography mass spectrometry quantification of α-solanine, α-chaconine, and solanidine in potato protein isolates. *Foods* 9:416.

Nigg, H.N., Ramos, L.E., Graham, E.M., Sterling, J., Brown, S. and Cornell, J.A. 1996.Inhibition of human plasma and serum butyrylcholinesterase (EC 3.1. 1.8) by α-chaconine and α-solanine. *Toxicological Sciences* 33:272–81.

Nishie, K., Norred, W.P. and Swain, A.P. 1975. Pharmacology and toxicology of chaconine and tomatine. *Research Communications in Chemical Pathology and Pharmacology* 12:657–68.

Omayio, D.G., Abong, G.O. and Okoth, M.W. 2016.A review of occurrence of glycoalkaloids in potato and potato products. *Current Research in Nutrition and Food Science* 4(3):195–202.

Ostry, V., Ruprich, J. and Skarkova, J. 2010. Glycoalkaloids in potato tubers: The effect of peeling and cooking in salted water. *Acta Alimentaria* 39:130–35.

Pan, Z., Qin, X.J., Liu, Y.P., Wu, T., Luo, X.D. and Xia, C. 2016. Alstoscholarisines H–J, indole alkaloids from Alstonia scholaris: Structural evaluation and bioinspired synthesis of alstoscholarisine H. *Organic Letters* 18:654–57.

Papathanasiou, F., Mitchell, S.H. and Harvey, B.M. 1998.Glycoalkaloid accumulation during tuber development of early potato cultivars. *Journal of the European Association for Potato Research* 41:117–25.

Percival, G.C., 1993. *Factors influencing accumulation of potato glycoalkaloids and their potential manipulation in tuber pathogen control.* PhD thesis, University of Strathclyde, SAC Auchincruive, UK.

Percival, G.C., Dixon, G.R. and Sword, A. 1996. Glycoalkaloid concentration of potato tubers following exposure to daylight. *Journal of the Science of Food and Agriculture* 71:59–63.

Paseshnichenko, V.A. and Guseva, A.R. 1956. Quantitative determination of potato glycoalkaloids and their preparative separation.*Biochemistry-Moscow* 21:606–11.

Patil, B.C., Sharma, R.P., Salunkhe, D.K. and Salunkhe, K. 1972. Evaluation of solanine toxicity. *Food and Cosmetics Toxicology* 10:395–98.

Peksa, A., Gołubowska, G., Rytel, E., Lisinska, G. and Aniołowski, K. 2002. Influence of harvest date on glycoalkaloid contents of three potato varieties. *Food Chemistry* 78:313–17.

Percival, G.C. and Dixon, G.R. 1997. Glycoalkaloids.In *Handbook of Plant and Fungal Toxins*, edited by J. P. Felix D'Mello (pp. 19–35). Boca Raton, FL: CRC Press.

Pezksa A, Golubowska G, Aniolowski K, Lisinska G. and Rytel. 2006. Changes of glycoalkaloids and nitrate contentin potatoes during chip processing. *Food Chemistry* 97:151–6.

Rayburn, J.R., Bantle, J.A. and Friedman, M. 1994. Role of carbohydrate side chains of potato glycoalkaloids in developmental toxicity. *Journal of Agricultural and Food Chemistry* 42:1511–15.

Reddivari, L., Vanamala, J., Safe, S.H. and Miller Jr, J.C. 2010. The bioactive compounds α-chaconine and gallic acid in potato extracts decrease survival and induce apoptosis in LNCaP and PC3 prostate cancer cells. *Nutrition and Cancer* 62:601–10.

Roddick, J.G. 1989. The acetylcholinesterase-inhibitory activity of steroidal glycoalkaloids and their aglycones. *Phytochemistry* 28:2631–34.

Rytel, E., Gołubowska, G., Lisinska, G., Peksa, A. and Aniołowski, K. 2005. Changes in glycoalkaloid and nitrate contents in potatoes during french fries processing. *Journal of the Science of Food and Agriculture* 85:879–82.

Rytel, E., Tajner-Czopek, A., Kita, A., Kucharska, A.Z., Sokoł-Łętowska, A. and Hamouz, K. 2018. Content of anthocyanins and glycoalkaloids in blue-fleshed potatoes and changes in the content of α-solanine and α-chaconine during manufacture of fried and dried products. *International Journal of Food Science and Technology* 53:719–27.

Schrenk, D., Bignami, M., Bodin, L., Chipman, J.K., Mazo, J., Hogstrand, C., Hoogenboom, L., Leblanc, J.C., Nebbia, C.S. and Nielsen, E. 2020.Risk assessment of glycoalkaloids in feed and food, in particular in potatoes and potato-derived products. *EFSA Journal* 18:06222.

Shin, J.S., Lee, K.G., Lee, H.H., Lee, H.J., An, H.J., Nam, J.H., Jang, D.S. and Lee, K.T. 2016. α-Solanine isolated from *Solanum Tuberosum* L. cv Jayoung Abrogates LPS-induced inflammatory responses via NF-κB inactivation in RAW 264.7 macrophages and endotoxin-induced shock model in mice. *Journal of Cellular Biochemistry* 117:2327–39.

Sinden SL. 1987. Potato glycoalkaloids. *Acta Horticulture* 207:41–48.

Sinden, S.L., Sanford, L.L. and Osman, S.F. 1980. Glycoalkaloids and resistance to the Colorado potato beetle in *Solanum Chacoense* Bitter. *American Potato Journal* 57:331–43.

Sinden, S.L., Sanford, L.L. and Webb, R.E. 1984. Genetic and environmental control of potato glycoalkaloids. *American Potato Journal* 61:141–56.

Smith, D.B., Roddick, J.G. and Jones, J.L. 1996. Potato glycoalkaloids: Some unanswered questions. *Trends in Food Science and Technology* 7:126–31.

Sotelo, A. and Serrano, B. 2000. High-performance liquid chromatographic determination of the glycoalkaloids α-solanine and α-chaconine in 12 commercial varieties of Mexican potato. *Journal of Agricultural and Food Chemistry* 48:2472–75.

Speroni, J.J. and Pell, E.J. 1980. Modified method for tuber glycoalkaloid and leaf glycoalkaloid analysis. *American Potato Journal* 57:537–42.

Sucha, L. and Tomsik, P. 2016. The steroidal glycoalkaloids from Solanaceae: Toxic effect, antitumour activity and mechanism of action. *Planta Medica* 82:379–87.

Sun, H., Lv, C., Yang, L., Wang, Y., Zhang, Q., Yu, S., Kong, H., Wang, M., Xie, J., Zhang, C. and Zhou, M. 2014. Solanine induces mitochondria-mediated apoptosis in human pancreatic cancer cells. *Bio Medical Research International* 2014:1–9.

Tajner-Czopek, A., Jarych-Szyszka, M. and Lisnska, G. 2008. Changes in glycoalkaloids content of potatoes destined for consumption. *Food Chemistry* 106:706–11.

Tajner-Czopek, A., Rytel, E., Aniołowska, M. and Hamouz, K. 2014. The influence of French fries processing on the glycoalkaloid content in coloured-fleshed potatoes. *European Food Research and Technology* 238:895–904.

Takagi, K., Toyoda, M., Fujiyama, Y. and Saito Y. 1990.Effect of cooking on the contents of a-chaconine and a-solanine in potatoes.*Shokuhin Eiseigaku Zasshi* 31:67–73.

Uluwaduge, D.I. 2018. Glycoalkaloids, bitter tasting toxicants in potatoes: A review. *International Journal of Food Science and Nutrition* 3:188–93.

Unverricht, W. 1937. Potatoes of high solanine content as the cause of illness. Clinical observations. *Ernahrung* 2:70–71.

Valkonen, J.P., Keskitalo, M., Vasara, T., Pietila, L. and Raman, K.V. 1996. Potato glycoalkaloids: A burden or a blessing? *Critical reviews in plant sciences* 15:1–20.

Wang, S.L., Bedford, C.L. and Thompson, N.R. 1972. Determination of glycoalkaloids in potatoes (S. tuberosum) with a bisolvent extraction method. *American Potato Journal* 49:302–8.

Widmann, N., Goian, M., Ianculov, I., Dumbrava, D. and Moldovan, C. 2008.Determination of the glycoalkaloids content from potato tubercules (*solanum tuberosum*). *Scientific Papers Animal Science and Biotechnologies* 41:807–13.

Wilson, G.S. 1959. A small outbreak of solanine poisoning. Monthly Bull. Ministry of Health & Pub.Health Lab. Service (directed by Medical Research Council) 18:207–10.

Yaksh, T.L. 1999. Spinal systems and pain processing: Development of novel analgesic drugs with mechanistically defined models. *Trends in Pharmacological Sciences* 20:329–37.

Yang, S.A., Paek, S.H., Kozukue, N., Lee, K.R. and Kim, J.A. 2006. α-Chaconine, a potato glycoalkaloid, induces apoptosis of HT-29 human colon cancer cells through caspase-3 activation and inhibition of ERK 1/2 phosphorylation. *Food and Chemical Toxicology* 44:839–846.

Yubin, J.I., Miao, Y., Bing, W. and Yao, Z. 2014.The extraction, separation and purification of alkaloids in the natural medicine. *Journal of Chemical and Pharmaceutical Research* 6:338–45.

Zwenger, C. and Kind, A. 1861.Ueber das Solanin und dessen Spaltungsproducte. *Justus Liebigs Annalen der Chemie* 118:129–51.

CHAPTER 5

# Oxalates

**Naveet Kaushal, Nitesh Sood, Talwinder Singh, Ajay Singh, Mandeep Kaur, and Mukul Sains**

## CONTENTS



DOI: 10.1201/9781003178446-5

## 5.1 INTRODUCTION

Oxalate is a naturally occurring substance or molecule which is normally found in some plant parts and humans. The previous term "oxalic acid" in addition to "oxalate" are preferred equivalently in nourishment studies. Humans can synthesize oxalate individually or attain it from foodstuffs. Although the metabolic role of oxalate in plants is vaguely known, it is proposed to be associated with germination of seed, calcium storage and their utilization, ion equilibrium, and structural strength of the living flora (Lane 1994). Calcium oxalate (CaOx) crystals are spread amongst the bottom liners of the autotrophic hierarchy, i.e., from minute algae to massive flowering plants. The plant cell that construct the pointed crystals are largely seen in the organelles named idioblasts (Foster 1956; Arnott 1982).

The name oxalic acid (ethanedioic acid) has been derived from the plant oxalis (wood sorrel) from it was originally derived (Liebman 2002). Calcium oxalate pictures were present on stone circles which were predicted by Justus Von Liebig in 1853 (Liebig et al. 1853). He investigated marble remains from the Parthenon (Athens, Greece) with the aim of obtaining a gloomy ochre shade, and revealed calcium oxalate stone to be a major fraction. He called this amalgam Theirschite, in honour of Friedrich Von Theirsch, the restorer of the scientific compilation of Bavaria who give him the limestone specimen. Thierschite and Whewellite were proved to be at par to each other (Frondel and Thierschite 1962).

The formation of natural crystal is the most primitive process connecting its roots to the formation, progression, and assurance of life on planet Earth. It is assumed that the life initiated with pyrite, which, once positively charged, can associate negatively charged bio molecules and consequently will get managed, resulting in huge natural chains in the evolution which will be converted into complex natural molecules (Wachtershauser 1988; Keller et al. 1994). Although the process with which crystal-originated life is not yet clear, it is true that the organisms of different kingdoms are regularly forming crystal diversification. Organisms have calcium salt crystals which are prevalent in birds, eggs shell algae, fungi, flora, and fauna; these are meant for sensing for support, defence, and protection, and the uniqueness of these crystal formationals is their association with protein mediation (Cuellar-Cruz 2017). There is a typical amount of inorganic-type crystals found mainly in the cellular structure within the cell wall, whose chemical composition is made from bimolecular-like proteins, carbohydrates, nucleic acids, and other minerals (Colfen 2010; Elejalde et al. 2020).

## 5.2 CHEMISTRY

Oxalate, which is a salt formed from oxalic acid, is a di-anion compound with an existing formula of $C_2O_4^{2-}$ (Gemede and Ratta 2014). It exists with two carbonyl groups in them and, based on

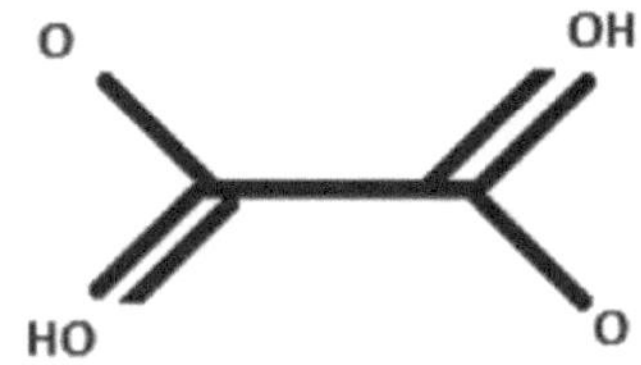


**Figure 5.1** Oxalate structure

dimension, it gives vibration motion with both on symmetrical and asymmetrical pattern (Colthrup 1990) (Figure 5.1).

Calcium oxalate crystals are extensive both in flowering monocotyledons and dicotyledons. Due to its variable shape, calcium oxalate is easily observable in young growing tissues. In monocotyledon, calcium oxalate mainly exists in raphide, styloid, and druse shapes. Anatomical investigations specified that the raphide biology and their development in precise locations inside the cell are hereditarily restricted (Horner and Wagner 1995). The main factors which are considered in differentiating raphide include dimensions, cross-section, and morphology, which are mainly affected by the taxonomical origin of the plant.

Structurally, raphides are mostly intracellular infinite, thin, enedacerate crystals, generally established in a particular structure (commonly known as idioblasts) of parenchymatous tissues. Although rare but extracellular crystals are also reported. (Barabé et al. 2004). Having specialized for the collection of the crystals in itself, idioblasts may show variations in size, shape, and composition even from the accompanying cells in the single tissue (Gallaher 1975; Sunell and Healey 1981). Idioblasts can be protective and non-protective in nature. The non-protective type has unorganized crystal arrangement as compared to the protective one (Sunell and Healey 1985). There are mainly four types of raphides:

1. **Type I:** Most prevalent in nature with four-sided single crystals having two balanced sharp edges (Figure 5.2).
2. **Type II:** These are tetragonal with a pointed end and one bidentate or branched terminal (Prychid and Rudall 1999). Being rare, it has been demonstrated only in the *Vitaceae* family (Cody and Horner 1983; Webb 1999). The bidentate end is created by crystal pairing (Figure 5.2) (Arnott and Webb 2000).
3. **Type III:** This third form can be hexagonal or octagonal in shape with regular acute ends. These are recognized in *Agavaceae* (Wattendorff 1976), *Typhaceae* (Horner et al. 1981), and *Dioscoreaceae* (Figure 5.2).
4. **Type IV:** The fourth type of raphide form involves paired crystals with H-shaped irregular terminals (Figure 5.2). Specifically, the first is wedge-shaped and the other is extremely pointed (Bradbury and Nixon 1998; Kostman and Franceschi 2000).

Moreover, the crystals are also present in the form of druses or styloids. Both Druses and styloids not often arise jointly except in *Araceae* in which all three types are recorded (Prychid and Rudall 1999). Calcium oxalate crystals mainly arise, moreover, in a monohydrate (whewellite) type or a di- (or tri-) hydrate (Weddellitte) form (Arnott 1981) (Figure 5.3).

Oxalate is also known by other names like ethanedioate, oxalate ion, and ethanedioic acid.

## 5.3 BIOSYNTHESIS

### 5.3.1 Biosynthesis of Soluble Crystals

To date, several pathways for the formation of oxalic acid have been proposed. In one process, this noxious organic acid can be produced through the oxidation of glycolate and glyoxylate by the

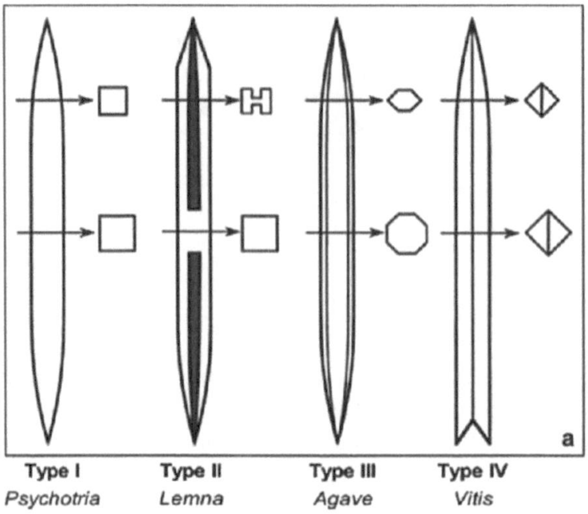


**Figure 5.2** Diagram showing the four basic types of raphide cross sections. (Reproduced from Saadi and Mondal 2012.)

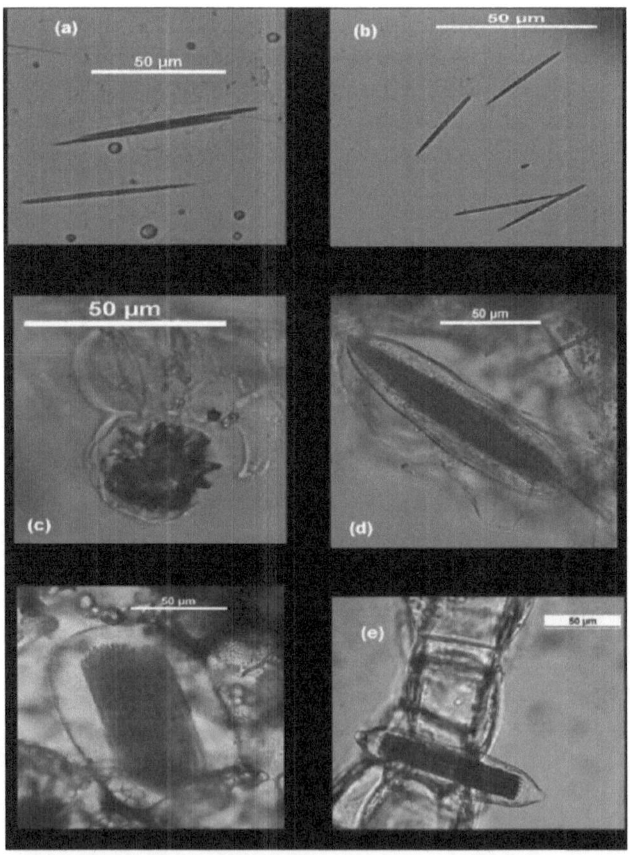


**Figure 5.3** (a) Calcium oxalate crystal (Raphide) of *Colocasia esculenta* from petiole; (b) Calcium oxalate crystal of *C. esculenta* from root; (c) Druse of *C. esculenta* from petiole; (d) Idioblast of *C. esculenta* from storage organ; (e) Idioblast of *C. esculenta* from petiole. (Reproduced from Saadi and Mondal 2012.)

action of enzyme, glycolate oxidase. These substrates may be produced as a by-product of photorespiration in photosynthetically active tissues, and glycolate oxidase, a peroxisomal enzyme, which is reasonably profuse in green tissues. Moreover, isocitrate lyase action on isocitrate and oxidation of oxaloacetate, are chiefly held responsible for the escalating levels of the oxalates. Although the enzyme involved in conversion of L-ascorbic acid into oxalate is unknown, the contribution of the vitamin cannot be denied. *Averrhoa carambola*, a member of *Oxalidaeae* family, has a high percentage of oxalic acid. After consuming, its direct relation has been confirmed with the development of acute renal injury (ARI) by the release of free radicals (Shimizu et al. 2017). The soluble forms (sodium, potassium, ammonium oxalate) and insoluble forms (calcium oxalate) are derived from oxalic acid in vegetation across the globe (Nguimezong et al. 2014).

### 5.3.2 Biosynthesis of Insoluble Oxalate

The non-dissolvable form of calcium, calcium oxalate (CaOx) crystals, is considered universal in the plants. CaOx crystals are deposited via bio-mineralization progression in several trends. The crystals are localized either in intra-vacuolar membrane or in idioblasts (Figure 5.4). The crystal development is directly concerned to membranes, compartments, or inclusion bodies present in the vacuole and proteins, specifically calsequestrin, which modulate the function of calcium of cytosol prior to its vacuolar storage (Prasad and Shivay 2017). Kinetically, after attaining the desired concentration of oxalic acid, oxalate oxidase gets charged and the oxalic acid load gets regulated, and hence contributes in crystal designing. These crystals have different surfaces, including druses,

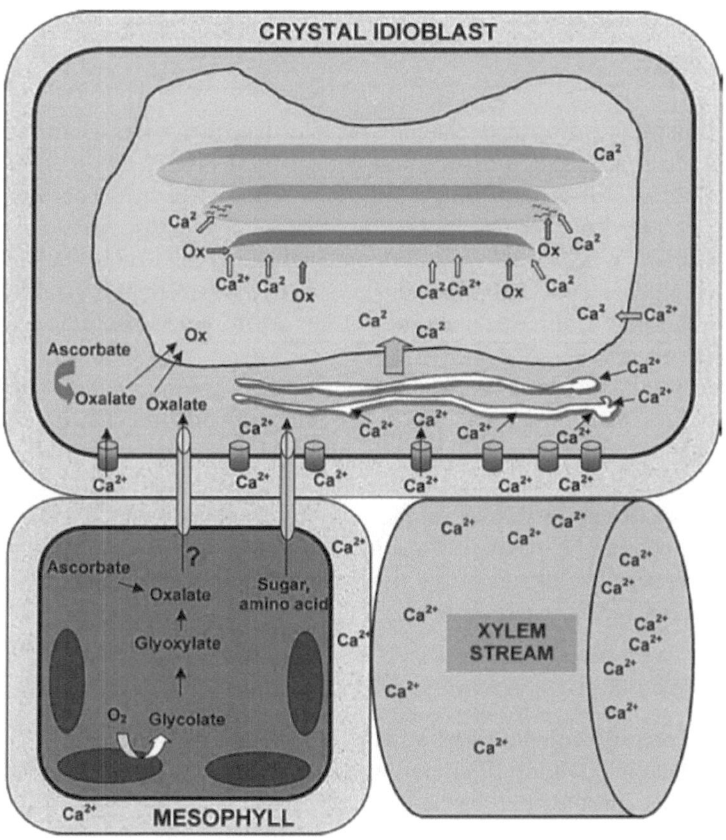


**Figure 5.4** Synthesis of calcium oxalate crystals in idioblasts. (Reprinted from Cruz et al. 2020.)

crystal, sand, styliods, etc. (Cadena et al. 2020). The overall functions of these crystals is to make the plant safe and secure from the external harmful agencies like grazing animals.

On the other hand, oxalates are also present in natural abundance.

### 5.3.3 Occurrence of Oxalate

Alkali and alkaline-earth oxalates that include natroxalate and ammonium oxalates are the common oxalates in nature.

#### 5.3.3.1 *Nitroxalate*

Being only naturally available as $Na_2(C_2O_4)$, its commercial production is ensured from the hemicellulosic component of sawdust, which is facilitated with NaOH. The decomposition of the resulting formate yield the oxalate, or by reaction of $CO_2$ with sodium amalgam (Baran 2014).

#### 5.3.3.2 *Ammonium Oxalate*

The fusion of this oxalate is very effortless, as it can be obtained by result of solutions of oxalic acid with aerated ammonium or bicarbonate. The configuration of the made $(NH_4)_2(C_2O_4) \cdot H_2O$ has been reported by unrelated authors in the past (Baran and Monje 2008; Hendricks and Jefferson 1936; Jeffrey and Parry 1952) and afterward polished by cold (30 K) diffraction dimensions (Robertson 1965), complemented by 3-D neutron and X-ray structural studies of both the protonated and deuterated forms (Taylor and Sabine 1972).

#### 5.3.3.3 *Whewellite*

The sandstone Whewellite, hydrated calcium oxalate, has the systemic formula $CaC_2O_4{\cdot}H_2O$. Because of its crude concentration association with natural origin, this matter is backed by its occurrence in coal and sedimentary lump. Still, it is reported in hydrothermal plants wherever a genetic relation is sceptical. For this motive, it could be classed as true sandstone. Whewellite is named after William Whewell (1794–1866), an English polymath, ornithologist, and scientist, professor of ethical thinking at Cambridge, and creator of the system of crystallographic indexing. It is normally established in three major types of lay down: near-surface/natural; digenetic, and hydrothermal occurrences.

Natural surfaces like snow peaks and genetic occurrences are reported to start with earth loam, crust, rocks, rusty ores, current sea, and non-aquatic deposits and manure. In all these media, the relationship of oxalate forms with organic matter has presented a comprehensible resource of oxalate existence.

In ancestral digenetic territory, Whewellite is closely associated with residue sequences rich in carbon such as coal beds and dark shells. In aquatic habitat, it occurs as a late-phase in aqua channels in which highly sensitive druses of the limestone become visible, often related to carbonates and sulfides (Hofmann and Bernasconi 1998).

#### 5.3.3.4 *Weddellitte*

It was first and foremost a minute-sized variety recognized at the bottom of the Weddell Sea (Antarctica) (Bannister and Discov 1936) and was soon exposed in whole from Western Australia, Southern England, and unusual areas of the United States of America. This crystal was formulated as $Ca\ (C_2O_4) \cdot (2 + x)\ H_2O$, where $0 < x \leq 0.5$, and the limited waters of hydration are of a catalyst nature (Baran and Monje 2008; Young and Brown 1982).

**Table 5.1 Major Classes of Natural Reserves of Different Oxalate with Different Name of Compositions**

| Mineral Name | Chemical Composition | Crystal System | Colour |
|---|---|---|---|
| Weddellite | $Ca(C_2O_4){\cdot}2H_2O$ | Tetragonal | Colourless to white, may be yellowish brown to brown from impurities |
| Whewellite | $CaC_2O_4{\cdot}H_2O$ | Monoclinic | Colourless, yellowish, brownish |
| Wheatleyite | $Na_2Cu^{II}(C_2O_4)_2{\cdot}2H_2O$ | Triclinic | Bright blue |
| Kyanoxalite | $Na_7[(Al_{5\text{-}6}Si_{6\text{-}7}O_{24})(C_2O_4)_{0.5-1}]{\cdot}5H_2O$ | Hexagonal | Pale bluish |
| Lindbergite | $Mn^{2+}(C_2O_4) \cdot 2H_2O$ | Monoclinic | White to greyish white |
| Moolooite | $Cu(C_2O_4) \cdot 0.4H_2O$ | Orthorhombic | ---------------- |
| Oxamite | $(NH_4)_2(C_2O_4){\cdot}H_2O$ | ---------------- | ---------------- |
| Caoxite | $Ca(C_2O_4) \cdot 3H_2O$ | Triclinic | Colourless |
| Natroxalate | $Na_2(C_2O_4)$ | Monoclinic | ------------- |
| Glushinskite | $Mg(C_2O_4) \cdot 2H_2O$ | Monoclinic | ---------------- |
| Humboldtine | $Fe^{2+}(C_2O_4) \cdot 2H_2O$ | Monoclinic | Yellow to amber-yellow |
| Stepanovite | $NaMgFe^{III}(C_2O_4)3{\cdot}8\text{–}9H_2O$ | Trigonal | Light green |
| Zhemchuzhnikovite | $NaMg(Al,Fe^{III})(C_2O_4)_3{\cdot}8H_2O$ | Trigonal | Smokey-green (daylight), violet (artificial light) |
| Coskrenite | $(Ce,Nd,La)_2(SO_4)_2(C_2O_4){\cdot}8H_2O$ | Triclinic | Usually pale pink under incandescent light, to cream-colored |

#### *5.3.3.5 Caoxite*

Its possible source was initially recognized in the Cerchiara pit near Faggiona, Eastern Liguria (Italy), connected with quartz, barite, and an anonymous manganese oxide (Basso et al. 1997; Jambor et al. 1998). Few other carboxylate raw materials, i.e., oxalate, formate, and acetate natural resources revealed the major class of unrefined reserves, and in middle, the oxalates are the main stream major assembly, with 14 unrelated kinds reported so far, along with 3 freshly reported sulfato–oxalates and 1 silico–aluminate–oxalato genus (Table 5.1).

Moreover, oxalates can be grouped into two classes on basis of solubility, i.e., soluble and insoluble oxalates.

## 5.4 DISTRIBUTION OF OXALATE

The oxalates are dispersed universally and their presence has been noticed in the following fields:

### 5.4.1 Atmosphere

The role of atmosphere in the itinerary of oxalic acid cannot be denied in whole. Being passive samplers, exposed architectural designs and its non-chosen areas ensnare all accumulated materials, such as oxalic acid, which is localized in the troposphere, in down pour and hail, and may be a photo-oxidation outcome of gas and vapour-hydro-carbons from vehicle pollution (Norton et al. 1983; Kawamura and Kaplan 1987; Martinelango et al. 2005). Oxalic and other dicarboxylic acids are fairly related with humidity, and consequently, an undeniable chelation on metallics is reported (Kawamura and Kaplan 1987). It was suggested that the origin of oxalic acid from non-renewable sources of energy ought to be retraced. Its reaction as a carbonate substratum in historic buildings contributes to calcium oxalate, that might be opted by the sulphates of the aerosols (Saiz-Jimenez 1989). Moreover, calcium oxalate presence was confirmed on the supports of the museum paintings facing the ocean as being non-carbonate, the acid held in air, have reacted with the calcium rich dust particles settled silicate supports (Casadio et al. 2013) (Tables 5.2a and 5.2b).

### 5.4.2 Food

Having the roots down in the ancient times, oxalic acid was originally cut off (separated) from timber sorrel. Oxalic acid salts are present in the roots of rhubarb plants. It is recognized for its curative properties (Sarma et al. 2010). The consumption of pomegranate is proven to have an inductive effect on the brain's oxidative harm caused by the oxalates and averts Giardiasis and obesity (Kochkoul et al. 2020). Pomegranate fruit remains a more different source of bioactive phenolic compounds, predominantly phenolic acids, flavonoids, anthocyanins, and tannins to counter the negative oxalates effects (Brighenti et al. 2016). The saturated and unsaturated oils are also the primary source in the seeds (Mena et al. 2012; Russo et al. 2018). The domestic supply of oxalate, embrace vitamin C, protein (from side to side assimilation of the amino acids hydroxylase, tryptophan, arginine, and hydroxyproline) and the instantaneous precursor of oxalate, such as L-glycerate

**Table 5.2a Insoluble Oxalates in Nature**

| S.no | Compound Name | Insoluble Formula | Reference |
|---|---|---|---|
| 1. | Aluminum Oxalate | $Al_2(C_2O_4)_3{\cdot}H_2O$ | Perry (2011) |
| 2. | Barium oxalate | $BaC_2O_4$ | Money and Davis (1938) |
| 3. | Bismuth oxalate | $Bi_2(C_2O_4)_3$ | Rumble et al. (2018) |
| 4. | Calcium oxalate | $CaC_2O_4$ | Rumble et al. (2018) |
| 5. | Cerous oxalate | $Ce(C_2O_4)_3{\cdot}9H_2O$ | Rumble et al. (2018) |
| 6. | Cobalt oxalate | $CoC_2O_4{\cdot}2H_2O$ | Rumble et al. (2018) |
| 7. | Cupric oxalate | $CuC_2O_4{\cdot}0.5H_2O$ | Rumble et al. (2018) |
| 8. | Ferrous oxalate | $FeC_2O_4{\cdot}2H_2O$ | Rumble et al. (2018) |
| 9. | Lanthanum Oxalate Hydrate | $La_2(C_2O_4)_3{\cdot}xH_2O$ | Perry (2011) |
| 10. | Lead oxalate | $PbC_2O_4$ | Rumble et al. (2018) |
| 11. | Magnesium oxalate | $MgC_2O_4$ | Rumble et al. (2018) |
| 12. | Manganese oxalate | $MnC_2O_4{\cdot}2H_2O$ | Rumble et al. (2018) |
| 13. | Mercury oxalate | $Hg_2C_2O_4$ | Rumble et al. (2018) |
| 14. | Nickle oxalate dehydrate | $NiC_2O_4{\cdot}2H_2O$ | Rumble et al. (2018) |
| 15. | Silver oxalate | $Ag_2C_2O_4$ | Rumble et al. (2018) |
| 16. | Strontium oxalate | $SrC_2O_4{\cdot}2H_2O$ | Rumble et al. (2018) |
| 17. | Stannous oxalate | $SnC_2O_4$ | Rumble et al. (2018) |
| 18. | Yttrium oxalate | $Y_2(C_2O_4)_3{\cdot}9H_2O$ | Perry (2011) |
| 19. | Zinc oxalate | $ZnC_2O_4{\cdot}2H_2O$ | Rumble et al. (2018) |

**Table 5.2b Soluble Oxalates in Nature**

| S.No | Compound Name | Soluble Formula | Reference |
|---|---|---|---|
| 1. | Beryllium Oxalate Trihydrate | $BeC_2O_4{\cdot}3H_2O$ | Rumble et al. (2018) |
| 2. | Chromium acetate hydrate | $CrC_2O_4{\cdot}H_2O$ | Rumble et al. (2018) |
| 3. | Iron oxalate | $Fe_2(C_2O_4)_3$ | Rumble et al. (2018) |
| 4. | Lithium oxalate | $Li_2C_2O_4$ | Rumble et al. (2018) |
| 5. | Potassium oxalate | $K_2C_2O_4$ | Rumble et al. (2018) |
| 6. | Sodium oxalate | $Na_2C_2O_4$ | Rumble et al. (2018) |
| 7. | Titanium sesquioxalate | $Ti_2(C_2O_4)_3{\cdot}10H_2O$ | Perry (2011) |
| 8. | Vanadyl oxalate | $VOC_2O_4$ | William (1972) |

glycolate and glyoxylate (Fargue et al. 2016). Both lethal and non-lethal toxin by rhubarb foliage is contemplation to be begin by lethal anthraxquin, one glycoside, rather oxalate. Moreover, there are a lot of types of food that contain extensive sum of oxalates like in spinach (0.320 to 1.29%), beet leaves (0.30% to 1.00%), tea (0.30% to 2.00%) and coco (0.50% to 0.90). Furthermore, some other foods own recognized to contain high quantities of oxalate concentrations with some nuts having 42–469 mg/100 g (Ritter and Savage 2007) and flour contains (37–269 mg/100 g) (Chai and Liebman 2005). Chocolate, kiwi fruits, wheat burns, strawberry have also known to be an noticeable exogenous supply of oxalates (Noonan and Savage 1999; Charriere and Imdorf 2002).

### 5.4.3 Meat

Oxalic acid absorption tendency is found elevated in the vegetarian options than in animal protein, that could be assumed as oxalate-free when low-oxalate diets are being planned for the patients (Massey et al. 1993). On the other hand, a species of snail (*Limicolaria aurora*), consumed in Nigeria, has been disclosed to have 381 mg/100 g dry weight (DW) of oxalate (Udoh et al. 1995). The mollusc, dog whelk (*Thaiscattifera*), carries an ever-superior level of oxalate, 1,686 mg/100 g DW (Udoh et al. 1995). Hence, the high consumption of the foresaid organisms can elevate the levels of oxalate in the body which is highly harmful for the consumer.

### 5.4.4 Plants

Foliar calcium oxalate, exists in two elemental states, associated with variation in the level of humidity. These two forms that are in fact two divergent mineral deposits: Whewellite, the monohydrated calcium oxalate, $CaC_2O_4.H_2O$, and Weddellitte, calcium oxalate dry out, $CaC_2O_4.2H_2O$ (Gaines et al. 1998). CaOx crystals are normally found in plants are made from endogenous integration of oxalic acid and exogenous calcium from the top loam that will get in touch with plant roots. To shape a crystal, the loam is supposed to be in unbalanced and supersaturated conditions. The series of structures of CaOx complexes is literally vast and holds block-like rhombohedra or prismatic crystals, which can be originated as single or in multiples per cell. The groups of pointed (acerose) raphides which are mentioned as crystal sand, and the broad multifarious crystals are included in druses (frequently single but numerous can also be present per cell). The hydration state of the crystal, the calcium/oxalate proportion and impurities play a pivotal role in the structural evolution of CaOx crystals (Guo et al. 2002; Ouyang et al. 2003; Ryall et al. 2000; Touryan et al. 2004). Involvement of an idioblast having a druse in the soft mesophyll, of a transactional illustration of a leaf of *Armeniaca manshurica* (*Prunus* genus) was confirmed (Dosuzeva 1969). Nine genus of *Prunus* in a survey of timber framework of Rosacea. Out of which eight lacked crystals; only in *P. ursina* he saw standard-sized druses, one per cell, specifically in axial parenchyma cells (Zhang 1992). Moreover, family *Cactaceae* is one of highest crystal accumulators of the plant kingdom. A variation in the composition and the variety of the crystals has been represented by it. The species under *Pereskioideae* and *Opuntioideae* sub-family form calcium oxalate monohydrate (COM, Whewellite), whereas the *Cereoideae* species form preferably calcium oxalate dihydrate (COD, Weddellitte) crystals whereas some species take the midway, i.e., they form mixed crystals of COM and COD (Hartl et al. 2007).

Plants may contain some amount of noxious elements that can cause illness or toxicity in any human and animals, are referred as venomous vegetation (Aplin 1976). Since the oxalate crystals are reported in vegetative, reproductive, storage space, meristems in photorespiration and non-photosynthetic tissues. Consequently, the toxicity may be in root, corm, tuber, stem, twigs, fruit, kernel, pollen, nectar, or sap. Oxalate rich foods are typically insignificant in earlier human diets but from time to time, are vital in regular diets. Timber sorrel, a high-oxalate eatable, is known to cause an injury to grazing livestock (Noonan and Savage 1999). In many plants, oxalate are metabolized very gradually or not static but infer a noxious effect when collective amounts are calculated (Franceshi and Horner 1980). Consequently, plants might opt for crystal development to eliminate excess of oxalate or calcium (Çaliskan 2000). Numerous tasks have been allocated to calcium oxalate crystals in plants such as contributing in calcium equilibrium, load space of calcium (Franceschi 1989), abrupt elemental withdrawal, light congregation along with mirror reflection (Franceschi and Horner 1980), and defence against insects and foraging fauna. These sharp structures guard plants with a considerable load of chemicals or (Rupali et al. 2012). Consequently, the consumption of such toxic flora can cause lethality to the grazing fauna. Conversely, receptiveness of fauna to toxin oxalate depends on factors such as compound form of the oxalate, maturity level of animal to scavenge oxalate-rich food, other dietary components (Rahman and Kawamura 2011)

### 5.4.5 Other Biological Systems

The existence of supplementary clinging oxalates is enormously unusual in genetic systems, even though the relevant copper, magnesium, and manganese complexes are found in rare lichens, while expected ammonium oxalate. Lately, guano remains have been reported to contain oxamite.

### 5.4.6 Fungi

Over one hundred years ago, Anton de Bary (1887) stated that "Calcium oxalate is a substance generally found in the fungi that it is unnecessary to enumerate the instances of its occurrence". He pointed out that the walls of *Agaricus campestris* were so encrusted that the mycelia appeared chalky. Shortly, Hein (1930) described the mycelia of *A. campestris* as having a broad covering of needle-shaped crystals. Moreover, *Aspergillus niger*, *Penicillium*, *Mucor*, *Boletus sulfurens*, and *Sclerotinia* can synthesize oxalic acid to an amount of 4–5 g/100 g dry weight (DW) (Fassett 1973; Gontzea and Sutzescu 1968). The giant mushroom (*Tricholoma giganteum*), an edible fungi, is stated to restrain 89 mg/100 g oxalic acid (Fujita et al. 1991). Numerous genus of mushrooms, like termite and ear mushrooms, were reported to be full of 80–220 g oxalate/1,000 g DW (Aletor 1995). It is fascinating to note that all the observation of calcium oxalate crystal and granule of many common fungi report their encrustation in hyphae but never report the occurrence of oxalate in the fruiting bodies, the edible portion of most of these fungi.

### 5.4.7 Insects and Microbes

Since the last two decades, bee keepers are experiencing major losses due to Colony Collapse Disorder (CCD) in which the bees are not able to form the comb. Initially, it was supposed that blood-sucker *Varroa destructor* (*V. destructor*, Varroa) mite is a chief force of honey bees' (*Apis mellifera*) settlement fatalities (Goulson et al. 2015). Consequently, the keepers were using oxalic acid as a potent miticite in order to kill this insect (Rosenkranz et al. 2010). But during last year, Varrora has shown the resistivity towards the treatment that has fumed the investigations of the responsible adaptability. As a result, it was investigated that one of the actinobacteria, *Bifidobacterium asteroides*, a common commensal in mite *A. mellifera* is oxalotrophous. Hence, the earlier treatment of these mites has now proved to be failed and the scientists are in the direction of finding more potent solution to control these destructors (Maddaloni and Pascual 2015).

## 5.5 MECHANISM OF ACTION OF OXALATE

Ethylene glycol oxidizes with glycolic acid which is in turn oxidized to oxalic acid which is toxic both for renal and coronary aspects. Renal lethality is associated with the fatal anabolism of oxalic acid, which settles down in the kidney in the shape of calcium oxalate crystals and is believed to exercise injury to the renal tubules. The examination of renal oxalate crystals in animal along with case studies of human being kidney and bladder gravel, confirmed their connection with dietetic oxalates and other oxalate precursors (Corley et al. 2005).

The crystals formed either in renal tubular solution or in the renal interstitial solution is pure with respect to its ingredients, which in turn may be a meaning of increased emission of stone-forming molecules, less urine quantity, an alteration in urine pH, or an amalgamation of these factors (Coe et al. 1992). The urine and, in all prospects, the tubular solution of stone formers is often added highly pure than that of standard healthy adults, with partiality nucleation and development of crystals (Lemann et al. 1996). Long-term build-up of additional elements, crystalline as well as natural medium, developed the clinical stones (Ratkalkar and Kleinman 2011). To be concise, urine in such situations is composed of tubular solution at some serious point in the nephron where the surgical procedures are the last resort (Ratkalkar and Kleinman 2011)

## 5.6 TOXICITY OF OXALATES

The intestinal pH does not allow the oxalate to get solubalize in its juice and it sticks to calcium to form calcium oxalate crystals. It hinders the absorption of calcium in animals resulting in diseases like Rickets and Osteomalacia.

While oxalic acid is a standard final product of mammalian anabolism, the ingestion of supplementary oxalic acid may result in stone development in the urinary tract when it is evacuated in the urine. The mean daily consumption of oxalate in the diet in the UK has been estimated to be 70–150 mg.

A diet with large intake of oxalate and low calcium and iron, is not recommended. Vegetarians and lactose intolerant persons are prone to kidney stones. The vegetarians being feeding on the plant based food, assimilate more oxalates, which may diminish calcium accessibility. The women are more prone to these clinical conditions particularly who require greater amounts of calcium in the diet. In dynamic individuals, the infrequent consumption of high-oxalate foods as fragment of a balanced diet does not stand any particular problem. Glycolate is an imperative ancestor of oxalic acid and its alteration to oxalate intensifies vitamin $B_6$ deficiency. Legumes like lentils, kidney beans, and white beans have been evaluated for oxalate. The maximum and minimum contents are present in Anasazi beans (80 mg, 100 g, 100 $g^{-1}$ wet weight) and black-eyed peas (4 mg, 100 g, 100 $g^{-1}$ wet weight).

The establishment of strong bonds among oxalic acid and various other minerals like calcium, magnesium, sodium, and potassium result in development of oxalate salts. The salts like calcium oxalate are unsolvable and thus have a propensity to participate, leading to formation of kidney stone. The oxalic acid results in formation of water soluble salts with $Na^+$, $K^+$, and $NH^+$ ions. Oxalic acid binds with $Ca^{2+}$, $Fe^{2+}$, and $Mg^{2+}$ resulting in its unavailability to the animals (Gemede and Ratta 2014). The oxidative stress can be held responsible the damage of all the essential bio compounds like proteins, DNA, and membrane lipids, and can result in cell death (Tandon et al. 2005). The superoxide ions have also been recognized as stimulators of oncogenes such as Jun and Fos genes (Rahman et al. 2012). Substantial calcium oxalate levels in kidneys are the most likely to be reason of the renal toxicity of ethylene glycol poisoning (Cruzan et al. 2004; Friedman et al. 1962; Jacobsen and McMartin 1986). The creation of free radicals and lipid per oxidation (Scheid et al. 1996; Thamilselvan and Khan 1998), resulting in cell necrosis and apoptosis, is also associated with oxalate poisoning (Khan et al. 1999; Miller et al. 2000). Being declared unstable by the US government in 2017, the two scrupulous oxalates-mercury oxalate and silver oxalate are to be placed in strict supervision (Bureau of Alcohol 2019). According to some experts, these oxalates are noted likely to explode as TNT (trinitrotoluene), RDX (hexogen), and HMX (octogen), but protection vulnerability; and harsh safety measures are big concerns.

## 5.7 RECOMMENDATIONS FOR OXALATE USAGE

Calcium oxalate crystals can gather in almost all the major vital organs causing severe damage and a whole consumption of 5–15 g of oxalic acid may cause fatality. 1 $mg/m^3$ with an 8-h time window is the suggested official limit for oxalic acid fumes. 500 $mg/m^3$ levels are extremely life threatening for the workers.

1. Skin or eye contact with oxalate results in pain and burning and the level of severities directly proportional to the duration of oxalate exposure.
2. Breathing can be coupled with swelling in oesophagus with persist and cough. Pneumonitis or pulmonary edema can also occur in severity.
3. Soluble oxalates, when infused cause weakness, tetany, convulsions, and cardiac arrest due to extreme levels of calcium depletion.
4. 10% calcium solution is prescribed as antidote to neutralize characteristic low calcium levels in the body.

## 5.8 IDENTIFICATION AND QUANTIFICATION

At present, a variety of reliable procedures are being announced to estimate oxalates in foodstuff. These embrace ion chromatography, gas chromatography, high-performance fluid chromatograph, enzymatic process, capillary electrophoresis, and chemiluminescence finding, etc. Few procedures are made available elevated consideration and specificity but also have drawbacks such as prolonged, complex act and them to quite large errors. The methods are:

### 5.8.1 Titration Using $KMnO_4$

Since this response is speedy, potassium permanganate ($KMnO_4$) is extensively considered as a reactant for estimation of oxalic acid (AOAC 1990). In acidic aqueous solution, $MnO_4^-$ with oxalic acid ($HO_2CCO_2H$) produces $Mn^{2+}$ and $CO_2$:

$$\underset{\text{Purple}}{MnO_4^-(aq)} + HO_2CCO_2H(aq) \rightarrow \underset{\text{Colorless}}{Mn^{2+}(aq)} + CO_2(g) + H_2O(l) \quad (5.1)$$

The oxalate was calculated by means of stoichiometric formula. The soluble oxalate was reduced from entirety oxalate to attain insoluble oxalate; both soluble and insoluble oxalates were expressed on dry weight basis (DW) (Kasimala et al. 2018). This method was used to estimate oxalate in *L. batatas* with the minimum of 20.3 mg/100 g FW whereas *Amarathus* sp. foliage has the maximum of 91.8 mg/100 g in it (Savage 2000). Although this was exploited for oxalate estimation since ancient times but high oxidation value of titrant, particularly in acidic medium, makes the researcher to give it a second thought. Thus, the food samples cannot be used as substrate in this procedure. Appearance of dark green coloration in the extract treated with few drops of glacial acetic confirms the presence of oxalates in the sample (Table 5.3).

### 5.8.2 Capillary Electrophoresis

Spinach, a widely used leafy vegetable, carries a large amount of oxalates, thus this vegetable has often been examined as a latent foundation in the determination of oxalates (Jaworska 2005a; b; Stagnari et al. 2007). It is probably a dominant practice for negative ions determination, because it enables fast estimation and fair organization price. Anions inserted into the capillary shift near the anode origin of their unresponsive accuse while electro osmotic flood (EOF) is usually headed towards the cathode, it is appropriate to undo it allowing anions' co-migration. This objective has been often attained by

**Table 5.3 Oxalate Content (mg/100g FW) of the Samples**

| S.No | Botanical name | Local Name | Oxalate (mg/100 g FW) |
|---|---|---|---|
| 1 | *Theobroma cacao* | Raw cocoa | 624 |
| 2 | *Camellia sinensis* | Tea | 300–2000 |
| 3 | *Solanum tuberosum* | Irish potato | 32.50 |
| 4. | *Ipomea batatas L.* | Sweet potato | 20.30 |
| 5 | *Discorea alta* | White yam | 24.30 |
| 6. | *Discorea rotundata* | Yellow yam | 33.80 |
| 7. | *Petroselinum crispum* | Parsley | 166 |
| 8. | *Triticum vulgare* | Wheat grain | 27.00 |
| 9. | *Soja hispida* | Soya bean | 85.10 |
| 10. | *Amarathus* | Spinach vegetable | 91.90 |

**Table 5.4 Quantitative Analysis of Oxalate in Vegetables**

| Vegetables | Oxalate Content (mg/g[1]-1) |
|---|---|
| Fresh spinach leaves | 15.229 |
| Ready-to-eat spinach | 19.765 |
| Frozen spinach | 9.777 |
| Fresh chard (leaves) | 16.022 |
| Frozen chard | 11.344 |

performing a covering of the capillary by the accumulating additives together the surroundings electrolyte (Chai et al. 2008). This outcome system has been abundantly implemented in investigation of special vegetables like spinach, chard, and carrot. The analysis of beet sugar, cane sugar, white refined cane sugar, grape sugar, dextrose, and the foods with large quantity of sugar, such as squash and cakes are blended with considerable amount of dietary fibers, can be possible base of nitrates' and oxalate ingestion that has never been estimated earlier. Since there are no recommended guidelines about' oxalate content in food items, it may denote a hazard when consumed by babies (Merusi et al. 2010) (Table 5.4).

Total oxalates' content estimated in all samples is with agreement with the literature (Conte et al. 2008; Jaworska 2005b).

### 5.8.3 Oxidation Method

Oxalic acid can be prepared in the lab by oxidation of sugar using nitric acid in the presence of catalytic vanadium pentoxide. On the other hand, it can be freely bought as the dehydrate or anhydrate, which it formed with mono or dihydration (Dollimore and Konieczay 1998). Water solubility is only expressed by alkali metal salts of oxalic acid. The capability of oxalic acid to form metal complexes is apparent in the precipitation of calcium oxalate, resulting in kidney stones formation. In the gas phase, metal oxalate groups are readily produced and bound with both indifferent and positive electro-spray collection spectrometry (Kim and Beauchamp 2007; Kim et al. 2006a, 2006b). In 2005, lithium oxalate anion was formulated and reported the evolution of $CO_2$ and CO by CID assortment spectrometry, making LiO, the sturdiest base known to date (Tian 2008).

### 5.8.4 Enzymatic Decarboxylation

A novel enzyme from the wood rot fungus *Cotybia velutipes*, that precisely decarboxylates oxalic acid to produce stoichiometric amounts of formic acid and carbon dioxide(Shimazono and Hayaishi 1957).

$$\begin{array}{l}\text{COOH}\\ |\\ \text{COOH}\end{array} \longrightarrow \text{HCOOH} + \text{CO}_2 \qquad (5.2)$$

The exceptional features of this enzyme are being maximally dynamic at pH 3.0 with highest stability at pH 4.5. However, like other oxalate decarboxylase in plants and bacteria, it does not require Adenosine Tri Phosphate, coenzyme A, thiamine pyrophosphate, acetate, magnesium ion, nor it is oxygen-dependent, though its catalytic action needs oxygen. Hydro quinine remains inactive in anaerobic conditions but it shoots the reaction by 60–100% in aerobic conditions. Mediator-cysteine and chelator EDTA, have next to nil effect up to range of 10 to 10 mol/litre. Oxalates in beer were determined by foresaid method in the year 1961 (Haas and Fleishman 1961).

Both white and brown rot fungi have intracellular oxalate decarboxylase which facilitates decarboxylation of oxalate to form $CO_2$.Moreover, *P. chrysosporium* decarboxylates oxalate is with the LiP (Lignin peroxidase) system. Lineweaver-Burk plot indicates that lignin degradation by LiP is greatly affected as long as both veratryl alcohol and oxalic acid are gathering in the common site, since $H_20_2$ is also depleted by this system Therefore, lignin degradation or veratryl alcohol oxidation is managed by the level of oxalate on one side and cleansing of the metabolite is affected by VAP or LiP activity on the other. Hence, VAP (veratryl alcohol peroxidase) or "Lip" plays an crucial physiological role in hunting toxic oxalate derived initially from wood carbohydrates during the white rot decay process (Akamatsu et al. 1990).

### 5.8.5 Chemiluminescence

The computerized methods have acknowledged superior attention, particularly in the investigation of biological materials. Various enzymatic and non-enzymatic flow injection (FI) fluorimetric and chemiluminescent (CL) detection methods are being used for determination of the oxalate content in biological systems. Most of the CL methods for oxalate involve either the reaction with the tris-(2,2 -bipyridyl) ruthenium(III) generated from the Ru(II) compound by chemical, electrochemical, and photochemical oxidation (Gerardi et al. 1991) or the formation of peroxy-oxalate (Albrecht et al. 1990). The amount of oxidation of methyl red by dichromate becomes more active with increasing oxalate concentrations, and that can be used for the kinetic determination of oxalate by measuring the reduction in the absorbance of the solution. However, the sensitivity can be enhanced by the use of an enormously sensitive procedure to detect the chromium (III) which is further quantified via $H_2O_2$. For kinetic estimation of oxalates, the following sequence of reactions can be referred.

$$\begin{aligned}&\text{Stain}(\text{red}) + \text{dichromate oxalate}^- \rightarrow \text{H}^+ \text{ stain}(\text{colorless}) + \text{chromium}(\text{III}) \quad (1)\\&\text{Luminol} + \text{hydrogen peroxide chromium}(\text{III})^- \rightarrow \text{OH}^- \text{ 3-aminophtalate} + \text{light} \quad (2)\end{aligned} \qquad (5.3)$$

The intensity of chemiluminescence is comparable to the oxalate concentration. A faint discharge appears at rocketed intensity and touches the extremes in fraction of time. This undoubtedly illustrates that the reagent of the reaction (Castro 1998) and the CL components ought to be mingled in a close vicinity of the detection flow cell. The recoveries attained by standard oxalates for frozen spinach, beet and beetroot leaves sample ranged between 94.0% and 98.6% (Perez-Ruiz et al. 2005). CL comes with much simpler detection equipment, along with high precision in results, even with minute sample loads. CL is often united with FI analysis or liquid chromatography (LC) which yields a low cost and reproducible set-up ensuring accurate estimation of the concerned elements (Burguera et al. 1980; Gerardi et al. 1999).

### 5.8.6 Advanced Chromatographic Techniques

Headspace gas chromatography (HS-GC) is an operational practice for the resolve of unstable species in the samples (Ioffe et al. 1984). It can moreover be used to secondarily to analyze some nonvolatile compounds that 86 can be transformed to their equivalent volatile species through chemical reactions (Chai et al. 2003). The present method is based on assessing headspace carbon dioxide which is consequently released in a reaction amongst oxalate and bromate at an acidic pH. The balanced equation is as follows:

$$3C_2O_4^{2-} + BrO_3^- + 6H^+ = Br^{-1} + 3H_2O + 6CO_2 \uparrow \quad (5.4)$$

The final amount of carbon dioxide released in the reaction can also be contributed by the other products of the food samples that are being kept in HS-GC for the estimation of oxalates in them. With the maximum estimation value of 1.95 µmol, it is a simple and applicable method which should be given a fair importance in the food industry (Li et al. 2014).

### 5.8.7 High-Performance Liquid Chromatography

It is a simple, fast, and cheap technique fortified with an anion investigation column (Shodex 1C SI-90 4E) and sodium hydrogen carbonate ($NaHCO_3$) as eluent. Oxalate can be estimated after withdrawal with water or 1 mol HCl (soluble form or total). Tough oxalates which are stuck between total and soluble forms can also be calculated. The total yield of oxalate after HPLC is near cent percent. However, certain considerations like pH 3 for acid extracts must be taken care of prior to run, along with instantaneous loading of 0.5% of oxalic acid is mandatory for a clear peak when the sample is feared to have less than 0.3%. The samples of Napier grass were found to have the lowest quantity of complex oxalates followed by guinea grass (Rahman et al. 2007).

## 5.9 EFFECT OF PROCESSING ON OXALATE

### 5.9.1 Fermentation

Only the limited studies demonstrated that cocoyam hold digestible starch, protein of good superiority, vitamin C, thiamin, riboflavin, niacin, and a good amount of amino acids. On the other hand, one chief restraining factor is the occurrence of oxalates that convey an acrid flavour or may lead to an experience of frustration for the eater. Moreover, these consumables can cause caustic effects, irritation to the intestinal tract, and even poisoning after absorption. A research to appraise the effect of fermentation on physicochemical properties and oxalate substance of cocoyam flour was conducted (Oke and Bolarinwa 2012). Firstly, the given pretreatments to flour, i.e., they were cleaned, washed, peeled, sliced into chips; white flesh cocoyam was aqua dipped and left to ferment for at least 24 h. Then, 48 h later, it was dried and milled into flour. Unfermented cocoyam underwent the same processing except fermentation and was used as a control. The oxalate content was analyzed by titrating an aliquot of extracts from the homogenized samples with 0.01 M $KMnO^4$ solution and the result indicated that the unfermented flour had $5.71 \pm 0^a$ % of the oxalate content. However, they observed a marked reduction of 58% ($2.38 \pm 0^b$ %) and 65% ($1.99 \pm 0^c$ %) after 24 h and 48 h of fermentation, respectively. This reduction is all attributed to usage of oxalates by growing micro flora and also through leaching phenomenon while in fermentation hours.

Cowpeas contain a rich amount of protein content and constitute the natural protein supplement to staple diets. Protein worth is synergistically enhanced in cereal-legume blends for the reason that the lysine contributed by the cowpea and methionine contributed by the cereals. A breadfruit, like some other legumes, has been known to hold some anti-nutrients which interfere with digestive processes and avoid resourceful consumption of their proteins. Still, they might be removing or compact by some processes such as soaking, dehulling, germination, and fermentation. Research was carried out to study the effect of fermentation on chemical composition of nutrient and anti-nutrient content of cowpea and breadfruit flour blend (Ojokoh et al. 2014). Six composite flour blends were formulated in ratios 100:0, 90:10, 80:20, 70:30, 60:40, and 50:50. Two batches each of fermented and unfermented samples were created using these blends while fermentation was carried out by adding 40 ml sterile water and keeping it aside for 72 h at room temperature. A noticeable decline in the amount of all the six fermented samples was observed when compared to unfermented flour and also, the amount of oxalates present per 100 g decreased with the reduction in the amount of breadfruit flour in the composite flour blend mix. Henceforth, the highest oxalate content was of the BcA unfermented (2.80 mg/100 g) and fermented sample (2.10 mg/100 g) out of all the six samples while BcF had the least value with 2.38 mg/100 g and 0.83 mg/100 g oxalate present in unfermented and fermented sample, respectively. However, the mean oxalates of fermented samples was 1.41 mg/100 g and unfermented was 2.65 mg/100 g. Leaching coupled with microbial action was responsible for the change in concentration of oxalates.

Kimchi, a fermented conventional food of Korea, has been eaten for a few centuries. Its preparation method implies prevention of food from spoilage. The photo-chemicals formed during the fermentation make it a practical food. As kimchi can be made from a range of vegetables and fruits, some kimchi may be formed from plants and spices which carry more amounts of oxalate. Silver Beet (*Beta vulgaris* var. Cicla) was utilized (stem and leaves) for the fermentation for kimchi preparation and then evaluated using HPLC for total, soluble, and insoluble oxalates (Wadamori et al. 2014). Main aim of this investigation was to reduce the oxalate development, thus pre-preparation slips were optimized where stems and leaves were dipped in 10% salt solution for 11 h, followed by cold tap water washing. The brine exposure reduces the oxalate amount significantly from 4,275.81 ± 165.48 mg/100 g to 3,709.49 ± 216.51 mg/100 g. Extension in fermentation time also contributed in the reduction of oxalates, i.e., 38.50% (total oxalates) and 22.86% (soluble oxalates). Point of benefit associated with this optimization tactic is the maintenance of the calcium level being the same as that available in fresh form. The losses of oxalates were all credited to the leaching of soluble oxalates due to washing, soaking in brine solution, and leaching of some water due to fermentation.

### 5.9.2 Baking

Oxalates, the anti-dietary substances reported in bread, can diminish the bioavailability of natural resources like calcium and iron and also diminish the protein digestibility. Yet, the bread manufacture stages, like fermentation and baking, are linked to lessening the oxalate amount. A study was conducted to assess the outcome on protein digestibility, mineral and oxalate content of wheat breads of baking at dissimilar temperatures fluctuation (160, 190, and 220°C) for different time frames (9, 12, 15, and 20 min) with and without steam (Bredariol et al. 2020). A significant decrease in the oxalate concentration was observed as the baking temperature and time increased in both cases, with or without steam. However, the lowest oxalate concentration at highest temperature and time was achieved in absence of steam with value of 30.4 mg/100 g extract while in presence of steam it settled around 33 mg/100 g of extract. The effect of baking temperature on oxalate content was even more clearer when baked in absence of steam, and throughout the result indicated on bar graphs the oxalate content in breads lay in the range of 30.4 to 44.0 mg/100 g of extract. High temperature of baking surpasses the melting point of oxalates, reducing the oxalates level.

Most taro cultivars have an acrid flavour and can result in swelling of the lips, mouth, and throat if taken uncooked. These severities are confirmed with the presence of needle-shaped calcium oxalate crystals, raphide, that can go through non-hard surfaces, especially skin. Afterward, an irritant near those needles, almost certainly a protease, results in uneasiness in the touched location. Mutually the root and the leaves may induce such a response, but repercussions can be hampered by cooking. An investigation was conducted on baked *Colocasia esculenta* var. Schott foliage to examine the oxalate concentrations (chemically and in-vitro) consumed with cow and coconut milk (Martensson and Savage 2008). Two varieties of taro leaves, Marori and Japanese, were baked in glass bowls covered with foil using domestic fans at150°C for 1.5 h and served as controls. For human findings of oxalates via urine samples, leaves baked with cow and coconut milk were used as a sample to analyze the increase in oxalate levels 6 h after consumption. Results showed that the total oxalates both Maori (524.2 ± 21.3 mg/100 g FW) and Japanese (525.6 ± 19.9 mg/100 g FW) are of similar level and have no significant difference. However, the soluble oxalates in Japanese leaves, 330.4 ± 28.3 mg/100 g FW, constituting 63% of the total was much higher than Maori leaves, 241.1 ±20.9 mg/100 g FW, constituting 46% of the total oxalates. Also, no significant increase in oxalate concentration was noted with both the samples cooked with milk. The statistics obtainable in this experiment advise that the adding up of calcium to the test meals by adding cow's milk or a combination of both has a little result in dropping of absorption of oxalate from said sample and its succeeding exclusion in urine. Although baking may decrease the amount of soluble oxalate, while using food wrappings, those oxalates may penetrate into the food stores in the leaves itself.

### 5.9.3 Frying

Oxalate is not even a major or important nutrient for the human body and, if eaten, it is not supposed be consumed in large quantities due to its fatal properties. Even though oxalates are found in various kinds of edible parts of vegetation, such as root stem portions, etc., in unreliable concentrations and, if consumed in large quantities, it may be injurious to human health; in some cases, it may even cause death or paralysis.

Determination of effect of wok-frying on oxalate contents of Fat Hen (*Chenopodium album*) leaves (Savage et al. 2018). In a preheated (170°C) canola oil, fresh leaves were added and cooked for 2 mins and then removed from the steel wok and are placed on absorbent kitchen paper to remove excess oil. Raw fresh leaves had higher total oxalates (1112.40 mg/100 g DM), soluble (866.31 mg/100 g DM) and insoluble oxalates (246.9 mg/100 g DM) then fried leaves. On the other hand, fried leaves had increased content of dry matter, 42.20 g/100 g WM, than fresh leaves having 20.06 g/100 g WM. The amount of total oxalates, soluble oxalates and insoluble oxalates present in wok-fried leaves were 883.57 mg/100 g DM, 472.14mg/100 g DM and 411.43 mg/100 g DM, respectively. Absorption of oil by leaves during stir frying resulted in loss of oxalates in the above research done.

The usually consumed foods such as silver beet, spinach, rhubarb, nuts, multi-grain flours, chocolate, black tea and parsley have high loads of oxalates particularly total and soluble one. Leafy vegetables such as spinach, amaranth and colocasia, are packed with oxalates while other frequently eaten vegetables and spices such as coriander, curry leaves, dill and fenugreek contain sensible amount of oxalates. Primarily, soluble oxalates get vanished with the steam while cooking. The soluble oxalate content of foods can also be lowered by components with high soluble calcium. Mixing of sour cream to baked yams, milk to cooked taro leaves and serving cooked spinach with milk, cream or cottage cheese and consuming ice cream with rhubarb are perfect to exemplify it. Silver Beet Leaves (*Beta Vulgaris Var. Cicla*) were used to prepare four samples (stir fried, soaked stir fried, boiled stir fried, and soaked and boiled stir fried) with added low and standard yoghurt for analyzing the oxalate contents (Teo and Savage 2011). The leaves were minced, boiling and soaking was done with tap water for 2 mins and at 12°C for 30 mins, respectively. In preheated canola oil at 200°C, all the soaked, boiled, soaked and boiled, and unprocessed silver beet leaves were stir fried for 2 mins with continuous stirring. The raw unprocessed silver beet leaves had 1,658 ± 114 mg/100 g dry matter (DM) of total oxalates, 954 ± 49 mg/100 g DM of soluble oxalates and 704 ± 98 mg/100 g DM insoluble oxalates. Pretreatments such as boiling and soaking before stir frying resulted in decrease of oxalates contents to a mean of 455 mg/100 g DM. Soaking and boiling reduces the soluble content of oxalates by leaching and also have been noted from the literature survey as well as the results of the research that administering calcium (yoghurt) with high oxalate foods does not affect human body adversely.

### 5.9.4 Boiling

Boiling the spinach leaves for two minutes can reduce the whole oxalate content of the cooked leaves, but the relative amount of soluble oxalate to the total oxalate content remained as it is the same as in the raw leaves (mean 75%). The total calcium content of the boiled leaves get ameliorated when the leaves were boiled and immediately mixed in the wok oil cooked leaves in cooking. An overall 2 mins of boiling can lead to a 36% reduction in the soluble oxalate content of the food sample.

The anti-nutrients present in three varieties of watermelon (*Citrullus lanatus*) seeds (namely; Sugar baby, Crimson sweet, and Kaolack) were determined by potassium permanganate titration method (Addo et al. 2018). The raw seeds were kept aside as control while the other was boiled at 100°C for 10 min and oven dried at 50°C for 12 h. These seeds were then milled into the flour which was then evaluated. Results showed that the raw seeds of Sugar baby and Kaolack, both have an oxalate content in the range of 0.43 to 0.48 g/100 g db while, Crimson sweet had 0.43–0.52 g of oxalates/100 g db. However, the results showed that the oxalate levels were lowered by 96.04%, 94.77%, and 92.5% for Sugar baby, Crimson sweet, and Kaolack watermelon seeds varieties, respectively. Boiling reduces the minor anti-nutrients present in watermelon seeds and it is also an effective method for reducing oxalates as they leaches out of seeds. The deteriorating effect of boiling temperature has also been seen in taro petioles and the leaves (*Alocasia odora*) and course ground nut samples, *Arachis hypogaea L.* (Hang et al. 2013; Mada et al. 2012). The impact of boiling on oxalate contents of Fat Hen (*Chenopodium album*) can be understood by an evident decrease in the total, soluble, and insoluble oxalates concentrations. Boiling led to leaching of soluble oxalates and the amount of locked calcium in insoluble oxalate can be decreased (Savage and Vanhanen 2019).

### 5.9.5 Soaking

Amongst the prominent forms of oxalates, i.e., solubility is the most affected by the process of soaking in food industry. An overnight soaking yields about 84% of the soluble oxalate content. Moreover, drenching for 18 h results in leaching of 26% of soluble oxalate into the tap water. The mean insoluble oxalate matter of the soaked leaves (168.35 mg/100 g WM) was almost alike to the insoluble oxalate of the raw tissue. Overall, it is unfortunate that immediately soaking is not an ordinary practice for taro leaves as the lessening of soluble oxalates would be a positive contribution (Savage 2000).

Conversely, it may be the fact that the released calcium from other food sources being cooked in the wok at the similar time would join the dissolvable type and rendered as insoluble calcium oxalate. Hence, soaking and cooking provide food with reasonable soluble oxalates but are nutritionally compromised compared to their raw form. Since such foods cannot be consumed raw, methods of cooking, along with their effects are the topmost points to be considered. Therefore, releasing is the chief factor which is accountable for the decrease in the earlier concentrations of oxalates while soaking (Handa et al. 2017).

### 5.9.6 Germination

Germination is an ordinary domestic skill approved out at little expenditure without the use of any complicated and pricey equipment. The bio-accessibility of iron and calcium was noticeably improved upon emergent. This higher bio-accessibility might be recognized to be diminished in anti-nutritional factors similar to phytate and oxalate as a consequence of germination. Alterations in mineral and anti-nutrient content all through development, led to considerable alterations in the anti-nutritional or mineral proportion that have an optimistic impact on the biological components. Soaking in running water before demonstrates the potential of millet in good iron and in turn, the mousy aroma of damp millet also gets eliminated (Gupta and Sehgal 1991). The impact of germination on pearl millet (*Pennisetum typhoideum*) using tap water, with an approach of improving mineral bio-accessibility to promote its consumption governed that the oxalate content affects the calcium bioavailability. Having extracted the oxalates through HCl and settled as calcium oxalate from the de-proteinized extracts, the concentrations in the samples drastically decreased and the cause for this must be due to the discharge of soluble oxalates during steeping, resulting in diminution of total oxalate content (Suma and Urooj 2011). Moreover, the light periods also do not have a substantial outcome on the presence of the oxalates in the horse gram, but the decrement in oxalates through germination was because of the establishment oxalate oxidase enzyme which causes breakdown of oxalic acid (Handa et al. 2017).

### 5.9.7 Roasting

Many researchers have been concerned with the evaluation of the effect of roasting on sesame seeds; these include: anti-oxidative progression of roasted sesame seed oil and the consequence of using the oil for frying (Fukuda et al. 1986), influence of seed roasting method on the changes in symphony and worth of sesame oil (Yen 1990), oxidative stability of sesame oil organized from sesame seed with dissimilar roasting temperatures (Yen and Shyu 1989). Being heat-labile, microwave roasting reduced oxalate content by 72.5%, with open pan roasting causing a further decrease (76.30%) in the activity of this anti-nutrient. The reduction of phytate concentration is an indication of the chemical poverty of phytate to minor inositol phosphates and inositol or cleavage of the phytate ring itself during roasting (Chen and Betty 2003).

*Senna occidentalis* seeds were utilized to examine the effect of different roasting temperatures (190, 210, and 230°C) with varying time (10, 15, and 20 mins) with respect to its phyto-chemical properties. The oxalates were determined using the titration method (Olapade and Ajayi 2016). The highest oxalate value was achieved at 210°C/20 min whereas the lowest oxalate levels were attained at 190°C/20 mins, which confirmed that the loss of oxalates was because of their destruction (as they are heat-labile).

### 5.9.8 Freezing

Freezing conditions have considerable impact on the biochemical changes occurring during storage. Leaves were washed with distilled water and frozen at - 4°C for 4 weeks, which demonstrated that the total oxalates were maximally affected by ultra-low temperatures; i.e., the lower the temperature, the lower the concentration of it. This trend is also true for the storage time in freezing conditions (Musa and Ogbadoyi 2013). The formation of ice crystals within the cell wall at high moisture content results in the loss of oxalates as the sharp edges of theses crystals lacerate the cell membrane, ultimately causing cell leakage.

### 5.9.9 Drying

Some vegetables can be consumed fresh or dried out and then used as a flavouring agent. Vegetables, being perishable, contribute to the major post-harvest loses of the nation. In order to increase their shelf life, an insert to the value of the produce are dried spices. The superiority of the dried product is totally linked to its drying situations.

The impact of various drying techniques (hot-air, freeze up, and vacuum drying) on the oxalate load of three rice paddy herbs (*phak-kha-yaeng* in Thai), *Limnophila aromatica* (*phak-kha-yaeng khao*), and *Limnophila geoffrayi* (*phak-kha-yaeng daeng*) showed that drying by hot air was very efficient in dropping the total oxalate content in *L. aromatica* (35.2 mg/g DW) *and L. geoffrayi* (29.66 mg/g DW), while in the case of freeze drying (40 mg/g DW) and vacuum drying

(39 mg/g DW) values remained the same for both varieties. The loss of oxalates can be due to their discharge while cooking in water (Wanyo et al. 2020). Cooking temperature is higher than the melting point of oxalates, and hence results in the decrease of overall oxalate content.

Likewise, the concentrations of oxalates in various drying techniques (sun, shade and oven drying) remained highest in shade drying, follow by sun and oven ventilation techniques, respectively (Mbah et al. 2012). Moreover, the raw elephant foot yam (*Amorphophallus paeoniifolius*) treated in a mixture of potassium metabisulphite, KMS + citric acid, and blanching for 30 mins have the higher amount of oxalates range for drying temp 40–70°C, whereas only KMS is at the onus to give the least amount of calcium oxalates at 70°C. The collapse of the cells due to high temperature causes the structural breakdown of calcium oxalate crystals in the cells.

### 5.9.10 Cooking

Like the abovementioned treatments, cooking coupled with boiling and other pretreatments like wilting and washing, resulted in the overall loss of oxalate levels by leaching. The effect of cooking on the oxalate level of three rice paddy herbs (*phak-kha-yaeng* in Thai), *Limnophila aromatica* (*phak-kha-yaeng khao*), and *Limnophila geoffrayi* (*phak-kha-yaeng daeng*) determined that the soluble oxalates for fresh and freeze dried *L. aromatica* increased after cooking, whereas it lowered in hot air and vacuum dried samples from 32.38% to 28.25% (4.76 mg/g DW) and 35.64% to 27.84% (7.62 mg/g DW), respectively (Wanyo et al. 2020). Hence, the potentially risky foods with much higher concentrations of oxalates can be consumed provided they are cooked properly in a considerable time.

## 5.10 FUTURE SCOPE OF OXALATES

Since oxalates are a potential toxin for humans when consumed, there are still several areas that need to be explored for their effective utilization.

### 5.10.1 Microbes Tailed to Degrade the Oxalates

GIT (gastrointestinal tract) is the key area for oxalate absorption and absorption of oxalate taken in diet can make a worthy share to urinary oxalate output. Different foods have their absorption rates varying from 2 to 15% and are dependent on myriad factors, particularly the intestinal ability to absorb, attendance of divalent cations with the intention to approach oxalate within the GIT, which consequently lowers the fraction of soluble oxalate, and of the utmost importance is the presence of oxalate-degrading bacteria, *Oxalobacter formigenes*. It is visualized that only a portion of soluble gastrointestinal oxalate has the ability to be absorbed. The point to be considered is whether the soluble oxalate content of the diet is similar to the proportion of soluble oxalate which is localized in intestinal lumen for absorption. Moreover, the potential of probiotics that raise bacteria with limiting the oxalate concentration to mitigate oxaluria, probably by alleviating oxalate load in absorption, have led to hopeful but varying outcomes. Now, studies with the vision to determine the severe consequences of oxalate excretion that may arise after ingesting probiotics should look into the following question: when these microbes are consumed with oxalate-rich food, does enhanced oxalate degradation in the gastrointestinal tract result? This probable consequence is left for future generations to confirm.

### 5.10.2 Nanoparticle Tracking Analysis

Crystalluria is a condition with kidney stone formation and can prevail when urine gets supersaturated with calcium, oxalate, and phosphate. The principal method used to diagnose urinary crystals is microscopy, with or without a polarized light source. This method can detect crystals above 1 mm in diameter (microcrystals). However, demonstration of calcium oxalates kidney stones has revealed that crystallite components in these calculi are 50–100 nm in diameter. It is also perceived that nanocrystals ( $< 200$ nm) impart more injury to renal cells than microcrystals. It is assumed that these nanocrystals can be detected and quantified by nanoparticle tracking analysis which will shed some light on the role of nanocrystals in crystallite and kidney stone formation (Kumar et al. 2020).

### 5.10.3 Industrial applications

The acidic properties, reducing power, and chelating potential of oxalic acid and oxalates provide a plethora of possibilities for application in industry. The potential of oxalic acid to get involved in the formation of metal oxalate complexes proves to be beneficial in tanning, blueprinting, electrolytic polishing, metal cleaning, electroplating, anodizing, protection against corrosion, ore-dressing, control of soil acidity. The list of applications given here is by no means exhaustive. Owing to its basic, reducing, and complexing agent properties, many more uses for the oxalates and oxalate complexes can be foreseen. Hence, the effective exploitation of oxalates not only will open the horizons for the medical field but also the commercial industries will profit in the near future.

## 5.11 CONCLUSION

Oxalates, one of the noxious acids, have been consumed in food since ancient times. Earlier reported in sorrel, it is in abundance in the commonly eaten vegetables spinach, rhubarb, cocoyam, and many more. After consumption of these vegetable, irritation and sometimes swelling can be reported in theatres, especially grazing livestock; these complications can be attributed to the crystal-like structures which are localized in the idioblasts. Chemically these crystals are composed of calcium oxalates and hence oxalates are meant to provide safety to the plants from the external sources. Being present in three main forms called raphide, styloid, and druse, the former is in abundance in nature. Biosynthetically, the self-synthesized oxalic acid of the plant gets reacted with root drawn calcium to form the crystal base which is calcium oxalate. Some other by products like glycolate, isocitrate, and oxaloacetate are also contributors as crystal synthesizers. Moreover, it is also prevailing in atmosphere, meat, biological systems, fungus, and even in some insects. Pathologically, the calcium oxalate crystals found accumulated in the kidney arising renal stones, which can turn into grave situations if left untreated. Several basic and advanced techniques have been discovered to estimate the oxalates in the food samples and all of the techniques have their own importance based on the cost of instrumentation, requirement of skilled personnel to operate, the amount of the sample to be loaded, different pretreatments that go before the loading of the sample, and last but not the least is the precision and accuracy of the results. Moreover, the various cooking methods like fermentation, boiling, soaking, germination, roasting, etc., have one common effect on the concentration of the food samples and that is a noticeable decrease in the initial concentration of the oxalates, because oxalates, being mostly soluble, elute out from the samples in the preparatory or operational cooking procedures. Although the oxalates have been labelled as notorious by the biologist community, the undiscovered potential of this toxic acid in the field of medicine and industry can open new avenues for patients and businessmen in the coming years, provided it is exploited in a better and effective way.

## REFERENCES

A.O.A.C. 1990. *Official Methods of Analysis* (15th ed.). Washington, DC: AOAC.

Addo, P. W., Agbenorhevi, J. K. and Adu-Poku, D. 2018. Antinutrient contents of watermelon seeds. *MOJ Food Processing and Technology* 6(2): 237–239.

Akamatsu, D.B., Higuchi, T. and Shimada, M. 1990. A novel enzymatic decarboxylation of oxalic acid by the lignin peroxidase system of white-rot fungus *Phanerochaete chrysosporium*. *FEBS Letters* 269(1): 261–263.

Albregts, E.E. and Howard, C.M. 1984. *Strawberry Production in Florida*, 841.

Aletor, V.A. 1995. Compositional studies on edible tropical species of mushrooms. *Food Chemistry* 54: 265–268.

Aplin, T.E. 1976. *Poisonous Garden Plants and Other Plants Harmful to Man in Australia*. Department of primary industries and regional development, Western Australia, *Perth Bulletin* 3964.

Arnott, H. J. 1982. *Three Systems of Biomineralization in Plants with Comments on the Associated Organic Matrix, Biological Mineralization and Demineralization*, G.H. Nancollas (Ed.), pp. 199–218.

Arnott, H..J. and Webb, M.A. 2000. Twinned raphides of calcium oxalate in grape (*Vitis*): Implications for crystal stability and function. *International Journal of Plant Science* 161: 133–142.

Barabé, D.C., Lacroix, M., Chouteau, M. and Gibernau, H. 2004. On the presence of extracellular calcium oxalate crystals on the inflorescences of Araceae. *Botanical Journal of Linnean Society* 146: 181–190.

Baran, E. J. and Monje, P. V. 2008. *In Biomineralization. From Nature to Application, Metal Ions in Life Sciences*, A. Sigel, H. Sigel, R. K. O. Sigel (Eds.), Vol. 4, pp. 219–254. Chichester: Wiley.

Basso, R., Lucchetti, G., Zefiro, L., Palenzona, A. and Jahrb, N. 1997. Ethnic tribes of Western Assam. *The Bioscan* 3: 613–625.

Bradbury, J.H. and Nixon, R.W. 1998. The acridity of raphides from the edible aroids. *Journal of the Science of Food and Agriculture* 76: 608–616.

Bredariol, P., Aparecida de Carvalho, R. and Maria Vanin, F. 2020. The effect of baking conditions on protein digestibility, mineral and oxalate content of wheat breads. *Food Chemistry*: 127399.

Bureau of Alcohol, Tobacco, Firearms, and Explosives, U.S. Department of Justice. 2017 Annual list of explosive materials. https://www.federalregister.gov/documents/2017/12/28/2017- 28010/commerce-in-explosives-2017-annual-list-of-explosivematerials (accessed Feb 17, 2019).

Burguera, A., Burguera, M. and Townshend, A. 1980. Determination of zinc and cadmium by flow injection analysis and chemiluminescence. *Analytica Chimica Acta* 127(1): 199–201.

Cadena, N.R., Cruz, M. and Moreno, A. 2020. The role of silica and alkaline earth metals with biomolecules in the biomineralization processes: The eggshells´s formation and the crystallization in vivo for x-ray crystallography. *Progress in Crystal Growth and Characterization of Materials* 66: 100473.

Çalışkan, M. 2000.The metabolism of oxalic acid. *Turkish Journal of Zoology* 24: 103–106.

Casadio, F., Miliani, C., Rosi, F., Roman, I. A., Anselmi, C., Brunetti, B., Sgamellotti, A., Andral, J. L. and Gautier, G. 2013. Scientific investigation of an important corpus of Picasso paintings in antibes: new insights into technique, condition, and chronological sequence. *Journal of the American Institute for Conservation* 52(3): 184–202.

Castro-Lopez, C., Ventura-Sobrevilla, J.M. and Gonzalez-Hernandez, M.D. 2017. Impact of extraction technique on antioxidant capacities and phytochemicals composition of polyphenols-rich extracts. *Food Chemisery* 237: 1139–1148.

Chai, W. and Liebman, M. 2005. Effect of different cooking methods on vegetable oxalate content. *Journal of Agricultural and Food Chemistry* 53: 2027–2030.

Chai, W., Liebman, M., Kynast-Gales, S. and Massey, L. 2004. Oxalate absorption and endogenous oxalate synthesis from ascorbate in calcium oxalate stone formers and non-stone formers. *American Journal of Kidney Diseases* 44(6): 1060–1069.

Chai, X.S., Hou, Q., Zhu, J., Chen, S.-L., Wang, S. and Lucia, L. 2003. Carboxyl groups in wood fibers. determination of carboxyl groups by headspace gas chromatography. *Industrial and Engineering Chemistry Research* 42: 5440–5444.

Charrière, J.D. and Imdorf, A. 2002. Oxalic acid treatment by trickling against Varroa destructor: Recommendations for use in Central Europe and under temperate climate conditions. *Bee World* 83: 51–60.

Chen, Q. and Betty, W. 2003. Separation of phytic acid and other related inositol phosphates by high-performance ion chromatography and its applications. *Journal of Chromatography* 1018: 41–52.

Cody, A.M. and Horner, H.T. 1983. Twin raphides in the Vitaceae and Araceae and a model for their growth. *Botanical Gazette* 144: 318–330.

Coe, F. L., Parks, J. H. and Asplin, J. R. 1992. The pathogenesis and treatment of kidney stones. *The New England Journal of Medicine* 327: 1141–52.

Colfen, H. 2010. Biomineralization: A crystal-clear view. *Nature Materials* 9: 960–961.

Colthrup, N. B., Daly, L. H. and Wiberley, S. E. 1990. *Introduction to Infrared and Raman Spectroscopy*, pp. 1–73. San Diego, CA: Academic Press.

Corley, R.A., Bartelz, M.J., Carney, E.W., Wertz, K.K., Soelberg J.J and Thrall, K.D. 2005. Development of a physiologically based pharmacokinetic model for ethylene and glycol and its development toxic metabolite glycocel acid in rats and humans. *Toxicology Science* 85(1): 476–490.

Cruz, M. 2017. Synthesis of inorganic and organic crystals mediated by proteins in different biological organisms. A mechanism of biomineralization conserved throughout evolution in all living species. *Progress in Crystal Growth and Characterization of Materials* 63: 94–103.

Cruz, M.C., Pérez, K.S., Mendoza, M.E. and Moreno, A. 2020. Biocrystals in plants: A short review on biomineralization processes and the role of phototropins into the uptake of calcium. *Crystals* 10: 591–594.

Cruzan, G., Corley, R. A., Hard, G. C., Mertens, J. J. W. M., McMartin, K. E., Snellings, W. M., Gingell and Deyo, J. A. 2004. Subchronic toxicity of ethylene glycol in Wistar and F344 rats related to metabolism and clearance of metabolites. *Toxicological Sciences* 81: 502–511.

De Bary, A. 1887. *Comparative Morphology and Biology of the Fungi, Mycetozoa and Bacteria*. Oxford: Clarendon Press. Department of Agriculture and Food, Western Australia, Perth. Bulletin 3964.

Dollimore, D. and Konieczay, J. L. 1998. The thermal decomposition of beryllium oxalate and related materials. *Thermochimica Acta* 318: 155–163.

Dosuzeva, T.V. 1969. Comparative-anatomical character of leaves of some species of the genus *Armeniaca Mill*. (Russ. w/Engtish summ.). *Scientific Bulletin of the Ozhgorod University* 2: 78–85.

Elejalde-Cadena, N. R., Cuéllar-Cruz, M. and Moreno, A. 2020. The role of silica and alkaline earth metals with biomolecules in the biomineralization processes: The egg shell's formation and the crystallization in vivo for x-ray crystallography. *Progress in Crystal Growth and Characterization of Materials* 66: 100473.

Fargue, S., Knight, J., Holmes, R.P., Rumsby, G. and Danpure, C. J. 1862. Effects of alanine: glyoxylate aminotransferase variants and pyridoxine sensitivity on oxalate metabolism in a cell based cytotoxicity assay. *Biochimica et Biophysica Acta* 1862(6): 1055–1062.

Fassett, D.W. 1973. Oxalates. In *Toxicants Occurring Naturally in Foods*, Washington, DC: National Academy of Sciences.

Foster, A.S. 1956. Plant idioblasts: remarkable examples of cell specialization. *Protoplasma* 46: 184–193.

Franceschi, V.R. 1989. Calcium oxalate formation is a rapid and reversible process in (*Lemna minor* L.). *Protoplasma* 148: 130–37.

Franceschi, V. R. and Horner, Jr. H. T. 1980. Calcium oxalate crystals in plants. *The Botanical Review* 4: 361–427.

Friedman, E. A., Greenberg, J. B., Merrill, J. P. and Dammin, G. J. 1962. Consequences of ethylene glycol poisoning. Report of four cases and review of the literature. *The American Journal of Medicine* 32: 891–902.

Frondel, C. 1962. Thierschite (Whewellite). *American Mineralogist* 47: 786.

Fujita, T. and Komemushis, Y. K. 1995. Content of amino acid, organic acid 5-nucleotides in tricholomagiganteum. *Journal of Science Food Agriculture* 55: 159–162.

Fukuda, Y., Nagata, M., Osawa, T. and Namika, M. 1986. Chemical aspects of the antioxidative activity of roasted sesame seed oil, and the effect of using the oil for frying. *Agricultural and Biological Chemistry* 50(4): 857–862.

Gaines, R.V., Skinner, H.C., Foord, E.E., Mason, B. and Rosenweig, A. 1998. *A Geological Magazine*. Cambridge: Cambridge University Press.

Gallaher, R.N. 1975. The occurrence of Calcium in plant tissue as crystals of calcium oxalate. *Communication in Soil Science and Plant Analysis* 6: 315–330.

Gemede, H.F. and Ratta, N. 2014. Antinutritional factors in plant foods: Potential healthbenefits and adverse effects. *International Journal of Nutrition and Food Sciences* 3(4): 284–289.

Gerardi, R.D., Barnett, N.W. and Lewis, S.W. 1991. Analytical applications of tris(2,2′-bipyridyl)ruthenium(III) as a chemiluminescent reagent. *Analytica Chimica Acta* 378: 1–8.

Gerardi, R. D., Barnett, N.W. and Lewis, S.W. 1999. *Analytica Chimica Acta* 378: 1.

Gontzea, I. and Sutzescu, P. 1968. *Natural Antinutritive Substances in Foodstuffs and Forages*. Basel: S Karger. DOI:10.1159/000389425.

Goulson, D., Nicholls, E., Botıas, C. and Rotheray, E.L. 2015. Bee declines driven by combined stress from parasites, pesticides, and lack of flowers. *Science* 347: 1255957.

Gregorc, A. and Planinc, I. 2002. The control of Varroa destructor using oxalic acid. *The Veterinay Journal* 163: 306–310.

Guo, S.W., Ward, M.D. and Wesson J.A. 2002. Direct visualization of calcium oxalate monohydrate crystallization and dissolution with atomic force microscopy and the role of polymeric additives. *Langmuir* 18: 4284–4291.

Gupta, C. and Sehgal, S. 1991. Development, acceptability and nutritional value of weaning mixture. *Plant Foods for Human Nutrition* 41: 107–116.

Haas, O.J. and Fleischman, A.I. 1961. The rapid enzymatic determination of oxalate in wort and beer. *Journal of Agricultural and Food Chemistry* 9: 451–456.

Handa, V., Kumar, V., Panghal, A., Suri, S. and Kaur J. 2017. Effect of soaking and germination on physicochemical and functional attributes of horsegram flour. *Journal of food Science and Technology* 54(13): 4229–4239.

Hang, D.T., Vanhanen, L. and Savage, G. 2013. Effect of simple processing methods on oxalate content of taro petioles and leaves grown in central Viet Nam. *Journal of Food Science and Technology* 50(1): 259–263.

Hart, P. n.d. Explosive properties of oxalate of peroxide of mercury. *American Journal of Pharmacology* 1860: 416.

Hartl, W.P., Klapper, H., Barbier, B., Ensikat, H.J., Dronskowski, R., Müller, P., Ostendorp, G., Tye, A., Bauer, R. and Barthlott, W. 2007. Diversity of calcium oxalate crystals in Cactaceae. *Canadian Journal of Botany* 85: 501–517.

Hendricks, S.B. and Jefferson, M. E. 1936. Electron distribution in (NH4)2C2O4–H2O and the structure of the oxalate group. *Jefferson Journal of Chemistry and Physics* 4: 102.

Hofmann, B.A., Bernasconi, S.M.. 1998. *Chemical Geology* 149: 127.

Horner, H.T. and Wagner, B.L. 1995. Calcium oxalate formation in higher plants. In *Calcium Oxalate in Biological Systems*, pp. 53–72. Boca Raton, FL: CRC.

Horner, H.T Jr., Kausch, A.P. and Wagner, B.L. 1981. Growth and change in shape of raphide and druse calcium oxalate crystals as a function of intracellular development in *Typha angustifolia*L. (Typhaceae) and *Capsicu*m annuumL. (Solanaceae). *Scanning Electron Microscopy* 34(4): 251–262.

Ioffe, B. V., Vitenberg, A. G. e., Gazovaya, V. and Ekstraktsiia, K. 1984. *Analyze head-space analysis and related methods in gas chromatography*, Vol. 222. New York: Wiley.

Jacobsen, D. and McMartin, K.E. 1986. Methanol and ethylene glycol poisoning. Mechanism of toxicity, clinical course, diagnosis and treatment. *Medical Toxicology* 1: 309–334.

Jambor, J. L., Grew, E. S. and Roberts, A. C. 1998. *American Mineralogist* 83: 185.

Jaworska, G. 2005a. Content of nitrates, nitrites, and oxalates in New Zealand spinach. *Food Chemistry* 89: 235–242.

Jaworska, G. 2005b. Effect of technological measures and storage time on the level of nitrates, nitrites, and oxalates in frozen and canned products of spinach and New Zealand spinach. *Food Chemistry* 93: 395–401.

Jeffrey, G. A and Parry, G.S. 1952. The crystal structure of sodium oxalate. *Journal of the Chemical Society* 5283–5286.

Kasimala, M.B., Tedros, B., Weldeyesus, M., Imru, H. and Negasi T.K. 2018. Determination of oxalates and investigation of effect of boiling on oxalate content from selected vegetables commonly grow in Eritrea. *Atoms and Molecules* 8(4): 1175–1180.

Kawamura, A.K. and Kaplan, I.R. 1987. Motor exhaust emissions as a primary source fordicarboxylic acids in Los Angeles ambient air. *Environmental Science and Technology* 21: 105–110.

Keller, M., Blochl, E., Wachtershauser, G. and Stetter, K.O. 1994. Formation of amide bonds without a condensation agent: Implications for the origin of life. *Nature* 368: 836–838.

Khan, S.R., Byer, K.J., Thamilvan, S., Hackett, R.L., McCormack, W.T., Benson, N.A., Vaughn, K.L. and Erdos,G.W. 1999. Crystal cell interaction and apoptosis in oxalate-associated injury of renal epithelial cells. *Journal of American Society of Nephrology* 10: 457–463.

Kim, I.H. and Beauchamp, J.L. 2007. Cluster phase chemistry: Collisions of vibrationally excited cationic dicarboxylic acid clusters with water molecules initiate dissociation of cluster components. *Journal of Physical Chemistry* 111: 5954–5967.

Kim, I.H., Goddard, A.W. and Beauchamp, J.L. 2006a. Cluster phase chemistry: Gas-phase reactions of anionic sodium salts of dicarboxylic acid clusters with water molecules. *Journal of Physical Chemistry A* 110: 7777–7786.

Kim, Y.E., Hong, S.H., Kim J.W. and Lee J.Y. 2006b. Evaluation of Fourier transform near-infrared spectrometer for determination of oxalate in standard urinary solution. *Journal of Preventive Medicine and Public Health* 39(2): 165–170.

Kochkoul, R., Housaini, T.S., Mohim, M., El Habbani, R. and Lahrichi, A. 2020. Chemical compounds identification and antioxidant and calcium oxalate anticrystallization activities of *Punica granatum* L. *Complementary and AlternativeMedicine* 4: 1–14.

Kostman, T.A. and Franceschi, V.R. 2000. Cell and calcium oxalate crystal growth is coordinated to achieve high-capacity calcium regulation in plants. *Protoplasma* 214: 166–179.

Kumar, P., Patel, M., Thomas, V., Knight, N., Holmes, R.P. and Mitchell, T. 2020. Dietary oxalate induces urinary nanocrystals in humans. *Kidney International Report* 5: 1040–1051.

Lane, B.G. 1994. Oxalate, germin, and the extracellular matrix of higher plant. *The FASEB Journal* 8(3): 294–301.

Lemann, J. Jr., Pleuss, J.A., Worcester, E.M., Hornick, L., Schrab, D. and Hoffmann,R.G. 1996. Urinary oxalate excretion increases with body size and decreases with increasing dietary calcium intake amonghealthy adults. *Kidney International* 49: 200–208.

Libert, B. and Creed, C. 1985. Oxalate content of seventy-eight rhubarb cultivars and its relation to some other characters. *Journal of Horticultural Sciences* 60: 257–61.

Liebman, M. 2002. The truth about oxalate answers to frequently asked questions. *The Vulvar Pain Newsletter.* Retrieved from http://www.thevpfoundation.org/vpfoxalate.htm. [Accessed 12 April, 2018].

Mada, S.B., Garba, A., Mohammed, A., Olagunju, A., and Mohammed, H.A. 2012. Effects of boiling and roasting on antinutrients and proximate composition of local and some selected improved varieties of *Arachishypogaea* L. (Groundnut). *International Journal of Food Nutrition and Safety* 1(1): 45–53.

Maddaloni, M. and. Pascual, D.W. 2015. Isolation of oxalo trophic bacteria associated with Varroa destructor mites. *Letters in Applied Microbiology* 61: 411–417.

Mårtensson, L. and Savage, G.P. 2008. Composition and bioavailability of oxalates in baked taro (Colocasia esculenta var. Schott) leaves eaten with cows milk and coconut milk. *International Journal of Food Science & Technology* 43(12): 2213–2218.

Martinelango, P. K., Dasgupta, P. K., and Al-Horr, R. S. 2007. Atmospheric production of oxalic acid/oxalate and nitric acid/nitrate in the Tampa Bay airshed: Parallel pathways. *Atmospheric Environment* 41(20): 4258–4269.

Massey, L.K., Roman-Smith, H. and Sutton, A.L. 1993. Effect of dietary oxalate and calcium on urinary oxalate and risk of formation of calcium oxalate kidney stones. *Journal of American Dietetic Association* 93(8): 901–906.

Mbah, B.O., Eme, P.E. and Ogbusu, O.F. 2012. Effect of cooking methods (boiling and roasting) on nutrients and anti-nutrients content of *Moringa oleifera* seeds. *Pakistan Journal of Nutrition* 11(3): 211–215.

Mena, P., Calani, L. and Dall'Asta, C. 2012. Rapid and comprehensive evaluation of (poly)phenolic compounds in pomegranate (*PunicagranatumL.*) juice by UHPLC-MSn. *Molecules* 17(12): 14821–14840.

Merusi, C., Corradini, C., Cavazza, A., Borromei, C. and Salvadeo, P. 2010. Determination of nitrates, nitrites and oxalates in food products by capillary electrophoresis with pH-dependent electroosmotic flow reversal. *Food Chemistry* 120: 615–620.

Miller, C., Kennington, L., Cooney, R., Kohjimoto, Y., Cao, L.C., Honeyman, T., Pullman, J., Jonassen, J. and Scheid, C. 2000. Oxalate toxicity in renal epithelial cells: Characteristics of apoptosis and necrosis. *Toxicology and Applied Pharmacology* 162: 132–141.

Money, R. W. and Davies, C. W. 1938. The solubility of barium oxalate in aqueous salt solutions. *Journal of the Chemical Society*: 2098–2100.

Musa, A. and Ogbadoyi, E.O. 2013. Levels of phytotoxins and nutrients in hibiscus sabdariffa as influenced by freezing storage. *Current Journal of Applied Science and Technology* 3(4): 799–812.

Nguimezong, B.N., Foba-Tendo, J., Yufanyi, D.M., Etape, E.P., Eko, J.N. and Ngolui, L.J. 2014. Averrhoacarambola: A renewable source of oxalic acid for the facile and green synthesis of divalent metal (Fe, Co, Ni, Zn, and Cu) oxalates and oxide nanoparticles. *Journal of Applied Chemistry* 14: 76–95.

Noonan, S.C. and Savage, G.P. 1999. Oxalate content of foods and its effect on humans. *Asia Paific Journal of Clinical Nutrition* 8(1): 64–74.

Norton, R.B., Roberts, J.M. and Huebert, B.J. 1983. Tropospheric oxalate. *Geophysical Reserach Letters* 10: 517–520.

Ojokoh, A.O., Fayemi, E.O., Ocloo, F.C.K. and Alakija, O. 2014. Proximate composition, antinutritional contents and physicochemical properties of breadfruit (*Treculiaafricana*) and cowpea (*Vignaunguiculata*) flour blends fermented with Lactobacillus plantarum. *African Journal of Microbiology Research* 8(12): 1352–1359.

Oke, M. O. and Bolarinwa, I. F. 2012. Effect of fermentation on physicochemical properties and oxalate content of cocoyam (Colocasiaesculenta) flour. *International Scholarly Research Notices*.

Olapade, A.A. and Ajayi, O.A. 2016. Effect of roasting regime on phytochemical properties of Sennaoccidentalis seeds. *International Journal of Food Studies* 5(2): 203–211.

Ouyang, J.M., Duan, L. and Tieke, B. 2003. Effects of carboxylic acids on the crystal growth of calcium oxalate nanoparticles in lecithin-water liposome systems. *Langmuir* 19: 8980–8985.

Perez-Ruiz, T., Martinem-Lozano, C., Tomas, V. and Fenoli, J. 2005. Chemiluminescent determination of oxalate based on its enhancing effect on the oxidation of methyl red by dichromate. *Analytica Chimica Acta* 552(2):147–151.

Perry, D.L. 2011. *Handbook of Inorganic Compounds* (2nd ed.). Boca Raton, FL: CRC Press. https://doi.org/10.1201/b10908.

Prasad, R., Singh-Shivay, Y. 2017. Oxalic acid/oxalates in plants: From self-defence to phytoremediation. *Current Science* 112: 1665–1667.

Prychid, C.J. and Rudall, P.J. 1999. Calcium oxalate crystals in monocotyledons: A review of their structure and systematics. *Annals of Botany* 84: 725–739.

Rahman, M. and Kawamura, O. 2011. Oxalate accumulation in forage plants: Some agronomic, climatic and genetic aspects. *Asian-Australasian Journal of Animal Sciences* 24: 439–448.

Rahman, M. M., Yamamoto, M., Niimi, M. and Kawamura, O. 2008a. Effect of nitrogen fertilization on oxalate content in Rhodes grass, Guinea grass and Sudan grass. *Asian-Australian Journal of Animal Science* 21(2): 214–219.

Rahman, T., Hosen, I., Towhidul Islam, M.M. and Shekhar, H.U. 2012. Oxidative stress and human health. *Advances in Bioscience and Biotechnology* 3: 997–1019.

Ratkalkar, V.N. and Kleiman, J G. 2011. Mechanisms of stone formation. *Clinical Reviews in Bone and Mineral Metabolism* 9: 187–197.

Ritter, M.. C. and Savage, G.P. 2007. Soluble and insoluble oxalate content of nuts. *Journal of Food Composition and Analysis* 20(3): 169–174.

Robertson, J. H.. 1965. *Acta Crystallogr.* 18: 410. Find online.

Rosenkranz, P., Aumeier, P. and Ziegelmann, B. 2010. Biology and control of Varroa destructor. *Journal of Invertebrate Pathology* 103(1, Supplement 1): 96–119.

Rumble, J.R., Lide, D.R., and Bruno, T.J. 2018. *CRC Handbook of Chemistry and Physics: A Ready-reference Book of Chemical and Physical Data*. Boca Raton, FL: CRC.

Rupali, T., Chavan, S. and Pandhure, N. 2012. Occurrence of chloride enriched calcium oxalate crystal in cissusquadrangularislinn. *International Journal of Pharmaceutics* 2(2): 337–340.

Russo, M., Fanali, C. and Tripodo, G. 2018. Analysis of phenoliccompounds in different parts of pomegranate (*Punicagranatum*) fruit by HPLC-PDA-ESI/MS and evaluation of their antioxidant activity: Application to different Italian varieties. *Analytical and Bioanalytical Chemistry* 410(15): 3507–3520.

Ryall, R.L., Fleming, D.E., Grover, P.K., Chauvet, M., Dean, C.J. and Marshall V.R. 2000. The hole truth: Intracrystalline proteins and calcium oxalate kidney stones. *Molecular Urology* 4: 391–402.

Saadi, S.M. and Mondal, A.K. 2012. Studies on the calcium oxalate crystals (Raphides) and idioblast of some selected memebers of Araceae in Eastern India. *African Journal of Plant Science* 6(9): 256–269.

Saiz-jimenez, C. 1989. Biogenic vs anthropogenic oxalic acid in the environment. In *The Oxalate Film: Origin and Significance in the Conservation of Works of aArt*, pp. 207–214.

Sarma,T.C., Sarma, I. and Patiri, B.N. 2010. Wild edible mushrooms used by some ethnic tribes of Western Assam. DO -10.13140/RG.2.1.3531.1842

Savage, G. and Vanhanen, L. 2019. Oxalate contents of raw, boiled, wok-fried and pesto and juice made from fat hen (Chenopodium album) leaves. *Foods* 8(1): 2.

Savage, M. 2000. Effect of cooking on the soluble and insoluble oxalate content of some New Zealand foods. *Journal of Food Composition and Analysis* 13(3): 201–206.

Scheid, C., Koul, H., Hill, W. A., Luber-Narod, J. and Kennington, L. 1996. Oxalate toxicity in LLC-PK1 cells: Role of free radicals. *Kidney International* 49: 413–419.

Shimazono, H. and Hayaishi, O. 1957. Enzymatic decarboxylation of oxalic acid. *Journal of Biological Chemistry* 227: 151–154.
Shimizu, M.H. Gois, P.H., Volpini, R.A., Canale, D., Luchi, W.M., Froeder, L., Heilberg, I.P., and Seguro, A.C. 2017. N-acetylcysteine protects against star fruit induced acute kidney injury. *Renal Failure* 39: 193–202.
Stagnari, F., Bitetto, V. and Pisante, M. 2007. Effects of N fertilizers and rates on yield, safety and nutrients in processing spinach genotypes. *Scientia Horticulurae* 114: 225–233.
Suma, P.F. and Urooj, A. 2011. Influence of germination on bioaccessible iron and calcium in pearl millet *(Pennisetumtyphoideum). Journal of Food Science and Technology.* 51(5): 976–981.
Sunell, L.A. and Healey, P.L. 1981. Scanning electron microscopy and energy dispersive x-ray analysis of raphide crystal idioblasts in taro. *Scanning Electron Microscopy* 81: 235–244.
Sunell, L.A. and Healey, P.L. 1985. Distribution of calcium oxalate crystal idioblasts in leaves of taro (*Colocasia esculenta*). *American Journal of Botany* 72: 1854–1860.
Tandon, V.R., Sharma, S., Mahajan, A. and Bardi, G.H. 2005. Oxidative stress: A novel strategy in cancer treatment. *Journal of Medical Education and Research* 7(1): 1–3.
Tampa Bay airshed: Parallel pathways. *Atmospheric Environment* 41(20): 4258–4269.
Taylor, J.C. and Sabine, T.M. 1972. *Acta Crystallographica Section B: Structural Science, Crystal Engineering and Materials* 28: 3340.
Teo, E. and Savage, G. 2011. Silver beet leaves (*Beta Vulgaris* Var. Cicla) with and without additions of yoghurt. *Journal of Food Research* 1(1): 126–131.
Thamilselvan, S. and Khan, S.R. 1998. Oxalate and calcium oxalate crystals are injurious to renal epithelial cells: Results of in vivo and in vitro studies. *Journal of Nephrology* 11(Supplement 1): 66–69.
Tian, Z., Chan, B., Sullivan, M.B., Radom, L. and Kass, S.R. 2008. Lithium monoxide anion: A ground-state triplet with the strongest base to date. *Proceeding of the Naional Academy of Science* 105: 7647–7651.
Touryan, L.A., Lochhead, M.J., Marquardt, B.J. and Vogel, V. 2004. Sequential switch of biomineral crystal morphology using trivalent ions. *Natural Material* 3: 239–43.
Udoh, A. P., Effiong, R. I. and Edem, D.O. 1995. Nutrient composition of dogwhelk. A protein source of human. *Tropical Science* 35: 64–67.
Wachtershauser, G. 1988. Pyrite formation, the first energy source for life: A hypothesis. *Systical Applied Microbiology* 10: 207–210.
Wadamori, Y., Vanhanen, L. and Savage, G.P. 2014. Effect of kimchi fermentation on oxalate levels in silver beet (*Beta vulgaris* var. cicla). *Foods* 3(2): 269–278.
Wanyo, P., Huaisan, K. and Chamsai, T. 2020. Oxalate contents of Thai rice paddy herbs (*L. aromatica and L. geoffrayi*) are affected by drying method and changes after cooking. *SN Applied Sciences* 2(5): 1–6.
Wattendorff, J. 1976. A third type of raphide crystal in the plant kingdom: Six-sided raphides with laminated sheaths in *Agave* (*Americana* L.). *Planta* 130: 303–311.
Webb, M.A. 1999. Cell-mediated crystallization of calcium oxalate in plants. *The Plant Cell* 11: 751–761.
William, N.S. 1972. Vanadyl Oxalate Compounds and Process for Producing Same. U.S. Patent US3689515A, 1972.
Yen, G.C. 1990. Influence of seed roasting process on the changes in composition and quality of sesame (*Sesamum indicum*) oil. *Journal of the Science of Food and Agriculture* 50: 563–570.
Yen, G.C. and Shyu, S.L. 1989. Oxidative stability of sesame oil prepared from sesame seed with different roasting temperatures. *Food Chemistry* 31: 215–224.
Young, R.A. and Brown, W.E. 1982. *Biological Mineralization and Demineralization*. Berlin: Springer Verlag.
Zhang, S.Y. 1992. Systematic wood anatomy of the Rosaceae. *Blumea Journal* 37: 81–158.

CHAPTER 6

# Goitrogens

**Sabeera Muzzaffar, Tuyiba Nazir, Mohd. Munaff Bhat, Idrees Ahmad Wani, and F.A. Masoodi**

## CONTENTS



## 6.1 INTRODUCTION

Goitrogens are naturally occurring compounds that can stand in the way of normal functioning of the thyroid gland, thereby causing hyperplastic goiter. They derive their name from the word "goiter", meaning growth or enlargement of the thyroid gland. Goitrogens suppress thyroid hormone synthesis and thus lower the hormone production. This suppression results in an elevated thyrotropin (thyroid-stimulating hormone) expression which, in turn, increases both the thyroid hormone secretion and thyroid cell development and eventually leads to an enlargement of the thyroid gland (a condition normally known as goiter). Goiter is typically the most visible symptom of iodine deficiency; however, it has more severe implications including its effect on brain, neurological delay,

DOI: 10.1201/9781003178446-6

reproductive dysfunction, and childhood death. It is now established that other factors also play a pivotal role in goiter formation as iodine supplementation has not been fully successful in eradicating this condition (Chandra, 2010). Thus, in addition to nutritional deficiency of iodine, naturally occurring goitrogenic compounds in diet and drinking water are factors which can also trigger the goiter endemics (Gaitan, 1989).

The findings of different experiments indicate that a variety of compounds that are or may be goitrogenic to humans and domesticated animals are found in many plants and their seeds. At least two distinct forms of compounds tend to exist, one inhibits the absorption of iodine by the thyroid, thus causing goiter (e.g., thiocyanates), and the other causes goiter by blocking the organic binding of protein (e.g., goitrin or L-5-vinyl-2-thio-oxazolidone) (Clements, 1960). Cassava, lima bean, linseed, cruciferous vegetables, soy, and millets are some of the examples of foodstuffs that contain goitrogens. Ironically, an excess of iodine may also become goitrogenic, probably by impeding the proteolysis of thyroglobulin and therefore hampering the secretion of thyroid hormone as hyperplastic goiter is seen in the case of foals of mares which are fed with seaweed or kelp as iodine supplements (Miller, 2017).

However, certain drugs such as rifampin, phenobarbital, etc., enhance degradation of $T_4$ and $T_3$ and hence are also considered as having goitrogenic potential. Goitrogens are typically only active where iodine is reduced and/or the intake of goitrogens is long-lasting (Zimmermann et al., 2008). Iodine is available in various chemical types in foods. Most of the iodine consumed is almost entirely absorbed into the duodenum. Iodine is primarily purged by the thyroid and kidney from circulation (Hess, 2013). Its primary role is synthesis of thyroid hormone, thyroxine (T4), and triiodothyronine (T3). For each T4 molecule, four iodine atoms are required, and three atoms are needed for each T3 molecule (Knust and Leung, 2017).

This chapter discusses the distribution of goitrogenic compounds, their identification, mechanism of action, toxicological effects, as well as the role of processing in reducing the toxic effects of goitrogens.

## 6.2 DISTRIBUTION

### 6.2.1 Dietary Sources of Goitrogens

- Cruciferous Vegetables: Cruciferous vegetables are part of the *Brassicaceae* (also known as *Cruciferae*) family of vegetables, which comprise a wide variety of vegetables, e.g., cabbage, broccoli, cauliflower, Brussels sprouts, radish, turnip, swede, rocket salad, wasabi, mustard, canola, rapeseed, and kale) (Holst et al., 2003). They contain glucosinolates, which are considered as potent goitrogens. They may also contain S-methycysteine sulfoxide (SMCO), tannins, and erucic acids (Griffiths et al., 1998).
- Fruits and starchy plants: Many tropical countries consider starchy fruits and tubers like banana, cassava, yam, and sweet potato to be staple foods (Wani et al., 2017; Satheesh and Solomon, 2019). World production of starchy fruits and tubers is 2.7 times lower than cereal production (FAOSTAT, 2017). Bamboo shoots, cassava, rice, lima beans, linseed, millet, peaches, almonds, pears, pine nuts, strawberries, sweet potatoes, and other products fall within this category. Cassava is a starchy root that is a favourite in many Latin American and Caribbean dishes.
- Soy-based foods: Soy has historically been used in food production as soybeans, tofu, miso, tempeh, etc., and its use is generally linked with a decrease in chronic illnesses owing to its antioxidant, anti-inflammatory, and anti-allergic features. Soy consists of a group of naturally occurring heterocyclic flavonoids. Experimental evidence has demonstrated that a significant number of flavonoids (genistein and daidzein) can inhibit thyroperoxidase production and decrease thyroid hormone synthesis (Santos et al., 2011). They may also be associated with the inhibition of activity of 5′-deiodinase, which results in decrease in conversion of $T_4$ to $T_3$. Such compounds can also cause the hepatic clearance of$T_3$ and $T_4$ (White et al., 2004).

Broadly, goitrogens can be classified into three groups:

1. Glucosinolates.
2. Cyanogenic glycosides.
3. Flavonoids.

## 6.3 CHEMISTRY OF GOITROGENS

### 6.3.1 Glucosinolates

Glucosinolates (alkyl aldoxime-O-sulphate esters with a β-D-thioglucopyranoside group) are sulphur-containing metabolites formed from amino acids because of secondary metabolism (Sønderby et al., 2010). They can be broken up into three classes based on their amino acid precursors: aliphatic glucosinolates (metabolized from methionine, alanine, leucine, isoleucine, valine, or glutamate); indole glucosinolates (synthesized from tryptophan), and benzenic glucosinolates (derived from phenylalanine and tyrosine) (Chhajed et al., 2020). Glucosinolates are widely present in the *Brassicaceae* family of plants, which include cabbage, kale, broccoli, etc., and are responsible for typical flavours of these vegetables. Species belonging to this group are widely used as a human food and livestock feed. Recently these compounds have received a lot of attention due to their health-promoting effects as well as their role in the plant defence system. All glucosinolates consist of the main core structure of a β-thioglucose residue, which is linked by a sulfur atom to a (*Z*)-*N*-hydroximinosulfate ester. Additionally, they have a variable side chain (R group), which is derived from an amino acid (Ettlinger and Lundean, 1956). The variation among individual glucosinolates appears according to the structure and configuration of the side chain. Glucosinolates are therefore classified based on their variable side groups R (VanEtten et al., 1969). The most significant glucosinolates are either direct (straight) or ramified (branched) carbon chains (Figure 6.1)

Plants can produce more than one kind of glucosinolates with most of them producing one to five GSLs. Glucosinolates can be hydrolyzed into different substances by myrosinase enzyme which are bound in the aqueous vacuoles in plants (McDanell et al., 1988). Thus, suggesting that the enzyme and substrate of intact plants exist in various sections of the plant. However, they can combine during chewing or pressing and grinding for oil extraction or upon any sort of plant damage. Thus, in the presence of water the process of conversion of glucosinolates into different breakdown products starts. Henceforth, the thioglucoside bond on glucosinolate is broken by myrosinase enzyme, resulting in glucose production and an intermediate aglucone product, which further breaks down into many toxicants, mostly isothiocyanates and nitriles, or even goitrin (Hill, 2003).

The widely accepted mechanism for glucosinolate biosynthesis includes 4 major steps and these are aglycone formation through initial N-hydroxylation, formation of aldoxime by oxidative decarboxylation, inclusion of sulphur to get thiohydroximic acid that experiences S glycosylation to the

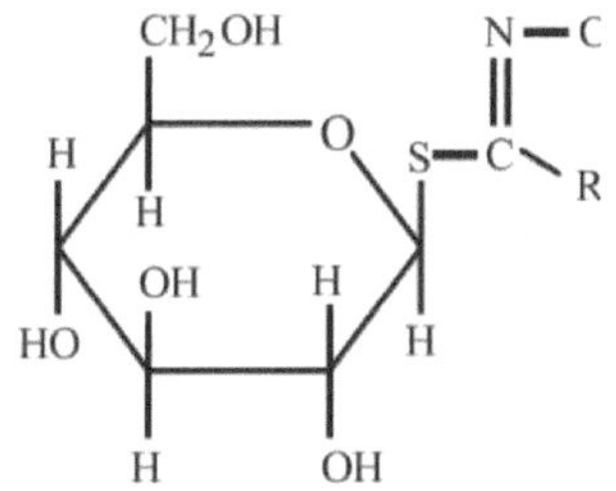


**Figure 6.1** Glucosinolate structure.

desulfoglucosinolate, and, lastly, sulfation. The observed structural variability of glucosinolates results from the alteration of the side chain involving oxidation, hydroxylation, and reduction (Holst et al., 2003). In brief, the typically recognized model for glucosinolate biosynthesis is described below:

- **Side chain elongation:** Methionine undergoes chain elongation before reaching the core structure route (Sønderby et al., 2010). At first, the mother amino acid is altered to form 2-oxo acid (Halkier and Gershenzon, 2006). Then the 2-oxo acid goes into a series of consecutive transitions: in the first transition there is condensation with acetyl-CoA using methylthioalkylmalate synthase (MAM), in the second transition there is isomerization using isopropyl malate isomerase (IPMI), and in the third transition there is oxidative decarboxylation using isopropyl malate dehydrogenase (IIPM-DH). The outcome of the above reactions is 2-oxo acid, lengthened by a single group of methylene (Sønderby et al., 2010), which condenses with acetyl-CoA into a substituted 2-malate derivative, which then (Agrawal et al., 2002) isomerizes through a 1,2- hydroxyl transition into a 3-malate derivative (Agrawal and Kurashige, 2003) while experiencing oxidation, which results in a 2-oxo acid, having one more methylene than its initial compound. After each turn of the loop, transamination of 2-oxo acid forms corresponding amino acid and initiates the second step of glucosinolate formation, else it can pass through further cycles of acetyl-CoA condensation, isomerization, and oxidation-carboxylation, leading to further extension. In plants, up to nine loops are reported (Fahey et al., 2001; Halkier and Gerzhenzon, 2006).
- **Glycone biosynthesis:** Glycone biosynthesis starts by the transformation of protein amino acids, e.g., alanine, methionine, valine, leucine, or isoleucine for the aliphatic glucosinolates; phenylalanine or tyrosine for the aromatic glucosinolates, and tryptophan for the indole glucosinolates (Mithen et al., 2000; Fahey et al., 2001). Various enzymes are responsible for the transformation of different amino acids, according to several reports. Cytochrome P450 monooxygenases (Mithen et al., 2000) which converts amino acids into aldoximes, are the enzymes most characterized (Du and Halkier, 1996). Fascinatingly, alike enzymes transform these amino acids into oxides as the early stages of cyanogenic glycoside biosynthesis (Halkier and Moller, 1991). Biosynthetic phases following the synthesis of aldoxime are assumed to include the conversion into the thiohydroximic acid, incorporation of thioglucoside sulphur from cysteine, *S. glycosyl* transfer from UDP-glucose (uracil-diphosphate glucose), and sulfation by 30-phosphoadenosine-50-phosphosulfate [PAPS] (Du and Halkier, 1998; Mithen et al., 2000). No biochemical proof has been attained for the possible intermediates between the production of aldoxime and thiohydroximic acid nor have several enzymes been purified and characterized in these stages. Thiohydroximic acid catalyzes S-Glycosylation of thiohydroximic acid leading to desulfoglucosinolate. Sulfation of desulfoglucosinolates is the final step in the formation of glycone. This happens by means of a soluble 30-phosphoadenosine 50-phosphosulfate (PAPS): desulfoglucosinolate sulfotransferase. This too has been refined and identified but it is incredibly unstable, and the specificity of its substrates is highly uncertain and choosy (Glendening and Poulton, 1988; Fahey et al., 2001).
- **Side chain modification:** The side chain may be subjected to different alterations following the biosynthesis of methyl thioalkyl glucosinolates (or probably desulphoglucosinolate or thiohydroximate) from methionine. The proposed route includes the starting oxidation of methylsulphinylalkyl, preceded by the deletion of methylsulphinyl group and desaturation leading to alkenyl glucosinolates and eventual hydroxylation to produce hydroxyalkenyl glucosinolates (Giamoustaris and Mithen, 1996; Mithen et al., 2000). Since branched chain, aromatic, and indole glucosinolates have a similar spectrum of structural complexity to aliphatic glucosinolates, they are likely to undergo similar hydroxylations, desaturations, and oxidations (Fahey et al., 2001) (Figure 6.2).

In certain tissues of Brassica vegetables (Rosa, 1997), the level of the glucosinolates in plants is roughly 1% dry weight basis (Kurilich et al., 1999) and can reach around 10% of the plant seed in which glucosinolates may constitute one half of the sulfur content of the seeds (Josefsson, 1970). Most of the plants have small amounts of glucosinolates. The concentration of studied glucosinolates fluctuate across plant organs, which have qualitative and quantitative variations among roots,

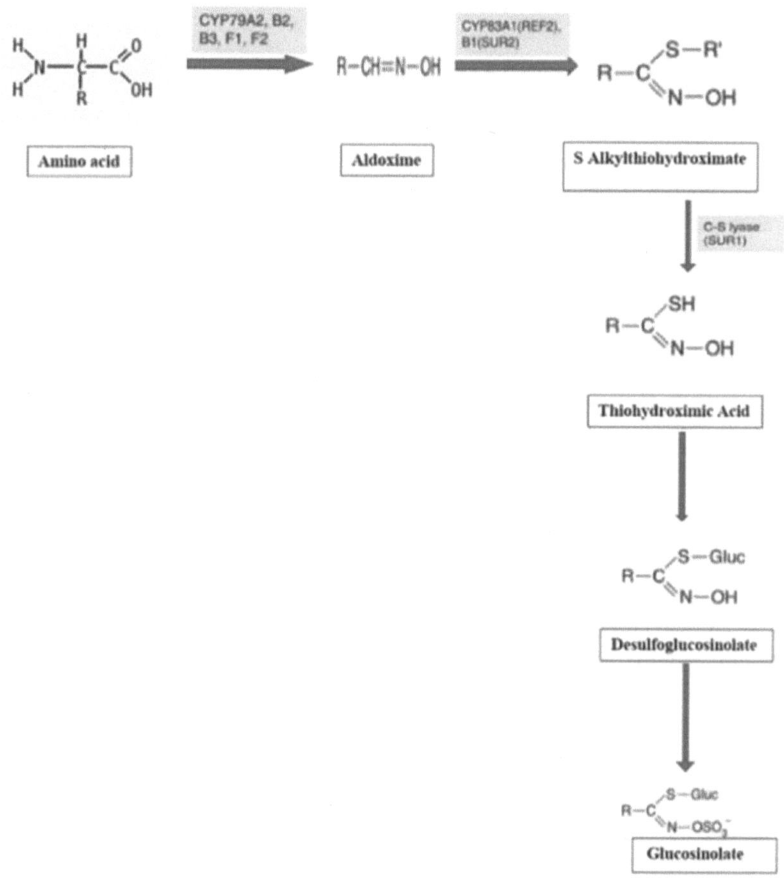


**Figure 6.2** Glucosinolate biosynthesis.

leaves, stems, and seeds (Fahey et al., 2001). The table below (see Table 6.1) lists some of the most common glucosinolates found in plants.

### *6.3.1.1 Glucosinolate: Hydrolysis Products*

Van Etten et al. examined the existence of natural glucosinolates and substances that may be produced from them by hydrolysis/autolysis (VanEtten et al., 1969; VanEtten and Tookey, 1979). These are hydrolysis derivatives, not intact glucosinolates, that are accountable for the bioactivities and organoleptic properties of cruciferous vegetables. Nearly all researchers agree that the glucosinolate hydrolysis involves only one enzyme (Nagashima and Uchiyama, 1959; VanEtten et al., 1969). The kinetics of myrosinase reaction are greatly different in plants and even in the same plant there can be many variants of the enzyme (James and Rossiter, 1991). Other than plant enzymes, there are fungal (Reese et al., 1958) and bacterial myrosinases (Tani et al., 1974) as well. Myrosinases are also commonly found in many humans and animal intestinal microflora (Rabot et al., 1993). The early report of myrosinase-like activities in mammalian tissue (Goodman et al., 1959) is likely to demonstrate the behaviour of the intestinal microflora, an observation supported by recent data from several labs (Rabot et al., 1993; Getahun and Chung, 1999). Myrosinase has been isolated and identified from many sources, particularly white mustard (*Sinapis alba*; Palmieri et al., 1986), cress (*Lepidium sativum*; Durham and Poulton, 1989), yellow mustard (*Brassica*

**Table 6.1 Common Glucosinolates Found in Some Plants**

| Common Name | Scientific Name | Glucosinolate Present | Structure | Reference |
|---|---|---|---|---|
| Field or Mustard turnip | *Brassicarapa* | Progoitrin | 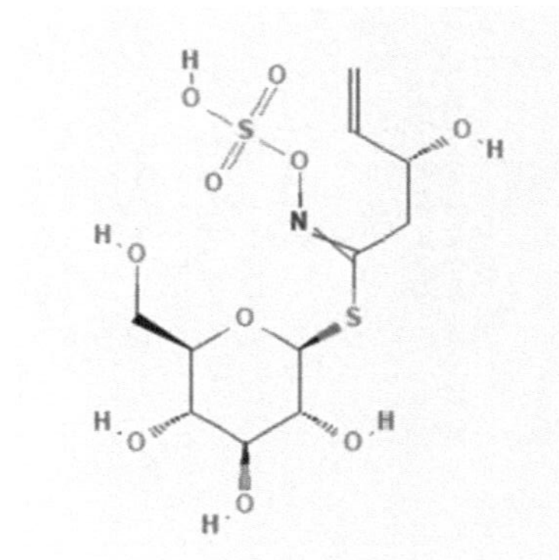 | Astwood et al. (1949) |
| Wild Cabbage | *Brassicaoleracea* | Sinigrin | 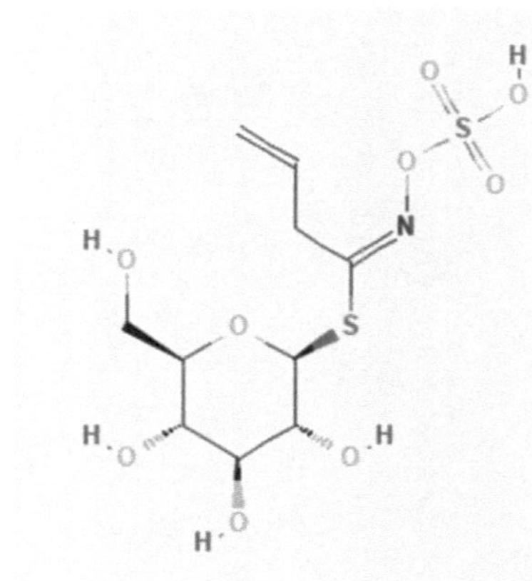 | Jensen et al. (1953) |

(*Continued*)

**Table 6.1 (Continued) Common Glucosinolates Found in Some Plants**

| Common Name | Scientific Name | Glucosinolate Present | Structure | Reference |
|---|---|---|---|---|
| Rutabaga or swede | *Brassica napobrass ica* | Glucobrassicin | 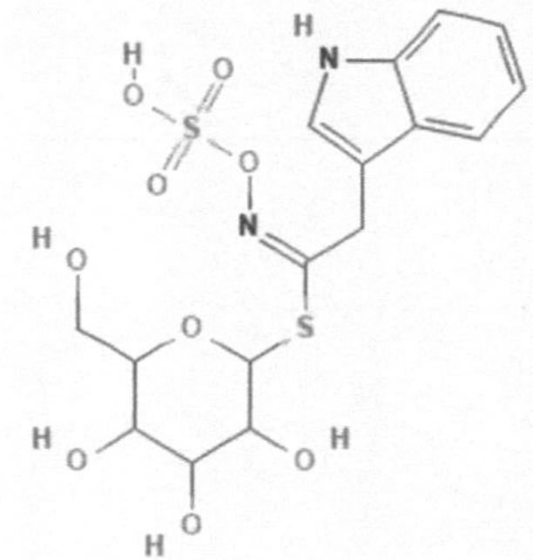 | Gmelin and Virtanen (1961) |
| Garden cress | *Lepidium sativum* | Glucotropaeolin | 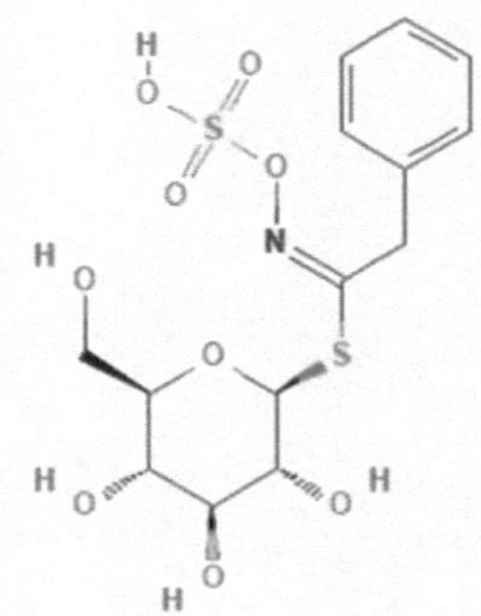 | Friis and Kjaer (1966) |

(*Continued*)

**Table 6.1 (Continued) Common Glucosinolates Found in Some Plants**

| Common Name | Scientific Name | Glucosinolate Present | Structure | Reference |
| --- | --- | --- | --- | --- |
| Horseradish | *Armoracia rusticana* | Gluconasturtiin | 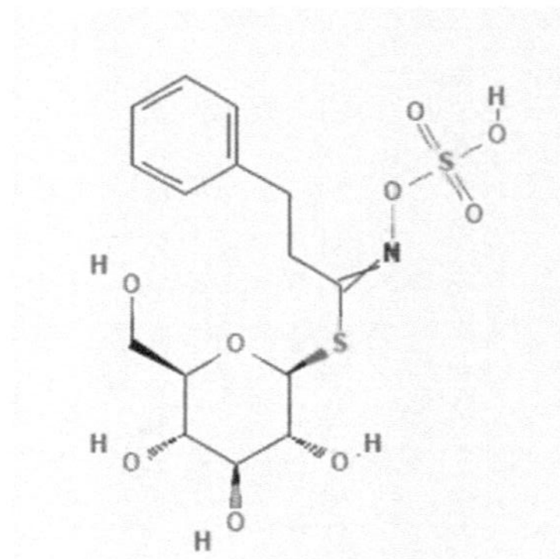 | Stoll and Seebeck (1948) |
| Ethiopian Mustard or Abyssinian mustard | *Brassica carinata* | epi-Progoitrin | 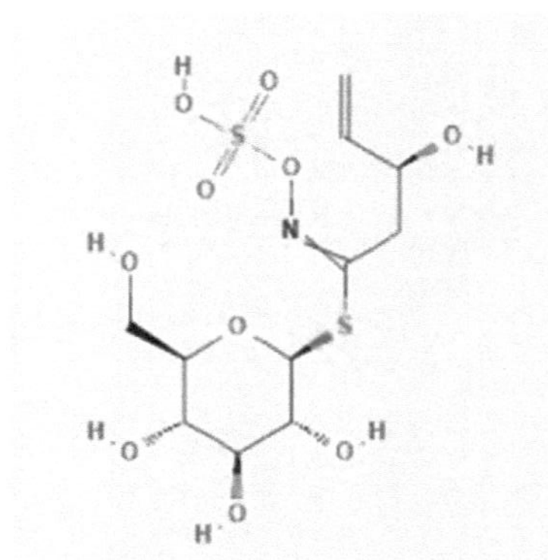 | Daxenbich ler et al. (1965) |

*juncea*; Bernardi et al., 2003), rapeseed (*Brassica napus*; Lonnerdal and Janson, 1973), and wasabi (*Wasabia japonica*; Ohtsuru and Kawatani, 1979). In different cruciferous plant sources, significant variations in myrosinase specific activity have been identified (Fahey et al., 2001). In several life forms the most popular glucosinolate hydrolysis products are Isothiocyanates, Nitrile, Epithionitrile, Oxazolidine2-thione, thiocyanate which rely on studied plant species, side chain replacement, cell pH, and concentration of cell iron (Fenwick et al., 1983) (Figure 6.3).

### 6.3.1.2 Thiocyanate and Isothiocyanates

Isothiothiocyanate is the most natural result of myrosinase hydrolysis produced from aglucone by a Lossen rearrangement (Fenwick et al., 1983). Just three glucosinolates, benzyl-, allyl- and 4-methyl-sulfinyl-butyl-glucosinolates, form thiocyanates which are all formed by stable side chains. The production of thiocyanate is linked to special protein factors (Hasapis and MacLeod, 1982), which

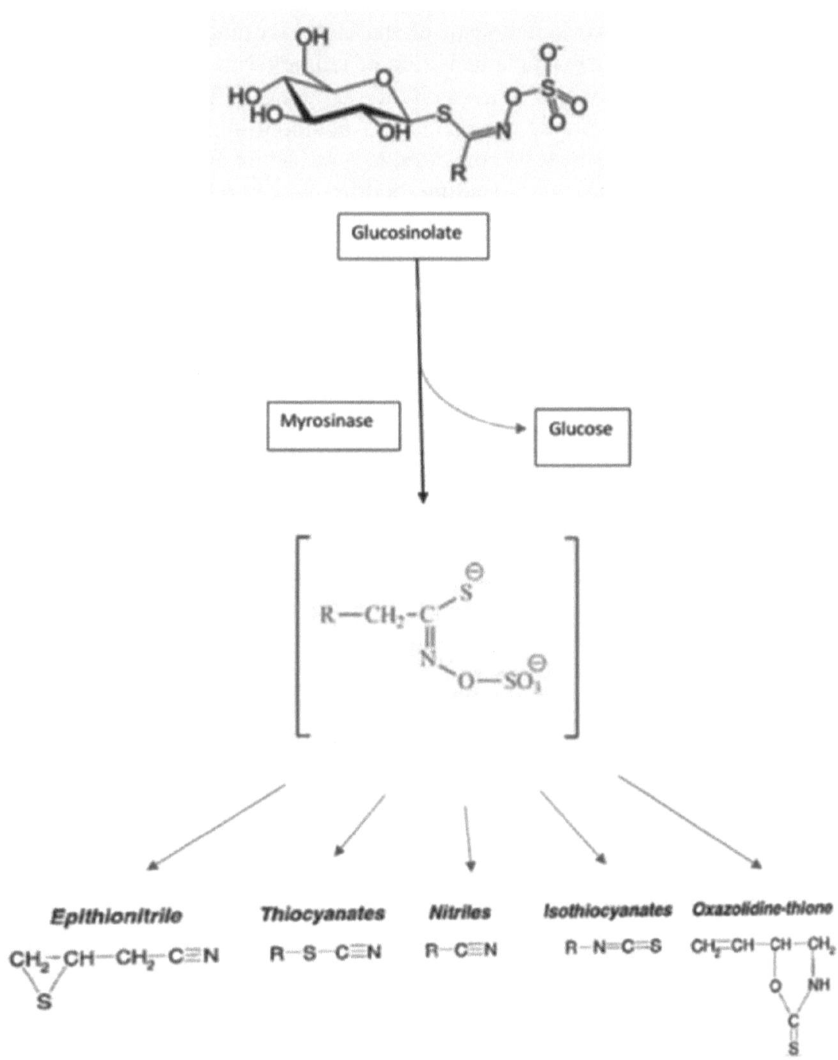


**Figure 6.3** Glucosinolates hydrolysis products.

have not been identified yet (Halkier and Gershenzon, 2006). The isothiocyanates, which are of natural origin, have a variety of anti-fungal (Virtanen, 1962), anti-bacterial (Dornberger et al., 1975) and anti-microbial (Zsolnai, 1966) behaviours likely to underlie the application of brassicas in traditional medicine (Fenwick and Heaney, 1983). Simultaneously, rats were fed normal doses of allyl isothiocyanate via gastric feeding tube at amounts comparable to their intake of mustard oil when they were on a high-cabbage content ration and it was seen that the rats have developed expanded thyroids. As the concentration of thiocyanates in the rat's blood and urine increased, the formation of thiocyanate from mustard oil was seen. In these studies, Langer and his colleagues have shown that goiter is possibly due to the thiocyanate ion and allyl isothiocyanate produced by glucosinolates in rats at a low level of iodine (Langer and Stolc, 1965). Thiocyanate and thiocyanate-related compounds interact with thyroid gland metabolism by lowering the levels of iodine (Ermans and Bourdoux, 1989). Furthermore, these impair the iodine accumulation function of thyroid gland by inhibiting unwitting clearance of iodine from the gland (Mitchell and O'Rourke, 1960). Thiocyanate prevents the absorption of iodide at low doses (Wolf, 1964); additionally, it prevents incorporation of iodine in thyroglobulin at higher doses (Ermans and Bourdoux, 1989). Isothiocyanates may have goitrogenic effects due to in vivo metabolism of the isothiocyanates (Langer and Greer, 1977), which can be related to the dietary supplementation of iodine (Fenwick et al., 1983). The real levels of thiocyanate and isothiocyanates in a specific food cannot reflect its true goitrogenic ability and the lack of such compounds does not preclude a potential anti-thyroid effect because, after consumption, inactive precursors may be converted to goitrogenic agents both in the plant and the animal body (Gaitan, 1986). Cassava is a leading food in many parts of the world, including in the Democratic Republic of Congo, where thiocyanate is expected to contribute towards high rates of goiter (Gaitan and Dunn, 1992). Another source of thiocyanate abundance is tobacco smoking. The risk of neonatal hypothyroidism in neonates from smoking mothers seems greater in a country with a borderline iodine deficiency (Vanderpas, 2003).

#### *6.3.1.3 Goitrin and Related Oxazolidinethiones*

They are also hydrolysis products of glucosinolates. Oxazolidine-2-thiones are suspected to have anti-nutritional influence by impairing thyroid hormone synthesis. One critical aspect of this action is that dietary iodine does not mitigate this effect (Langer and Greer, 1977). Langer and Michajlovskij (1969) demonstrated a substantial rise in thyroid size in rats after giving only 40μg of 5-vinyloxazolidine-2-thione for 20 days (Fenwick et al., 1983). Progoitrin, a thioglucoside, occurs in higher amounts in most *brassicaceous* species and in edible parts of some plants, notably in rutabaga and turnip. It is hydrolyzed to produce goitrin by myrosinase enzyme (Oginsky et al., 1965). Goitrin is a powerful goitrogen which has been shown to trigger glutathione S-Transferase (GST) action and to maximize detoxification of aflatoxins (Kelley and Bjeldanes, 1995). The goitrin inhibitor was first identified by the measurement of the decreased thyroid uptake of radioactive iodine (I131) in feeding (test) animals (Astwood et al., 1949). In goitrin-fed rats, hyperplasia and hypertrophy have been observed and the reaction is somewhat less than that of thiourea (Carroll, 1949).

#### *6.3.1.4 Other Glucosinolate Hydrolysis Products*

Nitriles represent a large proportion of glucosinolate hydrolysis outcomes in several plants (Cole, 1976). At pH less than 3, or when the $Fe^{2+}$ ions are present, nitrile formation in vitro is facilitated (Galletti et al., 2001). Also, protein factors like the epithiospecificator protein (ESP) may participate in nitrile in vivo formation (Bernardi et al., 2000). Thioglucoside nitriles can serve as goitrogens. In rabbits with regular doses of the substance, nitriles induce thyroid enlargement. The possible cause is the exfoliation of nitriles to thiocyanate ions (Greer, 1950). The latter workers could not, however, often validate the confirmed goitrogenic effects of organic nitriles. Simple nitriles are usually considered as less hazardous than isothiocyanates (Mumm et al., 2008).

### 6.3.2 Cyanogenic Glycosides

Cyanogenic glycosides are a form of substance present in food plants that has the potential to affect consumers. Cyanogenic glycosides are plant secondary metabolites that are chemically known as glycosides of α-hydroxy-nitriles (Australia et al., 2004) and emit hydrogen cyanide after consumption (Bolarinwa et al., 2016). The cyanogenic glycoside biosynthesis precursors are various hydroxylated L-amino acids i.e., N-hydroxyl-amino acid which are turned into aldoximes and transformed into nitriles and hydroxylated to α-Hydroxy-nitriles and finally glycosylated to cyanogenic glycosides (Vetter, 2000). The five hydrophobic amino acids tyrosine, phenylalanine, valine, leucine, and isoleucine are the precursors of most of the cyanogenic glycosides (Poulton, 1990). According to the molecular morphology of the aglycone, the cyanogenic glycosides can be easily classified into four classes:

1. Amygdalin type, glycosides obtained from 2-hydroxy-2-phenylacetonitrile (Bisset et al., 1969).
2. Linamarin type, glycosides resulting from aliphatic aglycones that are saturated (Abrol, 1967).
3. Acacipetalin type, glycosides having double bond in the aglycone (Blumenthal et al., 1968).
4. Gynocardins form, glycosides comprising an unsaturated, alicyclic aglycone (Blum and Woordring, 1962) (Figure 6.4).

Amygdalin is the best-known cyanogenic glycoside and is present in many *Rosaceae* members. It is a ß-glycoside of D (-) mandelonitrile or benzaldehyde cyanohydrin and on hydrolysis produces two moles of glucose with one mole each of benzaldehyde and HCN (Conn, 1969) (Figure 6.5).

At neutral pH, cyanogenic glycosides are stable chemical compounds. These can be hydrolyzed by acid at high temperatures into aldehyde or ketone, sugar, and HCN. Hydrogen cyanide development from cyanogenic glycosides is an enzymatic mechanism generally referred to as Cyanogenesis (Deshpande, 2002). The following table contains several well-known cyanogenic glycosides, their plant origins and hydrolysis products (Conn, 1973) (See Table 6.2):

#### *6.3.2.1 Dietary Sources of Cyanogenic Glycosides*

In so many tropical countries basic foods are starchy fruits and tubers, including cassava, yam, etc. (Satheesh and Solomon, 2019). These are often regarded as anti-obesity agents as there is less than 2% fat in them (Rinaldo, 2020). Bamboo shoots, cassava, corn, lima beans, linseed, millet, peaches, peanuts, pears, pine nuts, pears, strawberries, sweet potatoes, etc., are some of the representatives of this group. Cassava is an important element in many Latin American and Caribbean cuisines. Cassava encompasses poisonous substance known as cyanogenic glycosides, which disintegrates to form hydrogen cyanide. There are several types of cassava with different amounts of cyanide (Australia et al., 2004). Cassava intake can lead to cyanide toxicity when cyanogenic glucosides and their metabolic by-products are not properly separated from roots during processing. Cassava must therefore be boiled or pounded before being consumed because it is toxic in its native form (Choudhury et al., 2010). Further, when iodine intakes dip below the recommended daily ingest, the goitrogenic impact of thiocyanate overload from cassava just worsen iodine deficiency disorders (Delange et al., 1994). Some 25 known cyanogenic glycosides are present in foodstuffs, including apples, apricots, cherries, peaches, and quinces (particularly in the seed of those fruits).

They are also present in pome fruits, cassava, bamboo shoots, lima beans, coco yam, cassava, chickpeas, and kirsch (Haque and Bradbury, 2002). These foods thus constitute possible sources of hydrogen cyanide. The connection amongst humans and hydrogen cyanide (HCN) is complex: it

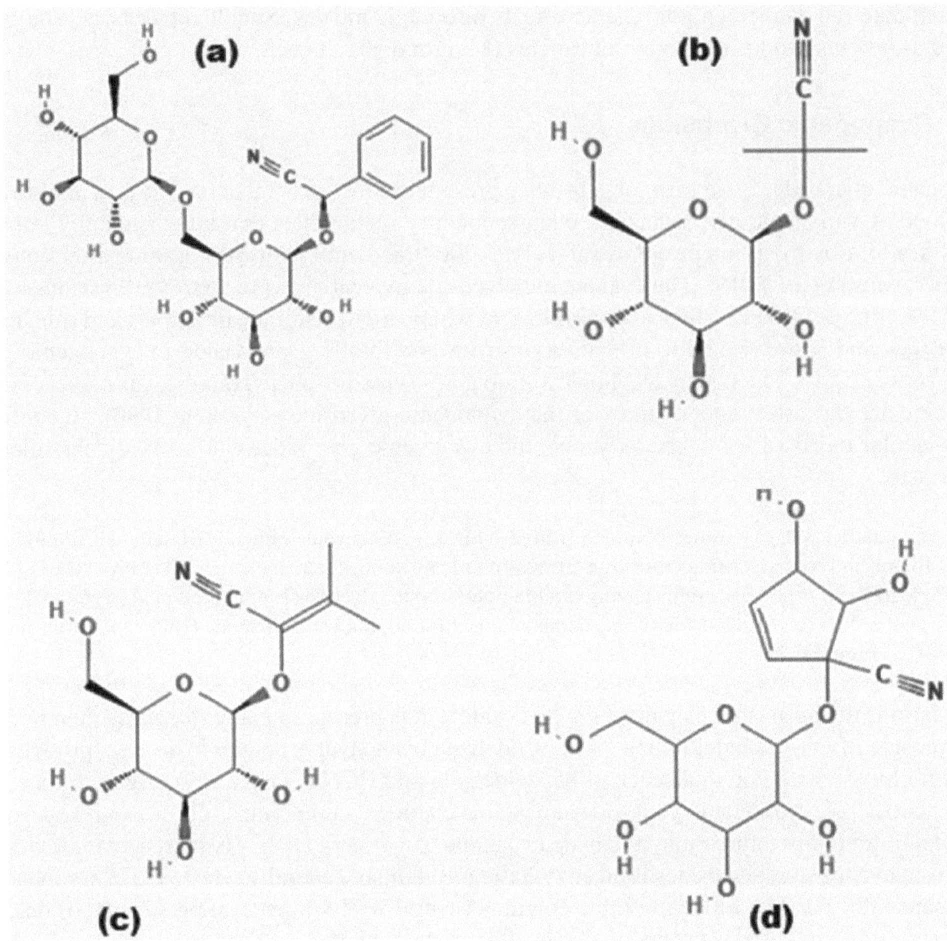


**Figure 6.4** Chemical structure of some widely recognized cyanogenic glycosides (a) amygdalin (b) linamarin (c) acacipetalin (d) gynocardins.

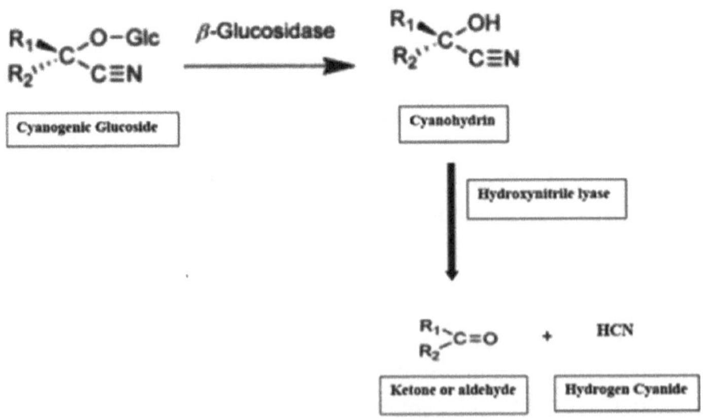


**Figure 6.5** Release of hydrogen cyanide.

**Table 6.2 Common Cyanogenic Glycosides Found in Some Plants**

| Common Name | Scientific Name | Glycoside Present | Hydrolysis Product | References |
|---|---|---|---|---|
| Rubber Tree | *Hevea brasiliensis* | Linamarin | d-glucose + HCN+ acetone | Australia et al. (2004) |
| Lima bean | *Phaseoluslunatus* | Lotaustralin | d-glucose+ HCN + 2Butanone | Ballhorn et al. (2009) |
| Pea | *Pisum sativum* | Prunasin | d-glucose + HCN+Benzaldehyde | Gilpin et al. (1997) |
| Eagle fern | *Pteridium aquilinum* | Dhurrin | d-glucose + HCN + p-Hydroxybenzaldehyde | Conn (1973) |
| Maize | *Zea mays* | Zierin | d-glucose + HCN + m-Hydroxybenzaldehyde | Jones (1998) |
| Sorghum | *Sorghumbicolor* | Dhurrin | d-glucose + HCN+p-Hydroxybenzaldehyde | Léder (2004) |
| Cassava | *Manihot esculenta* | Lotaustralin | d-glucose + HCN + 2-Butanone | Chandra et al., 2004 |

is poisonous, yet crops that cause HCN form a vital part of human menus (Conn, 1969). Research done in extreme endemic goiter regions in Zaire, Idjwi Island, Kivu, and Ubangi have shown the goitrogenic effect of cassava. Initially, these experiments were performed to adapt the thyroid system to iodine deficiency.

Bamboo shoot has also been established as a causative element in the continuance of endemic goiter in Manipur, India's northeastern province (Chandra, 2010). Related experiments on cabbage (*Brassica oleracea var. capitata Linn.*), cauliflower (*Brassica oleracea var. botrytis Linn.*), mustard (*Brassica juncea*), and maize (*Zea mays*) revealed that all these plant-based foods had effective anti-thyroid function even in the presence of iodine (Chandra et al., 2006).

### 6.3.3 Flavonoids

Flavonoids are a type of polyphenolic secondary metabolites obtained from plants that are widely included in diets. They come in a variety of forms, including aglycones, glycosides and methylated derivatives. Flavonoids have a 15-carbon backbone that consists of two phenyl rings (A and B) and a heterocyclic ring in general (C, which contains embedded oxygen) (Delage and Barbara, 2015). C6-C3-C6 is the shortened form for this carbon network. Flavonoids are categorized into subgroups based on the carbon of the C ring to which the B ring is connected, degree of unsaturation and oxidation of the C ring. These include flavones, flavonols, flavanones, isoflavonoids, neoflavonoids, flavan-3-ols or catechins, anthocyanins, chalcones. When ring B is attached to the third and fourth carbon of ring C, flavonoids are called isoflavones and neoflavanoids, respectively (Panche et al., 2016).

Flavonoids are essential natural components of many plants. They are common in vascular plants and a wide range of plant foods. They widely exist in the roots, stems, leaves, flowers, and fruits of higher plants and ferns (Bandele and Osheroff, 2007). Due to their wide distribution in plant foods (fruits, vegetables, grains, etc.), they are the significant components of a healthy diet (Gaitan, 1996). Major groups of flavonoids in human diets are:

1. Flavanols: It includes quercetin, kaempferol, quercetagetin.
2. Proanthocyanidins: It includes epicatechin, epicatechin gallate, epigallocatechin gallate epigallocatechin.
3. Isoflavonoids: It includes isoflavonoids and coumestrol.
4. Flavones: It includes apigenin, luteolin, quercetagetin.
5. Flavanones: It includes myricetin, naringin, naringenin.

The soy isoflavones genistein and daidzein have been shown to suppress thyroid peroxidase, an enzyme needed for thyroid hormone synthesis (Doerge and Sheehan, 2002), as well as 5'-deiodinase operations, resulting in a reduced T4 to T3 conversion. These compounds may also trigger hepatic enzymes that are mainly accountable for T3 and T4 clearance (White et al, 2004). They are present in lentils, chickpeas, soybeans, and other soy-based products such as tofu, miso, soy milk, and tempeh (Franke et al., 1995). Isoflavones, coumestans and lignans are non-steroidal substances with low estrogenic activity. These are usually referred to as "phytoestrogens". Soy, a possible dietary goitrogen, is widely used in commercial cat food as it is a rich source of vegetable protein. Coumestans, such as coumestrol, are abundantly present in alfalfa and clover (Franke et al., 1995), and are known to cause infertility in grazing herbivores. The flavones have no estrogenic function but the flavones, apigenin and luteolin, serve as powerful blockers of aromatase and 17β-hydroxysteroid oxidoreductase enzymes involved in estrogen metabolism (Le Bail et al., 1998). Research has also shown that the flavones and various glycocylflavones are strong goitrogens (Sartelet et al., 1996) (Table 6.3).

## 6.4 GOITROGENS: MECHANISM OF ACTION

For each group of chemical compounds, the process by which goitrogen blocks thyroid activity can vary.

Thiocyanate may not be found as a free ion in the plant but as a glycoside, transformed into a thiocyanate in the animal body. Thiocyanate and thiocyanate-like compounds derived from cyanogenic glycosides, glucosinolates, or thiocyanate impair thyroid iodine metabolism by suppressing iodide absorption, triggering iodide efflux, or swapping iodide with thiocyanate (Ermans and Bourdoux, 1989). In addition, thiocyanate and thiocyanate-like compounds primarily suppress the thyroid gland iodide-concentration system by inhibiting the unidirectional removal of iodide from the gland (Mitchell and O'Rourke, 1960). The main enzyme of thyroid hormone biosynthesis is thyroid peroxidase (TPO) which manages all the necessary reactions required in the thyroid gland to form thyroid hormones (T3 and T4) (Taurog, 1970).

Thiocyanate, which is a monovalent anion with a molecular size similar to that of iodine, inhibits iodide inclusion into thyroglobulin by participating with iodide at the level of the thyroid peroxidase (Ermans and Bourdoux, 1989). It prevents the oxidation of iodine by suppressing the action of TPO (Van Middlesworth, 1985). Thiocyanate prevents iodine uptake at low concentrations or doses, and at higher concentrations or doses thiocyanate prevents amalgamation of iodine into thyroglobulin (Ermans and Bourdoux, 1989). A meal high in thiocyanate (or glucosinolates) but low in iodide results in lower T3 and T4 levels (Lakshmy et al., 1995). Similarly, isothiocyanates predominantly affect the thyroid via their accelerated transformation to thiocyanate, and these not only follow the thiocyanate metabolic route but also respond instantaneously with thiourea-based amino groups that yield an anti-thyroid-like effect (Chandra, 2010). The existing thiocyanate or isothiocyanate content in a particular food cannot reflect its actual goitrogenic ability and neither does the lack of these substances prohibit a future anti-thyroid effect since inactive precursors in both plants and animals can be transformed into goitrogenic compounds after consuming it (Gaitan, 1986). By the action of a plant enzyme, myrosinase, mustard oil glycoside produces thiocyanate. In the absence of this enzyme, however, ingestion of pure progoitrin, a naturally occurring thioglucoside, evokes anti-thyroid action in rats and humans since it is gradually transformed in the animal body by intestinal microflora into the more active goitrin (Oginsky et al., 1965). Likewise, flavonoids, after ingestion, are hydrolyzed to flavonoid aglycans by intestinal microbial glycosidases that may be ingested and absorbed by the body and it is possible for B-ring hydroxylation and middle-ring fusion to further process intestinal microorganisms for the manufacture of different compounds, such as phenolic acids, phloroglucinol, and gallic acid. Many of these have significant anti-thyroid effects. Flavonoids not just suppress TPO behaviour but also impair deiodinase enzymes leading to the suppression of thyroid hormones from peripheral metabolism. Furthermore, flavonoid phloretin polymers interfere with the TSH, stopping it from acting on thyroid cells. As a result, these substances seem to have a profound effect on thyroid hormone activity (Gaitan, 1986; Chandra, 2010).

**Table 6.3 Flavonoid Source and Levels in Commonly Consumed Foods**

| Flavonoid | Common Name | Scientific Name | Structure | Levels (mg/kg Wet Weight) |
|---|---|---|---|---|
| Quercetin | Onion | *Allium cepa* | 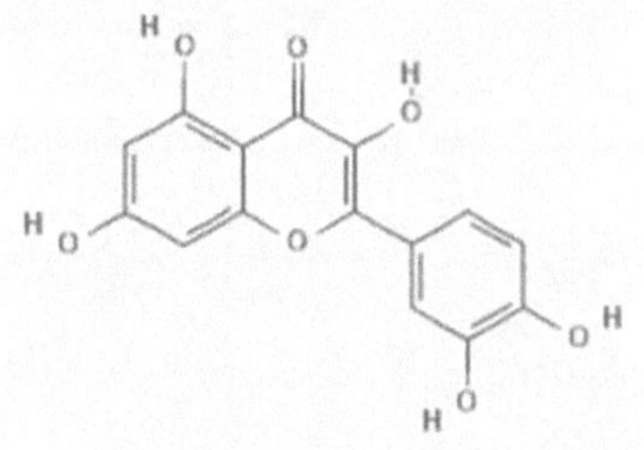 | 248–486 |
| | Kale | *Brassicaoleracea* | | 110 |
| | Apple | Malusdomestica | | 21–72 |
| Genistein | Tofu | | 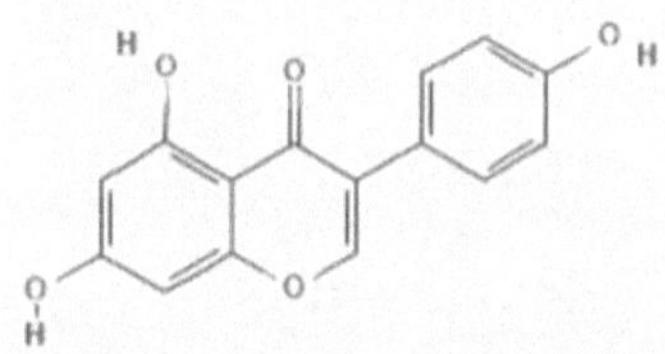 | 159–306 |
| Diadzein | Soy-milk formula | | 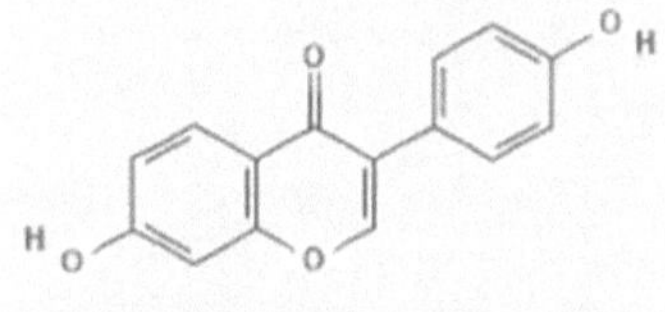 | 15–19 |
| Coumestrol | Alfalfa | *Medicago sativa* | 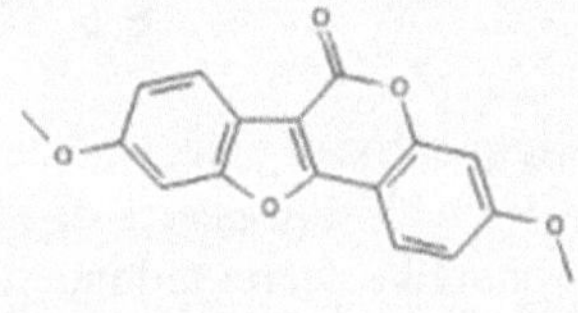 | 47 |
| | Clover | *Trifolium* | | 281 |

(*Continued*)

**Table 6.3 (Continued) Flavonoid Source and Levels in Commonly Consumed Foods**

| Flavonoid | Common Name | Scientific Name | Structure | Levels (mg/kg Wet Weight) |
|---|---|---|---|---|
| Apigenin | Millet | *Panicum miliaceum* | 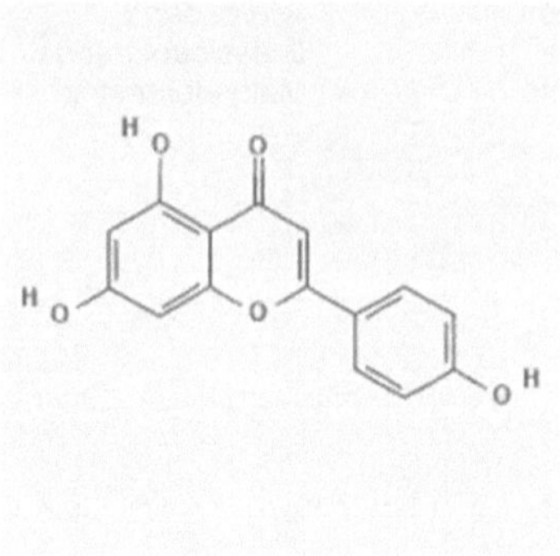 | 150 |
| Luteolin | Millet | *Panicum miliaceum* | 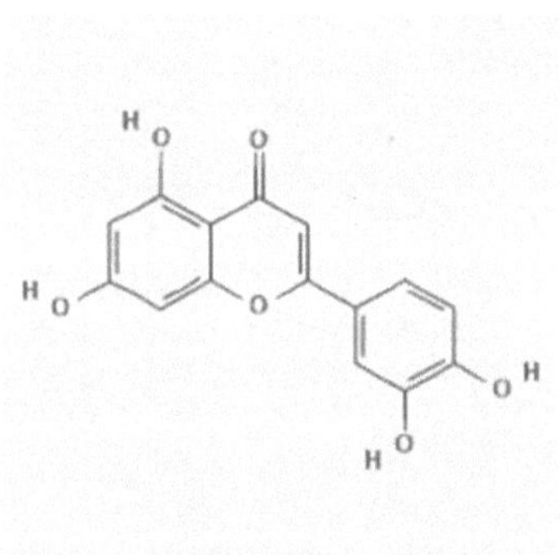 | 350 |
| Maringin | Grapefruit | *Citrus paradisi* | 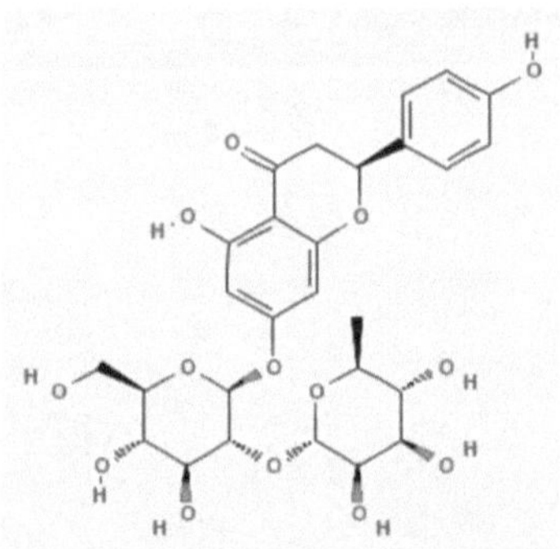 | 100–800 mg/L |

(Adapted and modified from Skibola and Smith, 2000)

## 6.5 TOXICOLOGY

The detrimental consequences of glucosinolates on animals are proportional to their level in the feed and the intensity varies with the species of animals involved. Several toxic effects are reported in animals feeding on them like decreased intake of feed, reduced growth, and reproduction (Bourdon et al., 1981). Kale has a high level of sulphur, which can hinder copper and selenium ingestion causing shortcomings in these essential nutrients (Taljaard, 1993; Bischoff, 2021). To determine the toxicity of the glucosinolates and their enzyme degradation products, a 24-h aquatic mortality experiment with *Caenorhabditis elegans* was done. It was observed that in absence of enzyme myrosinase it was reported that sinigrin, which is an allyl glucosinolate, was nontoxic at all the concentrations tested. However, water extract of *Crambe abyssinica* (freeze-dried, dialyzed) which contained about 26% of epi-progoitrin had 18.5 g/l $LC_{50}$ value. Further, the incorporation of the enzyme enhanced the sinigrin toxicity ($LC_{50}$) to 0.5 g/l, however the enzyme had little impact on *C. abyssinica* extract toxicity. Liquid chromatographic studies revealed that there is a possibility of sinigrin decomposition into allyl isothiocyanate. It can further be concluded that allyl isothiocyanate is nearly three times more toxic to *C. elegans* than the glucosinolate itself (Donkin et al., 1995).

There is little evidence of toxicity of individual glucosinolates and most of the cases arise from overall glucosinolates. For rapeseed meal or pressed cakes detailed animal feeding experiments were carried out in domestic animals, leading to the guidelines to minimize the amount of net glucosinolates to 1–1.5 mmol/kg in monogastric species and further decreased amount in case of early age animals (Assayed and Abd El-Aty, 2009). The carcinogenicity of various glucosinolates, including isothiocyanates, nitriles, 5-vinyl2, oxazolidinethiones, and indole-3-carbinol, in rodents were investigated by Nishie and Daxenbichler, 1980 and it was concluded that these were not teratogenic. While 2-propenyl isothiocyanate, 3-methylsulfinylpropyl isothiocyanate, and l-cyano-3,4-epithiobutane were found to be embryotoxic (Fenwick et al., 1983). Poisonings in all the leading life forms have been identified due to the ingestion of glucosinolate containing plants. In broad sense, after exposure to poisoning glucosinolates, typical clinical symptoms are found, and these are:

1. Changes in thyroid function and thyroid gland extension after consuming oxazolidinethiones and isothiocyanates (Spiegel et al., 1993).
2. Alkyl isothiocyanates lead to inflammation and localized tissue damage of the gastro-intestinal mucosa (Martland et al., 1984).
3. Suppression of growth (Schöne et al., 1997a).
4. Liver failure by enhanced enzyme discharge (Martland et al., 1984).
5. Fertility problems associated with prolonged access to glucosinolate rich plants (Taljaard, 1993).
6. Possibly due to isothiocyanates there are chances of temporary locomotive disability, cognitive adjustment, and blurred vision (rape blindness) (Rodriguez, 1997).

In humans, reduced iodine uptake by the thyroid gland was reported after daily ingestion of 500 g cabbage for 2 weeks (Langer, 1971) or after a single meal of 300 to 500 g swede or turnip (Greer and Astwood, 1948). However, a more recent study conducted by McMillan et al., (1986) revealed that daily consumption of 150 g Brussels sprouts for about 4 weeks did not lead to hypothyroidism in human volunteers. A few studies have been done to verify exactly which glucosinolate or its derivative results in glucosinolate toxicity. Increased liver hypertrophy in rats was the result of the incorporation of pure sinigrin or gluconapin to the diet. Progoitrin appears to have a higher toxicity potential; it has led to liver, kidney, and thyroid enlargement in rats (Vermorel et al., 1986). In terms of toxicity, goitrin (5-vinyloxazolidine-2-thione), one of the significant derivatives of progoitrin, is by far the most widely studied glucosinolate derivative. Goitrin appears to interact with the organic iodination of thyroxine precursors in the gland, resulting in goiter (Akiba and Matsumoto, 1977). Isothiocyanates and thiocyanates were blamed for related thyroid disorders (Langer, 1964). Sinigrin and glucoiberin isothiocyanate derivatives have been reported to cause embryo death in rats and the mechanism is not known yet (Nishie and Daxenbichler, 1980). The liver and kidneys appear to be the preferred sites of nitrile derivatives (Srivastava et al., 1975). The toxicity of nitriles occurs as hypertrophy of the target organ, leading to disruption of the liver's usual lobular structure and abnormal bile duct proliferation (VanEtten et al., 1969). The type and underlying mechanisms of toxic effects caused by glucosinolate derivatives often provide important data. It does not, however, consider the potential of the intestinal microflora to divide intact glucosinolates and its derivatives into metabolites, which remains to be fully elucidated. These results support the notion that, if the plant myrosinase in the diet is fully deactivated, the toxicity of glucosinolate would be determined solely by the balance of bacterial organisms with unique myrosinase-like behaviors. The toxic effects in traditional rats, whether developed by plant myrosinase or glucosinolate-rich but non-myrosinase diets, are generally identical. There are no different effects. Nonetheless, the risk of extra metabolites, toxic or non-toxic, being formed from intact glucosinolate or previously released derivatives cannot be eliminated. This, of course, adds to the challenge of determining the possible toxicity of a cruciferous vegetable diet based on its glucosinolate and glucosinolate derivative material.

Many researchers have hypothesized that the pesticidal impacts of glucosinolates are not caused directly by glucosinolates, but by the compounds mediated by their enzymes (Fenwick et al., 1983; Lazzeri et al., 1993). The key components of these derivatives are allyl isothiocyanate and allyl cyanide (i.e., nitrile), and their development is affected by pH, ferrous ion, and glucosinolate side chain configuration (Donkin et al., 1995). Bitterness is caused by isothiocyanates (Mithen et al., 2000), while nitriles have a negative impact on well-being (Tanii et al., 2004). Thiocyanates, thiourea, and oxazolidithione can impair thyroid activity by interfering with iodine supply (Brown et al., 2002). These have varying effects on the thyroid gland. Thiocyanate tends to block the thyroid gland's absorption of synthetic iodide in a selective fashion, as the suppression can be overturned with iodide supplementation (Fenwick, 1989). Once the iodine is embedded in the gland, it is oxidized to iodine and hormonal precursors of thyroxine (T4) or triiodothyronine (T3) are produced by the iodination of amino acid tyrosine and during this process goitrin and other thiouracil equivalents messes with the iodination procedure, eventually affecting the production of T4 and T3 precursors. Furthermore, reinforcement cannot undo this effect (Majak, 1992). Goitrogenicity (Schone et al., 1990), mutagenicity, hepatotoxicity, and nephrotoxicity (Tanii et al., 2004) are other detrimental consequences of glucosinolate derivatives. The detrimental impact of dietary glucosinolate on animal development and growth may be linked to the severe endocrine dysfunction by antinutritional factors (Ahlin et al., 1994). Also, there are chances that goitrogenic substances can be passed on to humans indirectly via milk of cows given brassica pasture (Fenwick et al., 1983). Arstila et al. (1969) discovered that milk from cows in goiter-endemic regions of Finland (where grasslands are polluted with brassica weeds) absorbs L-5-vinyl-2-thio-oxazolidine, which is missing from milk from other regions, and that this milk triggered goiter in rodents (Peltola and Krusius, 1960).

The thiocyanate ion formed by myrosinase-induced degradation of indole glucosinolates has been suspected to have additional negative effects on the thyroid (Agerbirk et al., 2009). The sodium/iodide symporter on the basolateral membrane of the thyroid follicular cell is competitively inhibited by the thiocyanate ion (Tonacchera et al., 2004). Thus, thiocyanate ingestion will minimize iodide absorption by the thyroid gland, eventually leading to reduced thyroid hormone synthesis (hypothyroidism).

Anti-TPO behaviour has been shown in processed and unprocessed cyanogenic plant foods such as cauliflower, cabbage, mustard, turnip, radish, bamboo shoot, and cassava. Furthermore, boiled extracts of these cyanogenic plant foods had the most anti-TPO activity, preceded by cooked and unprocessed extracts. Goitrin is an abundant goitrogen found in the seeds of brassica plants. However, cooking kills the progoitrin-goitrin activation enzyme, thereby minimizing its anti-thyroid strength. Goitrogenic foods, when ingested in large amounts, can lead to the production of goiter, but they are difficult to implicate as causative factors (Greer, 1957).

HCN, a potentially poisonous compound with the ability to interact with heme proteins, most prominently cytochrome oxidase, the enzyme that participates in the final stage of aerobic respiration, is emitted by cyanogenic plants (Møller, 1979a). At the concentrations of 0.5–3.5 mg/kg body weight, this HCN becomes deadly for humans and if multiple doses of HCN are taken at once, the concentration of 1–7 mg/kg body weight becomes deadly (Montgomery, 1969). Exposure to cyanide can also have repercussions other than serious harmful effects (Poulton, 1983). Cyanide can be inactivated by so many species. One mechanism that seems to be typical to mammals in this phase is the rhodanese enzyme system (Long and Brattsen, 1982), which participates in cyanide and thiosulfate reaction to yield thiocyanate and sulfite (Alexander and Volini, 1981) by utilizing sulfur and cysteine. Thiocyanate is steadily removed and much of the chronic symptoms of cyanide exposure are caused by thiocyanate (Møller, 1979a).

One finding confirmed the production of goiter and hypothyroidism in a 10-month-old baby who was given soybean product from birth, but the condition was reversed with soybean product removal and Lugol's iodine drops. Furthermore, after the removal of soybean products, the thyroid demonstrated a strong absorption of $I^{131}$. Adult surveys showed a substantial reduction in plasma bound $I^{131}$ when given soybean-based foods (Van Wykk et al., 1959). As a result, soybean-based foods appeared to contain a goitrogenic agent that interferes with normal functioning of thyroid gland. Though the soya protein and isoflavones do not really influence the natural thyroid function in people with adequate supply of iodine, still they can affect the absorption of synthetic thyroid hormone, requiring hypothyroid patients to take further medicine (Chandra et al., 2004). Furthermore, since flavonoids can bind nonheme iron, they are potentially toxic in vulnerable populations such as the elderly who are iron deficient (Corcoran et al., 2012).

## 6.6 IDENTIFICATION AND QUANTIFICATION OF GOITROGENS

From the past few decades, increased impetus is seen in knowing the safe levels of goitrogens present in various foods as there is a concern regarding their possible biological influence. So far, a number of analytical techniques in plant materials have been developed which can quantify the total as well as individual glucosinolates. However, an enzymatic assay wherein glucosinolates are hydrolyzed by widely accessible myrosinase is considered as the most popular and fastest method for estimating the amount of total glucosinolates. In the presence of hexokinase and glucose-6-phosphate dehydrogenase, the glucose generated through this operation is transformed into gluconate-6-phosphate. This process yields nicotinamide adenine dinucleotide phosphate (NADPH) (from $NADP^+$), which can be measured spectrophotometrically at 340 nm (Gardrat and Prevot, 1987) or 520 nm with additional redox coupling (Sørensen, 1990). The overall glucosinolate concentration is then typically represented as µmol glucose released per g of product and is calculated from the NADPH data.

For the complete identification of embedded glucosinolates, many procedures are accessible including thymol, palladium, or ELISA and glucose enzymes method. However, HPLC is by far the most precise method for identification of complete and specific glucosinolates, but it has a few drawbacks; for example, the costly devices and high quantity of solvents that are necessary to run it (Li et al., 2017). The International Organization for Standardization (ISO), the European Committee for Standardization (CEN), and the European Commission all advocate to use HPLC method for study of de-sulphoglucosinolates (enzymatically desulfated) as the approved method for rapeseed-specific glucosinolates. The IRMM (Institute for Reference Materials and Measurements) has reference data containing these de-sulphoglucosinolates (Institute for Reference Materials and Measurements) (Helboe et al., 1980).

For the assessment of glucosinolates and their equivalents, specialized chromatographic techniques including, ultra-high-performance liquid chromatography (UHPLC) anchored to numerous detectors such as diode array detectors (DAD) and UV detectors, and mass spectrometers have also been used in recent years (Smiechowska et al., 2010). Several glucosinolates (Sinigrin, gluconapin, glucocapparin, and glucoerucin) were isolated and evaluated using an HPLC-PDA/UV detector by Grosser and van Dam, 2017. Embedded glucosinolates in broccoli leaves were isolated, segregated, and measured by using water, methanol or 70% methanol at 70°C using water bath. Likewise, the system for chemical screening of supplement tablets derived from cruciferous vegetables with glucosinolates was generated based on ultra-high-performance liquid chromatography combined with tandem mass spectroscopy (Shi et al., 2017).

Cyanogenic glycosides were detected using the technique of the picrate-impregnated paper according to Harbone (1972). A brown-red colour appearing within 48 h indicated that the cyanogenic glycoside spontaneously released HCN without the action of enzyme. No colour change after 48 h indicated that the test was negative for cyanogenic glycoside (Francisco and Pinotti, 2000). Strategies for quantifying cyanide in living cells include hydrolysis of the cyanogenic glycosides and the liberation of HCN, retained in the basic solution and measured calorimetrically (Brinker and Seigler et al., 1989). Cyanide is often isolated using a method close to that defined by Pereira et al., (1981), which involves incubating plant tissue in Warburg flasks or small Erlenmeyer flasks (Brinker and Seigler, 1989). The specimen must be minutely smashed for maximum cyanide quantity. Cyanide quantities are greatest when the substance is crushed in liquid nitrogen, average when crushed in dry ice, and minimum when processed in a buffer at ambient temperature in a Waring mixer, mortar, or pestle (Torres et al., 1988). Some scientists have crushed samples in acidic or basic media to block beta glucosidases, then modified the pH to a level where the enzyme is functional before sealing the experimental flasks (Rosenthal and Berenbaum, 2012).

Since all flavonoids can absorb ultraviolet rays, UV detectors can detect them in most cases. For flavones, flavonols, and corresponding glycosides, it is generally detected in the range 254–280 nm or 340–360 nm, 520–540 nm for anthocyanidins and the corresponding glycosides, 250 nm for chromones. With the advancement in technology, a few new techniques for the detection and identification of flavonoids have been introduced, including silica gel chromatography, polyamide chromatography, and polydextran gel chromatography (Feng et al., 2017).

## 6.7 SAFETY, PRECAUTIONS, AND REGULATION OF GOITROGENS

Although goitrogens pose some health effects, especially their role in impairment of thyroid-related activities, but at the same time they also represent a class of foods, which are highly nutritious. So, restricting the diet rich in goitrogens seems to be illogical as we can take some other precautions while consuming such types of food like

1. Adding variety to our diet, i.e., taking both goitrogenic as well as non-goitrogenic food.
2. Applying different processing techniques like cooking, fermentation, or others, which reduce their toxic effects.
3. Supplementing iodine and or Selenium in our diet.

Glucosinolate level and formulation fluctuates depending on plant types, agricultural techniques, and environmental parameters. The glucosinolate levels of rapeseed meal cultivars cultivated in hot climates is typically greater than that of cooler climates. The glucosinolates found in rapeseed meal from southern India are mainly 3-butenyl, 2-propenyl and 4-pentenyl glucosinolates. Glucosinolate levels vary within rapeseed meal because of differing concentrations of glucosinolates hydrolysis products in different organisms. Ruminants have a lower susceptibility to glucosinolates in the diet. In comparison with rabbits, poultry, and fish, pigs are much more seriously influenced by glucosinolate in their diet. Tolerable ranges of total glucosinolates in ruminants, pigs, rabbits, poultry, and fish was assessed to be about 1.5–4.22; 0.78; 7.0, 5.4 and 3.6 μmol g–1 diet, respectively (Tripathi and Mishra, 2007).

The regular intake of cruciferous vegetables results in human glucosinolate exposure to several milligrams; 18 published reports, which included 140 assessments of 42 food products, provided sufficient information on the overall glucosinolate content of foods. Garden cress (*Lepidium sativum*) (3.89 mg/g) had the highest glucosinolate levels, while Pe-tsai Chinese cabbage (*Brassica rapa*) (0.20 mg/g) had the lowest glucosinolate content. A significant variation was noted in various experiments for the values of the same vegetables, with a median difference of 5.8-fold between the upper and lower limits. When comparing human exposure to glucosinolates derived from vegetable consumption (which ranges from 0.8 to 20 mmol/kg dry weight) (Kushad et al., 1999) to the possible exposure from milk (which contains thiocyanate at the concentration of 0.18 mmol/L and goitrin at 0.7 mmol/L), it is clear that animal-derived products will contribute quite little to human dietary exposure, even if the animal is accidentally given maximum rapeseed meal (EFSA, 2008)

No data have been generated on goitrin levels in human plasma after ingestion of brassica vegetables that would aid in setting the nutritional safety recommendations despite the production of high-performance liquid chromatography spectrometry techniques to measure goitrin and other glucosinolate derivatives in plasma (Song et al., 2005). One study looked at how recrystallized goitrin affected radioactive iodine absorption by the thyroid glands in humans. The researchers stated that 25 mg (194 μmol) of goitrin was the smallest dose needed to suppress radioiodine uptake; however, a smaller ingested amount of 10 mg (70 μmol), had no effect on uptake (Langer et al., 1971).

Influence of enzyme myrosinase on our health can be demonstrated using Brassica vegetables as example, eaten in their raw form. An 88-year-old Chinese woman, when brought to the emergency department by her family, reported that she had been lethargic and unable to walk or swallow for 3 days. On further inquiry, it came forth that she had been eating an estimated 1.0 to 1.5 kg of raw bok choy or Chinese white cabbage daily, for several months, in the belief that it would help control her diabetes. With no previous history of thyroid disease, the only problem here was her continuous consumption of a considerable amount of bok choy. The cooking process, which largely deactivates the myrosinase in these vegetables, was bypassed, proving deleterious to the old woman (Dekker et al., 2000).

Human fatal dosage of HCN as per reports is approximately 0.5 and 3.5 mg/kg body weight. For a 60-kg human, this equates to 30 to 210 mg. The gastrointestinal tract absorbs HCN

efficiently, producing identifiable effects including both chronic and acute stages of intake. Acute levels of HCN can also be transformed to thiocyanate, a popular goitrogen. While many food legumes produce only trace amounts of goitrogens, the transformation of cyanogens to goitrogens can contribute to the growth of goiter in some areas of the world (Deshpande, 2002).

The regular consumption of mixed flavonoids is reported to be between 500 and 100 mg, but after supplementing diets with flavonoids or flavonoid containing herbal preparations in USA, it can be more than several grams (Chandra, 2010). The average daily dietary intake of soy protein in heavy soy users, such as in Asian countries, is reported to be 20–80 g, while the average

Western dietary intake is 1–3 g approximately (Barnes et al., 1995).

A carryover effect of goitrogens (glucosinolates and their degradation products) into edible tissues, milk, eggs, etc., of farm animals feeding on goitrogen rich feed has also been studied and the results have revealed that this carryover rate is atypically low. It was further concluded that measurable limits in milk were about 0.1%, while in case of organs and muscle tissue the residues were even lower. It can be concluded that vegetables are the primary source of these compounds in the human diet as compared to animal derived products and therefore these types of products do not pose a serious threat to human health (Alexander et al., 2008).

## 6.8 EFFECT OF PROCESSING

Based on the reaction conditions, glucosinolate distortion may be enzymatic and/or nonenzymatic, as myrosinase co-occur with glucosinolates in plant tissues, and the hydrolysis only occurs when myrosinase is inactivated; for example, after cooking, or in case of high-acidic/basic conditions. Myrosinase isoenzymes and glucosinolates are located nearby but divided between the cells; glucosinolates are contained in the vacuole and the myrosinases in the cytoplasm (Holst et al., 2003). Operations including slicing, boiling, and freezing affect the degree of glucosinolate hydrolysis and the composition of the finished products. Pulping results in a higher degree of glucosinolate breakdown. Trimming, dicing, slicing, or peeling causes certain plant cells to fracture, causing myrosinase hydrolysis to proceed. Myrosinase expression is reported to stimulate with mild heat at temperatures close to 60°C, however it is inactivated near 100°C (Bjorkman and Lonnerdal, 1973).

Glucosinolates and a few of their hydrolysis components are water-soluble, and as they are heated, a portion of such metabolites are released into the mixture (Mullin and Sahasrabudhe, 1978). Based on the varieties and processing system of the cabbage, approximately 92% of the overall glucosinolates found in green cabbage were retrieved in processed product and boiling broth. The form of glucosinolate also influences recuperation (Rosa and Heaney, 1993).

The tendency for glucosinolates and hydrolysis products of glucosinolates recovered after cooking depends on the thermal stability of the particles. Sinigrin, for example, seems to be more thermostable than progoitrin or glucoiberverin; allyl isothiocyanate (from sinigrin) completely vanishes after boiling, whereas 5-vinyloxazolidine-2-thione (from progoitrin) and 3-methyl-sulphinylpropyl-isothiocyanate (from glucoiberin) can partially evade decomposition (de Vos and Blijleven, 1988). Yet again, ascorbigen seems to be the most common glucobrassicin derivative retrieved after cooking (McDanell et al., 1987).

Numerous processing approaches including microwaving and extrusion, treatment with water and metal solutions, solid state fermentation, heat treatment, water treatments, were attempted to eliminate or decrease glucosinolate content and to mitigate glucosinolate related negative effects on animal protection and betterment. The reduction of glucosinolate concentration was achieved by micronizing rapeseed meal for 90 seconds at 195°C. About 370 μmol/mmol gross glucosinolates, both isothiocyanates, and traces of oxazolidinethiones were eliminated by micronization (Fenwick et al., 1986). Extrusion of rapeseed meal outperformed microwaving in eliminating glucosinolates. Glucosinolates were reduced in the range of 193–428 μmol/mmol by dry extrusion of rapeseed meal (Smithard and Eyre, 1986). Quite a significant decrease (670 μmol/mmol) in overall glucosinolates content occurred from wet extrusion of high glucosinolate rapeseed meal with ammonia (50°C, 200 rpm, with 2% ammonia) (Huang et al., 1995).

Fermentation of cruciferous products (sauerkraut, salt fermented vegetables) promotes the rapid and absolute enzymatic hydrolysis of glucosinolates, thus there is an absence of such intact glucosinolates. Rapeseed meal fermentation utilizing *Rhizopus oligosporus* and *Aspergillus* species detoxified myrosinase, decreased gross glucosinolates by 431 μmol/mmol, and thiooxalidone by 340 mg/g–1 (Vig and Walia, 2001). Moreover, after 60–96 h of fermentation at 30°C, the glucosinolates were entirely deteriorated (Tripathi and Mishra, 2007).

Blanching and drying reduced the overall phenolic content of cabbage. Blanching cabbage for 30 seconds lowered the overall phenolic content from 5.70–4.79 mg/g DW. The depletion of phenolics may be because of phenolic leaching into cooking water. Meanwhile, the overall phenolic content of dried cabbages was smaller than that of fresh cabbage samples (Tao et al., 2019). Stir-frying is a common cooking method in European nations, and it is increasingly becoming one of the most popular food preparations around the world. The stir-fry method quickly reduces myrosinase activity while having little effect on glucosinolate (Song and Thornalley, 2007).

Freezing, dehydration, and irradiation are examples of storage methods that have gained even less publicity. Based on the few and often contradictory studies reported, it is reasonably concluded that, intact glucosinolates are preserved by dehydration process and at the same time processes as irradiation with U.V. or ionizing radiations trigger their breakdown (de Vos and Blijleven, 1988).

In China, industrial freezing is now among the most common broccoli manufacturing processes. A study on broccoli florets concluded that the glucosinolate content of frozen broccoli was lower than that of fresh broccoli. Chopping and cleaning practices had little effect on glucosinolate concentration, while blanching and freezing treatments resulted in significant decreases in glucosinolate concentrations (Cai et al., 2016).

Cassava intake may lead to cyanide exposure unless cyanogenic glucosides and their break-up products are adequately removed during processing from their roots. However, the goitrogenic effect of cassava overload only aggravates disorders of iodine deficiency when the iodine intake is less than the recommended daily intake (Delange et al., 1994). Sun-drying for blanched and raw chips is undertaken in southern India for preparing roots for utilization. Boiling and sun-drying eliminates approximately 80% of the glucosides, whereas frying, baking, and steaming eliminate just 20%. The enzyme decomposition of cyanogenic glucosides or the percolation of cyanogenic agents in water is responsible for lowering cyanogenic content. Smashing and grinding fresh roots, accompanied by sun-drying, removes up to 95% of the cyanogens. This is another immensely powerful approach for lowering the cyanogen level of cassava roots employed in India. Leaf boiling eliminates approximately 85% of the cyanogenic glucoside (Nambisan, 1994).

## 6.9 FUTURE SCOPE

Elaboration concerning safe levels of exposure to these substances is what stands pivotal to future studies. It is further to be put to note that not all vegetables have been accessed and experimented over to measure their levels of goitrogens. Also, what impact food processing and preparation have on glucosinolate content and aglucone formation is what needs to be investigated more. Overall, the results on goitrogenic content of foods and thus corresponding glucosinolate intake show that studies on their health impacts should include estimates of at least overall glucosinolate concentration and preferably individual GSL and hydrolysis products of the cruciferous vegetables used in the investigational diets. Furthermore, extensive data on processing of the cruciferous foods should be given; nutritionists and toxicologists should thus be able to receive more appreciated information from research that have inherently distinguished experimental diets. Although we have chromatographic tools as methods of identification and quantification of goitrogenic substances, still the technical know-how is not yet that advanced and skilled enough, to precisely identify every food product for its goitrogenic status. Investigations on accessing the toxicological and sensory aspects of such compounds as well their breakdown products must be carried out extensively as well.

## 6.10 CONCLUSION

The ability of a plant or its part used as a food to act as goitrogenic depends on the quantity of goitrogen present in active form in it. No doubt the main cause of endemic/sporadic goiter is iodine deficiency; however, the role of these naturally occurring goitrogens in causing thyroid malfunctioning cannot be overlooked. People already deficient in iodine should be more vigilant in making their food choices and over-consuming goitrogenic foods, especially in their raw state, should not be encouraged. Goitrogenic capacity of a food is determined not only by its content, but also by how it is consumed and the body's nutritional status. Moreover, processing of such foods by different methods, such as drying, fermentation, boiling, autoclaving, baking, freezing, frying, roasting, etc., should be encouraged to bring their goitrogenic levels down. Further, as there is a potential risk of adverse effects of high concentrations of glucosinolates, those forage crops should be selected for feeding animals which are of lower glucosinolate content (particularly rapeseeds), and processing of such goitrogenic crops before consumption should be taken as the efficient measures to prevent intoxications in farm animals, as well the undesirable effect in animal-derived products.

## REFERENCES


Abrol, Y. P. 1967. Studies on the biosynthesis of amygdalin, the cyanogenic glycoside of bitter almonds Prunus amygdalus Stokes. *Indian Journal of Biochemistry*, *4*:54–55.

Agerbirk, N., De Vos, M., Kim, J. H., and Jander, G. 2009. Indole glucosinolate breakdown and its biological effects. *Phytochemistry Reviews*, *8*:101.

Agrawal, A. A., and Kurashige, N. S. 2003. A role for isothiocyanates in plant resistance against the specialist herbivore Pieris rapae. *Journal of Chemical Ecology*, *29*:1403–1415.

Agrawal, A. A., Conner, J. K., Johnson, M. T., and Wallsgrove, R. 2002. Ecological genetics of an induced plant defense against herbivores: additive genetic variance and costs of phenotypic plasticity. *Evolution*, *56*:2206–2213.

Ahlin, K. Å., Emanuelson, M., and Wiktorsson, H. 1994. Rapeseed products from double-low cultivars as feed for dairy cows: effects of long-term feeding on thyroid function, fertility, and animal health. *Acta Veterinaria Scandinavica*, *35*:37–53.

Akiba, Y., and Matsumoto, T. 1977. Effects of graded doses of goitrin, a goitrogen in rapeseed, on synthesis and release of thyroid hormone in chicks. *Nippon Chikusan Gakkai-Ho*, *48*:757–765.

Alexander, K., and Volini, M. 1981, January. The different molecular forms of prokaryotic rhodanases. In Federation Proceedings Vol. 40, No. 6, pp. 1656–1656. 9650. Rockville pike Bethesda, MD: Federation American Society for Experimental Biolology.

Alexander, J., Auðunsson, G. A., Benford, D., Cockburn, A., Cravedi, J. P., Dogliotti, E., ... & Van, C. 2008. Glucosinolates as undesirable substances in animal feed Scientific Panel on Contaminants in the Food Chain. *European Food Safety Authority Journal*, *6*:590.

Assayed, M. E., and Abd El-Aty, A. M. 2009. Cruciferous plants: phytochemical toxicity versus cancer chemoprotection. *Mini Reviews in Medicinal Chemistry*, *9*:1470–1478.

Astwood, E. B., Greer, M. A., and Ettlinger, M. G. 1949. l-5-Vinyl-2-thiooxazolidone, an antithyroid compound from yellow turnip and from brassica seeds. *Journal of Biological Chemistry*, *181*:121–130.

Australia, F. S. A. N. Z., Zealand, F. N., and Zealand, A. N. 2004. Cyanogenic glycosides in cassava and bamboo shoots. Retrieved from https://www.foodstandards.gov.au/publications/documents/28_Cyanogenic_glycosides.pdf

Arstila, A., Krusius, F. E., and Peltola, P. 1969. Studies on the transfer of thio-oxazolidone-type goitrogens into cow's milk in goitre endemic districts of Finland and in experimental conditions. *European Journal of Endocrinology, 60*(4):712–718.

Bandele, O. J. and Osheroff, N. 2007. Bioflavonoids as poisons of human topoisomerase IIα and IIβ. *Biochemistry*, *46*:6097–6108.

Barnes, S., Peterson, T. G., and Coward, L. 1995. Rationale for the use of genistein-containing soy matrices in chemoprevention trials for breast and prostate cancer. *Journal of Cellular Biochemistry*, *59*:181–187.

Bernardi, R., Negri, A., Ronchi, S., and Palmieri, S. 2000. Isolation of the epithiospecifier protein from oil-rape Brassica napus ssp. oleifera seed and its characterization. *FEBS Letters*, *467*:296–298.

Bernardi, R., Finiguerra, M. G., Rossi, A. A., and Palmieri, S. 2003. Isolation and biochemical characterization of a basic myrosinase from ripe *Crambe abyssinica* seeds, highly specific for epi-progoitrin. *Journal of Agricultural and Food Chemistry*, *51*:2737–2744.

Bischoff, K. L. 2021. Glucosinolates. In *Nutraceuticals*, 903–909. Academic Press.

Bisset, F. H., Clapp, R. C., Coburn, R. A., Ettlinger, M. G., and Long Jr, L. 1969. Cyanogenesis in manioc: concerning lotaustralin. *Phytochemistry*, *8*:2235–2247.

Blum, M. S., and Woodring, J. P. 1962. Secretion of benzaldehyde and hydrogen cyanide by the millipede *Pachydesmus crassicutis* Wood. *Science*, *138*:512–513.

Blumenthal, S. G., Hendrickson, H. R., Abrol, Y. P., and Conn, E. E. 1968. Cyanide metabolism in higher plants: III. The biosynthesis of β-cyanoalanine. *Journal of Biological Chemistry*, *243*:5302s–5307.

Bolarinwa, I. F., M. O. Oke, S. A. Olaniyan, and A. S. Ajala 2016. A review of cyanogenic glycosides in edible plants. In *Toxicology–New Aspect to This Scientific Conundrum, Sonia Soloneski and Marcelo L. Larramendy.* Intech Open.

Brown, A. F., Yousef, G. G., Jeffery, E. H., Klein, B. P., Wallig, M. A., Kushad, M. M., and Juvik, J. A. 2002. Glucosinolate profiles in broccoli: variation in levels and implications in breeding for cancer chemoprotection. *Journal of the American Society for Horticultural Science*, *127*:807–813.

Brinker, A. M., and Seigler, D. S. 1989. Methods for the detection and quantitative determination Björkman, Rune, and Bo Lönnerdal. "Studies on myrosinases III. Enzymatic properties of myrosinases from Sinapis alba and Brassica napus seeds." *Biochimica et Biophysica Acta (BBA)-Enzymology* 327, no. 1 (1973): 121–131. of cyanide in plant materials. *Phytochem. Bull,* 21(2):24.

Ballhorn, D. J., Kautz, S., Heil, M., and Hegeman, A. D. 2009. Cyanogenesis of wild lima bean (*Phaseolus lunatus* L.) is an efficient direct defence in nature. *PLoS One*, 4(5):e5450.

Bourdon, D., Perez, J. M., and Baudet, J. J. 1981. Utilisation de nouveaux types de tourteaux de colza par le porc en croissance finition. Influence des glucosinolates et du depelliculage. *Revue de l'Alimentation Animale*, 343:27–38.

Cai, C., Miao, H., Qian, H., Yao, L., Wang, B., and Wang, Q. 2016. Effects of industrial pre-freezing processing and freezing handling on glucosinolates and antioxidant attributes in broccoli florets. *Food Chemistry, 210*:451–456.

Carroll, K. K. 1949. Isolation of an antithyroid compound from rapeseed Brassica napus. *Proceedings of the Society for Experimental Biology and Medicine, 71*:622–624.

Chandra, A. K. 2010. Goitrogen in food: cyanogenic and flavonoids containing plant foods in the development of goiter. In *Bioactive Foods in Promoting Health*, 691–716. Academic Press.

Chandra, A. K., Mukhopadhyay, S., Lahari, D., and Tripathy, S. 2004. Goitrogenic content of Indian cyanogenic plant food and their in vitro anti-thyroidal activity. *Indian Journal of Medical Research*, 119:180–185.

Chandra, A. K., Mukhopadhyay, S., Ghosh, D., and Tripathy, S. 2006. Effect of radish (Raphanus sativus Linn.) on thyroid status under conditions of varying iodine intake in rats. *Indian Journal of Experimental Biology, 44*:653–661.

Chhajed, S., Mostafa, I., He, Y., Abou-Hashem, M., El-Domiaty, M., and Chen, S. 2020. Glucosinolate biosynthesis and the glucosinolate–myrosinase system in plant defense. *Agronomy, 10*:1786.

Choudhury, D., Sahu, J. K., and Sharma, G. D. 2010. Biochemistry of bitterness in bamboo shoots. *Assam University Journal of Science and Technology, 6*:105–111.

Clements, F. W. 1960. Naturally occurring goitrogens. *British Medical Bulletin, 16*:133–137.

Cole, R. A. 1976. Isothiocyanates, nitriles and thiocyanates as products of autolysis of glucosinolates in Cruciferae. *Phytochemistry, 15*:759–762.

Conn, E. E. 1969. Cyanogenic glycosides. *Journal of Agricultural and Food Chemistry, 17*:519–526.

Conn, E. E. 1973. Cyanogenic glycosides: their occurrence, biosynthesis, and function. In *Chronic Cassava Toxicity*. IDRC.

Corcoran, M. P., McKay, D. L., and Blumberg, J. B. 2012. Flavonoid basics: chemistry, sources, mechanisms of action, and safety. *Journal of Nutrition in Gerontology and Geriatrics, 31*:176–189.

Daxenbichler, M. E., VanEtten, C. H., and Wolff, I. A. 1965. A new thioglucoside, R-2-hydroxy-3-butenylglucosinolate from Crambe abyssinica seed. *Biochemistry, 4*:318–323.

de Vos, R. H., and Blijleven, W. G. 1988. The effect of processing conditions on glucosinolates in cruciferous vegetables. *Zeitschrift für Lebensmittel-Untersuchung und Forschung, 187*(6), 525–529.

Dekker, M., Verkerk, R., and Jongen, W. M. 2000. Predictive modelling of health aspects in the food production chain: a case study on glucosinolates in cabbage. *Trends in Food Science and Technology, 11*:174–181.

Delage, B. 2015. *Flavonoids.* Linus Pauling Institute, Oregon State University. Retrieved on 2021-01-26.

Delange, F., Ekpechi, L. O., and Rosling, H. 1994. Cassava cyanogenesis and iodine deficiency disorders. In International Workshop on Cassava Safety, Vol. 375, pp. 289–294.

Deshpande, S. S. 2002. *Handbook of Food Toxicology.* CRC Press.

Doerge, D. R., and Sheehan, D. M. 2002. Goitrogenic and estrogenic activity of soy isoflavones. *Environmental Health Perspectives, 110*:349–353.

Donkin, S. G., Eiteman, M. A., and Williams, P. L. 1995. Toxicity of glucosinolates and their enzymatic decomposition products to Caenorhabditis elegans. *Journal of Nematology, 27*:258.

Dos Santos, M. C. D. S., Gonçalves, C. F. L., Vaisman, M., Ferreira, A. C. F., and de Carvalho, D. P. 2011. Impact of flavonoids on thyroid function. *Food and Chemical Toxicology, 49*:2495–2502.

Du, L., and Halkier, B. A. 1996. Isolation of a microsomal enzyme system involved in glucosinolate biosynthesis from seedlings of Tropaeolum majus L. *Plant Physiology, 111*:831–837.

Du, L., and Halkier, B. A. 1998. Biosynthesis of glucosinolates in the developing silique walls and seeds of Sinapis alba. *Phytochemistry, 48*:1145–1150.

Durham, P. L., and Poulton, J. E. 1989. Effect of castanospermine and related polyhydroxyalkaloids on purified myrosinase from Lepidium sativum seedlings. *Plant Physiology, 90*:48–52.

Dornberger, K., Böckel, V., Heyer, J., Schönfeld, C. H., Tonew, M., and Tonew, E. 1975. Investigations of the isothiocyanates erysolin and sulforaphan of Cardaria draba L. *Die Pharmazie*, 30(12):792–796.

Ermans, A. M., and Bourdoux, P. 1989. Antithyroid sulfurated compounds. In E. Gaitan (Ed.), *Environmental Goitrogens*, 15–31. CRC Press.

European Food Safety Authority (EFSA). 2008. Glucosinolates as undesirable substances in animal feed-Scientific Opinion of the Panel on Contaminants in the Food Chain. *EFSA Journal, 6*:590.

Ettlinger, M. G., and Lundeen, A. J. 1956. The structures of sinigrin and sinalbin; an enzymatic rearrangement. *Journal of the American Chemical Society*, 78(16): 4172–4173.

Fahey, J. W., Zalcmann, A. T., and Talalay, P. 2001. The chemical diversity and distribution of glucosinolates and isothiocyanates among plants. *Phytochemistry*, *56*:5–51.

FAOSTAT. (2017). Food and Agriculture Organization Statistics. Retrieved from http://www.org/faostat/fr/ on 22-01-2021.

Feng, W., Hao, Z., and Li, M. 2017. Isolation and structure identification of flavonoids. In Justino, G. C. (Ed.), *Flavonoids from Biosynthesis to Human Health*, pp. 17–43. Intech Open.

Fenwick, G. R., and Heaney, R. K. 1983. Glucosinolates and their breakdown products in cruciferous crops, foods and feeding stuffs. *Food Chemistry*, *11*:249–271.

Fenwick, G. R., Heaney, R. K., Mullin, W. J., and VanEtten, C. H. 1983. Glucosinolates and their breakdown products in food and food plants. *Critical Reviews in Food Science and Nutrition*, *18*:123–201.

Fenwick, G. R. 1989. Bracken (Pteridium aquilinum)—toxic effects and toxic constituents. *Journal of the Science of Food and Agriculture*, *46*(2):147–173.

Francisco, I. A., and Pinotti, M. H. P. 2000. Cyanogenic glycosides in plants. *Brazilian Archives of Biology and Technology*, *43*:487–492.

Franke, A. A., Custer, L. J., Cerna, C. M., and Narala, K. 1995. Rapid HPLC analysis of dietary phytoestrogens from legumes and from human urine. *Proceedings of the Society for Experimental Biology and Medicine*, 208:18–26.

Fenwick, G. R., Ann Spinks, E., Wilkinson, A. P., Heaney, R. K., and Legoy, M. A. 1986. Effect of processing on the antinutrient content of rapeseed. *Journal of the Science of Food and Agriculture* 37(8):735–741.

Friis, P. A. L. L. E., and Kjaer, A. 1966. 4-Methylthio-3-butenyl isothiocyanate, the pungent principle of radish root. *Acta Chemica Scandinavica*, *20*:73–91.

Gaitan, E. 1986. Environmental goitrogens other than iodine deficiency. *IDD Newsletter*, *2*:11–3.

Gaitan, E. 1989. *Environmental Goitrogenesis*. CRC Press.

Gaitan, E. 1996. Flavonoids and the thyroid. *Nutrition*, *12*:127–129.

Gaitan, E., and Dunn, J. T. 1992. Epidemiology of iodine deficiency. *Trends in Endocrinology and Metabolism*, *3*:170–175.

Galletti, S., Bernardi, R., Leoni, O., Rollin, P., and Palmieri, S. 2001. Preparation and biological activity of four epiprogoitrin myrosinase-derived products. *Journal of Agricultural and Food Chemistry*, *49*:471–476.

Gardrat, C. and Prevot, A. 1987. Quantitative determination of glucosinolates in rapeseeds and rapeseed meals by an enzymic method. *Revue Francaise des Corps Gras 34*:457–461.

Getahun, S. M., and Chung, F. L. 1999. Conversion of glucosinolates to isothiocyanates in humans after ingestion of cooked watercress. *Cancer Epidemiology and Prevention Biomarkers*, *8*:447–451.

Giamoustaris, A., and Mithen, R. 1996. Genetics of aliphatic glucosinolates. IV. Side-chain modification in Brassica oleracea. *Theoretical and Applied Genetics*, *93*:1006–1010.

Glendening, T. M., and Poulton, J. E. 1988. Glucosinolate biosynthesis: sulfation of desulfobenzylglucosinolate by cell-free extracts of cress Lepidium sativum L. seedlings. *Plant Physiology*, *86*:319–321.

Gmelin, Rolf and Virtanen, A. I. 1961. Glucobrassicin, der precursor von SCN^-, 3-indolylacetonitril und ascorbigen in Brassica oleracea species. *Annales Academiæ Scientiarum Fennicæ Series A*, *2* 107: 1–25.

Goodman, I., Fouts, J. R., Bresnick, E., Menegas, R., and Hitchings, G. H. 1959. A mammalian thioglycosidase. *Science*, *130*:450–451.

Greer, M. A. 1950. Nutrition and goiter. *Physiological Reviews*, *30*:513–548.

Greer, M. A. 1957. Goitrogenic substances in food. *The American Journal of Clinical Nutrition*, *5*: 440–444.

Greer, M. A., and Astwood, E. B. 1948. The antithyroid effect of certain foods in man as determined with radioactive iodine. *Endocrinology*, *43*:105–119.

Grosser, K., and van Dam, N. M. 2017. A straightforward method for glucosinolate extraction and analysis with high-pressure liquid chromatography HPLC. *Journal of Visualized Experiments: JoVE*, *121*. doi:10.3791/55425

McNaughton, S. A., and Marks, G. C.. 2003. Development of a food composition database for the estimation of dietary intakes of glucosinolates, the biologically active constituents of cruciferous vegetables. *British Journal of Nutrition, 90*(3):687–697.

Halkier, B. A., and Gershenzon, J. 2006. Biology and biochemistry of glucosinolates. *Annual Review of Plant Biology*, *57*:303–333.

Halkier, B. A., and Møller, B. L. 1991. Involvement of cytochrome P-450 in the biosynthesis of dhurrin in Sorghum bicolor L. Moench. *Plant Physiology*, *96*:10–17.

Haque, M. R., and Bradbury, J. H. 2002. Total cyanide determination of plants and foods using the picrate and acid hydrolysis methods. *Food Chemistry*, *77*:107–114.

Harborne, J. B. 1972. Cyanogenic glucosides and their function. In *Phytochemical Ecology*, pp. 104–123. Academic Press.

Hasapis, X., and MacLeod, A. J. 1982. Benzyl glucosinolate degradation in heat-treated Lepidium sativum seeds and detection of a thiocyanate-forming factor. *Phytochemistry*, *21*:1009–1013.

Helboe, P., Olsen, O. and Sørensen, H. 1980. Separation of glucosinolates by high-performance liquid chromatography. *Journal of Chromatography*, *197*:199–205.

Hess, S. Y. 2013. Iodine: physiology, dietary sources, and requirements. In S. Y. Hess (Ed.), *Encyclopaedia of Human Nutrition*, pp. 33–38. Elsevier.

Hill G. D. 2003. *Plant Antinutritional Factors. Encyclopedia of Food Science and Nutrition* (2nd ed.). Elsevier.

Holst, B., Fenwick, G. R., and Benjamin, C. 2003. Glucosinolates. In *Encyclopedia of Food Sciences and Nutrition*, pp. 2922–2930. Academic.

Huang, S., Liang, M., Lardy, G., Huff, H. E., Kerley, M. S., and Hsieh, F. 1995. Extrusion processing of rapeseed meal for reducing glucosinolates. *Animal feed science and technology*, 56(1–2):1–9.

James, D. C., and Rossiter, J. T. 1991. Development and characteristics of myrosinase in Brassica napus during early seedling growth. *Physiologia Plantarum*, *82*:163–170.

Josefsson, E. 1970. Glucosinolate content and amino acid composition of rapeseed Brassica napus meal as affected by sulphur and nitrogen nutrition. *Journal of the Science of Food and Agriculture*, *21*:98–103.

Jones, D. A. 1998. Why are so many food plants cyanogenic? *Phytochemistry*, 47(2):155–162.

Kelley, M. K., and Bjeldanes, L. F. 1995. Modulation of glutathione S-transferase activity and isozyme pattern in liver and small intestine of rats fed goitrin-and T3-supplemented diets. *Food and Chemical Toxicology*, 33:129–137.

Knust, K. S., and Leung, A. M. 2017. Iodine: basic nutritional aspects. In *Molecular, Genetic, and Nutritional Aspects of Major and Trace Minerals*, pp. 133–141. Academic Press.

Kurilich, Anne C., Grace J. Tsau, Allan Brown, Lenora Howard, Barbara P. Klein, Elizabeth H. Jeffery, Mosbah Kushad, Mathew A. Wallig, and John A. Juvik 1999. Carotene, tocopherol, and ascorbate contents in subspecies of Brassica oleracea. *Journal of Agricultural and Food Chemistry*, 47(4): 1576–1581.

Kushad, M. M., Brown, A. F., Kurilich, A. C., Juvik, J. A., Klein, B. P., Wallig, M. A., and Jeffery, E. H. 1999. Variation of Glucosinolates in Vegetable Crops of Brassica o leracea. *Journal of agricultural and food chemistry*, 47(4):1541–1548.

Kjaer, A., Conti, J., and Jensen, K. A. 1953. Isothiocyanates. 3. The volatile isothiocyanates in seeds of rape (*Brassica-napus* L). *Acta Chemica Scandinavica*, 7(9):1271–1275.

Lakshmy, R., Srinivas Rao, P., Sesikeran, B., and Suryaprakash, P. 1995. Iodine metabolism in response to goitrogen induced altered thyroid status under conditions of moderate and high intake of iodines. *Hormone and Metabolic Research*, *27*:450–454.

Langer, P. 1971. Extrathyroidal effect of thiocyanate and propylthiouracil: the depression of the protein-bound iodine level in intact and thyroidectomized rats. *Journal of Endocrinology*, *50*:367–372.

Langer, P., and Greer, M. A. 1977. *Antithyroid Substances and Naturally Occurring Goitrogens*, pp. 150–178. Karger Publishers.

Langer, P., Michajlovskij, N., Sedlak, J., and Kutka, M. 1971. Studies on the antithyroid activity of naturally occurring L-5-vinyl-2-thiooxazolidone in man. *Endokrinologie*, *57*(2), 225–229.

Langer, P., and Michajlovskij, N. 1969. Studies on the antithyroid activity of naturally occurring L-5-vinyl-2-thiooxazolidone and its urinary metabolite in rats. *European Journal of Endocrinology*, 62(1):21–30.

Langer, P. 1964. Relations between thiocyanate formation, and goitrogenic effect of foods. VI. Thiocyanogenic activity of allylisothiocyanate, one of the most frequently occurring mustard oils in plants. *Hoppe-Seyler's Z. Physiol. Chem*, 339:33.

Langer, P. A. V. E. L., and Stolc, V. 1965. Goitrogenic activity of allylisothiocyanate-a widespread natural mustard oil. *Endocrinology*, *76*:151–155.

Lazzeri, L., R. Tacconi, and S. Palmieri. 1993. In vitro activity of some glucosinolates and their reaction products toward a population of the nematode Heterodera schachtii. *Journal of Agriculture and Food Chemistry*, *41*:825–829.

Long, K. Y., and Brattsten, L. B. 1982. Is rhodanese important in the detoxification of dietary cyanide in southern armyworm (Spodoptera eridania Cramer) larvae? *Insect Biochemistry*, 12(4):367–375.

Le Bail, J. C., Laroche, T., Marre-Fournier, F., and Habrioux, G. 1998. Aromatase and 17β-hydroxysteroid dehydrogenase inhibition by flavonoids. *Cancer Letters*, *133*:101–106.

Li, L., Cheng, B., Zhou, R., Cao, Z., Zeng, C., and Li, L. 2017. Preparation and evaluation of a novel N-ben zyl-phenethylamino-β-cyclodextrin-bonded chiral stationary phase for HPLC. *Talanta*, *174*:179–191.

Lönnerdal, B., and Janson, J. C. 1973. Studies on myrosinases. II. Purification and characterization of a myrosinase from rapeseed (Brassica napus L.). *Biochimica et Biophysica Acta (BBA)-Enzymology*, *315*:421–429.

Léder, I. 2004. Sorghum and millets. *Cultivated plants, primarily as food sources*, 1:66–84.

Majak, W. 1992. Mammalian metabolism of toxic glycosides from plants. *Journal of Toxicology: Toxin Reviews*, 11(1):1–40.

Martland, M. F., Butler, E. J., and Fenwick, G. R. 1984. Rapeseed induced liver hemorrhage, reticulolysis and biochemical changes in laying hens: the effects of feeding high and low glucosinolate meals. *Research in Veterinary Science*, *36*:298–309.

McDanell, R., McLean, A. E. M., Hanley, A. B., Heaney, R. K., and Fenwick, G. R. 1987. Differential induction of mixed-function oxidase, MFO activity in rat liver and intestine by diets containing processed cabbage: correlation with cabbage levels of glucosinolates and glucosinolate hydrolysis products. *Food and Chemical Toxicology*, *25*:363–368.

McDanell, R., McLean, A. E. M., Hanley, A. B., Heaney, R. K., and Fenwick, G. R. 1988. Chemical and biological properties of indole glucosinolates,glucobrassicins: a review. *Food and Chemical Toxicology*, *26*:59–70.

McMillan, M., Spinks, E. A., and Fenwick, G. R. 1986. Preliminary observations on the effect of dietary brussels sprouts on thyroid function. *Human Toxicology*, *5*:15–19.

Miller, Margaret A. 2017. Endocrine system. In James F. Zachary (Ed.), *Pathologic Basis of Veterinary Disease* (6th ed.), pp. 682–723. Mosby.

Mitchell, M. L., and O'Rourke, M. E. 1960. Response of the thyroid gland to thiocyanate and thyrotropin. *The Journal of Clinical Endocrinology and Metabolism*, *20*:47–56.

Mithen, R. F., Dekker, M., Verkerk, R., Rabot, S., and Johnson, I. T. 2000. The nutritional significance, biosynthesis, and bioavailability of glucosinolates in human foods. *Journal of the Science of Food and Agriculture*, *80*:967–984.

Møller, B. L., and Conn, E. E. 1979. The biosynthesis of cyanogenic glucosides in higher plants. N-Hydroxytyrosine as an intermediate in the biosynthesis of dhurrin by Sorghum bicolor (Linn) Moench. *Journal of Biological Chemistry*, 254(17):8575–8583.

Montgomery, R. D. 1969. *Toxic constituents of plant foodstuffs*. ed. IE Liener.

Mullin, W. J., and Sahasrabudhe, M. R. 1978. An estimate of the average daily intake of glucosinolates via cruciferous vegetables. *Nutrition Reports International, USA*.

Mumm, R., Burow, M., Bukovinszkine'Kiss, G., Kazantzidou, E., Wittstock, U., Dicke, M., and Gershenzon, J. 2008. Formation of simple nitriles upon glucosinolate hydrolysis affects direct and indirect defense against the specialist herbivore, Pieris rapae. *Journal of Chemical Ecology*, *34*:1311–1321.

Nagashima, Z., and Uchiyama, M. 1959. Possibility that myrosinase is a single enzyme and mechanism of decomposition of mustard oil glucoside by myrosinase. *Journal of the Agricultural Chemical Society of Japan*, *23*:555–556.

Nambisan, B. 1994, March. Evaluation of the effect of various processing techniques on cyanogen content reduction in cassava. In International Workshop on Cassava Safety Vol. 375, pp. 193–202. Nigeria.

Nishie, K., and Daxenbichler, M. E. 1980. Toxicology of glucosinolates, related compounds, nitriles, R-goitrin, isothiocyanates and vitamin U found in Cruciferae. *Food and Cosmetics Toxicology*, *18*:159–172.

Oginsky, E. L., Stein, A. E., and Greer, M. A. 1965. Myrosinase activity in bacteria as demonstrated by the conversion of progoitrin to goitrin. *Proceedings of the Society for Experimental Biology and Medicine*, *119*:360–364.

Ohtsuru, M., and Kawatani, H. 1979. Studies on the myrosinase from Wasabia japonica: purification and some properties of wasabi myrosinase. *Agricultural and Biological Chemistry*, *43*:2249–2255.

Palmieri, S., Iori, R., and Leoni, O. 1986. Myrosinase from Sinapis alba L.: a new method of purification for glucosinolate analyses. *Journal of Agricultural and Food Chemistry*, *34*:138–140.

Panche, A. N., Diwan, A. D., and Chandra, S. R. 2016. Flavonoids: an overview. *Journal of Nutritional Science*, 5. https://doi.org/10.1017/jns.2016.41.

Peltola, P., and Krusius, F. E. 1960. Effect of cow's milk from the goitre endemia district of Finland on thyroid function. *European Journal of Endocrinology*, *33*:603–612.

Pereira, J. F., Seigler, D. S., and Splittstoesser, W. E. 1981. Cyanogenesis in sweet and bitter cultivars of cassava. *Hortscience, Ames*, 16(6):776–777.

Poulton, J. E. 1983. Cyanogenic compounds in plants and their toxic effects. *Handbook of natural toxins*, 1:117–157.

Poulton, J. E. 1990. Cyanogenesis in plants. *Plant Physiology*, *94*:401–405.

Rabot, S., Nugon-Baudon, L., Raibaud, P., and Szylit, O. 1993. Rape-seed meal toxicity in gnotobiotic rats: influence of a whole human faecal flora or single human strains of Escherichia coli and Bacteroides vulgatus. *British Journal of Nutrition*, *70*:323–331.

Reese, E. T., Clapp, R. C., and Mandels, M. 1958. A thioglucosidase in fungi. *Archives of Biochemistry and Biophysics*, *75*:228–242.

Rodriguez, R. A. 1997. Blindness in calves due to ingestion of turnip, Brassica campestris. *Veterinaria Argentina*, *14*:601–605.

Rosa, E. A. 1997. Daily variation in glucosinolate concentrations in the leaves and roots of cabbage seedlings in two constant temperature regimes. *Journal of the Science of Food and Agriculture*, *73*:364–368.

Rosa, E. A., and Heaney, R. K. 1993. The effect of cooking and processing on the glucosinolate content: studies on four varieties of Portuguese cabbage and hybrid white cabbage. *Journal of the Science of Food and Agriculture*, *62*:259–265.

Rosenthal, G. A., and Berenbaum, M. R. 2012. *Herbivores: Their Interactions with secondary Plant Metabolites: Ecological and Evolutionary Processes* Vol. 2. Academic Press.

Rinaldo, D. 2020. Carbohydrate and bioactive compounds composition of starchy tropical fruits and tubers, in relation to pre and postharvest conditions: a review. *Journal of Food Science*, 85:249–259.

Sartelet, H., Serghat, S., Lobstein, A., Ingenbleek, Y., Anton, R., Petitfrere, E., ... and Haye, B. 1996. Flavonoids extracted from fonio millet (Digitaria exilis) reveal potent antithyroid properties. *Nutrition*, *12*:100–106.

Satheesh, N., and Solomon, F. 2019. Review on nutritional composition of orange-fleshed sweet potato and its role in management of vitamin A deficiency. *Food Science and Nutrition*, *7*:1920–194.

Schone, F., Jahreis, G., Lange, R., Seffner, W., Groppel, B., Hennig, A., and Ludke, H. 1990. Effect of varying glucosinolate and iodine intake via rapeseed meal diets on serum thyroid hormone level and total iodine in the thyroid in growing pigs. *Endocrinol Experimentalis*, *24*:415–27.

Schöne, F., Rudolph, B., Kirchheim, U., and Knapp, G. 1997. Counteracting the negative effects of rapeseed and rapeseed press cake in pig diets. *British Journal of Nutrition*, *78*:947–962.

Shi, H., Zhao, Y., Sun, J., Yu, L. L., and Chen, P. 2017. Chemical profiling of glucosinolates in cruciferous vegetables-based dietary supplements using ultra-high performance liquid chromatography coupled to tandem high resolution mass spectrometry. *Journal of Food Composition and Analysis*, *61*:67–72.

Skibola, C. F., and Smith, M. T. 2000. Potential health impacts of excessive flavonoid intake. *Free Radical Biology and Medicine*, *29*:375–383.

Śmiechowska, A., Bartoszek, A., and Namieśnik, J. 2010. Determination of glucosinolates and their decomposition products—indoles and isothiocyanates in cruciferous vegetables. *Critical Reviews in Analytical Chemistry*, *40*:202–216.

Smithard, R. R., and Eyre, M. D. 1986. The effects of dry extrusion of rapeseed with other feedstuffs upon its nutritional value and anti-thyroid activity. *Journal of the Science of Food and Agriculture*, *37*: 136–140.

Sønderby, I. E., Geu-Flores, F., and Halkier, B. A. 2010. Biosynthesis of glucosinolates–gene discovery and beyond. *Trends in Plant Science*, *15*:283–290.

Song, L., and Thornalley, P. J. 2007. Effect of storage, processing, and cooking on glucosinolate content of Brassica vegetables. *Food and Chemical Toxicology*, *45*:216–224.

Song, L., Morrison, J. J., Botting, N. P., and Thornalley, P. J. 2005. Analysis of glucosinolates, isothiocyanates, and amine degradation products in vegetable extracts and blood plasma by LC–MS/MS. *Analytical Biochemistry*, *347*: 234–243.

Sørensen, H. 1990. Glucosinolates: structure-properties-function. In Shahidi, F. (Ed), *Rapeseed/Canola: Production, Chemistry, Nutrition, and Processing Technology*, pp. 149–172. Van Nostrand Reinhold Publisher, Chapter 9.

Spiegel, C., Bestetti, G. E., Rossi, G. L., and Blum, J. W. 1993. Normal circulating triiodothyronine concentrations are maintained despite severe hypothyroidism in growing pigs fed rapeseed presscake meal. *The Journal of Nutrition*, *123*:1554–1561.

Srivastava, V. K., Philbrick, D. J., and Hill, D. C. 1975. Response of rats and chicks to rapeseed meal subjected to different enzymatic treatments. *Canadian Journal of Animal Science*, *55*(3):331–335.

Stoll, A., and Seebeck, E. 1948. Allium compounds. I. Alliin the true mother compound of garlic oil. *Helvetica Chimica Acta*, *31*:189–210.

Taljaard, T. L. 1993. Cabbage poisoning in ruminants. *Journal of the South African Veterinary Association*, *64*:96–100.

Tani, N., Ohtsuru, M., and Hata, T. 1974. Isolation of myrosinase producing microorganism. *Agricultural and Biological Chemistry*, *38*:1617–1622.

Tanii, H., Takayasu, T., Higashi, T., Leng, S., and Saijoh, K. 2004. Allylnitrile: generation from cruciferous vegetables and behavioral effects on mice of repeated exposure. *Food and Chemical Toxicology*, *42*:453–458.

Taurog, A. 1970. Thyroid peroxidase and thyroxine biosynthesis. *Recent Progress in Hormone Research*, *26*:189–247.

Timmerman-Vaughan, G., Russell, A. C., Hill, A., Frew, T. J., and Gilpin, B. J. 1997. DNA markers for disease resistance breeding in peas (*Pisum sativum* L.). In Proceedings of the New Zealand Plant Protection Conference, vol. 50, pp. 314–315.

Tonacchera, M., Pinchera, A., Dimida, A., Ferrarini, E., Agretti, P., Vitti, P., ... and Gibbs, J. 2004. Relative potencies and additivity of perchlorate, thiocyanate, nitrate, and iodide on the inhibition of radioactive iodide uptake by the human sodium iodide symporter. *Thyroid*, *14*:1012–1019.

Tripathi, M. K., and Mishra, A. S. 2007. Glucosinolates in animal nutrition: a review. *Animal Feed Science and Technology*, *132*:1–27.

Van Middlesworth, L. 1985. Thiocyanate feeding with low iodine diet causes chronic iodine retention in the thyroid of mice. *Endocrinology*, *116*:665–670.

Van Wyk JJ, Arnold Mary B, Wynn J, Pepper F. 1959. The effects of a soybean product on thyroid function in humans. *Pediatrics*, *24*(5):752–60.

Vanderpas, J. 2003. Goitrogens and antithyroid compounds. In B. Caballero (Ed.), *Encyclopedia of Food Sciences and Nutrition*, pp. 2949–2957. https://doi.org/10.1016/B0-12-227055-X/00566-6

VanEtten, C. H., and Daxenbichler, M. E. 1977. Glucosinolates and derived products in cruciferous vegetables: total glucosinolates by retention on anion exchange resin and enzymatic hydrolysis to measure released glucose. *Journal of the Association of Official Analytical Chemists*, *60*:946–949.

Vanetten, C. H. and Tookey, H. L.. 1979. *Chemistry and Biological Effects of Glucosinolates in Herbivores.* G. A. Rosenthal and D. H. Janzen, Eds., pp. 471–500. Academic Press, New York.

VanEtten, C. H., Daxenbichler, M. E., and Wolff, I. A. 1969. Natural glucosinolates (thioglucosides) in foods and feeds. *Journal of Agricultural and Food Chemistry*, *17*:483–491.

Vermorel, M., Heaney, R. K., and Fenwick, G. R. 1986. Nutritive value of rapeseed meal: effects of individual glucosinolates. *Journal of the Science of Food and Agriculture*, *37*:1197–1202.

Vetter, J. 2000. Plant cyanogenic glycosides. *Toxicon*, *38*:11–36.

Vig, A. P., and Walia, A. 2001. Beneficial effects of Rhizopus oligosporus fermentation on reduction of glucosinolates, fibre and phytic acid in rapeseed (Brassica napus) meal. *Bioresource Technology*, *78*:309–312.

Virtanen, A. I. 1962. Some organic sulfur compounds in vegetables and fodder plants and their significance in human nutrition. *Angewandte Chemie International Edition in English*, *1*:299–306.

Wani, S. M., Amin, S., Javaid, I., Masoodi, A., Mir, S. A., Ganai, S. A., and Yildiz, F. 2017. Minimal processing of tropical and subtropical fruits, vegetables, nuts, and seeds. In F. Yildiz and R. C. Wiley (Eds.), *Minimally Processed Refrigerated Fruits and Vegetables* (2nd ed.), pp. 469–512. Food Engineering Series. Springer.

White, H. L., Freeman, L. M., Mahony, O., Graham, P. A., Hao, Q., and Court, M. H. 2004. Effect of dietary soy on serum thyroid hormone concentrations in healthy adult cats. *American Journal of Veterinary Research*, *65*:586–591.

Wolf, J. 1964. Transport of iodide and other anions in the thyroid gland. *Physiological Reviews*, *44*:45–90.

Zimmermann, M. B., Jooste, P. L., and Pandav, C. S. 2008. Iodine-deficiency disorders. *The Lancet*, *372*:1251–1262.

Zsolnai, T. 1966. The antimicrobial activity of thiocyanates and isothiocyantes. 1. *Arzneimittel-Forschung*, *16*:870–876.

# CHAPTER 7

# Gossypol

**Idrees Ahmed Wani and Sadaf Nazir**

## CONTENTS



## 7.1 INTRODUCTION

Cotton has long been known as a unique fibre plant of the genus *Gossypium*. The plant is widely grown in tropical and subtropical regions of the world. The world's production of cotton is about 88 million bales, with China as the largest producer. Almost three quarters of the world's production is accounted by United States, India, and Pakistan. About 22.3 to 34.8 million hectares of land is designated to its cultivation around the world. It is mainly grown for the cotton fibre which grows on the surface of seeds. Separation of cotton fibres results in the generation of cotton seeds (USDA, 2007). Besides fibre, the cottonseeds are valuable as they are rich sources of protein (~23%) and oil (~21%). The composition of seeds varies considerably depending on plant species, variety, and environment. Cottonseed meal is extensively used as an animal feed, and cotton oil is used for cooking purposes in some developing countries (Shahid et al., 2010). The cottonseeds are ovoid in shape.

DOI: 10.1201/9781003178446-7

The seeds are reported to possess high gossypol content which is reportedly known for its toxicity and now considered as a promising phytochemical.

Gossypol is a complex polyphenol which is a non-volatile and highly coloured yellow pigment (Kenar, 2008). The name "gossypol" is derived from the plant genus name prefixed with "ol" from phenol (Soto-Blanco, 2008). Gossypol is produced in the plant from two molecules of hemigossypol and is classified as a dimeric-sesquiterpenoid (Stipanovic et al., 1986). Gossypol and related sesquiterpene aldehydes in cotton function as the defence in the plant in response to insect herbivores and pathogens. However, it is an antinutritional compound in cottonseed products. Toxicity of cottonseed meal was suggested as early as 1915. It is well acknowledged that gossypol can be toxic to humans and monogastric animals such as fish, swine, poultry, and rodents (Zhang et al., 2007c). The degree of toxicity due to gossypol limits the applications of cottonseed oil and meal. Therefore, recommended regulations and limits (450 ppm FDA, 600 ppm FAO/WHO) have been set mandatory for human consumption.

Many studies have now reported that gossypol has biological activities including antioxidant (Wang et al., 2008), anticancer (Jin et al., 2015), antimicrobial (Vedehra et al., 1985), antiviral (Vander Jagt et al., 2000). However, these benefits are not reaped as its wide systemic toxicity limits its clinical uses (Francois et al., 2018).

## 7.2 STRUCTURE AND CHEMISTRY

Gossypol is complex polyphenolic compound with a chemical formula of $C_{30}H_{30}O_8$. It was first discovered and isolated as a crude pigment by Longmore (1886). Its scientific name is 1,1′, 6,6′, 7,7′-hexahydroxy, 3,3′- dimethyl, 5,5′-diisopropyl, 2,2′-binaphthyl, 8,8′-dialdehyde. Gossypol has a 518.55 Dalton molecular weight, and is a yellow pigment. It consists of two naphthalene rings joined by a single internaphthyl bond between the 2- and 2′-carbon atoms. Six hydroxyl groups are attached to the dimeric naphthalenic framework. The binapthalene structure makes it chemically reactive. Hydroxy groups at 1- and 1′ (peri positions) are more reactive than remaining four hydroxyl groups (6, 6′, 7, and 7′). Besides two aldehyde groups are attached at 8 and 8′ position. The two aldehyde groups lend a great deal of interesting chemistry, and are established to be the main contributor for gossypol's toxicity.

Gossypol is a mixture of two enantiomers, (–) gossypol and (+) gossypol (Kakani et al., 2010). The (–) gossypol enantiomer is the most biologically active form but is slowly eliminated. This results in its more toxicity than the (+) gossypol (Wu et al., 1986; Bailey et al., 2000). The Gossypium species produces both enantiomers in varied proportions, which is genetically determined (Lordelo et al., 2007; Scheffler et al., 2008). An enantiomeric excess of (+)-gossypol is usually found in plant species of *Gossypium arboreum*, *G. herbaceum*, *G. hirsutum*, *G. aboreum*, *G. mustelimum*, and *Thespesia populnea*, while (–)-gossypol was found in excess in *G. barbadens* (Figure 7.1).

Gossypol molecule has both hydrophilic and lipophilic groups. Two methyl and two isopropyl-groups at the 3,3′- and 5,5′-positions, respectively show gossypol's lipophilic region. The hydroxyl and aldehyde groups on the other side of the naphthalene ring exhibit the lipophobic region of the molecule (Vander Jagt et al., 2000).

The presence of eight polar groups in gossypol makes it soluble in most organic solvents such as glycol, methanol, butanol, ethanol, ethylene, carbon tetrachloride, ethers, acetates, phenols, naphthalene, pyridine, dimethyl sulfoxide, and vegetable oil at certain temperature but it remains less soluble in glycerin, petroleum ether, gasoline, cyclohexane, and benzene. However, it is insoluble in water due to the presence of dialkylnaphtalene groups in structure of gossypol (Xue et al., 1992; Francois et al., 2018).

Based on the AOCS (American Oil Chemists Society), official free gossypol (FG) is defined as gossypol and gossypol derivatives in cottonseed products that can be extracted by 70% aqueous

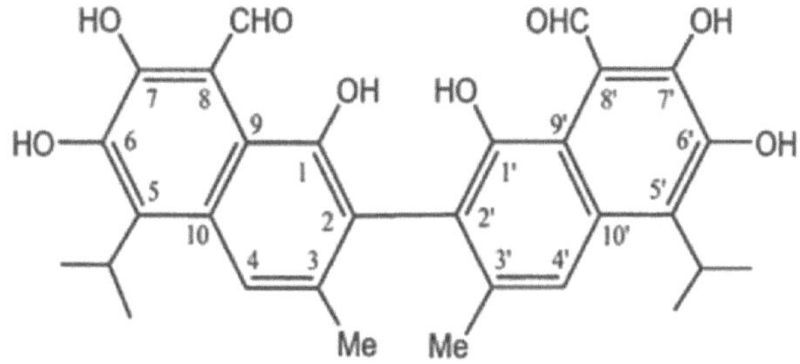


1

Formula: $C_{30}H_{30}O_8$
MW: 518.5

**Figure 7.1** Structure of Gossypol.

acetone (AOCS, Ba 7-58). Bound gossypol (BG), formed during cottonseed processing by reaction of gossypol with other compounds, is not soluble in aqueous acetone. Total Gossypol (TG) is defined as gossypol and gossypol derivatives, both FG and BG, which can react with 3-amino-1-propanol in dimethylformamide solution (Ba 8-78) (AOCS, 1987). FG and TG are determined empirically, and BG is determined mathematically by the equation

$$BG = TG - FG \quad (1)$$

A major concentration of gossypol exists as Schiff bases that are formed by the condensation between gossypol aldehydic groups with amino groups of proteins during cottonseed processing (Cater, 1968). Schiff's base confers a complex behaviour to gossypol. The Schiff's base is enhanced at alkaline pH and stabilized by reduction. Gossypol can get readily derivatized to form various structural forms. It can chelate with iron, oxidize to gossypolone/gossypolic acid/gossindane, and react with sodium hydroxide to form apogossypol (Wang et al., 2009).

## 7.3 DISTRIBUTION

Gossypol occurs in certain species of *Gossypium* (cotton). The genus includes many species distributed throughout the world, but only four species are grown for cotton fibre: *Gossypium hirsutum* L., *Gossypium barbadense* L., *Gossypium arboretum* L., and *Gossypium herbaceum* L. Among these species *G. hirsutum* is economically most important and is grown to produce 90% of the world's cotton (Borem et al., 2003). Gossypol is produced by pigment glands in cotton stems, leaves, seeds, and flower buds but is mostly in the seeds and root bark. The pigment glands in cotton plant are small black spots distributed throughout the plant with greatest concentration in the seeds (Alexander et al., 2008; Kenar, 2008). The seed of *G. barbadense* may contain up to 34 g of gossypol/kg (Percy et al., 1996). Gossypol accounts for about 20 to 40% of gland weight and 0.4 to 1.7% whole kernel. The gossypol content varies according to the species, variety and environmental conditions in which the cotton plant is grown (Markman, 1968).

Total gossypol production is affected by weather and species of cotton. Weather conditions like rainfall rate is positively correlated with gossypol production However, temperature is negatively correlated with its production (Pons et al., 1953). Among cotton species *G. barbadense* has high gossypol concentrations than *G. hirsutum* (Cass et al., 1991).

The free gossypol concentrations range from 0.02 to 6.64% in whole cottonseeds among many cotton varieties (Randel et al., 1992; Price et al., 1993). Cottonseed may contain concentrations greater than 14,000 mg/kg of total gossypol and 7,000 mg/kg of free gossypol have been reported in cottonseeds (Alexander et al., 2008). However, the concentration of gossypol decreases after oil extraction from the seeds. Concentrations up to 0.6% are available following solvent extraction, but approximately 0.06% is available, if the extraction process involves mechanical pressure and heat treatment (Nicholson, 2012).

## 7.4 TOXICITY

Gossypol toxicity occurs on consumption of cottonseed or oil and or meal derived out of it. Free gossypol is considered more toxic than bound gossypol to monogastric animals. The most common toxicity is known to occur due to cardiac irregularity that leads to death of animals due to the liberation of oxygen from oxyhaemoglobin. The toxicity due to gossypol is considered acute (circulatory failure), subchronic (pulmonary edema), and chronic (ill health and malnutrition) (Wang et al., 2008). Acute gossypol poisoning may take place on consumption of sufficient amount of cottonseed. Cumulative effects (chronic) of gossypol poisoning may however take place following intake period of two to three months. Gossypol toxicity has been reported in number of animal species including chicken (Henry et al., 2001), sheep (Morgan et al., 1988), pigs (Haschek et al., 1989), goat (East et al., 1994), and dogs (Uzal et al., 2005). Monogastric animals like pigs, birds, etc., are more prone to gossypol toxicity than ruminants. This is due to the reason that gossypol binds to proteins in the rumen, which renders it unavailable for absorption. However, free gossypol is lipid-soluble and readily absorbed from the intestine. Among the ruminants young animals are more sensitive to gossypol toxicity than adults. However, if the intake of gossypol exceeds the rumenal detoxification level, toxicity will result. Acute toxicity of gossypol produces different clinical signs among the farm animals, which include distress in respiration, weakness, anorexia, impaired body weight, and even death (Morgan et al., 1988; Fombad and Bryant, 2004). Post-mortem examination of ruminants affected by gossypol poisoning revealed necrosis in liver, hypertrophic cardiac fibre degeneration, swelling in lungs, yellowish liquid accumulation in chest, and gastroenteritis. Calves also showed kidney damage and cardiovascular damage (Holmberg et al., 1988; Morgan et al., 1988).

Animals fed with cottonseed/gossypol frequently show anaemia. This is due to reactivity of gossypol with minerals and amino acids. Gossypol form complex with iron and prevents its absorption. The deficiency of iron ultimately affects erythropoiesis-production of red blood cells. Moreover gossypol promotes increased erythrocyte fragility (Randel et al., 1996; Zhang et al., 2007a). Gossypol also stimulates the eryptosis due to increase in cytosolic $Ca^{2+}$ activity resulting in cell membrane scrambling and contraction, which further contributes to anaemia (Zbidah et al., 2012).

Thyroid metabolism is reported to be affected by gossypol. Studies with rats showed lower $T_4$ and $T_3$ concentrations in blood after gossypol dosing (Rikihisa and Lin, 1989; Lin et al; 1990). However there are also reports that doses of gossypol resulted in higher $T_3$ serum concentrations without affecting $T_4$ in rats and sheep (Tang and Wong, 1984; EL-Mokadem et al; 2012). The histological examination of thyroid glands from male rats dosed with gossypol showed follicular degeneration and atrophy (Rikihisa and Lin, 1989). Rats fed with gossypol showed hyperplasia, hypertrophy, and degranulation in thyrotropic cells in the pituitary gland (Udoh et al., 1992).

Gossypol is also reported as hepatotoxic (Kakani et al., 2010; El-Sharaky et al., 2009; Fonseca et al., 2013). In some rat studies rats which were given single dose intraperitoneal gossypol at a dose rate of 25–30 mg/kg body weight showed hepatocyte degeneration (Fonseca et al., 2013). Chickens fed a diet with free gossypol (0.1%) for a period of 21 days led to high plasma gamma glutamyltransferase activity and liver lipidosis (Blevins et al., 2010).

Gossypol has been reported to reduce fertility by affecting male and female gametogenesis. Gossypol toxicity for male reproduction has been reported by number of studies in rats (El-Sharaky et al., 2009), bulls (Hassan et al., 2004). Antifertility effect of gossypol is time- and dose-dependent.

Effective doses has shown infertility by inhibiting sperm motility, decreasing sperm concentrations, induce specific mitochondrial injury to the sperm tail, and damaging the germinal epithelium (Randel et al., 1992). These effects are reversible if gossypol is discontinued in the diet. Studies also reported decline in birth rate of humans in some areas of China due to consumption of cottonseed oil (Chang et al., 2011; Yu and Chan, 1998; Qian and Wang, 1984). Gossypol effect on female reproduction shows interference with the oestrous cycle, pregnancy, and early embryonic development (Randel et al., 1992, 1996). Lin et al. (1985) reported gossypol interfered with rodent oestrous cycles and Basini et al. (2009) observed pig granulosa cell function was negatively affected. It has been observed that ovaries from heifers fed cottonseed meal had fewer large follicles ( $>$ 5 mm) than heifers fed soybean meal.

Gossypol is also reported as immune toxic by some studies. It has been reported that gossypol effects leucocytes especially lymphocytes which may affect immune response of an organism (Braga et al., 2012). Mice treated with gossypol had decreased Ig M and Ig G production after sheep erythrocyte immunization (Sijun et al., 2012). Men treated with gossypol as a male contraceptive showed reduced Ig G titers which could be associated with altered lymphocytes (Xu et al., 1988).

## 7.5 MECHANISM OF ACTION OF TOXICITY

Gossypol is soluble in lipids and gets readily absorbed from the gastro-intestinal tract (Randel et al., 1992). The molecule has affinity of binding to amine groups of amino acids or proteins, and to iron-containing products (Nicholson, 2012). Gossypol renders amino acids unavailable by the formation of Schiff's base type derivatives and protein/gossypol interactions (Polsky et al., 1989). It interferes in enzymatic reactions which are essential for many biologic processes such as the ability of cells to respond to oxidative stress and inhibition of oxygen release from haemoglobin (Price et al., 1993). Conjugation, metabolism, and urinary excretion of gossypol is limited while most of it is eliminated in the faeces.

The biological activity of gossypol is mainly due to a disturbance of mitochondrial function. It may be due to modification of the mitochondrial concentration of $Ca^{2+}$, which is associated with membrane fluidity (Martinez et al., 1993), disruption of oxidative phosphorylation by inhibition of mitochondrial succinic dehydrogenase (Jiang et al., 2002), or by the release of cytochrome *c* from mitochondria into the cytosol causing a mitochondrial-mediated apoptotic mechanism (Oliver et al., 2005). It is the diversity of mitochondrial dysfunctions that keeps the problem of gossypol toxicity open. Arinbasarova et al. (2012) studied the effect of gossypol on the mitochondrial respiratory chain of *Yarrowia lipolytica*. The compound was shown to inhibit mitochondrial electron transfer and stimulate generation of reactive oxygen species.

## 7.6 IDENTIFICATION AND QUANTIFICATION

The quantitative determination of gossypol involves volumetric, gravimetric, polarographic, colorimetric, luminescent, and spectrophotometric methods. Literature studies report the use of gas chromatography mass spectroscopy (GC-MS) analysis, high-performance liquid chromatography (HPLC), near infrared reflectance, and electron impact-mass spectrometer (EI-MS) (Phillip et al., 1990). Such techniques provide a fingerprint mass spectrum and infra-red spectrum. The structural analysis of gossypol and its derivatives is successfully facilitated. However, HPLC has been widely used to detect gossypol quantitatively due to the presence of chromophoric groups with strong absorption power. Gossypol has been detected from cottonseed, leaves, flower buds, oils, and meals after derivatization (Chamkasem, 1988). With the advancement of research, studies demonstrated detection of gossypol without derivatization through HPLC. Non-derivatization methods involve the use of methanol-acetic acid aqueous solution (90:10, v/v) as mobile phase. Also, studies report the use of methanol-water (9:1) adjusted to pH 2.6 with phosphoric acid (Cai et al., 2004; Aoyama, 2008). The advancement of technology has led to more accuracy, sensitivity, and efficiency by the use of in-combination techniques. Recently, HPLC and in tandem mass spectrometry (LCMS) was used for the determination of gossypol. In addition, high-pressure liquid chromatography coupled with a triple quadrupole mass spectrometer has also been used for detection. Furthermore, the separation of gossypol enantiomers and their conversion to Schiff base diastereomers has been successfully implied for quantification by HPLC. Various chiral forms of gossypol, 6-methoxy gossypol, 6,6'-dimethoxy gossypol have been analysed via HPLC. Racemic mixtures of gossypol-acetic acid, gossypol-acetone at low temperature are also detected by HPLC (Dowd and Pelitire, 2008). Sprogoe et al. (2008) detected gossypol in crude extracts of *T. danis* by the use of combination technique involving HPLC, MS, and NMR.

Besides the advanced methods, standard procedures of AOCS are also used for gossypol determination. But, the methods lack sensitivity and are time-consuming. The lack of sensitivity is ascribed to the false readings that occur due to the reaction between aldehydic groups of gossypol and dye reagent (AOCS, 1987).

To overcome the shortcomings of advanced techniques and standard procedures of AOCS, immunochemical methods have been developed. ELISA-based biosensors that involve on monoclonal, polyclonal antibodies have been developed to detect gossypol. ELISA for gossypol generates an antibody–antigen-specific reaction that is sensitive and highly specific. This method has been demonstrated to detect gossypol at lower limits from crude extracts as well (Wang and Plhak, 2004).

## 7.7 SAFETY, PRECAUTIONS, AND REGULATION

Bioactive properties of gossypol have escalated an interest of its use as a functional ingredient. Clinical trials have been conducted to investigate the application of gossypol as a vital bioactive molecule. However, the concern about inadvertent exposure to gossypol remains still less relied upon. The use of gossypol as supplement is implied for livestock and aquaculture (Wang et al., 2009).

Gossypol is non-volatile and soluble in oils than water. Free form of gossypol is unstable and therefore will not persist processing conditions. Crude form of gossypol is only desired as a nutritional supplement in animal feed. The bioaccumulation and biomagnification of gossypol in food chain still stands unexplored. The pure form of gossypol finds use in orally ingested pharmaceuticals that are still under experimental trials. As a therapeutic drug, the exposure of gossypol could be regulated on allowable levels in edible foods. Clinical trials over rats show that on consumption of gossypol, it is distributed to most organs of the body. It disrupts gap junctions and cell to cell communication, inhibits microtubule assembly, and causes cytotoxicity. The alteration of DNA synthesis and cell cycle progression has also gained attention. The oral lethal doses of gossypol are estimated to be 2,300 mg/kg$^{-1}$. Exposures may cause irritation of skin, eyes, and respiratory tract. Therefore FDA- allowable limits of gossypol have been set to 0.045% or 450 ppm (FDA, 1974). The World Health Organization permits up to 0.6 μg/mg$^{-1}$ (600 ppm) in edible foods. No occupational or other specific standards are observed for gossypol. However, prudent safety practices are recommended when handling large quantities of gossypol experimentally in laboratory or while formulating therapeutic drugs (WHO, 2004).

## 7.8 EFFECT OF PROCESSING

Biodegradation of gossypol is observed under various processing conditions. Various studies on heat treatment of gossypol suggest degradability of gossypol at high temperatures. Heat treatment reduces the free concentration of gossypol in cottonseed meal. However, roasting is supposed to increase the bioavailability and absorption of gossypol in cottonseed meal. Grinding of cottonseed is also known to increase gossypol concentrations. Drying is found to have no effect on the concentrations of gossypol (Bernard et al., 1999).

Bressani et al. (1964) reported that an alkaline pH of cooking, associated with calcium ions, was effective in reducing FG and TG in cottonseed flour used for human foods. The addition of calcium increased the effectiveness of the gossypol–iron complex formation, resulting in full protection from gossypol toxicity. Nagalakshmi et al. (2002, 2003) also confirmed the effectiveness of calcium hydroxide for the gossypol detoxification.

Treatment of cottonseeds with solvents has been reported to reduce the gossypol content to lower levels. Organic solvents such as ethanol, hexane, aqueous acetone, acidic butanol, methylene chloride, aniline, and aliphatic amines have been reportedly reduced the gossypol levels (Wang et al., 2009). The processing of cottonseed to extract oil leads to the formation of Schiff bases from the condensation reaction between amino groups and aldehydes. This results in decreased availability of amino acids present in cottonseed meal and lowered digestibility. Such changes reduce nutritional value of cottonseed meal (Hron et al., 1996).

Microbial fermentation releases cellulolytic enzymes, amylase, protease, and lipolytic enzymes that cause in situ alkaline-catalyze transesterification which reduces FG and TG contents below the FAO standard (Qian et al., 2008).

## 7.9 BIOLOGICAL ACTIVITY OF GOSSYPOL

### 7.9.1 Insecticidal Activity

Gossypol is supposed to possess insecticidal activity. A research study on *Helicoverpa zea* larvae showed that a diet containing 0.16% gossypol was effective in pest control. The control is attributed to the inhibition of protease and lipid peroxidase activities as well as ATPase activity in larvae. Stronger activity of gossypol has been observed than the insecticide fenvalerate. Studies demonstrate that the activity is attributed to the changes caused in sterols, fatty acids to affect pests. Gossypol is complexed with metal cations and aza-derivatives so as to imply it for agricultural usage. The metal cations and aza-derivatives bind to aldehydic groups so as to reduce the toxicity of gossypol and make it safe for agricultural usage.

### 7.9.2 Antioxidant Activity

Gossypol is a polyphenolic compound and a potent natural antioxidant. Studies report gossypol inhibited carotene destruction (Hove, 1944). It is also observed that gossypol prevented microsomal peroxidation in rat liver. It was initiated by incubation with ferric ascorbate (Laughton et al., 1989). Gossypol bis (piperinoethylimine) and bis (morpholinoethylimine) demonstrate potent antioxidant activity in human blood serum and rat brain synaptosomes. At certain concentrations, these substances suppressed the peroxidation of lipids in enzymatic and nonenzymatic systems regarding the oxidation of rat liver microsomes (Dalimov et al., 1989).

### 7.9.3 Antifertility Activity

Gossypol has been studied extensively as a contraceptive agent through various in vivo models of rats, monkeys, rabbits, bulls, and hamsters (Wang et al., 2009). Oral administration in hamsters at 5 mg/kg body weight for 12 weeks induced sterility. At higher doses ( $>$ 20 mg) deleterious effects were observed (Chang et al., 1980). Studies report (–)-gossypol as the more active antifertility agent.

The mechanism of action exploited in rabbits for antifertility is blockage of T-type $Ca^{2+}$ currents and inhibition of hyaluronidase, β-glucuronidase, and acid phosphatase (Bai and Shi, 2002).

### 7.9.4 Anticancer Activity

Studies report in vitro inhibition of several cancer human cell lines by gossypol. In vitro studies have been observed for cell lines of colon, leukaemia, prostrate, breast (Huang et al., 2006). Antitumor activity was observed against several human cell lines by Band et al. (1989). Anticancer activity of gossypol is attributed to the inhibition of cytoplasmic and mitochondrial enzymes of cells, depletion of cellular ATP, and uncoupling of oxidative phosphorylation (Ueno et al., 1988; Keniry et al., 1989). Gossypol inhibits the key nuclear enzymes including DNA polymerase, topoisomerase responsible for DNA replication. Gossypol induced apoptosis in leukaemia cells at 50 μM for 6 h (Hou et al., 2004). At low dose (5 μM), gossypol induced apoptosis in human colon cancer cells. Human leukmia cells showed cell cytotoxicity at > 10 μM (Zhang et al., 2007b).

### 7.9.5 Antimicrobial Activity

Gossypol has reportedly antifungal activity with $LD_{50}$ values from 20 to 100 ppm of pure gossypol. Inhibitory effect on aerobic spore formers, lactobacilli, and some yeasts has been observed. Antibiotic activity was observed for *Staphylococuss aureus* (10 μg/mL), *Sarcina lutea* (25 μg/mL) *Bacillus polymyxa* (50 μg/mL), *Bacillus cereus* (50 μg/mL), *Leuconostoc mesentroides* (10 μg/mL) *Lactobacillus delbruckii* (20 μg/mL) *Escherichia coli* ( > 200 μg/mL) *Saccharomyces cerevisiae* ( > 200 μg/mL) *Saccharomyces carlsbergensis* ( > 200 μg/mL). The activity of gossypol has been seen to be more pronounced for gram positive microorganisms than gram negative microorganisms. Inhibition was observed on gram positive bacteria at levels of 100 ppm of gossypol. However, only few strains of gram negative bacteria showed inhibition at levels > 200 ppm. The fungi *Paecilomyces fumosoroeus* found to cause cutaneous and disseminated infections in cats and dogs was inhibited at levels of 1,000 ppm (Margalith, 1967; Wang et al., 2009).

### 7.9.6 Antiviral Activity

Reportedly, gossypol is known to inhibit human immunodeficiency virus type (HIV-I). Pronounced effect of (–)-gossypol is observed over (+)- gossypol. Activity is also observed against herpes virus, influenza virus, and para influenza virus. Several derivatives of gossypol including gossylic nitrile-1,10-diacetate, gossylic iminolactone, and gossylic lactone have shown inhibition towards the replication of HIV-1 in vitro (Vander Jagt et al., 2000).

### 7.9.7 Antiparasitic Activity

A series of gossypol derivatives with modified aldehydic and hydroxyl groups inhibit the growth of *Plasmodium falciparum* (Razakantoanina et al., 2000; Royer et al., 1986). Malaria which is a vector-borne infectious disease caused by protozoan parasites *Plasmodium falciparum*, *P. malariae*, *P. ovale*, *and P. vivax*. The activity of (–)-gossypol was seen to be more over (+)- gossypol. The inhibition was attributed to the inhibition of enzymes (lactate dehydrogenase-LDH), alcohol dehydrogenase and malic enzymes (Mendis et al., 2001).

### 7.9.8 Hypocholestromic Activity

Gossypol is known to reduce the levels of low-density lipoprotein (LDL) which is responsible for atherosclerosis and coronary heart disease. Research studies on cynomolgus monkeys administered gossypol orally (10 mg/kg/day) and observed a substantial decrease in total plasma cholesterol and low-density lipoprotein without any changes in the high-density lipoprotein (HDL) (Beynen and Liepa, 1987). The study inferred that gossypol reduces hepatic synthesis of LDL and its intestinal absorption. Similar results for reduction of cholesterol have been observed in rabbits. About 20 mg/kg body weight of gossypol was injected to rats for 4 weeks that resulted in lower levels of plasma cholesterol. However, the mechanism of action for reduction of cholesterol is not known (Akingbemi et al., 1995).

## 7.10 FUTURE SCOPE

Future scope of gossypol may be in the suppression of cancer cells. A synergistic effect of cancer inhibitor drugs and gossypol has been observed on cancer cell lines. Derivatized gossypol to form a Schiff base can be used as an antioxidant. Gossypol can act as a mimetic for apoptosis of lymphocytic leukaemia cells. Clinical trials for cancers of adrenal glands, brain gliomas at various stages show positive results for treatment with gossypol. Gossypol can be also used an antiviral drug against herpes. The multifaceted reactivity of gossypol confers it various biological activities which can be strived to form a fullerene hybrid, i.e., a nanoparticle-based therapeutic gossypol.

## 7.11 CONCLUSIONS

Gossypol is a polyphenolic aldehyde with versatile biological activity. The presence of six phenolic hydroxyl groups makes it chemically reactive. The two aldehydic groups present in the carbon chain of gossypol are responsible for the toxicity of gossypol. The toxicity is substantially reduced by fermentation, solvent extraction, and high temperatures. Recently, studies report enantiomers of gossypol exhibiting different biological activities. The biological activities involve various antioxidant, antivirus, antimicrobial, and anticancer activities. However, due to its toxicity there is limitation on the application of gossypol. The toxicity of gossypol depends upon its dose and the toxicity is categorized as acute (circulatory failure), subchronic (pulmonary edema), and chronic (ill health and malnutrition). Future prospectus of gossypol may be in the suppression of cancer cells.

## REFERENCES


Akingbemi, B. T., Ogwuegbu, S. O., Onwuka, S. K., Oke, B. O. and Aire, T. A. 1995. The effects of protein malnutrition and experimental infection with Trypanosoma brucei on gossypol treatment in the rat: Haematological and serum biochemical changes. *Journal of Comparative Pathology* 112: 361–371.

Alexander, J., Benford, D., Cockburn, A. et al. 2008. Gossypol as undesirable substance in animal feed. *EFSA Journal* 908: 1–55.

Aoyama, K. 2008. Determination of gossypol in feeds by HPLC. *Journal of the Food Hygienic Society of Japan* 49: 303–307.

Arinbasarova, A. Y., Medentsev, A. G. and Krupyanko, V. I. 2012. Gossypol inhibits electron transport and stimulates ROS generation in *Yarrowia lipolytica* mitochondria. *The Open Biochemistry Journal* 6: 11–15.

Bai, J. and Shi, Y. 2002. Inhibition of T-type Ca(2þ) currents in mouse spermatogenic cells by gossypol, an antifertility compound. *European Journal of Pharmacology* 440: 1–6.

Bailey, C. A., Stipanovic, R. D., Ziehr, M. S., Haq, A. U., Sattar, M., Kubena, L. F., Kim, H. L. and Vieria, R. 2000. Cottonseed with a high (+)- to (–)-gossypol enantiomer ratio favorable to broiler production. *Journal of Agricultural and Food Chemistry* 48(11): 5692–5695.

Band, V., Hoffer, A. P., Band. H., Rhinehardt, A. E., Knapp, R. C., Matlin, S. A. and Anderson D. J. 1989. Antiproliferative effect of gossypol and its optical isomers on human reproductive cancer cell lines. *Gynecologic Oncology* 32(3): 273–274.

Basini, G., Bussolati, S., Baioni, L. and Grasselli, F. 2009. Gossypol, a polyphenolic aldehyde from cotton plant, interferes with swine granulosa cell function. *Domestic Animal Endocrinology* 37(1): 30–36.

Bernard, J. K., Freeman, D. W., Waldner, D. and Lane, G. T. 1999. Review: Effect of processing whole cottonseed on nutrient digestion, performance of lactating dairy cows, and gossypol bioavailability. *The Professional Animal Scientist* 15(4): 224–229.

Beynen, A. C. and Liepa, G. U. 1987. Dietary cottonseed protein and cholesterol metabolism. *Ernahrungswiss* 26: 219–225.

Blevins, S., Siegel, P. B., Blodgett, D. J., Ehrich, M., Saunders, G. K. and Lewis, R. M. 2010. Effects of silymarin on gossypol toxicosis in divergent lines of chickens. *Poultry Science* 89(9): 1878–1886.

Borem, A., Freire, E. C., Cesar, J., Penna, V. and Vianna, P. A. 2003. Considerations about cotton gene escape in Brazil: A review. *Crop Breeding and Applied Biotechnology* 3(4): 315–332.

Braga, A. P., MacIel, M. V., Guerra, D. G. F., Maia, I. S. A. S., Oloris, S. C. S. and Soto-Blanco B. 2012. Extruded-expelled cottonseed meal decreases lymphocyte counts in male sheep. *Revue de MedecineVeterinaire* 163(3): 147–152.

Cai, Y., Zhang, H., Zeng, Y., Mo, J., Bao, J., Miao, C., Bai, J., Yan, F. and Chen, F. 2004. An optimized gossypol high-performance liquid chromatography assay and its application in evaluation of different gland genotypes of cotton. *Journal of Bioscience* 29: 67–71.

Cass, Q. B., Tritan, E., Matlin, S. A. and Freire, E. C. 1991. Gossypol enantiomer ratios in cotton seeds. *Phytochemistry* 30: 2655–2657.

Cater, C. M. 1968. Studies on the reaction products of gossypol with amino acids, peptides, and proteins. Dissertation. Texas A & M University, College Station, TX.

Chamkasem, K. 1988. Gossypol analysis in cottonseed oil by HPLC. *Journal of the American Oil Chemists' Society* 65: 1601–1605.

Chang, M. C., Gu, Z. P. and Saksena, S. K. 1980. Effects of gossypol on the fertility of male rats, hamsters and rabbits. *Contraception* 21: 461–469.

Chang, S., Condon, B., Graves, E., Uchimiya, M, Fortier, C., Easson, M. and Wakely, P. 2011. Flame retardant properties of triazine phosphonates derivative with cotton fabric. *Fiber and Polymers* 12(3): 334–339.

Dalimov, D. N., Mukhamedzhanova, E. N., Shneivais, V. B., Biktimirov, L., Isamilov, A. I. and Kamaev, F. G. 1989. Synthesis, structure, and action of some gossypol derivatives on the peroxidation of the lipids of biosubstrates. *Khimiya. Prirodnykh. Soedinenii* 5: 707–712.

Dowd, M. K. and Pelitire, S. M. 2008. HPLC preparation of the chiral forms of 6-methoxy-gossypol and 6, 60-dimethoxy-gossypol. *Journal of Chromatography B: Biomedical Sciences* 867: 69–77.

East, N. E. Anderson, M. and Lowenstine, L. J. 1994. Apparent gossypol-induced toxicosis in adult dairy goats. *Journal of the American Veterinary Medical Association* 204(4): 642–643.

EL-Mokadem, M. Y., Taha, T. A., Samak, M. A. andYassen, A. M. 2012. Alleviation of reproductive toxicity of gossypol using selenium supplementation in rams. *Journal of Animal Science* 90(9): 3274–3285.

El-Sharaky, A. S., Newairy, A. A., Elguindy, N. M. and Elwafa, A. A. 2009. Mutual anti-oxidative effect of gossypol acetic acid and gossypol–iron complex on hepatic lipid peroxidation in male rats. *Food and Chemical Toxicology* 47: 2735–2741.

Fombad, R. B., Bryant, M. J. 2004. An evaluation of the use of cottonseed cake in the diet of growing pigs. *Tropical Animal Health and Production* 36(3): 295–305.

Fonseca, N. B. S., Gadelha, I. C. N., Oloris, S. C. S. and Soto-Blanco, B. 2013. Effectiveness of albumin-conjugated gossypol as an immunogen to prevent gossypol-associated acute hepatotoxicity in rats. *Food and Chemical Toxicology* 56: 149–153.

Food and Drug Administration (FDA) 1974. Food Drug Cosmetic Law. 56, 518.94, 172.894.

Francois, M., Luhong, T, Clement, M. O. and Honghua, W. 2018. Insights on synthesis and potential applications of gossypol, a promising multipurpose contraceptive and antiinfections agent: A review. *Journal of Emerging Technologies and Innovative Research* 5(10):768–798.

Haschek, W. M., Beasley, V. R., Buck, W. B. and Finnell, J. H. 1989. Cottonseed meal (gossypol) toxicosis in a swine herd. *Journal of the American Veterinary Medical Association* 195(5): 613–615.

Henry, M. H., Pesti, G. M. and Brown, T. P. 2001. Pathology and histopathology of gossypol toxicity in broiler chicks. *Avian Diseases* 45(3): 598–604.

Holmberg, C. A., Weaver, L. D., Gutterbock, W. M., Genes, J. and Montgomery, P. 1988. Pathological and toxicological studies of calves fed a high concentration cotton seed meal diet. *Veterinary Pathology* 25(2):147–153.

Hou, D. X., Uto, T., Tong, X., Takeshita, T., Tanigawa, S., Ima-mura, I., Ose, T.andFujii, M. 2004. Involvement of reactive oxygen species-independent mitochondrial pathway in gossypol-induced apoptosis. *Archives of Biochemistry and Biophysics* 428: 179–187.

Hove, E. L. 1944. Gossypol as a carotene-protecting antioxidant, in vivo and in vitro. *Journal of Biological Chemistry* 156: 633–642.

Hron, R. J., Wan, P. J. and Kuk, M. S. 1996. Ethanol vapor deactivation of gossypol in cottonseed meal. *Journal of American Oil Chemical Society* 73: 1337–1339.

Huang, Y. W., Wang, L. S., Chang, H. L., Ye, W., Dowd, M. K., Wan, P. J. and Lin, Y. C. 2006. Molecular mechanisms of (-)-gossypol-induced apoptosis in human prostate cancer cells. *Anticancer Research* 26(3A): 1925–1933.

Jiang, J., Ghosh, P., Kulp, S., Sugimoto, Y., Liu, S., Czekajewski, J., Chang, H. and Lin, Y. 2002. Effect of gossypol on $CO_2$ consumption and $CO_2$ production in human prostate cancer cells. *Anticancer Research* 22: 1491–1496.

Jin, C., Chen, M., Wang, Y., Kang, X., Han, G.and Xu, S. 2015. Preparation of novel (-)-gossypol nanoparticles and the effect on growth inhibition in human prostate cancer Pc-3 cells in vitro. *Experimental and Therapeutic Medicine* 9: 675–78.

Kakani, R. Gamboa, D. A., Calhoun, M. C., Haq, A. U. and Bailey C. A. 2010. Relative oxicity of cottonseed gossypol enantiomers in broilers. *Open Toxicology Journal* 4: 26–31.

Kenar, J. A. 2008. Reaction chemistry of gossypol and its derivatives. *Journal of American Oil Chemists Society* 83(4): 269–302.

Keniry, M. A., Hollander, C. and Benz, C. C. 1989. The effect of gossypol and 6-aminoni- cotinamide on tumor cell metabolism: A $^{31}$P-magnetic resonance spectroscopic study. *Biochemical and Biophysical. Research Communications* 164: 947–953.

Laughton, M. J., Halliwell, B., Evans, P. J. and Hoult, J. R. 1989. Antioxidant and pro- oxidant actions of the plant phenolics quercetin, gossypol and myricetin. Effects on lipid peroxidation, hydroxyl radical generation and bleomycin-dependent damage to DNA. *Biochemical Pharmacology* 38: 2859–2865.

Lin, Y. C., Chitcharoenthum, M. andRikihisa, Y. 1990. Effect of gossypol on thyroid hormones in young female rats. *Contraception* 41(4): 431–440.

Lin, Y. C., Pathmanayaki, R. and Rikihisa, Y. (1985). Inhibition of embryo implantation in the unilaterally gossypol-treated uterine horn of pregnant rats. *Biology of Reproduction* 32(Suppl. 1): 143.

Longmore J. 1886. Cotton seed oil: Its colouring matter and mucilage, and description of a new method of recovering the loss occurring in the refining process. *Indian Journal of Chemistry 5*: 200–206.

Lordelo, M. M., Calhoun, M. C., Dale, N. M., Dowd, M. K.and Davis, A. J. 2007. Relative toxicity of gossypol enantiomers in laying and broiler breeder hens. *Poultry Science* 86(3): 582–590.

Margalith, P. 1967. Inhibitory effect of gossypol on microorganisms. *Applied Microbiology* 15: 952–953.

Markman, L. 1968. *Gossypol Derivatives*, D. Greenberg, ed., The U. S. Department of Agriculture and the National Science Foundation, Washington, DC.

Martinez, F., Milan, R., Espinosa-Garcia, T. and Pardo, J. P. 1993.The anti-fertility agent, gossypol, releases calcium from rat liver mitochon-dria. *Comparative. Biochemistry and. Physiology* 104: 165–169.

Mendis, K., Sina, B. J., Marchesini, P. and Carter, R. 2001. The neglected burden of plasmodium vivax malaria. *American Journal of Tropical Medicine and Hygiene* 64(1–2): 97–106.

Morgan, S., Stair, E. L., Martin, T., Edwards, W. C. and Morgan, G. L. 1988. Clinical, clinicopathologic, pathologic, and toxicologic alterations associated with gossypol toxicosis in feeder lambs.*American Journal of Veterinary Research* 49(4): 493–499.

Nagalakshmi, D., Sastry, V. and Pawde, A. 2003. Rumen fermentation patterns and nutrient digestion in lambs fed cottonseed meal supplemental diets. *Animal Feed Science and Technology* 103: 1–14.

Nagalakshmi, D., Sastry, V. R. B. and Agrawal, D. K. 2002. Detoxification of undecorticated cottonseed meal by various physical and chemical methods. *Animal Nutrition and Feed Technology* 2(2): 117–126.

Nicholson, S. S. 2012. Cottonseed toxicity. In *Veterlnary Toxicology: Basic and Clinical Principles*, R. C. Gupta, ed., pp. 1161–1165. Academic Press, London, UK, 2nd edition.

Official Methods and Recommended Practices of the American Oil Chemists' Society. 1987b. *Total Gossypol. Ba, 8-78*, D. Firestone, ed., p. 61821, American Oil Chemists' Society, Champaign, IL.

Oliver, C. L., Miranda, M. B., Shangary, S., Land, S., Wang, S.and Johnson, D. E. 2005. (-)-Gossypol acts directly on the mitochondria to overcome Bcl-2- and Bcl-X(L)-mediated apoptosis resistance. *Molecular Cancer Therapeutics* 4: 23–31.

Percy, R. G., Calhoun, M. C., Kim, H. L.1996. Seed gossypol variation within *Gossypium barbadense* L. cotton. *Crop Science* 36(1): 193–197.

Phillip, V. A. and Hedin, P. A. 1990. Spectral techniques for the structural analysis of the cotton terpenoid aldehydes gossypol and gossypolone. *Journal of Agricultural and Food Chemistry* 38: 525–528.

Polsky, B., Segal, S. J., Baron, P. A., Jonathan, W. M. G., Uen, H. and Armstrong, D. 1989. Inactivation of human immunodeficiency virus in vitro by gossypol. *Contraception* 39(6): 579–587.

Pons Jr., W. A., Hoffpauir, C. L. and Hopper, T. H. 1953. Gossypol in cottonseed: Influence of variety of cottonseed and environment. *Journal of Agricultural and Food Chemistry* 1(18): 1115–1118.

Price, W. D., Lovell, R. A. and Mc Chesney, D. G. 1993. Naturally occurring toxins in feedstuffs: Center for veterinary medicine perspective. *Journal of Animal Science* 71(9): 2556– 2562.

Qian, J., Wang, F., Liu, S. and Yun, Z. 2008. In situ alkaline transesterification of cottonseed oil for production of biodiesel and nontoxic cottonseed meal. *Bioresources. Technology* 99: 9009–9012.

Qian, S.-Z. and Wang, Z.-G. 1984. Gossypol: A potential antifertility agent for males. *Annual Reviews of Pharmocology and Toxicology* 24: 329–360.

Randel, R. D., Chase Jr. C. C. and Wyse, S. J. 1992. Effects of gossypol and cottonseed products on reproduction of mammals. *Journal of Animal Science* 70(5): 1628–1638.

Randel, R. D., Willard, S. T., Wyse, S. J.and French, L. N. 1996. Effects of diets containing free gossypol on follicular development, embryo recovery and corpus luteum function in brangus heifers treated with bFSH. *Theriogenology* 45(5): 911–922.

Razakantoanina, V., Nguyen Kim, P. P. and Jaureguiberry, G. 2000. Antimalarial activity of new gossypol derivatives. *Parasitol Research* 86: 665–668.

Rikihisa, Y. and Lin, Y. C. 1989. Effect of gossypol on the thyroid in young rats. *Journal of Comparative Pathology* 100 (4): 411–417.

Royer, R. E., Deck, L. M., Campos, N. M., et al. 1986. Biologically active derivatives of gossypol: Synthesis and antimalarial activities of peri-acylated gossylic nitriles. *Journal of Medical Chemistry* 29: 1799–801.

Scheffler, J. A. and Romano, G. B. 2008. Breeding and genetics: Modifying gossypol in cotton (*Gossypium hirsutum*L.): A cost effective method for small seed samples. *Journal of Cotton Science* 12(3): 202–209.

Shahid L. A, Saeed M. A. and Amjad, N. 2010. Present status and future prospects of mechanized production of oilseed crops in Pakistan: A review. *Pakistan Journal of Agriculture Research* 23: 83–93.

Sijun, D., Pawlak, A., Pozniak et al. 2012. Effects of gossypol acetic acid on cellular and humoral immune response in nonimmunized and SRBC-immunized mice. *Central-European Journal of Immunology* 37(1): 11–19.

Soto-Blanco, B. 2008. Gossipol-e-fatoresantinutricionais da soja. In *Toxicologia Aplicada: A Mediclna Veterlnaria*, Spinosa, H. S., Gorniak, S. L. and Neto, J. P., eds., pp. 531–545, Manole, Barueri, Brazil.

Sprogoe, K., Staek, D., Ziegler, H. L., Jensen, T. H., Holm-Moller, S. B. and Jaroszewski, J. W. 2008. Combining HPLC-PDA-MS-SPE-NMR with circular dichroism for complete nat- ural product characterization in crude extracts: Levorotatory gossypol in Thespesia danis. *Journal of Natural Products* 71: 516–519.

Stipanovic, R., Stoessl, A., Stothers, J. B., et al. 1986. The stereochemistry of the biosynthetic precursor of gossypol. *Journal of Chemical Society Chemical Communications* 2: 100–102.

Tang, F., Wong and P. Y. D. 1984. Serum potassium and aldosterone levels in gossypol-treated rats. *International Journal of Andrology*7(2): 149–153.

Udoh, P., Patil, D. R. and Deshpande, M. K. 1992. Histopathological and biochemical effects of gossypol acetate on pituitary-gonadal axis of male albino rats.*Contraception* 45(5): 493– 509.

Ueno, H., Sahni, M. K., Segal, S. J. and Koide, S. S. 1988. Interaction of gossypol with sperm macromolecules and enzymes. *Contraception* 37: 333–341.

USDA. 2007. World oilseed production. http://www.soystats.com/2008/page_29.html.

Uzal, F. A., Puschner, B., Tahara, J. M. and Nordhausen, R. W. 2005 Gossypol toxicosis in a dog consequent to ingestion of cottonseed bedding. *Journal of Veterinary Diagnostic Investigation*17(6): 626–629.

Vadehra D. V., Kalla N. R. and Saxena, M., et al. 1985. Antimicrobial activity of gossypol acetic acid. *IRCS Medicinal Science* 13: 10–11.

Vander Jagt, D. L., Deck, L. M. and Royer, R. E. 2000. Gossypol: Prototype of inhibitors targeted to dinucleotide folds, *Current Medicinal Chemistry* 7: 479–498.

Wang, X. and Plhak, L. C. 2004. Monoclonal antibodies for the analysis of gossypol in cottonseed products. *Journal of Agricultural and Food Chemistry* 52: 709–712.

Wang, X., Beckham, T., Morris, J., et al. 2008. Bioactivities of gossypol, 6-methoxy gossypol and 6,60 - dimethoxy gossypol. *Journal of Agricultural Food Chemistry* 56: 4393–4398.
Wang, X., Howell, C. P., Chen,F., Yin, J. and Jiang,Y. 2009. In: Chapter 6. *Gossypol-A Polyphenolic Compound from Cotton Plant Advances in Food and Nutrition Research*, 58. Elsevier, Amsterdam.
World Health Organization (WHO) 2004. *The World Health Report: Changing History*. WHO, Geneva.
Wu, D. F., Yu, Y. W., Tang, Z. M. and Wang, M. Z. 1986. Pharmacokinetic of (±)-, (+)-, and (–)-gossypol in humans and dogs. *Clinical Pharmacology and Therapeutics* 39(6): 613–618.
Xu, D., Cai, W.-J., Zhu, B.-H., Dong, C.-J., Zheng, Z.-C. and Gao, Z.-Q.1988. Clinical safety of long-term administration of gossypol in 32 cases. *Contraception* 37(2): 129–135.
Xue, H., Z. Guo, A. Kon and Wu, G. 1992.The synthesis of unsymmetric analogs of gossypol. 6-*O*-methylgossypol. *Chinese Chemical Letters* 3: 165–166.
Zbidah, M., Lupescu, A., Shaik, N. and Lang, F. 2012. Gossypolinduced suicidal erythrocyte death. *Toxicology* 302(2–3): 101–105.
Zhang, H. P., Wang, X., Chen, F., Androulakis, X. M. and Wargovich, M. J. 2007a. Anticancer activity of limonoid from Khaya senegalensis. *Phytotherapy Research* 21: 731–734.
Zhang, M., Liu, H., Tian, Z., Huang, J., Remo, M. and Li, Q. Q. 2007b. Differential growth inhibition and induction of apoptosis by gossypol between HCT116 and HCT116/Bax (/) colorectal cancer cells. *Clinical and Experimental Pharmacology and Physiology* 34: 230–237.
Zhang, W. J., Xu, Z. R., Pan, X. L., Yan, X. H., Wang, Y. B. 2007b. Advances in gossypol toxicity and processing effects of whole cottonseed in dairy cows feeding. *Livestock Science*111(1–2): 1–9.

CHAPTER 8

# Erucic Acid

**Idrees Ahmed Wani, Zanoor ul Ashraf, and Sabeera Muzzaffar**

## CONTENTS



## 8.1 INTRODUCTION

Antinutritional constituents are the organic compounds present in natural foodstuffs such as legumes, edible crops, and animal feeds. They are produced by the healthy metabolism of plant species and have harmful effects on humans. They are classified on the basis of their activity and chemical nature, such as nitrogenous compounds, erucic acid, saponins, tannins, glucosinolates, and phenolic compounds, etc. These antinutrient factors have substantial effect on the nutritive value of foods as they decrease the nutrient value of foods, which is responsible for malnutrition of micronutrients and mineral deficiencies. Furthermore, decreased nutritive bioavailability and increased antinutritive factor can be toxic when available in higher concentration (Reddy and Pierson, 1994). Hence, reduction in the amount of antinutritional elements in legumes, edible crops, and animal feed is an interesting field of exploration because of the necessity to inhibit its toxicity and other related health diseases (Gemede and Ratta, 2014).

Erucic acid is chemically a monounsaturated fatty acid containing a double bond at the Omega-9 position (Akoh and Min, 2008). It is derived from a Latin word *eruca*, which signifies arucola/*Eruca sativa* (garden rocket), a flowering plant of the family of *Brasicaceae*. Erucic acid is the main constituent of rapeseed and mustard oils. Broccoli and Brussels sprouts also constitute

DOI: 10.1201/9781003178446-8 

about 40–50% of erucic acid. Besides their role in reducing several nutrients and minerals, they are reported to cause toxicity in humans when consumed in higher proportion in the diet. Consumption of erucic acid-rich foods has harmful effects on health (Abbott et al., 2003). Large amounts of this acid in the diet has been linked to heart disease such as myocardial lesions, accumulation of triacylglycerols in the heart (Bremer and Norum, 1982; Chow Ching, 2008). So, overcoming the health hazards of erucic acid is paramount and attention-grabbing. New breeds (*Brassica napus* and *Brassica rapa*) of rapeseed have been cultivated which contain low amounts of erucic acid, up to 2% by weight. Also, technological and traditional methods which involve soaking, germination debranning, roasting, fermentation, cooking, and milling have been employed for decreasing the antinutritional constituents in food products. Therefore, the key purpose of this chapter is to discuss the erucic acid, its health hazards, and also to evaluate the role of different processing methods to reduce its concentration.

## 8.2 CHEMISTRY OF ERUCIC ACID

Erucic acid is a non-branched, fatty acid which occurs naturally. It consists of 22 carbons with a cis-configurated double bond on the C-13 position. It is chemically known as cis-13-docosenoic acid (see Figure 8.1).

It is an unsaturated fatty acid with a lone *cis* double bond from the methyl end at an Omega-9 (ω-9) position. From carbon 20 atoms onwards it belongs to the sub-group known as very long-chain fatty acids (VLCFA). Oleic acid is the elongation product of erucic acid in animals. However, erucic acid present in food can be retro-converted to oleic acid having a molecular formula of $C_{22}H_{42}O_2$ and an IUPAC name of (Z)-docos-13-enoic acid. It is found in oils and seeds mostly as triglycerides which comprise a glycerol molecule where all the three OH, groups (hydroxyl groups) labelled as sn-1, sn-2, and sn-3 are esterified by fatty acids. The position of fatty acids on the glycerol backbone varies with respect to plant species (Belitz et al., 2009). In some plant species of seed oils containing erucic acid, the sn-2 site is not preferentially esterified with erucic acid, whereas in other species there is a balanced distribution of erucic acid at three sn sites of triacylglycerol molecule. For example, the amount of erucic acid is very low at the sn-2 site in rapeseed oil; however, in seed oil of *Tropaeolum majus* and *B. oleracea* there are equal amounts of erucic acid at the three sn sites

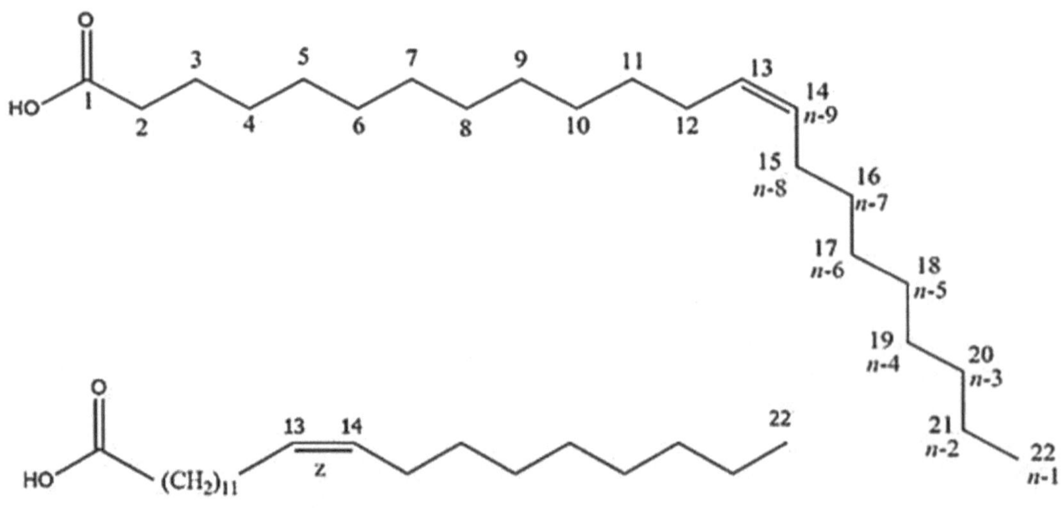

**Figure 8.1** The chemical structure of erucic acid.

(Taylor et al., 1994). These changes may affect the nutraceutical viewpoint. Also, the main factor of metabolic pathway which fatty acids will follow during digestion and absorption depends on the chain length and stereospecificity of fatty acids at the three sn sites (sn-1, sn-2, and sn-3) of triacylglycerols (Karupaiah and Sundram, 2007). Moreover, besides triacylglycerol, erucic acid is also present in fatty diacylglycerols, sterol esters, phospholipids, and glycolipids.

Erucic acid is a monounsaturated Omega-9 fatty acid, denoted by 22:1ω9, having a molecular weight of 338.57 g/mol and a chemical formula of $CH_3(CH_2)_7CH{=}CH(CH_2)_{11}COOH$. It has a boiling point of 265°C at 15 mm Hg and a melting point of 33.8°C with a density of 0.860 at 55°C/4°C (Lide, 2005; O'Neil, 2006). It is soluble in $CCl_4$-carbon tetrachloride, ethanol, and very soluble in ethyl ether and methyl alcohol (Lide, 2005).

## 8.3 DISTRIBUTION

Erucic acid is found in the seed oils of numerous *Brassicaceae*, such as mustard (*Brassica juncea* and *Brassica nigra*), rapeseed (*Brassica napus*), Brussels sprouts, seed oils (e.g., rapeseed oil), and wallflower as glycerol esters. Seeds from vegetable varieties such as kale, turnips, and cabbages, etc., contain erucic acid. The plant seeds of other members of the *Brassicaceae* family contain a high concentration of erucic acid, although mustard species and rapeseed contain a higher amount of erucic acid, commonly greater than 40% of the entire fatty acids in their natural form. However, new cultivars of rapeseed bred for human consumption have as low as 0.5% of erucic acid, but high erucic acid rapeseed (HEAR) cultivars which are composed of higher erucic acid are still cultivated for their use in the chemical industry. Nasturtium seeds (*Tropaeolum spp.*) of the family Tropaeolaceae also contain erucic acid up to 80% of the total fatty acids. Marine food sources/oils like fish contain a small amount of erucic acid. Food products prepared or processed using the oils/seeds containing erucic acid may also contain erucic acid depending on the content of oils/oil bearing seeds in it.

## 8.4 MECHANISM OF ACTION

Erucic acid is an unsaturated fatty acid with a lone double bond at the Omega-9 position (Akoh and Min 2008). The oil source (triacylglycerols) containing erucic acid on ingestion is digested by pancreatic lipases, resulting in the release of fatty acids (erucic and other fatty acids) and glycerol. The liberated fatty acids are absorbed by intestinal cells and reach circulation via lymph. The fatty acids are then distributed to tissues as they represent the fuel for skeletal and heart muscles. In the cells, the oxidation and breakdown of fatty acids mostly take place in the mitochondria. Initially, fatty acids are transported to the mitochondria, which is a transporter-dependent process using carnitine followed by its degradation that takes place by the release of acetyl coenzyme A (acetyl–CoA), which are two-carbon segments and the whole process is known as β-oxidation. An enzyme responsible for the β-oxidation system is either inhibited or has low activity. As a result, erucic acid is not oxidized by the mitochondrial β-oxidation system (Sauer and Kramer, 1980). On the other hand, Clouet et al. (1974) reported that heart mitochondria in humans break down erucic acid more slowly than oleic acid, which confirms that the proportion of erucic acid oxidation is very low in humans or similar to experimental animals. Furthermore, the β-oxidation rate of the other fatty acids decreases in the existence of erucic acid. As a result, lipids get accumulated in the heart, and to a minor amount in the liver, and heart tissue is not able to oxidize erucic acid properly.

However, in the liver, the perioxisomal β-oxidation system gets induced in the presence of erucic acid, resulting in a higher proportion of erucic acid oxidation compared to oleic and palmitic acid short-chain fatty acids, which gets metabolized by the mitochondrial β-oxidation system

(Thomassen et al., 1982). Also, concentration of erucic acid in liver tissue gets reduced with the initiation of the peroxisomal β-oxidation system, which is responsible for inhibiting the oxidation of other fatty acids.

## 8.5 TOXICOLOGICAL DATA

Erucic acid is an unsaturated fatty acid, which is digested, metabolized, and absorbed in a similar manner as fatty acids. As soon as fatty acids are absorbed they get dispersed to tissues. Also, fatty acids signify the main energy source of the skeletal and cardiac muscles. β-oxidation enzymes poorly use erucic acid as a substrate in the mitochondrial β-oxidation system. Similarly, the heart muscle is also poor at oxidizing erucic acid. Also, erucic acid seems to constrain an oxidation of fatty acid by the mitochondria. Further, in the liver, erucic acid acts to encourage peroxisomal β-oxidation system, causing delay in the erucic acid build-up and further decreases the inhibition of fatty acid oxidation. Also, some concentration of un-metabolized erucic acid can be found in the faeces. Erucic acid produces a toxic effect on human health, such as a higher prevalence of heart disease focal myocardial lesions. A literature survey has reported that a specific level of vegetable oils is responsible for myocardium lesions (Grice and Heggtveit, 1983). In another study, a survey in Calcutta was held where edible mustard oil contained erucic acid (40–44%), whereas in Madras, the main edible oils were sesame and peanut oil. In Calcutta and Madras, hearts were studied which detected substantial concentration of erucic acid in the myocardium (range of 0.9–9.9%) from Calcutta, whereas in Madras, no noticeable concentration of erucic acid in the myocardium was found, signifying consumption of dietary erucic acid is imitated in the levels of fatty acids in the myocardium (Grice and Heggtveit, 1983).

## 8.6 IDENTIFICATION AND QUANTIFICATION

Identification and quantification of erucic acid in plant materials/oils involves extraction of oil by mechanical means or by using suitable solvents like hexane or petroleum ether. If the lipids are to be extracted from animal tissues, solvent blends like chloroform-methanol (2:1v/v) may be used as the lipids are associated with other non-lipid moieties like proteins or carbohydrates. The extracted lipids are further purified and analyzed using suitable techniques. Various techniques can be used for quantification such as gas chromatography with flame ionization detection (GC-FID), infrared diffuse reflectance spectrometry, HPLC (high-performance liquid chromatography) with fluorescence detection at 350 nm (excitation) and 530 nm (emission), HPLC with ultraviolet detection at 242 nm, and Raman spectroscopy.

### 8.6.1 Gas Chromatography-Derived Methods

The best technique for quantification and identification of erucic acid (fatty acid profile) of fats and oils involves derivatization, and later separation and identification by gas chromatography (GC) (Wendlinger et al., 2014). Derivatization involves the transesterification of the COOH (carboxylic acid) group of fatty acids. In this process, triacylglycerol molecules are treated with an alcohol, mostly methanol, in the presence of a strong acid or base as catalyst. This results in the formation of a mixture of fatty acid methyl ester (FAMA) (using methanol), glycerol and mono- and di-glycerides.

The mixture is then injected into the capillary column of gas chromatograph with polar polyester coatings of low to medium polarity. FAME is separated in the column on the basis of their chain length, number of double bonds, position of double bond, and also the cis/trans-configuration of double bonds. Erucic acid identification is done by equating the retention time of the sample with the analytical standard. Flame ionization detectors (FID) are mostly used in fatty acid analysis (Dijkstra et al., 2007). Mass spectroscopic analysis is sometimes performed for confirmatory identification.

### 8.6.2 High-Performance Liquid Chromatography-Derived Methods

The high-performance liquid chromatography-derived method is also used in analysis for fatty acid, which usually recovers some portions of fatty acid aimed for further characterization. HPLC has an advantage over other techniques as it allows the decreased chance of isomerization of unsaturated fatty acids. The analysis can be done with or without derivatization of fatty acids, using an UV (ultraviolet-visible) photodiode array detector (Makahleh et al., 2010).

### 8.6.3 Nuclear Magnetic Resonance Spectroscopy

Nuclear magnetic resonance (NMR) spectroscopy is an influential technique to explain the structural properties of fatty acids. Both $^{1}H$- and $^{13}C$ NMR spectroscopy can be used to detect fatty acids including erucic acid (Dijkstra et al., 2007). Barison et al. (2010) reported NMR technique for analyzing fatty acid composition of oil. Kok et al. (2017) reported an analytical method for the estimation of erucic acid content in edible oils by quantitative $^{13}C$ NMR.

### 8.6.4 Attenuated Total Reflection Fourier-Transform Infrared Spectroscopy (FTIR)

FTIR is a secondary method designed for determining the fatty acid profile that needs standardization using laboratory data delivered by a primary technique, usually GC analysis (Kolackova et al., 2014). FTIR is less precise than the GC technique: it accumulates an estimation error to its own analytical error. However, the advantage lies in fast investigation without any kind of sample preparation.

## 8.7 SAFETY PRECAUTIONS AND REGULATIONS

Mustard and rapeseed contain erucic acid as an antinutritional factor and hence is undesirable for human consumption. A large amount of this acid has been linked to heart disease such as myocardial lesions, accumulation of triglycerides in the heart due to insufficient oxidation. It mostly enters the food chain once mustard or rapeseed oil is used in home cooking and the food processing industry. The European Food Safety Authority (EFSA) in 2016 proposed 2% erucic acid content in edible oils (instead of 5%) and also suggested a tolerable daily intake of 7 mg erucic acid per kg of body weight. For infant formulation, its limit was set five times lower than that for other food formulations. In 2020, the Food Safety and Standards Authority of India also regulated the maximum permissible erucic acid in mustard/rapeseed oil at 2% level. Food Standards Australia set an interim allowable daily consumption of 500 mg/day of erucic acid for adults. The intake of erucic acid by an individual at or below the maximum permissible daily intake limit is safe and no health risks are linked with it.

## 8.8 FUTURE SCOPE

Mustard, canola, rapeseed oil, fish/seafood are primary sources of erucic acid. Higher consumption of this acid has been linked to heart disease such as myocardial lesions, and the accumulation of triglycerides in the heart due to insufficient oxidation of this acid. Research findings related to effect of processing- like hydrogenation, heating (frying, cooking, etc.) on the content of erucic acid are not available. So, to fill this gap, research in this direction is needed. Interesterfication of oils rich in erucic acid is another possibility where erucic acid in the fat can be exchanged with other fatty acids. Genetic improvement of traditional cultivars for low erucic acid content and the replacement of traditional germplasm with the improved one will also benefit.

## 8.9 CONCLUSION

Erucic acid is an unsaturated fatty acid with a 18-carbon backbone. It is considered as an antinutritional agent in seeds and oils of the *brassica* family. Its consumption beyond prescribed daily limits may lead to accumulation of fat in the heart and myocardial lesions. Further research is needed to evaluate the effect of processing on erucic acid content of oils. Moreover, further genetic interventions need to be taken to bred cultivars which have low erucic acid content, especially in developing countries.

## REFERENCES

Abbott, P., Baines, J., Fox, P., Graf, L., Kelly, L., Stanley, G., and Tomaska, L. 2003. Review of the regulations for contaminants and natural toxicants. *Food Contamination* 14: 383–389.

Akoh, C.C. and Min, D.B. 2008. *Food Lipids: Chemistry, Nutrition, and Biotechnology*. 3th ed. CRC Press, Boca Raton, FL. P10

Barison, A., Pereira da Silva, C.W., Campos, F.R., Simonelli, F., Lenz, C.A., and Ferreira, A.G. 2010. A simple methodology for the determination of fatty acid composition in edible oils through H-1 NMR spectroscopy. *Magnetic Resonance in Chemistry* 48: 642–650.

Belitz, H.D., Grosch, W. and Schieberle, P. 2009 *Food Chemistry*. 4th Edition, Springer-Verlag, Berlin, p 654

Bremer, J. and Norum, K.R. 1982. Metabolism of the very long-chain monounsaturated fatty acids (22:1) and the adaption to the presence in the diet. *Journal of Lipid Research* 23: 243–256.

Chow Ching, K. 2008. *Fatty Acids in Foods and Their Health Implication*. 3th ed. CRC Press.

Clouet, P., Blond, J. & Bézard, J. 1974. *[Comparison of erucic and oleic acids oxidation by human heart mitochondria]. Comptes rendus hebdomadaires des séances de l'Académie des sciences*. Série D: Sciences naturelles. 279. 1003-6

Dijkstra, A.J., Christie, W.W., and Knothe, G. 2007. Analysis. In: *The Lipid Handbook* (Gunstone, F.D., Harwood, J.L., and Dijkstra, A.J., eds). 3rd ed. CRC Press, New York 1472.

Gemede, H. F and Ratta, N. 2014. Antinutritional factors in plant foods: Potential health benefits and adverse effects. *International Journal of Nutrition and Food Sciences* 3: 284–289.

Grice, H.C. and Heggtveit, H.A. 1983. The relevance of humans of myocardial lesions induced by rats by marine and rapeseed oils. In: *High and Low Erucic Acid Rapeseed Oils Production, Usage, Chemistry, and Toxicological Examination* (J. K. G. Kramer, F.D. and W.J. Pigden, eds). Academic Press, Toronto, Canada 551–562.

Karupaiah, T and Sundram, K. 2007. Effects of stereospecific positioning of fatty acids in triacylglycerol structures in native and randomized fats: a review of their nutritional implications. *Nutrition and Metabolism* 4: 16. Doi: 10.1186/1743-7075-1184-1116

Kok, W. M. 2017. Positional distribution of fatty acids in natural edible oils and structured lipids / Kok Wai Ming. Masters thesis, University of Malaya.

Kolackova, P, Ruzickova, G, Gregor, T and Sisperova E. 2014. Quick method (FT-NIR) for the determination of oil and major fatty acids content in whole achenes of milk thistle (Silybum marianum (L.) Gaertn.). *Journal of the Science of Food and Agriculture* 95: 2264–2270.

Lide, D.R. 2005. *CRC Handbook of Chemistry and Physics*. 86th Edition 2005-2006. CRC Press, Taylor & Francis, Boca Raton, FL 3–224.

Makahleh, A., Saad, B., Siang, G.H., Saleh, M.I., Osman, H., and Salleh B. Talanta. 2010. Determination of underivatized long chain fatty acids using RP-HPLC with capacitively coupled contactless conductivity detection. *National Library of Medicine* 81: 20–24.

O'Neil, M.J. (ed). 2006. *The Merck Index: An Encyclopedia of Chemicals, Drugs, and Biologicals.* Merck and Co., Inc, Whitehouse Station, NJ 629.

Reddy, N. R. and Pierson, M. D. 1994. Reduction in antinutritional and toxic components in plant foods by fermentation. *Food Research International* 27: 281–290.

Sauer, F. D. and Kramer, J. K. G. 1980. The metabolism of long-chain monoenoic fatty acids in heart muscle and their cardiopathogenic implications. In: Draper H (ed.). Advances in Nutritional Research. Springer, USA. p 207–230.

Taylor, D.C., Mackenzie, S.L., McCurdy, A.R., McVetty, P.B.E., Giblin, E.M., Pass, E.W. et al. 1994. Stereospecific analyses of seed triacylglycerols from high-erucic acid Brassicaceae: detection of erucic acid at the sn-2 position in Brassica oleracea L. genotypes. *Journal of the American Oil Chemists Society* 71: 163–167.

Thomassen, M.S., Christiansen, E.N., and Norum, K.R. 1982. Characterization of the stimulatory effect of high fat diet on peroxisomal b–oxidation in rat liver. *Journal of Biochemistry* 206: 195–202.

Wendlinger, C., Hammann, S., and Vetter, W. 2014.Various concentrations of erucic acid in mustard oil and mustard. *Food Chemistry* 153: 393–397.

# CHAPTER 9

# Saponins

**Usma Bashir, Nafia Qadir, and Idrees Ahmed Wani**

## CONTENTS



## 9.1 INTRODUCTION

Saponins are the secondary metabolites of a glycosidic nature with a characteristic foaming ability. They are particularly synthesized by plants, small aquatic fauna, and some microorganisms as a natural defence system (Riguera, 1997; Yoshiki et al., 1998). The word "saponin" has been derived from plant *Saponaria*, whose roots were utilised for developing soap in ancient times (Latin "*sapo*" means soap) (Augustin et al., 2011). Hence, the term saponin has been granted to this class of secondary metabolites due to their foaming ability upon agitation in aqueous medium. Chemically, saponins are glycosidic substances with high molecular weights, which have a glucan molecule associated with an aglucan moiety, termed as genin or sapogenin (Hostettmann and Marston, 2005). Saponins are divided into two groups: steroids and triterpenoid glycosides. The steroidal saponins are abundant in monocotyledonous plants of *Agavaceae*, *Liliaceae*, and *Discoreaceae* families. On the other hand, triterpenoid saponins are dominant in dicotyledonous plants of *Leguminosae*, *Araliaceae*, and *Caryophyllaceae* families, respectively (Sparg et al., 2004). The difference in functional and biological attributes of saponins is mainly due to the variation in their molecular structure. Such functional attributes of saponins are widely utilised both for traditional (manufacture of soap, fish poisons, etc.) and industrial purposes (Price et al., 1987; Oakenfull & Sidhu, 1989; Hostettmann & Martson, 1995). Saponins have versatile properties due to which they can either be beneficial or harmful for humans upon consumption. Saponins protect plants against attacks by microorganisms, herbivorous animals, pests, insects, molluscs, etc. (San Martin & Briones, 1999).

DOI: 10.1201/9781003178446-9

Saponins are the antinutritional entities in foods (Thompson, 1993). Some foods containing saponins are not used extensively due to the bitter taste developed after consumption (Ridout et al., 1991). From the past few decades, saponins from different sources have been extensively studied due to the revelation of several health benefits associated with their consumption, such hypocholesterolemia, anticarcinogenic properties, etc. (Gurfenkel & Rao, 2003; Kim et al., 2003). Saponins have been identified as active substances in herbal medicine (Alice et al., 1991, Liu & Henkel, 2002). They have been found to be responsible for health promoting properties of soyabeans (Oakenfull, 2001; Kerwin, 2004) and garlic (Matsuura, 2001). Re-designing of previous processing techniques (Muir et al., 2002) as well as development of new ones is going on for extraction of saponins from different sources because of their widespread applications (Rickert et al., 2004) (Figure 9.1).

## 9.2 CHEMISTRY

Saponin is an amphillic substance wherein a glucan molecule (pentose, hexose, or uronic acid) is associated with a hydrophobic moiety (sapogenin). The hydrophobic moiety of saponin is either a sterol or a triterpene (Kitagawa & Kobayashi, 1977). Sapogenin is further divided into neutral saponin and acid saponin. The neutral saponin is a derivative of sterol with spiroketal side chains that are abundant in monocotyledonous plants. On the other hand, acid saponin is composed of a triterpenoid structure and is found in dicotyledonous plants (Sparg et al., 2004).

Saponins have a polycyclic aglycone structure which can either be a choline steroid or a triterpenoid. The aglycone moiety consists of either one or several C-C linkages. In some saponins, an oligosaccharide chain exists at the C3 position (monodesmosidic), while in others an additional glucan moiety exists either at C26 or at C28 atom of aglycones (bidesmodic). The structural diversity of saponins exists mainly due to structural disparities in aglycone moiety, the form of side linkages and the functional groups associated with them (Francis et al., 2002). The ability of saponins to develop foam is due to the association of hydrophobic moiety with the hydrophilic side linkage (Morrissey & Osbourn, 1999). Both the sapogenins involve the same pathway and include the head

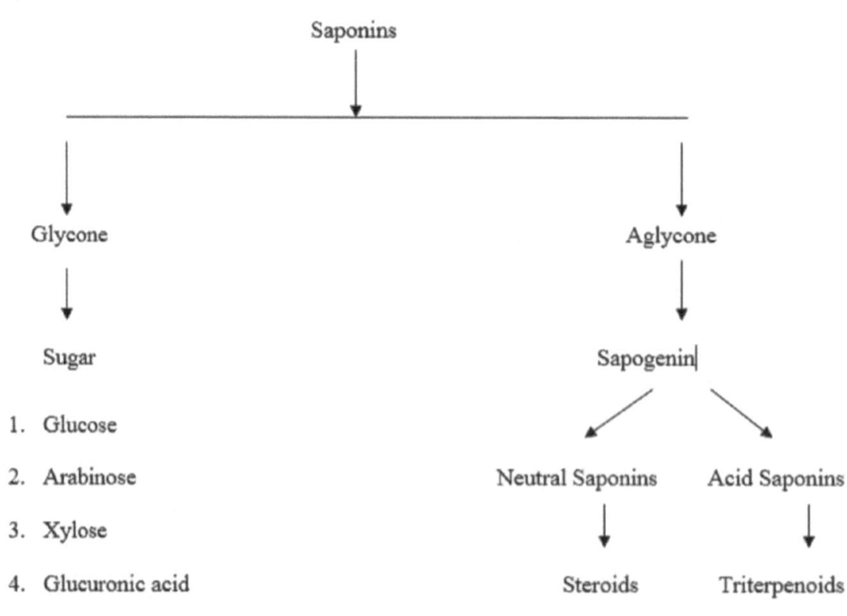


**Figure 9.1** Classification of saponins.

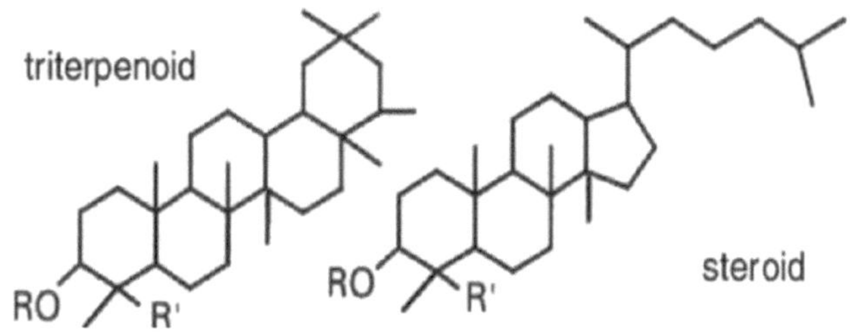


**Figure 9.2** Structure of saponins.

to tail coupling of acetate units. After the formation of triterpenoid hydrocarbon sequence, a branch is formed which takes the steroid in one direction and the cyclic terpenoids in the other direction (Misawa, 2011) (Figure 9.2).

## 9.3 DISTRIBUTION

Saponins are abundantly found in angiospermic plants of kingdom plantae. Saponins are distributed in several geographical zones around the world mainly in the form of herbs, shrubs, trees, etc., grown as wild and cultivated plants. They are grouped into two categories: triterpenoids and steroidal saponins (Vincken et al., 2007). Triterpenoid saponins are generally present in dicotyledonous crops like soyabean, pea, quinoa, tea seeds, etc. On the other hand, steroidal saponins exist in monocotyledenous plants and natural herbs (Nguyen et al., 2020). Each individual plant part differs in the amount of saponin present. For example, the quantity of saponin in cortex of yam tuber was about 2.55 times more than that of its flesh (Lin & Yang, 2008). Abundance of saponins in cereal grains and grasses is generally low, with the exception of oats, quinoa, etc. Both triterpenoid and steroidal saponins are found in oats (Osbourn, 2003). The active form of oat saponin (avenacin) is present in root portion while the inactive forms (avenacoside A and B) are abundant in the leaf and grain portion of the oat plant. Out of the gross saponin content of grain, nearly 60% is present as Avenacosides A. On the other hand, up to 55.2% and 49.0% of the total saponin content of grain and husk exists as Avenacosides B (Pecio et al., 2013). Triterpenoid saponins are also present in seeds of edible legumes such as soyabean, pea, beans etc. Triterpenoid saponins present in soyabean are of oleanen type where a $-CH_3$ group is present at C28 position and a glucuronic acid at C3 position (Berhow et al., 2002). Among legumes, kidney beans, butter beans, lentil and peas contain soya saponin I (Bb) whereas soya saponin βg is present in chickpeas (Serventi et al., 2013). The saponin content of soyabean and chickpeas ranges between 1.0–5.6 g/100 g on dry weight basis (Kerem et al., 2005). Monodesmoside saponins were reported in dry peas (Tsurumi et al., 1992). Saponin compounds have also been reported in quinoa where they mostly occupy the hull portion of seed. Until now, nearly 40 saponin compounds have been identified from *Chenopodium* seed (Hazzam et al., 2020). The seeds of wild *Chenopodium* varieties contain approximately 0.14–2.30% triterpenoids (Mastebroeket al., 2000). On commercial scale, saponins are obtained from *Quillaja saponeria* and *Yucaa schidigera* (Haralampidis et al., 2002). There are several plants in which saponin synthesis occurs in roots. In plants such as *Glycorrhiza glabra* (liquorice), *Panax ginseng* (ginseng), and *Polygala tenuifolia*, synthesis of saponins-glycyrrhizin (*G. glabra*), ginsenosoides (*P.ginseng*), and senegenin-derived saponins (*P. tenuifolia*) takes place in root and or rhizome of the plant (Park et al., 2005; Seki et al., 2008; Teng et al., 2009). Approximately 40 saponins have been identified from *Panax ginseng*, broadly classified into three categories: protopanaxadiol, protopanaxatriol, and oleanolic acid (Yu et al., 2009; Cheng et al., 2008). Glycyrrhizin saponin is present in liquorice in large amounts. Out of the total saponins in liquorice, 83% is composed of glycyrrhizin whose concentration varies between 19–70 mg/g (Tao et al., 2013). Saponins in tea plant are mainly triterpenoids of oleanolic acid and pentacyclic nature (Guo et al., 2018). Saponin compounds have also been identified from fruits and vegetables such as tomato, onion, bitter gourd, etc., α-tomatine, a saponin, occupies up to 500 mg/Kg of unripe tomato fruit (Friedman, 2002). Several saponin compounds ( > 100) have been identified and characterized from the bitter gourd plant, some of those which occupy the fruit portion are momordicoside I, momordicoside F2 and momordicoside F1 (Wang et al., 2008). In addition to this, alfalfa, which is a forage legume from the *Fabaceae* family, has been reported to be rich in triterpenoid compounds (Massiot et al., 1988). Steroidal saponins have been reported in herbs such as asparagus, fenugreek, etc. The root portion of asparagus is rich in steroidal saponins. Saponin compounds in asparagus are collectively termed as shatavarins (Asmari et al., 2004). On the other hand, a steroidal saponin called dioscin has been reported in fenugreek seed. Fenugreek is grown in Asia and North Africa where it is used as one of the essential spices in foods (Chaudary et al., 2018).

## 9.4 BASIC STRUCTURES OF SAPOGENINS

Saponin synthesis in plants takes place through the isoprenoid pathway. This pathway involves a sequential series of enzymatic reactions for the production of several compounds. Both terpenoids and steroidal saponins are synthesized from a precursor, squalene which is a 30 carbon intermediate. Squalene in turn is synthesized from the mevalonate and non-mevalonate [2-C-methyl-D-erythritol-4-phosphate (MEP)] pathways. These pathways proceed through a series of enzymatic reactions involving different enzymes at each step: geranyl diphosphate synthase (GDS), squalene synthase, etc. (Misawa, 2011). After the synthesis of squalene, an enzyme called squalene epioxidase converts it to 2,3-oxidosqualene. 2,3-oxidosqualene (OSCs) undergoes cyclization and produces tetracyclic sterols by cycloartenol formation (CS). Furthermore, during the phytosterol pathway downstream cycloartenol formation, steroidal saponins are thought to be formed as intermediates (Vincken et al., 2007). Triterpene steroid formation separates from phytosterol pathway by an apparent cyclization of 2,3-oxisqualene by the activity of an enzyme such as β-amyrin synthase (βAS), α-amyrin synthase (αAS), lupeol synthase (LuS), dammarenediol synthase (DDS) (Haralampidis et al., 2002; Vincken et al., 2007). The existence of hydrophobic aglycone and hydrophilic glucan moieties in the basic structure is responsible for the amphillic nature of saponin. The amphillic nature makes them potent surfactants with good wettability, and results in their emulsifying and foaming properties (Ibanoglu & Ibanoglu, 2000; Sarnthein-Graf & La Mesa, 2004; Wang et al., 2005).

## 9.5 TOXICOLOGY AND ITS MECHANISM OF ACTION

Toxicological testing is essential for understanding either threshold toxicity limits or safety of new compounds. In spite of several therapeutic effects of saponins on humans, their toxicological studies are very important because of their diverse distribution. Polygalae radix (PR), a plant of family *Polygalaceae* is distributed in north Asian nations and has been used for improving intellectual ability since ancient times (Jiang et al., 2016). But saponin compounds isolated from this herb have been known to induce gastrointestinal toxicity in animals (Guan et al., 2012). In a study, raw sample (R) and isolated saponins (IS) of PR were administered to mice for acute toxicity tests and it was observed that R and IS samples had $LD_{50}$ of 15.31 g/Kg and 212 mg/Kg, respectively in subjects. Further, a study led by Guan et al. (2012) investigated the toxicity of alcoholic extracts of PR products and noticed that with increase in concentration of saponins, the toxicity effect increased. The reason behind toxicity of GI tract of mice by R and IS samples might have been associated with the attack of saponins on GI cells of Cajal (Jin et al., 2014). The intestinal cells of Cajal are useful for regulating gastrointestinal motility.

In another study, Al-Ashban et al. (2010) observed that upon administration of alcoholic extracts of fenugreek (100 mg/Kg bw/day) to mice for 3 months, sperm abnormality developed. The same conclusion was drawn after treatment of mice with 305 and 610 mg/Kg bw/day doses of fenugreek seed (Al-Yahya, 2013). It was observed that high doses of fenugreek seed resulted in low sperm count and highly abnormal sperms that ultimately were responsible for sterility in mice. Another investigation was performed to study the safety of a standardized saponin-rich extract of fenugreek seed. Acute (2,500 mg/Kg bw for 2 weeks) and sub chronic (250–1,000 mg/Kg bw for 3 months) investigations were carried out on Wistar rats. It was observed that no toxicological effect was observed in rats treated with saponin-rich extract of fenugreek. Even the highest dose receiving rats had no harmful effects on their health. On the basis of this study, no observed adverse effect (NOAEL) of the extract was set at 1,000 mg/Kg bw/day (Sureshkumar et al., 2018). In spite of the toxicity of fenugreek extracts detected in past experiments, the reason for forgetting contrary results in this study might have been due to the presence of other phytochemical compounds in the extract that would have overshadowed the harmful effects of saponins.

Glycyrrhizin is a highly abundant saponin present in liquorice root (6-10%). The gut microbiota have the ability to dissociate it into an aglycone molecule (glycyrrhetinic acid) and a glucan sub-unit, both of which are absorbed (Hatori et al., 1983). Administration of liquorice in high concentrations is associated with development of hypertension in individuals. The harmful effect of liquorice is mainly because of the effect of glycyrrhetinic acid. Regular consumption of liquorice root (greater than 3g/day for > 6 weeks) or glycyrrhizin (greater than 100 mg/day) results in retention of $Na^+$ and water in the body, causing high blood pressure (Nazari et al., 2017). People suffering from high blood pressure are more prone to this effect because of their high sensitivity to the inhibition of 11-β-hydroxysteroid-dehydrogenase by glycyrrhenitic acid (Tanahashi et al., 2002). 11-β–hydroxysteroid-dehydrogenase is an enzyme that plays an important role in regulation of blood pressure.

In another study, rats were administered with saponins from tea seeds for 90 days. The NOAEL and the lowest observed adverse effect level (LOAEL) were observed to be 50 mg/Kg/day and 150 mg/Kg/day, irrespective of sexes (Kwaguchi et al., 1994). In another study, mice were orally administered with *Camellia sasanqua* seed saponins for acute and sub-chronic toxicity testing. The NOAEL for acute toxicity studies was found to be 125 mg/Kg bw. For sub-chronic toxicity testing, mice were administered with tea seed saponins at 100–400 mg/Kg bw for 6 weeks. Mice that were administered with the highest dose had severe abdominal swelling and died during experimentation (Yoshikawa et al., 1996).

*Yucca schidigera* is an arid plant that grows in south-west parts of USA and Mexico. This plant finds its applications in food, feed, pharmaceutical and cosmetic industries. Glycosides of sarsasapogenin and smilagenin are the predominant saponin substances in *Yucca shidigera* (Cheeke, 1998). Juice of this plant was administered at doses of 1.5 g and 3.0 g/Kg live weight to 30 lambs for 21 days. Twelve lambs died during experimentation while fifteen were killed towards the completion of study and histological examination of their body tissues was carried out. Kidney and liver of dosed animals were found to contain saponins. Death of lambs might have happened because of saponins in administered juice. The reason for saponin toxicity of organs might have happened due to alteration in activity of gut microbiota that might have prevented hydrolysis of saponins, promoting their direct absorption (Wisloff et al., 2008).

In another study, rats of both sexes were treated with four doses (1.0, 2.15, 4.64, and 10 g/Kg bw) of saponins isolated from *Chenopodium* husk. After experimentation, it was observed that the median lethal dose of *Chenopodium* saponins was higher than 10 g/Kg. However, when they were forcibly given a saponin-rich diet, the animals suffered from stomach irritation. It was concluded that saponin administration could be the reason for stomach irritation in rats (Lin et al., 2021). Absorption of saponins in the intestine is very low and they accumulate there for longer time periods. The gut microbiota is able to convert small amount of saponins into sapogenin, which is acidic and causes intestinal irritation (Strauss-Grabo et al., 2011) (Figure 9.3).

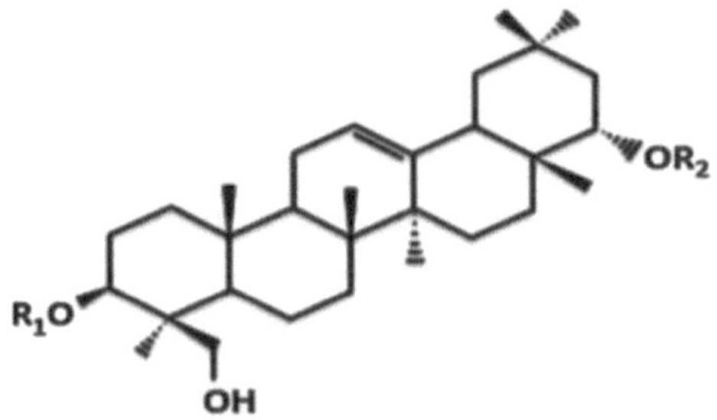

Structure 1: $R_1$=$R_2$=H
Structure 2: $R_1$= α-Rha-1→ 2-β-Gal-1→2-β-GlcA; $R_2$=H
Structure 3: $R_1$= α-Rha-1→ 2-β-Gal-1→2-β-GlcA; $R_2$=α-Glc

**Figure 9.3** Structure of purified GTS isolated from *Pisumsativum*.

## 9.6 IDENTIFICATION AND QUANTIFICATION

Qualitative identification of saponins involves taking plant sample (1–2 g) in a test tube and adding water to it. This is followed by vigorous shaking of tube contents for 2 min. Development of stable foam after shaking confirms presence of saponins in the sample (Ncube et al., 2011). However, quantification of saponins is generally done by spectrophotometric and chromatographic techniques. Spectrophotometric technique provides information about the quantity of saponin in given sample while as the chromatographic technique provides information about both the quantity as well as the type of saponin present.

*Spectrophotometric method*: The most extensively used method for spectrophotometric quantification of plant saponins is the Vanillin-sulfuric acid assay. However, quantification of saponins by this method should be done only after thorough understanding of certain factors such as choice of standard, wavelength, etc. This method is based on the reaction between the oxidized triterpene saponins and vanillin (Li et al., 2010). Generally, triterpenoid saponins are oxidised with the help of $H_2SO_4$, which results in development of purple colour (Hiai et al., 1976). But per chloric acid can also be used as an oxidising agent (Chen et al., 2007; Li et al., 2010). Total steroidal sapogenin is estimated by taking 40 μg of the crude extract in a test tube and adding 2 mL of ethyl acetate to it for dissolution. Then, the contents of the tube are treated with reagent A (0.5 mL of anisaldehyde and 99.5 mL of ethyl acetate) and 1 mL of reagent C (50 mL of conc. $H_2SO_4$ and 50 mL of ethyl acetate). The contents of the tube are incubated at 60°C in water bath for 10 min for appropriate colour development. The test tube is taken out from the water bath and cooled to ambient conditions before measurement of absorbance at 430 nm with a spectrophotometer.

Another spectrophotometric method used for quantification of plant saponins is the hemolytic method (Barve et al., 2010). This method is based on the reaction between saponin compounds and a blood reagent which releases oxy-haemoglobin, producing a remarkable colour for spectrophotometric quantification. This method has been applied for quantification of saponins from several varieties of bitter gourd. Saponin content of bitter gourd varieties came to be low (0.25 %) after quantification by hemolytic method (Habicht et al., 2011). In this method, the saponin-rich extract is mixed with distilled water. Then, 100 μL of aliquot is taken and reacted with 1 mL of fresh EDTA- blood at 30°C. Reaction mixture is centrifuged for 10 min and supernatant is collected. The concentration of haemoglobin in the supernatant is quantified at 545 nm with a spectrophotometer.

*Chromatographic method*: Saponins are first extracted for their estimation by chromatography. Several researchers have used chromatographic techniques for identification and quantification of saponins (Adao et al., 2011; Liu et al., 2012). The most common chromatographic methods used for quantification and identification of saponins are HPLC – High Performance Liquid chromatography (Bi et al., 2012; He et al., 2012; Liu et al., 2012; Mostafa et al., 2013) and TLC – Thin Layer

Chromatography (Adão et al., 2011; Liu et al., 2012; Patel et al., 2012). Besides these techniques, UPLC – Ultra pressure liquid chromatography (Foubert et al., 2010; Verza et al., 2012; Serventi et al., 2013;Ha et al., 2014) is also in used to quantify saponins.

## 9.7 EFFECT OF PROCESSING

Foods are subjected to different processing techniques to reduce the amount of saponins. The presence of saponin compounds in the seed coat of *Chenopodium* reduces its commercial applicability (Chauhan et al., 1992). The traditional processing method used for the isolation of saponin compounds from quinoa seeds is washing them in running water. But the main drawbacks of this method are the requirement of water in abundance and pollution of water bodies (Ruales, 1998). To prevent contamination of water bodies, several other methods are practised for removal of saponins from quinoa seeds. One such method involves removal of saponins by physical abrasion of seed. A study based on the effect of physical abrasion of quinoa seed at two polishing degrees (20 and 30%) was investigated (Gomez-Caravaca et al., 2014). From the study, it was observed that saponin content of polished (20%) quinoa seeds reduced to 129.8 mg/100 g d.w. which was 50% higher than the saponins in unpolished seeds (244.3 mg/100 g d.w.). Moreover, higher polishing degree (30%) led to further reduction in saponin concentration (50.88 mg/100 g d.w.). After a couple of years, another investigation was carried out to check the impact of polishing level on saponin content of quinoa seeds. Upon successive increase in milling (8.45%, 15.89%, 21.17%, and 27.37%), the saponin content of polished seeds reduced by 12.9%, 36.7%, 39.9%, and 41.8%, respectively (Han et al., 2019).

Another method for the removal of saponins from food grains and legumes is sprouting. Sprouting is a processing technique that improves the bioactive profile, vitamins, mineral content, etc., of seeds with simultaneous loss of antinutritional factors (Lemmens et al., 2019). Sprouting of quinoa seeds was carried out for evaluating the impact of sprouting on quinoa saponins. The quinoa seeds were immersed in water for 12, 24, 48, and 72 h at 22°C and dried at 55°C for 6 h. Mass spectroscopic analysis of sprouted samples revealed that with progress in sprouting time (12–72 h), the saponin content of sprouted seeds reduced from 0.4–0.05 g/100 g (Suarez-Estrella et al., 2021).

Another processing technique that lowers saponin content of foods is steaming. Le et al. (2015) studied the effect of steaming (105°C and 120°C for 2–20 h) on saponin concentration in Vietnamese ginseng. From the study, it was concluded that increase in temperature from 105–120°C resulted in a three-fold reduction in ginsenoside content of ginseng. Another processing technique to lower saponin content of foods is the application of microwaves. An investigation by Zhong et al. (2015) studied the effect of microwave treatment on saponin content of black soyabean. It was observed that application of microwave treatment to black soyabean resulted in a 22% reduction in its saponin content. The reduction in saponin content of black soyabean after application of microwaves might have been due to heat-induced structural modifications (Badifu, 2001). Another investigation studied the effect of three treatments – soaking, cooking, and pressure cooking on sapogenol contents of kidney beans. There was 6.2% and 9.1% reduction in sapogenol A and B contents of beans after soaking. More pronounced reduction in sapogenol A was observed after cooking of beans. However, pressure cooking of pre-soaked beans resulted in 90.1% reduction in sapogenol B content of beans. Complete removal of sapogenol B was observed after pressure cooking of beans (Vasishtha & Srivastava, 2014). In another study, the effects of heat treatment on saponin content of alcoholic extracts of bitter gourd were evaluated. Heating of bitter gourd extracts was performed in a water bath at 30, 60, and 100°C for 5, 10, and 20 min. Autoclaving of control samples were performed at 121°C for 20 min. It was concluded from the study that alcoholic extracts of bitter gourd heated at 100°C for 20 min had the lowest saponin content among the heat treated samples. Similarly, high reduction in saponin content was observed in autoclaved samples (Liu et al., 2020). Application of processing techniques – boiling and steaming – on amount of saponins in quinoa seeds was evaluated. From the study, it was observed that the boiling process was more effective in lowering saponin content (0.06%) of quinoa seeds than that of the steaming process (0.2%). Higher loss of saponins after boiling of quinoa seeds might have been because of the release of saponin compounds into boiling water (Hostettmann & Marston, 2005). However, there was no direct contact between seeds and water during steaming and soluble saponins leached slowly from seeds. Hence, removal of saponin compounds from the seeds was limited (Mhada et al., 2020).

In another study, five types of processing treatments – washing, washing plus hydration, cooking (with or without pressure), and toasting – on amount of saponins in quinoa seeds were investigated (Nickel et al., 2016). By washing, saponin concentration of seeds decreased. It might have happened because of the leaching of saponin in water due to the presence of hydrophilic moiety in its structure which makes it water-soluble. There was not much difference in the saponin contents of quinoa seeds cooked at ambient conditions, under pressure and toasting. On the other hand, combined treatments of washing plus hydration resulted in further reduction in amount of saponins. Hydration treatment might have allowed quick penetration of water into the seeds, facilitating greater release of saponin compounds by diffusion (Vega-Galvez et al., 2010). Oat saponins (Avenacosides A and B) were given two heat treatments (100°C and 140°C) under different pH conditions (4–7). It was observed that heat treatment of 100°C at varying pH (4–7) for 3 h was insufficient to degrade the saponins. On the other hand, high heat treatment caused degradation of saponin compounds as the pH increased from 4–6 (Onning et al., 1994).

## 9.8 FUTURE SCOPE

In ancient times, saponin was thought to be an antinutritional substance due to its toxicological effects. Saponins include a large group of substances that are mistakenly known as toxins, although few of them are toxic. In the middle of the twentieth century, the use of saponins started to decline due to their harmful effects on livestock (Lindahl et al., 1957). But later on, new studies described the positive role of saponins on mankind. Saponin compounds were found to lower serum cholesterol levels (Oakenfull and Sidhu, 1990; Carroll and Kurowska, 1995), boost immune system (Kenarova et al., 1990; Wu et al., 1990), and provide protection against carcinogens (Kikuchi et al., 1991; Tokuda et al., 1991). It was discovered that saponins helped in boosting immune response of mammals, because of which they could be considered as vaccine adjuvants (Sun et al., 2009). Saponin compounds activate Thl immune response and produce the cytotoxic T-lymphocytes (CTLs) against antigens, making them potent vaccine candidates. Saponins have hypo-cholesterolemic effect as, after consumption, these metabolites associate with bile acids and form mixed micelles which promote excretion, improve cholesterol metabolism in liver and cause reduction in serum cholesterol levels (Oakenfull, 1986). Saponins from different sources should be extensively studied to derive maximum benefit from this class of secondary metabolites.

## 9.9 CONCLUSION

Saponins are the secondary metabolites having widespread distribution in the plant kingdom. From ancient times, saponin-rich plants have been widely used as herbs because of their health-promoting properties. Therefore, it is important to study this class of phytochemicals so as to understand the mechanism of action behind their therapeutic properties. Further research is required in this area to identify the toxicity thresholds of saponin compounds and side effects associated with long-term consumption of such substances. Each processing technique cannot be completely effective in reducing saponins in food matrix. However, the application of combined processing treatments has proven to be successful in lowering the amount of saponins in foods. It would be better to develop and optimise new processing techniques so as to keep saponin concentration below its threshold toxicity limit. Moreover, for reduction of saponins in foods, researchers should focus on selection of such processing conditions that would not lead to depletion of other constituents of the food matrix.

## REFERENCES


Adão, C. R., da Silva, B. P. and Parente, J. P. (2011). A new steroidal saponin with anti inflammatory and anti-ulcerogenic properties from the bulbs of *Allium ampeloprasum* var. *porrum*. *Fitoterapia* 82: 1175–1180.

Al-Ashban, R. M., Barrett, D. A. and Shah, A. H. (2010). Toxicity studies on *Trigonella foenumgraecum L.* seeds used in spices and as a traditional remedy for diabetes. *Oriental Pharmacy & ExperimentalMedicine* 10: 66–78.

Alice, C. B., Vargas, V. M. F., Silva, G. A. A. B., de Siqueira, N. C. S., Schapoval, E. E. S., Gleye, J., Henriques, J. A. P. and Henriques, A. T. (1991). Screening of plants used in south Brazilian folk medicine. *Journal of Ethnopharmacology* 35: 165–171.

Al-Yahya, A. A. (2013). Reproductive, cytological and biochemical toxicity of fenugreek in male Swiss albino mice. *African Journal of Pharmacy & Pharmacology* 7: 2072–2080.

Asmari, S., Zafar, R. and Ahmad, S. (2004). Production of sarsasapogenin from tissue culture of *A. racemosus* and its quantification by HPTLC. *Iranian Journal of Pharmaceutical Research* 2: 66–67.

Augustin, J. M., Kusina, V., Anderson, S. B. and Bak, S. (2011). Molecular activities, biosynthesis and evolution of triterpenoid saponins. *Phytochemistry* 72: 435–457.

Badifu, G. I. O. (2001). Effect of processing on proximate composition, antinutritional and toxic contents of kernels from Cucurbitaceae species grown in Nigeria. *Journal of Food Composition & Analysis* 14: 153–61.

Barve, K. H., Laddha, K. S. and Jayakumar, B. (2010). Extraction of saponins from Safed Musli. *Pharmacognosy Journal* 2: 561–564.

Berhow, M. A., Cantrell, C. L., Duval, S. M., Dobbins, T. A., Maynes, J. and Vaughn, S. F. (2002). Analysis and quantitative determination of group B saponins in processed soybean products. *Phytochemical Analysis* 13: 343–8.

Bi, L., Tian, X., Dou, F., Hong, L., Tang, H. and Wang, S. (2012). New antioxidant andantiglycation active triterpenoid saponins from the root bark of *Aralia taibaiensis*. *Fitoterapia* 83: 234–240.

Carroll, K. K. and Kurowska, E. M. (1995). Soy consumption and cholesterol reduction: Review of animal and human studies. *Journal of Nutrition* 125(Supplement): 594–597.

Chaudhary, S. A., Chaudhary, P. S., Syed, B. A., Misra, R., Bagali, P. G., Vitalini, S., et al. (2018). Validation of a method for diosgenin extraction from fenugreek (*Trigonella foenum-graecum* L.). *Acta Scientiarum Polonorum Technologia Alimentaria* 17: 377–385.

Chauhan, S., Eskin, N. A. M. and Tkachuk, R. (1992). Nutrients and antinutrients in quinoa seeds. *Cereal Chemistry*, 69: 85–88.

Cheeke, P. R. (1998). Toxins intrinsic to forages. In: Cheeke, P. R. (Ed.), *Natural Toxicants in Feed, Forages and Poisonous Plants*. Interstate Publishers, Danville, pp. 275–324.

Chen, J., Li, W., Yang, B., Guo, X., Lee, F. S. C. and Wang, X. (2007). Determination of four major saponins in the seeds of *Aesculus chinensis* Bunge using accelerated solvent extraction followed by high-performance liquid chromatography and electrospray-time of flight mass spectrometry. *Analytica Chimica Acta* 596: 273–280.

Cheng, L. Q., Na, J. R., Bang, M. H., Kim, M. K. and Yang, D. C. (2008).Conversion of major ginsenoside Rb1 to 20(S)-ginsenosideRg3 by microbacterium sp. GS514. *Phytochemistry* 69: 218–224.

El Hazzam, K., Hafsa, J., Sobeh, M., Mhada, M., Taourirte, M., et al. (2020). An insight into saponins from quinoa (*Chenopodium quinoa* Willd.): A review. *Molecules* 25: 1059. doi: 10.3390/molecules25051059.

Foubert, K., Cuyckens, F., Vleeschouwer, K., Theunis, M., Vlietinck, A., Pieters, L., et al. (2010). Rapid quantification of 14 saponins of *Maesa lanceolata* by UPLC–MS/MS. *Talanta* 81: 1258–1263.

Francis G., Kerem, Z., Makkar, H. P. S. and Becker, K. (2002). Thebiological action of saponins in animalsystems. *British Journal of Nutrition* 88: 587–605.

Friedman, M. (2002). Tomato glycoalkaloids: roles in the plant and in the diet. *Journal of Agricultural and Food Chemistry* 50:5751–5780.

Gómez-Caravaca, A., Iafelice, G., Verardo, V., Marconi, E. and Caboni, M. F. (2014). Influence of pearling process on phenolic and saponin content in quinoa(*Chenopodium quinoa*Willd.). *Food Chemistry* 157: 174–178.

Guan, S. J., Yan, X. P. and Lin, J. K. (2012). Study on acute toxicity test of different processed products of *Radix Polygalae. Chinese Journal of Integrated Traditional & Western Medicine* 32: 398–401.

Guo, N., Tong, T., Ren, N., Tu, Y. and Li, B. (2018). Saponins fromseeds of genus Camellia: Phytochemistry and bioactivity. *Phytochemistry* 149: 42–55.

Gurfinkel, D. M. and Rao, A. V. (2003). Soyasaponins: The relationship betweenchemical structure and colon anticarcinogenic activity. *Nutrition & Cancer* 47: 24–33.

Ha, T. J., Lee, B. W., Park, K. H., Jeong, S. H., Kim, H. T., Ko, J. M., et al. (2014). Rapid characterisationand comparison of saponin profiles in the seeds of Korean Leguminousspecies using ultra performance liquid chromatography with photodiode array detectorand electrospray ionisation/mass spectrometry (UPLC–PDA–ESI/MS) analysis. *Food Chemistry* 146: 270–277.

Habicht, S. D., Kind, V., Rudloff, S., Borsch, C., Mueller, A. S., Pallauf, J., et al. (2011). Quantificationof anti-diabetic extracts and compounds in bitter gourd varieties. *Food Chemistry* 126: 172–176.

Han, Y., Chia, J., Zhang, M., Zhang, R., Fan, S., Dong, L., et al. (2019). Changes in saponins, phenolics and antioxidant activity of quinoa(*Chenopodium quinoa* willd) during milling process. *LWT: Food Science and Technology* 114: 108381.

Haralampidis, K., Trojanowska, M., Osbourn, A. E. (2002). Biosynthesisof triterpenoid saponin in plants. *Advances in Biochemical Engineering/Biotechnology* 75: 31–49.

Hattori, M., Sakamoto, T., Kobashi, K. et al. (1983). Metabolism of glycyrrhizin by human intestinal flora. *Planta Medica* 48: 38–42.

He, H., Xu, J., Xu, Y., Zhang, C., Wang, H., He, Y., et al. (2012). Cardioprotective effects of saponinsfrom *Panax japonicas* on acute myocardial ischemia against oxidativestress-triggered damage and cardiac cell death in rats. *Journal of Ethnopharmacology* 140: 73–82.

Hiai, S., Oura, H. and Hakajima, T. (1976). Colour reaction of some sapogenins and saponinswith vanillin and sulphuric acid. *Planta Medica* 29: 116–122.

Hostettmann, K. A. and Marston, A. (1995). *Saponins: Chemistry and Pharmacology of Natural Products.* Cambridge University Press, Cambridge, UK.

Hostettmann, K. and Marston, A. (2005). *Saponins.* Cambridge University Press, Cambridge, UK.

Ibanoglu, E. and Ibanoglu, S. (2000). Foaming behavior of liquorice (*Glycyrrhizaglabra*) extract. *Food Chemistry* 70: 333–336.

Jiang, H. J., Liu, T., Li, L., Zhao, Y., Pei, L. and Zhao, J. C. (2016). Predicting the potential distribution of *Polygala tenuifolia*Willd. under climate change in China. *PLoS One* 11:e0163718

Jin, Z. L., Gao, N., Zhang, J. R., Li, X. R., Chen, H. X., Xiong, J., Li, Y. F. and Tang, Y. (2014). The discovery of Yuanzhi-1, atriterpenoid saponin derived from the traditional Chinese medicine, has antidepressant-like activity. *Progress in Neuro-Psychopharmacology & Biological Psychiatry* 53: 9–14.

Kawaguchi, M., Kato, T., Kamada, S. and Yahata, A. (1994). Three-month oral repeatedadministration toxicity study of seed saponins of *Thea sinensis* L. (Ryokucha saponin) in rats. *Food & Chemical Toxicology* 32: 431–442.

Kenarova, B., Neychev, H., Hadjiivanova, C. and Petkov, V. D. (1990). Immunomodulatingactivity of ginsenoside Rg1 from *Panax ginseng. Japanese Journal of Pharmacology* 54: 447–454.

Kerem, Z., German-Shashoua, H. and Yarden, O. (2005). Microwave assisted extraction of bioactive saponins from chickpea (*Cicer arietinum* L.). *Journal of the Science of Food & Agriculture* 85: 406–412.

Kerwin, S. M. (2004). Soy saponins and the anticancer effects of soybeans andsoy-based foods. *Current Medicinal Chemistry: Anti-Cancer Agents* 4: 263–272.

Kikuchi, Y., Sasa, H., Kita, T., Hirata, J. and Tode, T. (1991). Inhibition of humanovarian cancer cell proliferation in vitro by ginsenoside Rh2 andadjuvant effects to cisplatin in vivo. *Anti-Cancer Drugs* 2: 63–67.

Kim, S. W., Park, S. K., Kang, S. I., Kang, H. C., Oh, H. J., Bae, C. Y. and Bae, D. H. (2003). Hypocholesterolemic property of *Yucca schidigera* and *Quillajasaponaria* extracts in human body. *Archives of Pharmacal Research* 26: 1042–1046.

Kitagawa, I. and Kobayashi M. (1977). On the structure of the major saponin from *Acanthaster planci. Tetrahedron Letters* 2:859–862.

Le, T. H. V., Lee, S. Y., Lee, G. J., Nguyen, N. K., Park, J. H. and Nguyen, M. D. (2015). Effects of steaming on saponin compositions and antiproliferativeactivity of Vietnamese ginseng. *Journal of Ginseng Research* http://dx.doi.org/10.1016/j.jgr.2015.01.006

Lemmens, E., Moroni, A. V., Pagand, J., Heirbaut, P., Ritala, A., Karlen, Y., et al. (2019). Impact of cereal seed sprouting on its nutritional and technological properties: A critical review. *Comprehensive Reviews in Food Science and Food Safety* 18: 305–328.

Li, J., Zu, Y. G., Fu, Y. J., Yang, Y. C., Li, S. M., Li, Z. N., et al. (2010). Optimization ofmicrowave-assisted extraction of triterpene saponins fromdefatted residue of yellowhorn (*Xanthoceras sorbifolia* Bunge.) kernel and evaluation of its antioxidant activity. *Innovative Food Science and Emerging Technologies* 11: 637–643.

Lin, B., Qi, X., Fang, L., Zhao, L., et al. (2021). *In vivo* acute toxicity and mutagenic analysis of crude saponins from *Chenopodium quinoa* Willd husks. *RSC Advance* 11: 4829.

Lin, J. T. and Yang, D. J. (2008). Determination of steroidal saponins in different organs of yam (*Dioscorea pseudojaponica* Yamamoto). *Food Chemistry* 108: 1068–1074.

Lindahl, I. L., Shalkop, W. T., Whitmore, G. E., Davis, R. E. and Tertell, R. T. (1957). Toxicity of saponins when administered to ruminants. *Technical Bulletin US Department of Agriculture* 1161: 53–60.

Liu, J. and Henkel, T. (2002). Traditional Chinese Medicine (TCM): Are polyphenolsand saponins the key ingredients triggering biological activities? *Current Medicinal Chemistry* 9: 1483–1485.

Liu, Y., Lai, Y., Wang, R., Lo, Y. and Chiu, C. (2020). The effect of thermal processing on the saponin profiles of *Momordica charantia* L. *Journal of Food Quality* 2020. https://doi.org/10.1155/2020/8862020

Liu, Y. W., Zhu, X., Lu, Q., Wang, J. Y., Li, W., Wei, Y. Q. and Yin, X. X. (2012). Total saponins from Rhizoma Anemarrhenae ameliorate diabetes-associated cognitive decline in rats: involvement of amyloid-beta decrease in brain. *Journal of Ethnopharmacology* 139(1):194–200.

Massiot, G., Lavaud, C., Guillaume, D. and Le Men-Olivier, L. (1988). Re-investigation of thesapogenins and prosapogenins from alfalfa (*Medicago sativa*). *Journal of Agricultural & Food Chemistry* 36: 902–909.

Mastebroek, H. D., Limburg, H., Gilles, T. and Marvin, H. J. (2000). Occurrence of sapogenins in leavesand seeds of quinoa (*Chenopodium quinoa* Willd). *Journal of the Science of Food & Agriculture* 80: 152–6.

Matsuura, H. (2001). Saponins in garlic as modifiers of the risk of cardiovascular disease. *Journal of Nutrition* 131: 1000S–1005S.

Mhada, M., Metougui, M. L., El Hazzam, K., El Kacimi, K. and Abdelaziz Yasri, A. (2020).Variations of saponins, minerals and total phenolic compounds due to processing and cooking of quinoa (*Chenopodium quinoa* Willd.) seeds. *Foods* 9. doi:10.3390/foods9050660

Misawa, N. (2011). Pathway engineering for functional isoprenoids. *Current Opinion in Biotechnology* 22: 627–633.

Morrissey, J. P. and Osbourn, A. E. (1999). Fungal resistance to plant antibiotics as a mechanism of pathogenesis. *Microbiological & Molecular Biological Reviews* 63: 708–724.

Mostafa, A., Sudisha, J., El-Sayed, M., Ito, S. I., Yamauchi, N., Shigyo, M., et al. (2013). Aginoside saponin, a potent antifungal compound, and secondary metabolite analysesfrom *Allium nigrum* L. *Phytochemistry* 6: 274–280.

Muir, A. D., Paton, D., Ballantyne, K. and Aubin, A. A. (2002). Process for recoveryand purification of saponins and sapogenins from quinoa (*Chenopodiumquinoa*). US Patent 6,355,249.

Nazari, S., Rameshrad, M. and Hosseinzadeh, H. (2017). Toxicological effects of *Glycyrrhiza glabra* (liquorice): A review. *Phytotherapy Research* 31: 1635–1650.

Ncube, B., Ngunge, V. N. P., Finnie, J. F. and Staden, J. V. (2011). A comparative study of theantimicrobial and phytochemical properties between outdoor grown andmicropropagated *Tulbaghia violacea* Harv. plants. *Journal of Ethnopharmacology* 134: 775–780.

Nguyen, L. T., Fărcas, A. C., Socaci, S. A., Tofană, M., Diaconeasa, Z. M., et al. (2020). An overview of saponins: A bioactive group. *Bulletin UASVM Food Science and Technology* 77: 25–36.

Nickel, J., Spanier, L. P., Botelho, F. B., Gularte, M. A. and Helbig, E. (2016). Effect of different types of processing on the total phenolic compoundcontent, antioxidant capacity, and saponin content of *Chenopodiumquinoa* Willd grains. *Food Chemistry* 209: 139–143.

Oakenfull, D. (2001). Soy protein, saponins and plasma cholesterol. *Journal of Nutrition* 131: 2971.

Oakenfull, D. and Sidhu, G. S. (1989). Saponins. In: Cheeke, P. R., Ed., *Toxicants of Plant Origin, Vol II Glycosides*. CRC Pres, Inc., Boca Raton, FL, pp. 97–141.

Oakenfull, D. and Sidhu, G. S. (1990). Could saponins be a useful treatment forhypercholesterolemia? *European Journal of Clinical Nutrition* 44: 79–88.

Oakenfull, D. G. (1986). Aggregation of bile acidsand saponins in aqueous solution. *Australian Journal of Chemistry* 39: 1671–1683.

Onning, G., Juillerat, M. A., Fay, L. and Asp, N. G. (1994). Degradation ofoat saponins during heat processing-Effect of pH, stainless steel, and iron atdifferent temperatures. *Journal of Agricultural & Food Chemistry* 42: 2578–2582.

Osbourn, A. E. (2003). Saponins in cereals. *Phytochemistry* 62: 1–4.

Park, J. D., Rhee, D. K. and Lee, Y. H. (2005). Biological activities and chemistryof saponins from Panax ginseng C. A. Meyer. *Phytochemistry Reviews* 4: 159–175.

Patel, P. K., Patel, M. A., Vyas, B. A., Shah, D. R. and Gandhi, T. R. (2012). Antiurolithiatic activityof saponin rich fraction from the fruits of *Solanum xanthocarpum* Schrad. &Wendl. (Solanaceae) against ethylene glycol induced urolithiasis in rats. *Journal of Ethnopharmacology* 144: 160–170.

Pecio, L., Wawrzyniak-Szolkowska, A., Oleszek, W. and Stochmal, A. (2013). Rapid analysisof avenacosides in grain and husks of oats by UPLC-TQ-MS. *Food Chemistry* 141: 2300–2304.

Price, K. R., Johnson, I. T. and Fenwick, G. R. (1987). The chemistry and biologicalsignificance of saponins in food and feeding stuffs. *CriticalReviews in Food Science & Nutrition* 26: 27–135.

Rickert, D. A., Meyer, M. A., Hu, J. and Murphy, P. A. (2004). Effect of extractionpH and temperature on isoflavone and saponin partitioning and profile duringsoy protein isolate production. *Journal of Food Science* 69: C623–C630.

Ridout, C. L., Price, K. R., DuPont, M. S., Parker, M. L. and Fenwick, G. R. (1991). Quinoa saponins: Analysis and preliminary investigations into theeffects of reduction by processing. *Journal of the Science of Food & Agriculture* 54: 165–176.

Riguera, R. (1997). Isolating bioactive compounds from marine organisms. *Journal of Marine Biotechnology* 5: 187–193.

Ruales, J. (1998). *Increasing the Utilisation of Sorghum, Buckwheat, Grain Amaranth Andquinoa for Improve Nutrition.* Institute of Food Research, Norwich, UK.

San Martin, R. and Briones, R. (1999). Industrial uses and sustainable supply ofQuillaja saponaria (Rosaceae) saponins. *Economic Botany* 53: 302–311.

Sarnthein-Graf, C. and La Mesa, C. (2004). Association of saponins in water andwater-gelatine mixtures. *Thermochimica Acta* 418: 79–84.

Seki, H., Ohyama, K., Sawai, S, et al. (2008). Liquorice beta-amyrin 11-oxidase, a cytochrome P450 with a key role in the biosynthesis of thetriterpene sweetener glycyrrhizin. *Proceedings of the National Academy of Sciences USA* 105: 14204–14209.

Serventi. L., Chitchumroonchokchai, C., Riedl, K. M., Kerem, Z., Berhow, M. A. and Vodovotz, Y. (2013). Saponins from soy and chickpea: Stability during beadmaking and in vitro bioaccessibility. *Journal of Agricultural & Food Chemistry* 61: 6703–6710.

Sparg, S. G., Light, M. E. and Van Staden, J. (2004). Biological activities and distribution of plant saponins. *Journal of Ethnopharmacology* 94: 219–243.

Strauss-Grabo, M., Atiye, S., Warnke, A., Wedemeyer, R. S., Donath, F., and Blume, H. H. (2011). Observational study on tolerability and safety of film coated tablets containing ivy extract (Prospa Cough Tablets) in the treatment of colds accompanied by coughing. *Phtyomedicine* 18: 433–436.

Suárez Estrella, D., Borgonovo, G., Buratti, S., Ferranti, P., et al. (2021). Sprouting of quinoa (*Chenopodium quinoa* Willd.): Effect on saponin content and relation to the taste and astringency assessed by electronic tongue. *LWT-Food Science & Technology* 144: 111234.

Sun, H. X., Xie, Y. and Ye, Y. (2009). Advances in saponin-based adjuvants. *Vaccine* 27: 1787–1796.

Sureshkumar, D., Begum, S., Johannah, N. M., Maliakel, B. and Krishnakumar, I. M. (2018). Toxicological evaluation of a saponin-rich standardized extractof fenugreek seeds (FenuSMART*TM*): Acute, subchronic and genotoxicity studies. *Toxicology Reports*, 5: 1060–1068 https://doi.org/10.1016/j.toxrep.2018.10.008

Tanahashi, T., Mune, T., Morita, H., et al. (2002). Glycyrrhizic acid suppresses type 2 11 beta-hydroxysteroid dehydrogenase expression in vivo. *Journal of Steroid Biochemistry & Molecular Biology* 80: 441–447.

Tao, W., Duan, J., Zhao, R., et al. (2013). Comparison of three officinal Chinese pharmacopoeia species of *Glycyrrhiza* based on separation and quantification of triterpene saponins andchemometrics analysis. *Food Chemistry* 141: 1681–1689.

Teng, H. M., Fang, M. F., Cai, X. and Hu, Z. H. (2009). Localization and dynamic change of saponin in vegetative organs of *Polygala tenuifolia*. *Journal of Integrative Plant Biology* 51: 529–536.

Thompson, L. U. (1993). Potential health benefits and problems associated withantinutrients in foods. *Food Research International* 26: 131–149.

Tokuda, H., Konoshima, T., Kozuka, M. and Kimura, T. (1991). Inhibition of 12-O-tetradecanoyl phorbol-13-acetate–promoted mouse skin papilomaby saponins. *Oncology* 48: 77–88.

Tsurumi, S., Takagi, T. and Hashimotoq, T. (1992). A gamma pyronyl triterpenoid saponin from *Pisum sativum*. *Phytochemistry* 31: 2435–2438.

Vasishtha, H. and Srivastava, R. P. (2014). Processing effect on saponins of rajmash beans (*Phaseolus vulgaris*). *Current Advances in Agricultural Sciences* 6: 28–30.

Vega-Gálvez, A., MartÍn, R. S., Sanders, M., Miranda, M. and Lara, E. (2010). Characteristics and mathematical modeling of convective drying of quinoa *Chenopodium* quinoa Willd.): Influence of temperature on the kineticparameters. *Journal of Food Processing and Preservation* 34: 945–963.

Verza, S. G., Silveira, F., Cibulski, S., Kaiser, S., Ferreira, F., Gosmann, G., et al. (2012). Immunoadjuvant activity, toxicity assays, and determination by UPLC/Q-TOF-MS oftriterpenic saponins from *Chenopodium quinoa* seeds. *Journal of Agricultural & Food Chemistry* 60: 3113–3118.

Vincken, J. P., Heng, L., de Groot, A. and Gruppen, H. (2007). Saponins,classification and occurrence in the plant kingdom. *Phytochemistry* 68: 275–297.

Wang, Y. H., Avula, B., Liu, Y. and Khan, I. A. (2008). Determinationand quantitation of five cucurbitane triterpenoids in*Momordica charantia* by reversed-phase high-performanceliquid chromatography with evaporative light scattering detection. *Journal of Chromatographic Science* 46: 133–136.

Wang, Z. W., Gu, M. Y. and Li, G. Z. (2005). Surface properties of gleditsiasaponin and synergisms of its binary system. *Journal of Dispersion Science & Technology* 26: 341–347.

Wisloff, H., Uhlig, S., Scheie, E., Loader, J., Wilkins, A. and Flaoyen, A. (2008). Toxicity testing of saponin-containing *Yucca schidigera* Roetzl.juice in relation to hepato- and nephrotoxicity of *Narthecium ossifragum* (L.) Huds. *Toxicon* 51: 140–150.

Wu, J., Lin, L. and Chau, L. (2001). Ultrasound-assisted extraction of ginseng saponinsfrom ginseng roots and cultured ginseng cells. *Ultrasonics Sonochemistry* 8: 347–352

Wu, R. T., Chaing, H. C., Fu, W. C., Chein, K. Y. and Chung, Y. M. (1990). Formosanin-C, an immunomodulator with antitumor activity. *International Journal ofImmunopharmacology* 12: 777–786.

Yoshikawa, M., Murakami, T., Yoshizumi, S., Murakami, N., Yamahara, J. and Matsuda, H. (1996). Bioactive saponins and glycosides. V. acylated polyhydroxyolean-12-enetriterpene oligoglycosides, camelliasaponins A1, A2, B1, B2, C1 and C2, fromthe seeds of Camellia japonica L.: Structures and inhibitory activity on alcoholabsorption. *Chemical Pharmacology Bulletin* 44: 1899–1907.

Yoshiki Y., Kudou S. and Okubo K. (1998). Relationship between chemicalstructures and biological activities of triterpenoid saponins from soybean. *Bioscience Biotechnology & Biochemistry* 62: 2291–2299.

Yu, H., Liu, Q., Zhang, C., Lu, M., Fu, Y., et al. (2009). Anew ginsenosidase from Aspergillus strain hydrolyzing 20-Omulti-glycoside of PPD ginsenoside. *Process Biochemistry* 44: 772–775.

Zhong, Y., Wang, Z. and Zhao, Y. (2015). Impact of radio frequency, microwaving, and high hydrostatic pressure at elevated temperature on the nutritional and antinutritional components in black soybeans. *Journal of Food Science* 80: C2732–C2739.

CHAPTER 10

# Cyanogenic Glycosides

**Nadira Anjum, Mohd Aaqib Sheikh, Charanjiv Singh Saini, Fozia Hameed, Harish Kumar Sharma, and Anju Bhat**

## CONTENTS



## 10.1 INTRODUCTION

Plant toxins are naturally occurring secondary metabolites that are widely distributed among the species of the plant kingdom such as fruits and vegetables. Many plants protect themselves against predators, including herbivores, insects, pathogens etc., by employing an extraordinary array of defensive chemical compounds (toxic compounds) to deter them (Yulvianti and Zidorn, 2021). One such protection system of plants is the ability to synthesize cyanogenic glycosides: a chemical weapon that has the potential to generate toxic hydrogen cyanide. Currently, more than 2,650 plant

DOI: 10.1201/9781003178446-10

species are known to contain cyanogenic glycosides, of which a number of species are used as food substances in different parts of the world (Bolarinwa et al., 2014). Cyanogenic glycosides are an important and widespread class of anti-nutrients which are classified as phyto-anticipins. They are water-soluble, heat-stable secondary metabolites, structurally less diverse than classes of natural products and related to bitterness (Yulvianti and Zidorn, 2021). So far, more than 112 naturally occurring cyanogenic glycosides have been reported in the phyto-chemical literature. The major cyanogenic glycosides are found in the edible parts of plants including cassava, bamboo shoots, coco yam, sorghum, chick peas, linseeds, lime beans, flaxseeds, bitter almonds, apples, quinces peach, pear, apricots, plums, particularly in the seeds of such fruits. They are often located in plant vacuoles and the amount of cyanogenic glycosides in plants is usually related to the quantity of releasable hydrogen cyanide (Goverde et al., 2008). They are stable bioactive compounds, but when chewed, digested, or enzymically hydrolyzed, they release hydrogen cyanide, which can be potentially poisonous to the consumers. Some of these plants are commonly consumed as food and may pose potential risks to consumers (animals or humans). Cyanogenesis is the ability of some plant species to biosynthesize and accumulate cyanogenic glycosides via a common biosynthetic process. Depending upon a variety of environment conditions, plants contain different levels of cyanogenic glycosides (Gonzalez-Garcia et al., 2014). The plant species that contains cyanogenic glycosides also has a corresponding hydrolytic enzyme (β-glucosidase). Cyanogenic glycosides are not toxic when intact, but they become toxic when enzymes (endogenous or exogenous, such as β-glycosidase and α-hydroxynitrilelyases) come into contact with them, producing hydrogen cyanide, which causes tissue damage after bruising or chewing (Goverde et al., 2008). They are a unique class of amino acid-derived metabolites featuring a nitrile moiety, which upon enzymatic hydrolysis releases hydrocyanic acid. Upon the disruption of plant tissues due to maceration or in presence of water, cyanogenic glycosides are degraded or hydrolyzed by the catabolic intracellular enzyme β–glucosidase into a benzaldehyde or ketone compound, a glucose molecule, and a cyanohydrin compound which quickly decompose to the toxic hydrogen cyanide. The potential toxicity for animals consuming edible parts containing cyanogenic glycosides depends primarily on certain factors, including potential of plant species to produce hydrogen cyanide, size of animal, percentage of β-glucosidases, length of time between tissue disruption and ingestion, and the presence and nature of other components in the meal.

In humans, cyanogenic glycosides have been categorized as having both adverse and health-promoting benefits. For example, consumption of cyanogenic seeds can be potentially dangerous because can undergo hydrolysis to produce hydrogen cyanide and cause sub-acute cyanide poisoning with symptoms including anxiety, headaches, dizziness, and confusion (Shi et al., 2019). Health-promoting benefits of cyanogenic glycosides have been well-documented over the years, including anti-fibrosis, anti-inflammation analgesia, auxiliary anticancer, immune-regulation, anti-atherosclerosis; they also have the potential to treat neurodegenerative diseases (He, et al., 2020). To be specific, the lower doses have been shown to reduce the risks of degenerative diseases, proved to be beneficial for health, while the higher dose is responsible for deleterious effects, such as cyanide poisoning-like symptoms, including headache, nausea, vomiting, and dizziness (Shi et al., 2019). Depending upon the chemical structure, different cyanogenic compounds release different amounts of hydrogen cyanide, such as amygdalin release 59 mg HCN/g cyanogenic compound (EFSA CONTAM Panel, 2019). The maximum limits for HCN of 50 mg/kg have been established by Commission Regulation (EU) (2017/123712) for nougat, marzipan, or its substitutes, or 5 mg/kg in canned stone fruits and of 35 mg/kg in alcoholic beverages (EFSA CONTAM Panel, 2019). Despite having unique medicinal properties like anti-cancer, anti-asthmatic, anti-neoplastic, and analgesic effects (Saleem et al., 2018), utilization of edible parts of plants containing cyanogenic glycosides for human nutrition requires adequate detoxification to attain the reduction under the allowed limits as set by the European Commission Regulation (EU) (2017/ 123712).

## 10.2 DISTRIBUTION

Cyanogenic glycosides are widely distributed among the species of the plant kingdom, whereas in animals they are mainly restricted to arthropods and Lepidoptera, more common in moths and butterflies (Zagrobelny and Moller, 2011). In plantae, they are commonly present in one of the oldest terrestrial plants (known as ferns), as well as in angiosperms and gymnosperms (Moller, 2010). Cyanogenic glycosides present in angiosperms contain aromatic or aliphatic amino acids, whereas cyanogenic glycosides in gymnosperms are derived from aromatic amino acids only (Zagrobelny et al., 2008). Around 2,500–3,000 different plant species which belong to more than 100 families of flowering plants have been reported to contain cyanogenic glycosides, thus representing almost 10–12% of the cultivated plant species tested. Humans have been cultivating the cyanogenic plants in the course of history either due to their resistance against herbivores or because of the need to process the plants before consumption makes them less attractive to trespassers (Gleadow and Moller, 2014). Among the 112 cyanogenic glycosides reported to the present date, Linamarin and lotaustralin are the most common cyanogenic glycosides found in the families of higher plants, including Linaceae, Papilionaceae, Euphorbiaceae, and Papaveraceae (Zagrobelny et al., 2008). Another cyanogenic glycoside, namely prunasin, which was recently included in the list has been reported to be widespread in the families of Rosaceae, Myrtaceae, Myoporaceae, Polypodiaceae, Scrophulariaceae, and Saxifragaceae. Similarly, sambunigrin – a cyanogenic glycoside somehow similar in structure to prunasin – is only found in the families of Caprifoliaceae, Oleaceae, and Mimosaceae, vicianin is restricted to the Papilionaceae and Polypodiaceae families, whereas amygdalin is solely present in the Rosaceae family. On the other hand, dhurrin is the only cyanogenic glycoside occurring in the family of Gramineae (Francisco and Pinotti, 2000).

## 10.3 CHEMISTRY

Cyanogenic glycosides identified so far consist of mainly three parts, an aglycone, a sugar moiety, and a nitrile group (Figure 10.1). The basic structure of cyanogenic glycosides is shown in Figure 10.1. Due to the presence of this nitrile moiety, cyanogenic glycosides are also termed as α-hydroxynitrile glycosides. Enzymatic hydrolysis of this nitrile moiety present in any natural product results in the production of hydrogen cyanide or prussic acid (Yulvianti and Zidorn, 2021). The nitrile group is either linked to aromatic or aliphatic, cyclic or heterocyclic amino acids, which include valine, tyrosine, leucine, isoleucine, phenylalanine, as well as some nonproteinogenic amino acids such as 2-(2′-hydroxy-3′-cyclopentenyl)-glycine and 2-(2′-cyclopentenyl)-glycine (Gleadow and Moller, 2014). These amino acids are mainly responsible for biosynthesis of the aglycone part of cyanogenic glycosides. Hydroxylations (single or multiple) of the amino acids present in the cyanogenic glycosides, particularly those derived from leucine and isoleucine, also define their core

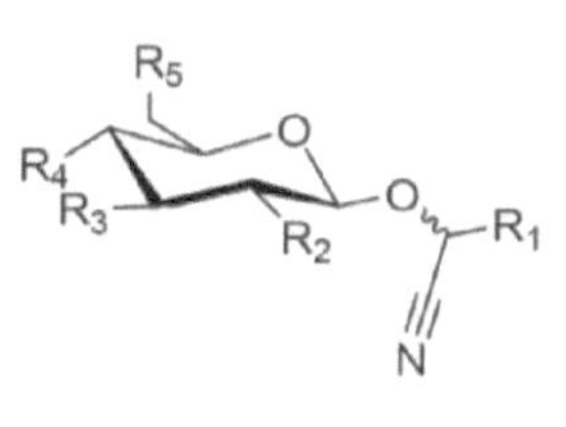


**Figure 10.1** Basic structure of cyanogenic glycoside, where $R_1$ represents the aglycone group, $R_2$, $R_3$, $R_4$, and $R_5$ represent the positions of substituents connected to the glucose moiety, and N represents the nitrile moiety.

structure (Nielsen et al., 2002). Some research studies have also reported that the hydroxylation process resulted in the breakage of aromatic amino acids as observed during the biosynthesis of triglochinin (Nielsen and Moller, 1999).

The sugar moiety is usually made of monoglycosides, in particular glucose; however, some compounds have also been reported to contain di and triglycosides, e.g., apiose, arabinose, allose, rhamnose, and xylose (Miller et al., 2006). Structurally, the sugar moiety is linked to the aglycone group with help of an oxygen molecule which in turn is connected to the α-carbon atom of the nitrile moiety. When the plant tissue containing cyanogenic glycosides gets damaged by any means, enzymes, particularly β–glucosidases present in the plants, act upon the cyanogenic glycosides and hydrolyze their structure (Yulvianti and Zidorn, 2021). Hydrolysis can also result from dilute acids or bases. After splitting off the aglycone from the sugar moiety because of the enzymatic degradation of β-glycosidic bond, the aglycone moiety is further hydrolyzed, either in vitro or by the action of enzyme, namely (s)-hydroxynitrilelyase, therefore producing hydrogen cyanide. This process is known as cyanogenesis (Yulvianti and Zidorn, 2021).

## 10.4 MECHANISM OF ACTION

Cynogenic biosynthesis is catalyzed by multi-enzyme complex and is derived from L-amino acids. Dhurrin biosynthesis was seen in microsomal membrane preparation. During the initial steps of biosynthesis, hydroxylation of L-amino acids occurs by the enzyme L-amino acid N-monooxygenase. The N-hydroxyl S-L- amino acid is converted to an aldoxime upon oxidative decarboxylation. The aldoxime thus formed is converted to a nitrile by the action of enzyme aldoximedehydratase. Nitrile monooxygenase hydroxylates the nitrile at $C_2$-position to produce an intermediate 2-hydroxy nitrile (or cyanohydrins). Further, lucosyltransferase acts on an activated glucose, i.e., UDP-glucose, to yield 3-glucoside. In many cases herbivores or other organisms cause an injury to plants, which results in breakdown of the cellular compartmentation. This breakdown causes the cyanogenic glycosides to come in contact with an active /5-glucosidase, which gets further hydrolyzed in order to yield 2-hydroxynitrile (cyanohydrin). The cyanohydrin thus formed forms an aldehyde or ketone and hydrogen cyanide by the action of enzyme hydroxynitrilelyase. In case of cyanolipids, enzyme esterase causes the hydrolysis of fatty acids to 2-hydroxynitrile which further yields aldehyde and hydrogen cyanide (Nielsen and Møller, 1999). The hydrogen cyanide is considered toxic for both humans and microorganisms. The dosage of hydrogen cyanide considered lethal for humans is 1.52 mg/kg after oral application. Death of humans as well as animals has been reported by the consumption of plants which contained about 500 mg HCN/100 g seeds (Wittstock and Gershenzon, 2002). Foods such as manihot (Cassava esculenta) have been known to contain cyanogenic glycosides. Consumption of manihot has resulted in intoxications as well as deaths in humans and animals. A number of herbivores have been found to tolerate hydrogen cyanide. Animals cause rapid detoxification of some amounts of cyanogenic glycosides by rhodanese. Besides the formation of cyanogenic glycosides in cytoplasm, their storage occurs in the central vacuole. Storage of these toxic substances in sorghum leaves is tissue-specific and thus takes place in epidermal vacuoles. Due to the polar nature of cyanogenic glycosides they do not diffuse through the biological membranes by the process of simple diffusion and thus the transfer of such compounds from cytoplasm to the vacuole is carrier-mediated. The cyanogenic glycosides as such, or the aldehydes and ketones produced from their hydrolysis, are considered as feeding deterrents. These compounds are active and potent chemical defence compounds.

## 10.5 TOXICOLOGY OF CYANOGENIC GLYCOSIDES

The plants containing cyanogenic glycosides upon consumption result in a number of diseases in humans as well as animals. About 2,500 species of plants are known to contain cyanogenic glycosides and these plants belong to families like Leguminoseae, Rosaceae, Gramineae, Poaceae, Araceae, Euphorbiaceae, Compositeae, and Passifloraceae. Cyanogenic glycosides are actually the secondary metabolites of plants. The process by which plants as well as other living organisms produce hydrogen cyanide from the hydrolysis of cyanogenic glycosides is called as cyanogenesis. About 25 cyanogenic glycosides have been reported to be present in the plants. The ability of a cyanogenic glycoside to produce hydrogen cyanide determines its toxicity. The presence of cyanogenic glycosides in diet causes a number of chronic diseases in humans (Monago and Akhidue, 2002). Improperly processed cassava has resulted in diseases like tropical ataxic neuropathy (TAN) disease, and konzo (Mlingi et al., 1992). Toxicity of plants containing cyanogenic glycosides is determined by their ability to produce hydrogen cyanide in concentrations lethal to the human body. During maceration or processing of the cyanogenic plants, the conversion of cyanogenic compounds to hydrogen cyanide is triggered. The unconsumed cyanogenic compounds get broken down in the intestinal tract to release hydrogen cyanide which is considered as the major reason for cyanide toxicity in humans (Rosling, 1994). Cellular enzymes can detoxify low amounts of cyanogenic compounds. Thiosulphates present in some plant tissues convert hydrogen cyanide to thiocyanate which is relatively a harmless compound (Salkowski and Penney, 1994). Hydrogen cyanide affects central nervous system, endocrine, respiratory, and cardiovascular system in humans, and the symptoms of cyanide poisoning are a decrease in blood pressure, headache, vomiting, diarrhoea etc., the poisoning in severe cases may lead to coma and death of the individual. Various reports have shown that consumption of cassava containing about 10–50 mg/kg cyanogenic glycosides causes swelling of thyroid glands (Wink, 1988).

## 10.6 IDENTIFICATION AND QUANTIFICATION OF CYANOGENIC GLYCOSIDES

About 75 cyanogenic glycosides have been identified in plants including those used as a food for humans like lima beans, tapioca, sorghum, and few foods from the assifloraceae family. So far various methods have been developed to identify and quantify the cyanogenic glycosides. The major techniques used are discussed below:

### 10.6.1 Pyridine-Barbituric Acid Colorimetry

In this method the sample is first hydrolyzed with the help of an acid, after hydrolysis of the sample distillation is carried out and the liberated hydrogen cyanide is quantified. The sample (5–30 g) is first suspended in water (200 ml). To the mixture of about 10% tartaric acid and 10% lead acetate are added in 1:1 ratio. After addition of antifoam A (0.1 ml), about 20 ml of 1 N sulphuric acid is added to the mixture. The mixture is heated properly for a specific period of time. After heating, distillation is carried out to remove the hydrogen cyanide from the mixture. Distillates thus formed are first trapped in primary receiver (30 ml of 0.25 N NaOH) and finally in secondary receiver, i.e., 1030 ml of 0.25 N NaOH (Winkler, 1958). The distillate obtained is transferred to the test tubes to which about 1.5 ml of 1 N acetic acid-NCS reagent is added (1:1) At last the barbituric acid reagent (1ml) is also added to the distillate. The tubes are allowed to stand for a period of 10 minutes after stirring properly. Absorbance of the mixture is then taken at580 nm against a standard using a spectrophotometer (Honig et al., 1983).

### 10.6.2 Feigl-Anger or Sodium Picrate Paper

These methods of cyanogen determination doesn't require any equipment and are considered as simple as well as reliable. For preparation of sodium picrate paper, a filter paper is dipped into an aqueous solution of 0.5% picric acid and 5% $Na_2CO_3$ for a specific time. The filter paper is then dried but it should be moistened prior to use. This type of paper is used in situations where water is present and has a detection limit of 0.001–0.002% HCN by weight. For preparation of Feigl-Anger paper, pieces of filter paper are dipped in a solution made by combining equal amount of tetrabase and copper ethylacetoacetate solutions (1% prepared in $CHCl_3$). Drying of the paper strips is then done in fume hood. This type of paper is more sensitive than sodium picrate paper and is the most common type of paper used for cyanide determination. Fresh sample is crushed in a vial or test tube. In case the sample is dry a few drops of liquid or a buffer of pH 6.8 are added to the sample. The paper used for cyanide determination is then suspended over the sample present; the vial and the change in colour of paper will indicate the presence of hydrogen cyanide in the sample. In case of picrate paper, the colour changes from yellow to orange or red, while in case of Feigl-Anger paper the colour change occurs from pale blue green to bright blue or purple (Brinker and Seigler, 1989).

### 10.6.3 Use of Ion Selective Cyanide Electrodes

This technique for cyanide determination is simple and is based on the use of ion selective electrodes (ISE). The ion selective electrode used for direct determination of cyanides generally involves the use of a membrane made of $Ag/Ag_2S$- or Ag/AgI. The membrane remains in contact with the electrode and the principle for detection actually is based on the potentiometric Nernstian selectivity of the membrane. This method has the drawback of being functional only in highly alkaline medium (Jovanovic et al., 1987).

### 10.6.4 Use of Biosensoric System

A biosensoric system involving the use of ammonia electrode as well as a cyanide catalyzing enzyme (cyanidase). It is considered as an effective analytical method for determination of cyanides as compared to the ion selective cyanide electrodes. The enzymes catalyse hydrogen cyanide into ammonium and formiate (Ipatov et al., 2002). The sensor for detection of cyanogenic compounds is usually based on a pH-sensitive electrolyte/insulator/semiconductor-structure (EIS). Selection of a suitable hydrogen cyanide catalyzing enzyme is a prerequisite for development of such sensors. For determination of cyanides, extracts prepared from plant materials are used. This technique is usually based on two steps. First step involves conversion of cyanogenic compounds into hydrogen cyanide by the action of plant enzymes upon disintegration of plant tissues. The second step involves action of cyanidase on hydrogen cyanide, which produces ammonia and formiate and that ammonia is detected with the help of an electrode (Sandstrom et al., 2000).

### 10.6.5 Micellar Capillary Electrophoresis

The use of capillary electrophoresis has given good results in detection of saccharides and other secondary metabolites present in plants, but an attempt to use Micellar capillary electrophoresis in determination of cyanogenic glycosides in apple and peach seeds was made by Campa et al. (2000). Two cyanogenic compounds (amygdalin and prunasin) were identified along with their isomeres (neoamygdalin and sambunigrin). The extraction of samples was done using aqueous methanol in an ultrasonic bath, the samples after filtration were concentrated using a rotary vacuum evaporator. The samples before use were dissolved in 0.5 ml distilled water. It was observed that use of Micellar capillary electrophoresis (MCEK) with UV detection at 214 nm provided promising results in separation of relevant cyanogenic compounds. The anionic micelles (SDS) resulted in providing a higher resolution of amygdalin and prunasin from their isomers without the addition of chiral agents in the separation buffer.

### 10.6.6 High Performance Liquid Chromatography (HPLC)

In HPLC analysis of cyanogenic glycosides a known amount of sample is ground and then a solvent like ethanol is added to it. After giving a specific time and temperature for extraction, the extract is then filtered through filter paper (whatman No.1). After centrifugation, the residues obtained are discarded. The solvent is removed from the supernatant part using rotary vacuum evaporator. Mostly reversed-phase HPLC consisting of a pump, degasser, and diode array detector is used for identification of the cyanogenic glycosides. The standards of the cyanogenic glycosides are dissolved in water to prepare a stock solution of 100 µg/ml. the diode array detector is set at a wavelength required to identify the cyanogenic compounds once the sample is run through the column. The mobile phase consists of methanol and water (25:75 v/v). Before use, the gas bubbles are properly removed from the mobile phase (Amjadian et al., 2020).

### 10.6.7 Liquid Chromatography and Mass Spectrometry (LCMS)

The extracts prepared from the plant samples are first diluted using acetronitrile, water, and acetic acid in a vial. The diluted extract is vortexed for about 30 seconds before injection through a LC-MS system. After identification of the cyanogenic compound's quantification can be done using different analytical techniques. HPLC is the most commonly used method for quantification of such compounds (Malachova et al., 2014).

## 10.7 SAFETY, PRECAUTIONS AND REGULATION

Cyanogenic glycosides are responsible for multiple diseases in humans as well as in animals. These contribute for about 90% of the wider group of plant toxins. Commonly containing plant genera are wild cherry, black cherry, bitter almonds, sorghum, mushroom, etc. (Osuntokun, 1981). These glycosides have harmful effect on humans but their presence in the plants acts as a defence against the insects and pests (Wittstock and Gershenzon, 2002). Significant reduction in the cynogenic compounds can be achieved by the adopting the technique of genetic modification in the crops. One possible strategy to reduce root linamarin (a type of cyanogenic glycoside) content is to divert symplastically loaded linamarin from storage in roots vacuole towards assimilation into asparagine via CN production and assimilation into cyanoalanine by the action of enzyme cyanoalanine synthase (Okafor and Ejiofor, 1986). The adverse effects of cyanogenic glycosides can be avoided by proper preparation and processing of food plants. When fruits are processed into juices, the seeds obtained as waste should be removed before they are crushed, s crushing of seeds may lead to formation of hydrogen cyanide which in turn causes cyanide poisoning.

All those plant foods like cassava, almonds etc., which contain the cynogenic glycosides must be minimally processed before consumption. Minimal processing includes drying by different methods such as oven freeze and sun drying, boiling, cooking, soaking, wetting, fermentation. Use of superheated steam is another method to reduce cyanide poisoning. During processing the air and water used result in disintegration of hydrogen cyanide. No safety limit has been set for the cyanogenic glycosides, but the regulatory limits of total hydrocyanic acid in some food products set by the Australia New Zealand Food Standards Code are given below:

(i) Confectionery: 25 mg/kg.
(ii) Stone fruit drinks: 5 mg/kg
(iii) Marzipan: 50 mg/kg.
(iv) Alcoholic beverages: 1 mg/kg per 1% alcohol content

## 10.8 EFFECTS OF DIFFERENT PROCESSING TECHNIQUES ON CYANOGENIC GLYCOSIDES

In order to prevent cyanide toxicity, processing methods like roasting, soaking, peeling, pounding, fermenting, grating, grinding, boiling, and drying have been used over the years to slack off the cyanide content before consumption through the loss of water-soluble glycoside (Gonzalez-Garcia et al., 2014). Degradation of toxic compounds by enzymes can lead to the production of hydrogen cyanide, when cyanogen-containing substances are macerated or crushed. The heat treatments such as autoclaving, extrusion, and microwave roasting are usually used for reduction of cyanogenic glycosides (Wu et al., 2008). Miao et al. (2013) studied cyanogenic glycosides present in apricot kernels *(Armeniacasibirica L)* and reported that, to facilitate the exploitation and use of prunus kernels, it is necessary to determine the cyanogen concentration present within the kernels because it is potentially dangerous as it produces hydrogen cyanide which causes poisoning. Several studies have been conducted to remove cyanogens from prunus kernels. The conventional methods including soaking, autoclaving, fermenting, and boiling have been used to reduce the potential for toxicity to the safe limits (Bolarinwa et al., 2014). Appropriate processing methods prior to consumption are needed to reduce cyanogenic glycosidases.

### 10.8.1 Effect of Soaking

It is a simple and quite effective traditional practice to eliminate cyanogenic glycosides from edible substances. Soaking has been reported by several studies to cause considerable reduction in cyanogenic glycosides of the processed foods. Iwuoha et al. (2013) reported that the reduction of cyanogenic glycosides during soaking might be attributed to enhanced hydrolysis of cyanogenic glycosides due to cellular damage as a result of grating, which brought both cyanogenic glycosides and endogenous enzymes in contact. Since cyanogenic glycosides are water-soluble in nature and the loss during soaking is attributed to the leaching of water-soluble compounds into the soaking medium. EL-Adawy and Kadousy (1994) reported that the soaking of peach kernel meal in water exhibited a marked reduction in cyanogenic glycoside and the reduction of cyanogenic glycosides during soaking depends upon certain factors such as temperature, time, and soaking medium. Sheikh et al. (2021) studied detoxification of plum kernels by hydrothermal treatment and demonstrated that optimized hydrothermal treatment of soaking temperature of 45 °C and soaking time of 9 h, could be an effective tool for neutralizing the toxic effect of cyanogenic glycosides. Cyanogens from apricot kernels were removed by soaking the kernels either in water or 2% sodium hydroxide at 60°C with a ratio of soaking medium to kernel of 2:1 (Tuncel et al., 1990). The reduction level in cyanogenic glycosides was more than 99% and the water absorption was at higher level than un-detoxified meal. Apart from reduction in anti-nutritional factors, amino acid profile, especially essential amino acids, improved due to detoxification treatment. The reduction of cyanogenic glycosides by soaking showed no effect on the limiting amino acids (El-Adawy and Kadousy, 1994). Moreover, detoxified sample exhibited a decrease in fat absorption, foam capacity, emulsification capacity, and lowest foam stability. Finer particles in general result faster degradation of glycosides. Thus finely ground seeds contain no glycosides after 0.5 h of soaking. Sharma et al. (2010) also reported that boiling of apricot kernel meal in water removed 89.3% cyanogenic toxins. Tuncel et al. (1994) studied the effect of soaking and grinding on the amygdalin content of apricot kernel and reported a considerable reduction as well as accumulation of non-glycosides in the soaking medium.

### 10.8.2 Effect of Microwave Heating

Heating generally increases palatability of food substances by enhancing flavour through non-enzymatic reactions. It converts micronutrients as well as macronutrients into a more palatable form, i.e., changes structure and chemical composition. Generally, nuts are roasted to improve the colour, flavour, texture, and taste (Bagheri et al., 2016). Various methods of heating, including microwaving, have been used to improve the nutritional value of beans (Hernande-Infante et al., 1998). Heating with microwaves has recently become the most adaptable method for reducing the anti-nutritional factors. In microwave heating, heat is generated volumetrically inside the food in a short period of time due to greater penetration depth. It is a possible alternative and additional processing technique for reducing both heat-stable and heat-labile anti-nutrients such as phytic acid, hydrogen cyanide, total oxalate, trypsin inhibitor activity, oligosaccharides and phyto-haemagglutinating activity (Kala and Mohan, 2012). Feng et al. (2003) reported that prolonged exposure to microwave heating promotes a greater reduction in cyanogenic glycoside compounds of flaxseed and the application of high temperature (extrusions) can be used as a successful tool to reduce the cyanogenic glycosides in the flaxseed. Microwave heating at 500W for 9 min after soaking for 1 h is sufficient for complete degradation of toxic compound (Ahmad et al., 2015). It effectively reduce some anti-nutrients (tannins, phytic acid, and trypsin inhibitor activity) and improve protein quality in selected common beans (Emire and Rakshit, 2007). Microwave power of 400W for4 min and 50 s caused a reduction in hydrogen cyanide content under allowed limits (230 mg/kg of linseed) (Ivanov et al., 2012). Emire and Rakshit (2007) studied the effect of microwave heating in the reduction of anti-nutrients of selected common bean and concluded that microwave heating effectively reduced some anti-nutrients (tannins, phytic acid, and trypsin inhibitor activity) and improved protein quality. The impact of microwave heating on anti-nutritional compounds and protein quality of selected legume seeds and reported that microwave heating constitutes an adequate method for destroying hemagglutinins and trypsin inhibitors without affecting protein quality of legumes (Hernande-Infante et al. (1998).

### 10.8.3 Effect of Fermentation

Fermentation is a widely employed and quite effective processing technique to eliminate cyanogenic glycosides from the various food forms. During fermentation, plant material is exposed for various periods of time to the action of fermenting microflora (non-pathogenic microorganisms) which naturally inoculate the medium and degrade the hydrolytic enzymes (beta-glycosidase) thus reducing the HCN formation. Sarangthem and Hoikhokim (2010) reported that the fermentation of bamboo shoot could be an effective technique to decrease the cyanogen content below the human toxic level. Similarly, Iwuoha et al. (2013) reported that prolonged fermentation (5–6 days) and favourable pH (4.0–4.5) of freshly soaked and grated cassava tuber is an excellent technique to reduce the cyanogen content below toxic level.

### 10.8.4 Effect of Drying

Drying is a mass transfer process which reduces moisture content from the food substances by evaporation. Drying methods such as sun, oven, freeze, and superheated steaming has proven to be an appropriate processing technique to reduce cyanogenic glycosides under the allowed limits. Drying of food grains at high temperature for short time causes faster removal of water, enhances shelf life, crispness, and overall consumer acceptability. The efficiency of cyanogen reduction during drying is dependent on moisture percentage of the substance, rate of moisture removal, and the cellular damage of the food substance. Since food processing techniques generally disintegrate the cyanogen content and lead to the production of cyanide from cyanogen-containing food substances. Further processing techniques such as drying will volatilize the remaining cyanogen content to minimum levels because drying temperatures are above the boiling point of hydrogen cyanide (26°C). Ndubuisi and Chidiebere (2018) reported that prolonged drying of high moisture content foods results to the higher reduction of cyanogen content.

## 10.9 CONCLUSION

Cyanogenic glycosides are a widespread class of anti-nutrients distributed among edible plants. They are phyto-toxins which occur in more than 2,650 plant species, of which a number of species are used as food substances in different parts of the world. The potential toxicity of cyanogenic plants is mostly dependent on their ability to release lethal concentrations of hydrogen cyanide when exposed to humans. Human exposure to cyanide by the consumption of improperly processed cyanogenic plants can lead to chronic and acute health problems. To prevent adverse effects of cyanogenic glycosides, various conventional methods, including soaking, autoclaving, fermenting, and boiling have been used to reduce the potential toxicity below the acceptably safer limits. It is recommended that plant foods containing cyanogenic glycosides should be properly detoxified before consumption to avoid cyanide poisoning.

## REFERENCES


Ahmed, A. Abd El-Rahman, El-Hadary, Abdalla E., and Abd El-Aleem, Mohammed I. 2015. Detoxification and nutritional evaluation of peach and apricot meal proteins. *Journal of Biological Chemistry and Environmental Sciences*, 10: 597–622.

Amjadian, O.A., Arji, I., Changizi, M., Khaghani, S., and Salehi, H.R. 2020. Determination of cyanogenic glycosides in endemic species of wild almond seeds in the Zagros Mountains. *Brazilian Journal of Botany*, 43: 697–704.

Bagheri H., Kashaninejad M., Ziaiifar A.M., and Aalami M. 2016. Novel hybridized infrared-hot air method for roasting of peanut kernels. *Innovative Food Science and Emerging Technologies*, 37, 106–114.

Bolarinwa, I.F., Orfila, C., and Morgan, M.R.A. 2014. Development and application of an enzyme-linked immunosorbent assay (ELISA) for the quantification of amygdalin, a cyanogenic glycoside, in food. *Journal of Agricultural and Food Chemistry*, 62: 6299–6305.

Brinker, A.M. and Seigler, D.S. 1989. Methods for the detection and quantitative determination of cyanide in plant materials. *Phytochemical Bulletin*, 21: 24–31.

Campa, C., Kopplin, P.S., Cataldi, T.R.I., Bufo, S.A. Freitag, D., and Kettrup, A. 2000. Analysis of cyanogenic glycosides by micellar capillary electrophoresis. *Journal of Chromatography B*, 739: 95–100.

EFSA CONTAM Panel (EFSA Panel on Contaminants in the Food Chain), Schrenk, D., Bignami, M., Bodin, L., Chipman, J.K., delMazo, J., Grasl-Kraupp, B., et al. 2019. Scientific opinion on the evaluation of the health risks related to the presence of cyanogenic glycosides in foods other than raw apricot kernels. *EFSA Journal*, 17(4): 5662, 78 pp. https://doi.org/10.2903/j.efsa. 2019.5662.

El-Adawy T.A. and El-Kadousy S.A. 1994. Changes in chemical composition, nutritional quality, physico-chemical and functional properties of peach kernel meal during detoxification. *Food Chemistry*, 52: 143–148.

Emire S.A. and Rakshit S.K. 2007. Effect of processing on antinutrients and in vitro protein digestibility of kidney bean (Phaseolus vulgaris L.) varieties grown in East Africa. *Food Chemistry*, 103: 161–172.

Feng, D., Shen, Y., and Chavez, E.R. 2003. Effectiveness of different processing methods in reducing hydrogen cyanide content of flaxseed. *Journal of the Science of Food and Agriculture*, 83: 836–841.

Francisco, I.A. and Pinotti, M.H.P. 2000. Cyanogenic glycosides in plants. *Brazilian Archives of Biology and Technology*, 43(5): 487–492.

Gleadow, R.M. and Møller, B.L. 2014. Cyanogenic glycosides: Synthesis, physiology, and phenotypic plasticity. *Annual Reviews in Plant Biology*, 65: 155–85.

Gonzalez-Garcia, E., Marina L.M., and Garcia C.M. 2014. Plum (PrunusDomestica L.) by product as a new and cheap source of bioactive peptides: Extraction method and peptides charcterization. *Journal of Functional Foods*, 11: 428–437.

Goverde, M., Bazin, A., Kéry, M., Shykoff, J.A., and Erhardt, A. 2008. Positive effects of cyanogenic glycosides in food plants on larval development of the common blue butterfly. *Oecologia*, 157: 409–418.

He, X.Y., Wu, L.J., and Wang, W.X. 2020. Amygdalin: A pharmacological and toxicological review. *Journal of Ethnopharmacology*, 254: 112717. doi: 10.1016/j.jep.2020.112717.

Hernande-Infante M., Sousa V., Montalvo I., and Tena E. 1998. Impact of microwave heating on hemagglutinins, trypsin inhibitors and protein quality of selected legume seeds. *Plant Foods for Human Nutrition*, 52, 199 –208.

Honig, D.H., Hockridge, M.E., Gould, R.M., and Rackis, J.J. 1983. Determination of cyanide in soyabeans and soyabean products. *Journal of Agricultural and Food Chemistry*, 31: 271–275.

Ipatov, A., Ivanov, M., Makarychev-Mikhailov, S., Kolodnikov, V., Legin, A., and Vlasov, Y. 2002. Determination of cyanide using flow-injection multisensor system. *Talanta*, 58: 1071–1076.

Ivanov D., Kokic B., Brlek T., Colovic R., Vukmirovic D., Levic J., and Sredanovic S. 2012. Effect of microwave heating on content of cyanogenic glycosides in linseed. *Ratarstvo and Povrtarstvo*, 49: 63–68.

Iwuoha, G.N., Ubeng, G.G., and Onwuachu, U.I. 2013. Detoxification effect of fermentation on cyanide content of cassava tuber. *Journal of Applied Sciences and Environmental Management*, 17: 567–570.

Jovanovic, V.M., Sak-Bosnar, M., and Jovanovic, M.S. 1987. Determination of low levels of cyanide with a silver/silver sulphide wire electrode. *AnalyticaChimicaActa*, 196: 221–227.

Kala, B.K. and Mohan, V.R. 2012. Effect of microwave treatment on the antinutritional factors of two accessions of velvet bean, *Mucunapruriens (L.)D. C.* var. utilis (Wall. ex Wight) Bak. exBurck. *International Food Research Journal*, 19: 961–969.

Malachova, A., Sulyok, M., Beltran, E., Berthiller, F., and Krska, R. 2014. Optimization and validation of a quantitative liquid chromatography-tandem mass spectrometric method covering 295 bacterial and fungal metabolites including all regulated mycotoxins in four model food matrices. *Journal of Chromatography A*, 1362: 145–156.

Miao X., Zhao Z., Zhu H., Li M., and Zhao Q. 2013. Comparison of second-derivative spectrophotometry and HPLC for determination of amygdalin in wild apricot kernels. *Science Asia*, 39: 444–447.

Miller, R.E., McConville, M.J., and Woodrow, I.E. 2006. Cyanogenic glycosides from the rare Australian endemic rainforest tree *Clerodendrumgrayi*(Lamiaceae). *Phytochemistry*, 67: 43–51.

Mlingi, N., Poulter, N.H., and Rosling, H. 1992. An outbreak of acute intoxications from consumption of insufficiently processed cassava in Tanzania. *Nutrition Research*, 12(6): 677–687.

Møller, B.L. 2010. Functional diversifications of cyanogenic glucosides. *Current Option in Plant Biology*, 13: 337–347.

Monago, C.C. and Akhidue, V. 2002. Cyanide poisoning. *Journal of Applied Sciences and Environmental Management*, 6(1): 22–25.

Ndubuisi, N.D. and Chidiebere, A.C.U. 2018. Cyanide in Cassava: A review. *International Journal of Genomics and Data Mining*, 2: 1–10.

Nielsen, J.S. and Møller, B.L. 1999. Biosynthesis of cyanogenic glucosides in *Triglochinmaritima*and the involvement of cytochrome P450 enzymes. *Archives of Biochemistry and Biophysics*, 368: 121–30.

Nielsen, K.A., Olsen, C.E., Pontoppidan, K., and Møller, B.L. 2002. Leucine-derived cyanoglucosides in barley. *Plant Physiology*, 129: 1066–75.

Okafor, N. and Ejiofor, M.A.N. 1986. The microbial breakdown of linamarin in fermenting pulp of cassava (ManihotesculentaCrantz). *Journal of Microbiology and Biotechnology*, 2: 327–338.

Osuntokun, B.O. 1981. Cassava diet, chronic cyanideintoxication and neuropathy in the Nigerian Africans. *World Review of Nutrition and Dietetics*, 36: 141–173.

Rosling H. 1994. Measuring effects in humans of dietary cyanide exposure from cassava. *Acta Horticulturae*, 375(375): 271–284.

Saleem, M., Asif, J., Asif, M., and Saleem, U., 2018. Amygdalin from apricot kernels induces apoptosis and causes cell cycle arrest in cancer cells: An updated review. *Anti-cancer Agent M. E.* 18: 1650–1655.

Salkowski, A.A. and Penney, D.G. 1994. Cyanide poisoning in animals and humans: A review. *Veterinary and Human Toxicology*, 36(5): 455–466.

Sandstrom, K.J.M., Newman, J., Sunesson, A.L., Levin, J.O., and Turner, A.P.F. 2000 Amperometric biosensor for formic acid in air. *Sensors and Actuators B: Chemical*, 70: 182–187.

Sarangthem, K, and Hoikhokim. 2010. Cyanogen content in bamboo plants. *Asian Journal of Bio Science*, 5: 178–180.

Sharma, P.C., Tilakratne, B.M., and Gupta, A.K. 2010. Utilization of wild apricot kernel press cake for extraction of protein isolate. *Journal of Food Science and Technology*, 47, 682–685.

Sheikh, M. A., Saini, C. S., & Sharma, H. K. (2021). Analyzing the effects of hydrothermal treatment on antinutritional factor content of plum kernel grits by using response surface methodology. *Applied Food Research*, 100010.

Shi, J., Chen, Q., Xu, M., Xia, Q., Zheng, T., Teng, J., Li, M., and Fan, L. 2019. Recent updates and future perspectives about amygdalin as a potential anticancer agent: A review. *Cancer Medicine*, 8, 3004–3011.

Tuncel, G., Nout, M.J., Brimer, L., and Goktan, D. 1990. Toxicological, nutritional and microbiological evaluation of tempe fermentation with Rhizopusoligosporusof bitter and sweet apricot seeds. *International Journal of Food Microbiology*, 11: 337–344.

Wink, M. 1988. Plant breeding importance of secondary metabolites for production against pathogens and herbivores. *Theoretical and Applied Genetics*, 75(2): 225–233.

Winkler, W.O. 1958. Report of methods for glucosidal HCN in lima beans. *Journal of the Association of Official Agricultural Chemists*, 41: 282–287.

Wittstock, U. and Gershenzon, J. 2002. Constitutive plant toxins and their role in defense against herbivores and pathogens. *Current Opinions in Plant Biology*, 5: 300–307.

Wu, M., Li, D., Zhou, Y.G., Brooks, M.S.L., Chen, X.D., and Mao, Z.H. 2008. Extrusion detoxification technique on flaxseed by uniform design optimization. *Separation and Purification Technology*, 61: 51–59.

Yulvianti, M. and Zidorn, C. 2021. Chemical diversity of plant cyanogenic glycosides: An overview of reported natural products. *Molecules*, 26: 1–19.

Zagrobelny, M. and Møller, B.L. 2011. Cyanogenic glucosides in the biological warfare between plants and insects: The Burnet moth-Birdsfoot trefoil model system. *Phytochemistry*, 72: 1585–1592.

Zagrobelny, M., Bak, S., and Møller, B.L. 2008. Cyanogenesis in plants and arthropods. *Phytochemistry*, 69: 1457–1468.

CHAPTER 11

# Phytohaemagglutinins

**Jasmeet Kour, Monika Hans, Hitesh Chopra, Renu Sharma, Breetha Ramaiyan, and Bharti Mittu**

## CONTENTS



## 11.1 INTRODUCTION

Phytohaemagglutinins (PHA) are the lectins found in red kidney beans, *Phaseolus vulgaris*, chemically belonging to carbohydrate-binding proteins (Banwell et al., 1983, 1985; Shi et al., 2007; Zhang et al., 2008). They are mainly present in seeds, and are toxic; therefore they are generally cooked at higher temperature for human consumption (*Eating Raw, Undercooked Dry Beans Can Be Unpleasant | Archives | Hpj.Com*, n.d.). Lectins can be defined as the proteins having more than two binding sites, which can form crosslinking and forms agglutinate with cells bearing the target carbohydrates (Mishra et al., 2019; Nathan Sharon, 2007; Nathan Sharon & Lis, 1997). Initially they were identified as compounds that agglutinate blood cells, so they were named accordingly.

Pharmacologically they induce cells to enter the mitotic cell division phase, which may be by acting as a cross-linker to cell surface receptors that are directly or indirectly involved in cell activation (Berchtold & Villalobo, 2014; Kennedy & Nager, 2006; Movafagh et al., 2011). Upon exposure of lymphocytes from mammals to PHA, the mitosis starts for T lymphocytes and can be applied in the form of T cell mitogen in human immunology. When PHA is injected to animal tissues, they are designated as harmful. The series of steps involving the cell activation, destruction, and infiltration

DOI: 10.1201/9781003178446-11

starts as PHA is injected into the human body. The immediate response is local inflammation and rise in blood pressure levels along with cellular infiltration.

PHA consists of two closely related proteins such as leucoagglutinin (PHA-L) and Pha-E. PHA-E plays a major role in erythrocytic clumping and PHA-L clumps the leukocytes (Fitches et al., 2001; Nagae et al., 2014; Shi et al., 2007). PHA consists of carbohydrate-binding site, which consists of galactose, N-acetylglucosamine, and mannose. In legumes, the concave face has shallow cleft on the loops for carbohydrate binding. In case of legumes, the principal binding site for carbohydrate is having a slight cleft on the loops associated with the concave face. In case of Man/Glc and Gal/GalNAc type of lectins, five loops (A–E) are present, which have various residues (Loris et al., 2000, 2003; Manoj & Suguna, 2001; Rao et al., 1998) form.

PHA contains two polypeptide chains called as E and L, having possible combination as E4, E3L, E2L2, EL3, and L4 (Herzig et al., 1997; Voelker et al., 1986). These two subunits carry out the erythroagglutining and leucoagglutinin action of PHA moiety. The presence of N-acetylglusosamine is important for the binding and two Gal residues on the arm must be present. Also the interaction requires the galactosylation of the Manα1-6 arm. But the presence of Manα1-3 arm is not necessary for same. Researchers have reported that, at low temperature, weak binding of nonbisected and galactosylated N-glycans takes place (*Walker: The Protein Protocols Handbook* – Google Scholar, n.d.).

PHA-E has been used in a primary role as a biochemical detection tool for GlcNAc- and Gal-bearing proteins (Chen et al., 2020; Xie et al., 2020). Though PHA-L and E resemble for 70% with structural reference to each other but are highly specific in their binding affinity. Recombinant variants of lectin isoforms have been developed by heterogeneous expression system. Yeast has been found to one of the best hosts for expressions of PHA-E, as isolectin subunits of *Phaseolus vulgaris* has one N-linked high mannose and one complex N-linked sugar side chain (Mishra et al., 2019; Nagae et al., 2014; Vitale et al., 1984). Yeast has inherent capacity to produce the glycosylating proteins and modulated proteins with suitable biological activity (Burnett & Burnett, 2020; Vieira Gomes et al., 2018).

Initially the PHA-L was tried to be expressed in *Saccharomyces cerevisiae* but produced the poor yields and incorrect processed proteins (Tague & Chrispeels, 1987). So later researchers tried on methylotrophic yeast *Pischiapastoris* that can be used for expression purpose of PHA-L and has advantages on *Saccharomyces cerevisiae* in regard to higher levels of heterologous gene expression (Baumgartner et al., 2002).

## 11.2 CHEMISTRY

Structurally PHA consists of four subunits defined as A, B, C, and D (Hamelryck et al., 1996; Sharma et al., 2017). The root mean square differences between the α-carbon of subunits vary from 0.11 to 0.16 Å. It has been observed that the PHA-L monomer had 233 amino acid residues out of total 252 residues and no electron density observed at the 19-C-terminal residue. Due to flexibility of glycan moieties, the core GlcNAc residues linked to mannose glycan is attached to Asn-12, which can be observed easily during the electron density study.

PHA-L is tetramer with dimensions of 40 × 60 × 80 Å, and has four subunits as structural units. Each monomeric unit faces two interface monomer-monomer units (Loris et al., 1998). The first interface is composed of β-sheet, creating a continuous curved anti-parallel 12-stranded sheet spanning between two monomers. While other interface involves weak forces such as Van der Waals forces. PHA-L tetramer has 222 as type of internal symmetry. The two canonical dimers in PHA-L get packed in such a way that two outmost strands of the 12-strand sheets of both dimers have close contact with each other. The Van der Waal forces act as cross-linking for the side chains mainly involved in residues of 181 to 192. The dimers get oriented in such a way that two chains face towards the inside of monomer and towards the interface. Protruding chains are intercalated in a zipper-like fashion. β-side of the packing is not generally present in face to face orientation, but the side chain present may be separated by plane and their interface is entirely smooth. The back boning atoms providing main structural power are located at a distance of 6.5 Å from each other. A total of eight H-bonds are present between each interface of two dimers and involve the side chain of two serine residues with hydroxyl groups and lysine as main chain oxygen atom. At the end of β-side, there lies the lysine with 184 residues, positioned in parallel with the β-strand, via formation of weak Van der Waal forces. The two dimers get packed in such a manner that a central channel is formed in the central core with 12 β-strands facing each other and are about 18 Å apart (Loris et al., 1998).

The lectins generally possess two bound metallic ions, such as calcium and one belonging to d and f block elements per monomer near to the sugar-binding site (Bianchet et al., 2010; Sharon & Ofek, 2007; Singh & Walia, 2018). These two metal ions are needed for the sugar-binding capability of legume lectins. These two metallic ions are further lined up with the four molecules of water along with six amino acid residues. In case of PHA-L, $Mn2^{+}$ ions takes the central seat and coordinates itself with His-137, Glu-122, Asp-124, and Asp-132. While $Ca^{2+}$ ions coordinate with Leu-126, Asp-124, Asn-128, and Asp-132. The Ca2+ interacts via water molecules, with oxygen atom present at the side chain of Asp-86, which further stabilizes the Ala-85, Asp-86 cis-peptidal bond. Treatment with trypsin and human erythrocytes resulted in release of glycopeptides which can further bind with PHA, thus inhibiting the process of agglutination of erythrocytes.

## 11.3 DISTRIBUTION OF PHYTOHAEMOGLUTINNINS

Grain legumes inhabit a substantial place in human nutrition as these are one of the important staple foods. These exhibit a distinctive nutritive importance owing to the presence of abundant amounts of proteins, carbohydrates, dietary fiber, and various micronutrients including vitamins and minerals (Tharanathan and Mahadevamma, 2003; Osorio-Díaz et al., 2003). Amongst the frequently consumed legumes, dried beans (*Phaseolus vulgaris* L.) are reported to be extensively consumed throughout the world.

Seeds contained in common beans (*Phaseolus vulgaris*) that produce lectin and have sugar-binding and hemagglutinating characteristics are termed as phytohaemagglutinins (PHA) (Chrispeels & Raikhel, 1991). Phytohaemagglutinins (PHAs), carbohydrate-binding proteins, are able to interact with membrane receptors that agglutinate cells (Banwell et al., 1983; Imran et al., 2013). The primary PHA was revealed in semen ricini extract (Barondes, 1988; Peumans, & Van Damme, 1995). PHA is identified in several varieties of beans, but its maximum concentration is reported in red kidney beans. The PHA concentration is determined as hemagglutinating unit abbreviated as HAU, which is related to hemagglutination properties of red blood cells. Uncooked or raw kidney beans comprising enormous quantities of PHA have concentration varied from 20,000 to 70,000 HAU, while completely cooked kidney beans possess lesser PHA concentrations around 200 and 400 HAU. About one-third of PHA concentration existing in red kidney beans is known to be found in white kidney beans (McNeil, 2014).

PHA is quite abundant in bean seeds and constitutes about 5–10% of the seed protein. The seeds are well recognized for having two homologous polypeptides, PHA-E and PHA-L, with varying sugar specificities and biological characteristics. PHA-E agglutinates RBCs, whereas PHA-Lagglutinates lymphocytes. Theselectin polypeptides are synthesized simultaneously in the seed and leads to the formation of homo- as well as hetero-tetramers. PHA-L is a potent mitogen and is employed as a tool in sustaining lymphocyte cultures, detection of cancer, and cell biology (Licastro et al., 1993; Van Damme et al., 1998).

Various research studies reported that roots of leguminous plants release lectins into the rhizosphere which are reported to be identical with the well-characterized lectins contained within the seeds (Diaz et al., 1986; Vodkin & Raikhel, 1986). Similar amino acid sequence was identified in both cases. In light of their capacity to discriminate among various saccharides, lectins are appropriate to assume a part in recognition processes. Kjemtrup et al. (1995) reported the targeting and discharge of phytohaemagglutinins (PHA-E) from bean seedling roots. They observed that roots of bean seedlings produce authentic phytohaemagglutinins into the surrounding culture medium. This PHA-E stores in root vacuoles in the meristem tissue of the primary roots which is an indicator of correct targeting, whereas the elongated cells possess PHA only in their cell wall which indicates the poor recognition of the target signal. They suggested that PHA of cell wall is the basis of the PHA present in the culture medium.

Sun et al. (2019) examined the dispersion of phytohaemagglutinins (PHAs) in various cultivars of fresh kidney bean as well as in their different parts. In their study, PHA concentration was measured in different parts such as entire pod, hull, side rib, and seeds of six kidney bean cultivars. Critical variations in distribution PHA among the hull, seed and side rib were noticed. They concluded that seeds contained abundant PHA in contrast to side rib. The outcome of the study was sensible because proteins are ordinarily put away in seeds. In the same study, it was also seen that harvest maturity exhibits significant effect on PHA concentration. It seems to be diminishing with ripeness. PHA is a sort of naturally derived toxin safeguarding plants against insect impairment. A high PHA concentration in plants is generally observed during their growth period.

## 11.4 MECHANISM OF ACTION

PHA is resistant to enzymatic digestion and denaturation due to protease inhibitors present in the legumes (Lajolo & Genovese, 2002). This enables PHA to comfortably get across the digestive enzymes from the stomach and related parts of the gut. After entering the intestine and reaching the lumen, PHA will be attracted towards the sugar groups along the outer surface of a cell wall. To be precise, PHA has affinity with respect to the sugars like galactose, N-acetylglucosamine, and mannose. After the successful binding with the intestine wall, PHA is quite impervious to removal and this enables the obstruction of nutrient uptake, especially sodium, potassium, and water. Also, PHA will attach itself to or congest the receptors that are responsible for the intestinal epithelium and produce the secretion in the lumen (Nader et al., 2015). This concept was raised based on the complications related to lectins with malnutrition and diarrhoea. On the other hand, PHA will parallel be endocytosed inside the cellular cytoplasm. PHA will proceed along the epithelial areas and invade the intercellular extent. At this instant, PHA will begin an immune response where the excess fluids get transported between the lumen of the intestines and escalate the destruction of gut lining and the complications increase the risks of diarrhoea.

Similar studies were conducted where various cell lines including human (Intestine-407) and rat intestinal epithelial cell lines IEC-6 and IEC-18 were invigorated with PHA. Phytohaemagglutinins (0.1 μg/ml) significantly accelerated proliferation of all the accessed cell lines post 48–72 hours. The activation MAPK was observed after 15–30 minutes of administration, and after 15–30 minutes of it was found the initiation of c-fos mRNA expression (Otte et al., 2001).

It was observed that the binding properties of PHA to epithelial cell lining of intestine can alter the glycosylation patterns on the surface layers of epithelial lining. Along with this, PHA can result in degranulation of intestinal mast cells and increases the chances of vascular permeability. This condition enables the serum proteins to infiltrate across the intestinal cavity. In a separate study conducted, it was reported that PHA could result in decline in body weight and the lipid weight fraction, leading to suppressed rat growth (Bardocz et al., 1996). Thus, PHA is considered to be accountable for the maximum toxicologic manifestations to humankind, such as gastroenteritis, nausea, and diarrhoea.

## 11.5 TOXICOLOGY OF PHYTOHAEMAGGLUTININS

Bean lectins were initially characterized as carbohydrate-binding proteins because of their capacity in carbohydrates precipitation, but devoid of any enzymatic action on carbohydrate ligand molecules (Nciri et al., 2015). They additionally play out an assortment of biological properties, including anti-tumor (Pusztai, 1998), immunomodulatory (Abdullaev & Gonzalez, 1997), anti-fungal (Rubinstein et al., 2004), anti-human immunodeficiency virus (HIV) (Herre et al., 2004), and anti-insect activities (Barrientos & Gronenborn, 2005). Also, seeds belonging to common beans (*Phaseolus vulgaris*) produce lectin-possessing, sugar-binding potential and showing hemagglutinization action, called phytohaemagglutinins (PHA) (Chrispeels & Raikhel, 1991).

Now a days, more than seventy types of phytohaemagglutinins have been identified and isolated from numerous leguminous plants (Sun et al., 2019). PHAs are plentiful in several kidney bean cultivars, but red kidney beans are found to have significant concentrations of PHAs. The intake of red kidney beans which are crude or imperfectly cooked holds the credit for one of the vital elements for outbreaks. However well-drenched and cooked beans have no such antagonistic impact (Nciri et al., 2015). The phytohaemagglutinins (PHAs) consumed through crude or improperly cooked kidney beans may act as poison for monogastric animals like humans which can be related to transient gastrointestinal instabilities (Rodhouse et al., 1990). In animals, PHAs toxicity might result in reduction in the intake of food, impairment in weight gain, and even death in some cases (Grala et al., 1998; Lajolo & Genovese, 2002). Amongst various danger factors, PHAs in kidney beans were discovered to be accountable for various human toxicologic expressions, such as nausea, diarrhoea, and gastroenteritis (Sun et al., 2019).

Literature studies reported that the harmfulness caused by PHA is exceptionally predominant in the UK. Because of the large occurrence of PHA toxicity, protective procedures have been suggested by the public health laboratory services (PHLs), Colindale, UK with respect to intake of beans (FDA, 2004). Furthermore, the import of some kidney beans, especially red kidney beans, has been banned in South Africa due to the toxic effects of PHA on human population (De Mejia & Valadez-Vega, 2005; Kumar et al., 2013). The intake of PHAs can exhibit various anti-nutritive properties (Bardocz et al., 1996) and affect animal metabolism and growth parameters such as small intestine growth (Bardocz et al., 1995; Pusztai et al., 1991) and intestinal microflora ecology (Pusztai et al., 1991; Sun et al., 2019). The primary indications of PHA poisoning are nausea, vomiting, and diarrhoea (Nciri et al., 2015). People generally feel they are recovering within 3–4 hours after the symptoms initiated (Filipic, 2014). The optimum protection of beans must be cultivated through appropriate and focused research.

## 11.6 IDENTIFICATION AND QUANTIFICATION

PHAs are the types of vegetable lectin, proteinaceous in nature, which bind to carbohydrates interacting with membrane receptors that bind cells (Imran et al., 2013). To date, many plants and legumes have been found. More than 70 PHAs were separated from legume plants and purified. PHAs may also be anti-microbial and have an impact on animal growth and metabolism parameters; for example, small intestine growth and ecological bowel flora. In many cultivars of kidney beans, PHAs are abundant. PHAs were deemed to be attributed for human toxicological conditions in the form of gastroenteritis and diarrhoea, among the linked risk factors in kidney beans (Sun et al., 2019). A protein must meet three fundamental requirements to be classified as a lecithin, independent of its origin. They must a) bind the carbs, b) differ in immunoglobulins, and c) not biochemically change the carbs they bind. Tannins, certain lipids, carbohydrate-specific antibodies, glycosyltransferases, glycosidases, and other enzymes that bind and change carbohydrates can all be excluded using these criteria (Rudiger & Gabius, 2001).

A family of five isolectin red kidney bean lectins consists of a complex of four units that are not covalently bounded. There are different proportions of E and L subunits in the isolectins, which are also called erythroagglutinin, PHA-E and leukoagglutinin, PHA-L. They can be characterized by their N-terminal, isoelectric point, and, most importantly, biological features despite extensive sequence similitudes. PHA-L is a strong mitogen in the lymphocytes and has strong affinity for cell lymphocytes but the affinity for red blood cells, whereas PHA-E shows a strong erythrocyte affinity (Baumgartner et al., 2002).

A significant work carried out by Badri Nath et al. (2015) to prepare phytohaemagglutinins (PHA) from seed of 70% ethanol in the red kidney and 100 mL sterile Ringer seeds. It was used to prepare the working solution and stored at - 20°C and different stock solutions. Different chemical tests such as thin layer chromatography of the pHA solutions were conducted (TLC). For the probes, the chloroform (20:80, 30:70, 40:50, and 50:50 ratio) has been used in different ratios of methanol. The UV visible spectroscopy can be identified and defined in these PHA solutions. Samples were recorded in the water in the 200–800 nm range of the absorption spectrum. Characterization of the PHA solutions was also done by FTIR spectroscopy. The samples were subjected to freeze drying for lyophilization. The lyophilized samples were mixed with potassium bromide (KBr) and broken into very thin pellets and then analyzed for infrared spectra to form a very fine powder. A Schimadzu IR Affinity-1 Spectrophotometer was recorded in FT-IR Spectra. The PHA was also characterized by NMR spectroscopy. The samples were freeze-dried and active fractions were collected, dissolved in $D_2O$, and used for NMR, $^{13}C$ NMR, and DEPT analysis of protons. In $D_2O$, $CDCl_3$ and DMSO-$d^6$ solutions, $^1H$ and $^{13}C$ NMR spectra were determined using Bruker Ascend Model400 MHz respectively.

Nader et al. (2015) conducted a pivotal research on white kidney beans. A centrifugal retrieval at 328 g was made in proteins fractions for 30 minutes, dialyzed and electrophoresed on sodium dodecyl sulphate-polyacrylamide gels and to the Tris-NaCl buffer (pH 8) dialysis tubed in 10 kDa (SDS-PAGE). For further usage, the samples were kept at - 20°C.

SDS-PAGE was carried out in a reducing environment. Standard proteins with molecular weight of 14.00, 20.00, 30.10, 43.00, 67.00, and 94.00 kDa were used for A-lactalbumin, trypsin inhibitor, carbonic anhydrase, ovalbumin, albumin, and phosphorylase respectively. PHA purified and phaseoline pH 4.2 and 5.5 were extracted from the Beldia beans for 5 minutes in a Tris-HCL (pH 6.8) buffer of 10% SDS, 10% glycerol, and 0.1% Blue Bromophenol at 100°C. SDS-PAGE aimed mainly at the visualization in the crude extracts of white Beldia beans of a 33 kDa molecular weight and results found were consistent (Rui et al. 2011).

A crude bean (*Phaseolus vulgaris L.*) extract agglutination has been carried out in the red blood cells as previously outlined by Confalonieri et al. (1992). The best semi-quantitative method to determine whether lectins are present in legumes is HA method (Cuadrado et al. 2002). The HT has been defined as the reciprocal dilution leading to agglutination as stated before. CBBE with agglutination generated 1:512 for an HT of 512 is the highest dilution. These findings have shown that in raw Beldia beans bioactive PHAs are present in significant quantities.

## 11.7 SAFETY, PRECAUTIONS, AND REGULATIONS

According to safety issues, phytohaemagglutinins have various risk factors. They are responsible for some of the health related issues. Some studies and experiments have been conducted to check the effects of the phytohaemagglutinins and also various have been included to lower their effectiveness. Kidney beans have high levels of phytohaemagglutinins, which is a protein that can mess with cell walls metabolism. Furthermore, PHA-induced intoxication is very prevalent in the United Kingdom. It is owing to high PHA toxicity in kidney beans, various safety guidelines have been issued by the public health laboratory services (PHLS), Colindale UK.

To establish a method to determine PHA concentrations, standard sampling comprising five different PHA concentrations were evaluated for hemagglutinating activity, The relationship between hemagglutinating activity (*Y*) and PHA concentration (*X*) was established based on the following coefficient, $R^2 = 0.999$), which indicated that the method used for the determination of PHA concentrations.

$$Y = 0.017X - 0.8$$

The PHA concentration of tested samples was calculated using following equation:

$$C = S_0 \times H \times V / H_0 \times M$$

where $S_0$ and $H_0$ were the PHA concentration and hemagglutinating activity of the standard sample, respectively and *H, V,* and *M* were the hemagglutinating activity, volume and weight of the tested sample respectively.

For example, the safe level of PHA when fed to rats is 1,250 μg/g. However, there are few published reports on the safety profile of PHA with respect to humans. Thus, for safety evaluations and risk assessments regarding the consumption of PHA in daily human life, it is necessary to determine safe levels in future. If we follow the safe limits of the PHA, it will not affect the humans.

"Precaution is always better than cure". So it important that we have to avoid the consumption of the phytohaemagglutinins to avoid the bad effects. High intake of PHA can be toxic resulting in nausea, vomiting and diarrhoea apart from "leaky gut" and serious health issues such as food sensitivity autoimmune response, and inflammation.

The PHA skin test can be done on infants and children but pregnant women should not ingest or use due to lack of safety data. This type of food poisoning occurs as a result of consuming raw or undercooked kidney beans. So in order to prevent this from happening, the following precautions should be followed:

- Soaking of red kidney beans for up to 8 hours followed by draining and rinsing.
- Boiling these beans at least for 10 minutes to destroy the toxins followed by simmering for an hour to lessen its harmful effects.
  Cooking is of one the methods to reduce the toxic effects of the phytohaemagglutinins. If these beans are not properly cooked and are still hard in the centre then cook them for longer until they have soften.

## 11.8 EFFECT OF PROCESSING (DRYING, FERMENTATION, BOILING, AUTOCLAVING, BAKING, BROILING, COOKING, FREEZING, FRYING, ROASTING, GERMINATION)

Processing of foods has its own effect on the overall palatability and also the disintegration of natural matrices of any specific foods. Based upon the type of process involved the outcome varies (Fardet, 2018). Various cooking processes including stir-frying between 3–18 minutes and braising for 30 minutes using the fresh kidney beans were assessed by Guzel and Sayar (2012). It was observed that the variation in cooking methods had significant effects on PHA levels in fresh kidney beans. Profoundly, the PHA levels were significantly decreased with the increase in cooking duration. This states that the PHA concentrations are inversely proportional to the duration of cooking or processing (Guzel & Sayar, 2012). Furthermore, stir-frying for 18 minutes or braising for 10 minutes altered the PHA concentrations from fresh kidney beans to take a drop than the detection range (200 μg/g). This denotes that the denaturation of protein requires appropriate temperature and time. Stir-frying requires a higher duration of time to ameliorate PHA while compared to braising. The better justification for this reason could be that fresh kidney beans show poor uniformity in heating while stir-frying. Since PHA concentrations can be effectively removed by braising for 10 minutes.

Although heating is the most conventional processing method to remove the toxicity of PHA, it is proven that the PHA is resistant to thermal denaturation, thus taking long processing time in inactivating the PHA (Sun et al., 2019). Alternatively, ultra-high pressure treatment (UHP), is a relatively recent processing technology and has the advantage of reduced energy consumption and keeps the nutrients intact. Fresh kidney beans were subjected to ultra-high pressure (UHP) treatment including 150, 250, 350, 450 MPa. The purified form of PHA and its haemagglutination activity had significantly reduced post treating with 450 MPa treatment. The mechanism of UHP works on altering the molecular volume via ultra-high pressure, which results in the destruction of chemical bonds present in the protein molecules. Hence, UHP can activate the changes in secondary and tertiary structures of the protein molecules thus making the inactivation of PHA swift.

## 11.9 FUTURE SCOPE

These extracted phytohaemagglutinins may be utilized in the developing countries such as India owing to its inexpensiveness and longer shelf life at storage temperature of 20°C where various cytogenetic tests are carried out in hospitals and in research (Badari Nath et al., 2015). Plant derived lectins are known to perform plethora of functions, most prominently encompassing imparting protection from predators as well as pathogens, exhibiting symbiotic association between plants acting as microbes such as mycorrhizal fungi and nitrogen-fixing rhizobia (Movafagh et al., 2013).

Hailing from a varied group of proteins bounded to carbohydrate, the phytohaemagglutinins exist in close association with organisms from various living kingdoms (Movafagh et al., 2013). Lectins modulate the cell substratum interactions and bring about the normal differentiation along with rigorous growth of all multicellular animals. Lectins are also promisingly known as cell proliferators inducing cell death, morphogenesis of various pivotal organs, spread of tumour cell due to leukocytes, dermal analysis for immunological assessment response (Movafagh et al., 2011). The end of the 19th century has been able to gather evidences for the detection of proteins which had the potential to agglutinate erythrocytes which were later called as phytoagglutinins being derivatives of plants (Movafagh et al., 2013).

Over the years, the isolation and characterization of various lectins possessing various in vivo and in vitro anti-cancerous properties have been carried out (Movafagh et al., 2013). The prominent areas where phytohaemagglutinins can find their applications in the medical field in the form of surgical pins, sutures, blood vessel replacement, along with drug carriers. Apart from this, these plant toxins also find their prevalence in industries in the form of biodegradable agents which carry several fungicides, fertilizers, and packaging containers (Badari Nath et al., 2015). Some crucial studies need to be undertaken to unravel molecular mechanism involved in various allergic reactions induced by these phytohaemagglutinins. Owing to their physiological role, investigators have generated their focus on plant lectins. Lectins were also speculated to act as antibodies which could impart protection to plants from harmful soil bacteria. Lectins work as recognition molecules not only inside cells but also on cell surfaces and in physiological fluids. It was in the year 1978 when the biological function of lectins got evolved (Movafagh et al., 2013). The phytohaemagglutinins has been seen in membrane-induced fusion in human oocytes (Tesarik et al., 2000). There was a beginning of the association of bacterial lectins to initiate infection and to utilize carbohydrates for anti-adhesion therapy of such diseases. These phytohaemagglutinins also find their powerful biological application as a potent biochemical warfare agent ricin as well as these have been able to receive considerable attention is in the field of cancer biology owing to their impeccable anti-tumorous nature (Movafagh et al., 2013). Various studies have also demonstrated that the proliferation of cells is diminished due to these lectins inhibiting cell proliferation (De Mejía et al., 2005).

These molecules are of physiological importance due to their ubiquitous distribution in the plant world. The characteristic property of lectins is their ability to bind to specific carbohydrate structure leading to a basis of biologically reliable recognition (Doltchinkova & Angelova, 2017). One of the most exhaustive lectins derived from legumes belong to the family of simple lectins with the maximum proportion derived from plant seeds (Sharon & Lis, 1989). Lectins from plants are also involved in blood typing, thus playing a major role in a clinical setting (Movafagh et al., 2013). The proliferative activity of leukemic cells has been also credited to these lectins. Phytohaemagglutinins work as model to evaluate the recognizability of proteins towards carbohydrates due to their easy availability and diversified sugar specificities (Movafagh et al., 2013). Apart from the well-established effect of phytohaemagglutinins on mitotic stimulation, these toxins are also being useful to develop novel pharmaceuticals (Movafagh et al., 2011).

Phytohaemagglutinins (PHA) from the red kidney bean (*Phaseolus vulgaris*) can be one of promising factors in the medical field with respect to biological recognition phenomena involving cells and proteins for their mitotic stimulation to human lymphocytes apart from producing novel pharmaceuticals in health care services and phytomedicine research (Movafagh et al., 2013). These lectins have been also discovered as antibodies which could impart immense protection to plants against harmful soil bacteria as well as aid in controlling seed germination.

## 11.10 CONCLUSIONS

Phytohaemagglutinins belong to one of the most intensively studied simple lectins isolated from plant seeds. These are the plant lectins which are carbohydrate-binding proteins interacting with membrane receptors leading to agglutination of the cells. There are about 70 different types of phytohaemagglutinins which have been separated and purified from leguminous plants. These compounds have indeed been able to acquire various biological properties out of which the most prominent and universal function of these is in their recognition of molecules.

## REFERENCES

Abdullaev, F.I. and Gonzalez de Mejia, E., 1997. Antitumor effect of plant lectins. *Natural Toxins* 5(4): 157–163.

Bad Bug Book FDA, 2004. *Handbook of Foodborne Pathogenic Microorganisms and Natural Toxins*, 2nd edition, Center for Food Safety and Applied Nutrition (CFSAN) of the Food and Drug Administration (FDA), USA, 254–256.

Banwell, J.G., Boldt, D.H., Meyers, J. and Weber Jr, F.L., 1983. Phytohaemagglutinins derived from red kidney bean (*Phaseolus vulgaris*): a cause for intestinal malabsorption associated with bacterial overgrowth in the rat. *Gastroenterology* 84(3): 506–515.

Banwell, J.G., Howard, R., Cooper, D. and Costerton, J.W., 1985. Intestinal microbial flora after feeding Phytohaemagglutinins lectins (*Phaseolus vulgaris*) to rats. *Applied and Environmental Microbiology* 50(1): 68–80.

Bardocz, S., Ewen, S.W., Grant, G. and Pusztai, A., 1995. Lectins as growth factors for the small intestine and the gut. *Lectins: Biomedical Perspectives* 4: 103–116.

Bardocz, S., Grant, G., Pusztai, A., Franklin, M.F. and Carvalho, A.D.F., 1996. The effect of phytohaemagglutinins at different dietary concentrations on the growth, body composition and plasma insulin of the rat. *British Journal of Nutrition* 76(4): 613–626.

Barondes, S.H., 1988. Bifunctional properties of lectins: lectins redefined. *Trends in Biochemical Sciences* 13(12): 480–482.

Barrientos, L.G. and Gronenborn, A.M., 2005. The highly specific carbohydrate-binding protein cyanovirin-N: structure, anti-HIV/Ebola activity and possibilities for therapy. *Mini Reviews in Medicinal Chemistry* 5(1): 21–31.

Baumgartner, P., Raemaekers, R.J., Durieux, A., Gatehouse, A., Davies, H. and Taylor, M., 2002. Large-scale production, purification, and characterisation of recombinant *Phaseolus vulgaris* Phytohaemagglutinins E-form expressed in the methylotrophic yeast Pichia pastoris. *Protein Expression and Purification* 26(3): 394–405.

Berchtold, M.W. and Villalobo, A., 2014. The many faces of calmodulin in cell proliferation, programmed cell death, autophagy, and cancer. *Biochimica et Biophysica Acta (BBA)-Molecular Cell Research* 1843(2): 398–435.

Bianchet, M.A., Odom, E.W., Vasta, G.R. and Amzel, L.M., 2010. Structure and specificity of a binary tandem domain F-lectin from striped bass (Morone saxatilis). *Journal of Molecular Biology* 401(2): 239–252.

Burnett, M.J. and Burnett, A.C., 2020. Therapeutic recombinant protein production in plants: challenges and opportunities. *Plants, People, Planet* 2(2): 121–132.

Chen, Q., Tan, Z., Guan, F. and Ren, Y., 2020. The essential functions and detection of bisecting GlcNAc in cell biology. *Frontiers in Chemistry* 8: 511.

Chrispeels, M.J. and Raikhel, N.V., 1991. Lectins, lectin genes, and their role in plant defense. *The Plant Cell* 3(1): 1.

Confalonieri, M., Bollini, R., Berardo, N., Vitale, A. and Allavena, A., 1992. Influence of Phytohaemagglutinins on the agronomic performance of beans (*Phaseolus vulgaris* L.). *Plant Breeding* 109(4): 329–334.

Cuadrado, C., Hajos, G., Burbano, C., Pedrosa, M.M., Ayet, G., Muzquiz, M., Pusztai, A. and Gelencser, E., 2002. Effect of natural fermentation on the lectin of lentils measured by immunological methods. *Food and Agricultural Immunology* 14(1): 41–49.

De Mejía, E.G. and Prisecaru, V.I., 2005. Lectins as bioactive plant proteins: a potential in cancer treatment. *Critical Reviews in Food Science and Nutrition* 45(6): 425–445.

De Mejia, E.G., Valadez-Vega, M.D.C., Reynoso-Camacho, R. and Loarca-Pina, G., 2005. Tannins, trypsin inhibitors and lectin cytotoxicity in tepary (Phaseolus acutifolius) and common (*Phaseolus vulgaris*) beans. *Plant Foods for Human Nutrition* 60(3): 137–145.

Diaz, C.L., Van Spronsen, P.C., Bakhuizen, R., Logman, G.J.J., Lugtenberg, E.J.J. and Kijne, J.W., 1986. Correlation between infection by Rhizobium leguminosarum and lectin on the surface of *Pisum sativum* L. roots. *Planta* 168(3): 350–359.

Doltchinkova, V. and Angelova, P.R., 2017. Phytohaemagglutinins and light-induced charge density effects on plasma membrane of plectonemaboryanum. *Journal of New Developments in Chemistry* 1(1): 11.

Fardet, A., 2018. Characterization of the degree of food processing in relation with its health potential and effects. *Advances in Food and Nutrition Research* 85: 79–129.

Fitches, E., Ilett, C., Gatehouse, A.M.R., Gatehouse, L.N., Greene, R., Edwards, J.P. and Gatehouse, J.A., 2001. The effects of *Phaseolus vulgaris* erythro-and leucoagglutinating isolectins (PHA-E and PHA-L) delivered via artificial diet and transgenic plants on the growth and development of tomato moth (*Lacanobia oleracea*) larvae; lectin binding to gut glycoproteins in vitro and in vivo. *Journal of Insect Physiology* 47(12): 1389–1398.

Filipic, M. (2014). *Dry kidney beans need to be boiled.* Chow Line. www.extension.osu.edu.

Grala, W., Verstegen, M.W.A., Jansman, A.J.M., Huisman, J. and Van Leeusen, P., 1998. Ileal apparent protein and amino acid digestibilities and endogenous nitrogen losses in pigs fed soybean and rapeseed products. *Journal of Animal Science* 76(2): 557–568.

Güzel, D. and Sayar, S., 2012. Effect of cooking methods on selected physicochemical and nutritional properties of barlotto bean, chickpea, faba bean, and white kidney bean. *Journal of Food Science and Technology* 49(1): 89–95.

Hamelryck, T.W., Dao-Thi, M.H., Poortmans, F., Chrispeels, M.J., Wyns, L. and Loris, R., 1996. The crystallographic structure of Phytohaemagglutinins-L. *Journal of Biological Chemistry* 271(34): 20479–20485.

Herre, J., Willment, J.A., Gordon, S. and Brown, G.D., 2004. The role of Dectin-1 in antifungal immunity. *Critical Reviewsin Immunology* 24(3):193–203.

Herzig, K.H., Bardocz, S., Grant, G., Nustede, R., Fölsch, U.R. and Pusztai, A., 1997. Red kidney bean lectin is a potent cholecystokinin releasing stimulus in the rat inducing pancreatic growth. *Gut* 41(3): 333–338.

Hong, S.B., Uhm, S.J., Lee, H.Y., Park, C.Y., Gupta, M.K., Chung, B.H., Chung, K.S. and Lee, H.T., 2005. Developmental ability of bovine embryos nuclear transferred with frozen-thawed or cooled donor cells. *Asian-Australasian Journal of Animal Sciences* 18(9): 1242–1248.

Imran, M., Anjum, F.M., Butt, M.S., Siddiq, M. and Sheikh, M.A., 2013. Reduction of cyanogenic compounds in flaxseed (*Linum usitatissimum* L.) meal using thermal treatment. *International Journal of Food Properties* 16(8): 1809–1818.

Kennedy, M.W. and Nager, R.G., 2006. The perils and prospects of using phytohaemagglutinin in evolutionary ecology. *Trends in Ecology & Evolution* 21(12): 653–655.

Kjemtrup, S., Borkhsenious, O., Raikhel, N.V. and Chrispeels, M.J., 1995. Targeting and release of Phytohaemagglutinins from the roots of bean seedlings. *Plant Physiology* 109(2): 603–610.

Kumar, S., Verma, A.K., Das, M., Jain, S.K. and Dwivedi, P.D., 2013. Clinical complications of kidney bean (*Phaseolus vulgaris* L.) consumption. *Nutrition* 29(6): 821–827.

Lajolo, F.M. and Genovese, M.I., 2002. Nutritional significance of lectins and enzyme inhibitors from legumes. *Journal of Agricultural and Food Chemistry* 50(22): 6592–6598.

Licastro, F., Davis, L.J. and Morini, M.C., 1993. Lectins and superantigens: membrane interactions of these compounds with T lymphocytes affect immune responses. *International Journal of Biochemistry* 25(6): 845–852.

Loris, R., De Greve, H., Dao-Thi, M.H., Messens, J., Imberty, A. and Wyns, L., 2000. Structural basis of carbohydrate recognition by lectin II from Ulex europaeus, a protein with a promiscuous carbohydrate-binding site. *Journal of Molecular Biology* 301(4): 987–1002.

Loris, R., Hamelryck, T., Bouckaert, J. and Wyns, L., 1998. Legume lectin structure. *Biochimica et Biophysica Acta (BBA): Protein Structure and Molecular Enzymology* 1383(1): 9–36.

Loris, R., Imberty, A., Beeckmans, S., Van Driessche, E., Read, J.S., Bouckaert, J., De Greve, H., Buts, L. and Wyns, L., 2003. Crystal structure of Pterocarpus angolensis lectin in complex with glucose, sucrose, and turanose. *Journal of Biological Chemistry* 278 (18): 16297–16303.

Manoj, N. and Suguna, K., 2001. Signature of quaternary structure in the sequences of legume lectins. *Protein Engineering* 14(10): 735–745.

McNeil, P.L., 2014. Medical College of Georgia, USA 2007. www.accessibility.com.au/news (accessed April 2014).

Mishra, A., Behura, A., Mawatwal, S., Kumar, A., Naik, L., Mohanty, S.S., Manna, D., Dokania, P., Mishra, A., Patra, S.K. and Dhiman, R., 2019. Structure-function and application of plant lectins in disease biology and immunity. *Food and Chemical Toxicology* 134: 110827.

Movafagh, A., Ghanati, K., Amani, D., Mahdavi, S.M., Hashemi, M., Abdolahi, D. Z and Zamani, M., 2013. The structure Biology and Application of Phytohaemagglutinins (PHA) in Phytomedicine: with special up-to-date references to lectins. *Archives of Advances in Biosciences* 4:126–141.

Movafagh, A., Hajifathali, A. and Zamani, M., 2011. Secondary chromosomal abnormalities of de novo acute myeloid leukemia: a first report from the Middle East. *Asian Pacific Journal of Cancer Prevention* 12(11): 2991–2994.

Movafagh, A., Heydary, H., Mortazavi-Tabatabaei, S.A. and Azargashb, E., 2011. The significance application of indigenous Phytohaemagglutinins (PHA) mitogen on metaphase and cell culture procedure. *Iranian Journal of Pharmaceutical Research* 10(4): 895.

Nader, N., Hanen, B.I., Fatma, B.A.F. and Namjun, C., 2015. In vitro assessment of *Phaseolus vulgaris* L. lectins activities against various pathogenic and beneficial microbes. *Research Journal of Biotechnology*10: 11.

Nagae, M., Soga, K., Morita-Matsumoto, K., Hanashima, S., Ikeda, A., Yamamoto, K. and Yamaguchi, Y., 2014. Phytohaemagglutinins from *Phaseolus vulgaris* (PHA-E) displays a novel glycan recognition mode using a common legume lectin fold. *Glycobiology* 24(4): 368–378.

Nath, A.B., Sivaramakrishna, A., Marimuthu, K.M. and Saraswathy, R., 2015. A comparative study of phytohaemagglutinin and extract of *Phaseolus vulgaris* seeds by characterization and cytogenetics. *Spectrochimica Acta Part A: Molecular and Biomolecular Spectroscopy* 134: 143–147.

Nciri, N., Cho, N., Mhamdi, F.E., Ismail, H.B., Mansour, A.B., Sassi, F.H. and Aissa-Fennira, F.B., 2015. Toxicity assessment of common beans (*Phaseolus vulgaris* L.) widely consumed by Tunisian population. *Journal of Medicinal Food* 18(9): 1049–1064.

Osorio-Díaz, P., Bello-Pérez, L.A., Sáyago-Ayerdi, S.G., Benítez-Reyes, M.D.P., Tovar, J. and Paredes-López, O., 2003. Effect of processing and storage time on in vitro digestibility and resistant starch content of two bean (*Phaseolus vulgaris* L) varieties. *Journal of the Science of Food and Agriculture* 83(12): 1283–1288.

Otte, J.M., Chen, C., Brunke, G., Kiehne, K., Schmitz, F., Fölsch, U.R. and Herzig, K.H., 2001. Mechanisms of lectin (Phytohaemagglutinins)-induced growth in small intestinal epithelial cells. *Digestion* 64(3): 169–178.

Peumans, W.J. and Van Damme, E.J., 1995. Lectins as plant defense proteins. *Plant Physiology* 109(2): 347.

Pusztai, A. 1998. Effects of lectin ingestion on animal growth and internal organs. In *Lectin Methods and Protocols*, Rhodes JM, Milton JD, eds., Human Press, Totowa, NJ, 485–494.

Pusztai, A., Watt, W.B. and Stewart, J.C., 1991. A comprehensive scheme for the isolation of trypsin inhibitors and the agglutinin from soybean seeds. *Journal of Agricultural and Food Chemistry* 39(5): 862–866.

Rao, V.S.R., Lam, K. and Qasba, P.K., 1998. Architecture of the sugar binding sites in carbohydrate binding proteins: a computer modeling study. *International Journal of Biological Macromolecules* 23(4): 295–307.

Rodhouse, J.C., Haugh, C.A., Roberts, D. and Gilbert, R.J., 1990. Red kidney bean poisoning in the UK: an analysis of 50 suspected incidents between 1976 and 1989. *Epidemiology & Infection* 105(3): 485–491.

Rubinstein, N., Ilarregui, J.M., Toscano, M.A. and Rabinovich, G.A., 2004. The role of galectins in the initiation, amplification and resolution of the inflammatory response. *Tissue Antigens* 64(1): 1–12.

Rüdiger, H. and Gabius, H.J., 2001. Plant lectins: occurrence, biochemistry, functions and applications. *Glycoconjugate Journal* 18(8): 589–613.

Rui, X., Boye, J.I., Ribereau, S., Simpson, B.K. and Prasher, S.O., 2011. Comparative study of the composition and thermal properties of protein isolates prepared from nine *Phaseolus vulgaris* legume varieties. *Food Research International* 44(8): 2497–2504.

Sharma, P.K., Munir, R.I., Blunt, W., Dartiailh, C., Cheng, J., Charles, T.C. and Levin, D.B., 2017. Synthesis and physical properties of polyhydroxyalkanoate polymers with different monomer compositions by recombinant Pseudomonas putida LS46 expressing a novel PHA synthase (PhaC116) enzyme. *Applied Sciences* 7(3): 242.

Sharon, N., 2007. Lectins: carbohydrate-specific reagents and biological recognition molecules. *Journal of Biological Chemistry* 282(5): 2753–2764.

Sharon, N. and Lis, H., 1989. Lectins as cell recognition molecules. *Science* 246(4927): 227–234.

Sharon, N. and Lis, H., 1997. Microbial lectins and their glycoprotein receptors. *New Comprehensive Biochemistry* 29: 475.

Sharon, N. and Ofek, I., 2007. Microbial lectins. *Comprehensive Glycoscience* 623–659.

Shi, J., Xue, S.J., Kakuda, Y., Ilic, S. and Kim, D., 2007. Isolation and characterization of lectins from kidney beans (*Phaseolus vulgaris*). *Process Biochemistry* 42(10): 1436–1442.

Singh, R.S. and Walia, A.K., 2018. Lectins from red algae and their biomedical potential. *Journal of Applied Phycology* 30(3): 1833–1858.

Sun, Y., Liu, J., Huang, Y., Li, M., Lu, J., Jin, N., He, Y. and Fan, B., 2019. Phytohaemagglutinins content in fresh kidney bean in China. *International Journal of Food Properties* 22(1): 405–413.

Tague, B.W. and Chrispeels, M.J., 1987. The plant vacuolar protein, Phytohaemagglutinins, is transported to the vacuole of transgenic yeast. *The Journal of Cell Biology* 105(5): 1971–1979.

Tesarik, J., Nagy, Z.P., Mendoza, C. and Greco, E., 2000. Chemically and mechanically induced membrane fusion: non-activating methods for nuclear transfer in mature human oocytes. *Human Reproduction* 15(5): 1149–1154.

Tharanathan, R.N. and Mahadevamma, S., 2003. Grain legumes: a boon to human nutrition. *Trends in Food Science & Technology* 14(12): 507–518.

Van Damme, E.J., Peumans, W.J., Pusztai, A. and Bardocz, S. 1998. *Handbook of Plant Lectins: Properties and Biomedical Applications*, Wiley, New York, 466.

Vieira Gomes, A., Souza Carmo, T., Silva Carvalho, L., Mendonça Bahia, F. and Parachin, N. 2018. Comparison of yeasts as hosts for recombinant protein production. *Microorganisms* 6(2): 38.

Vitale, A., Ceriotti, A., Bollini, R. and Chrispeels, M.J., 1984. Biosynthesis and processing of Phytohaemagglutinins in developing bean cotyledons. *European Journal of Biochemistry* 141(1): 97–104.

Vodkin, L.O. and Raikhel, N.V., 1986. Soybean lectin and related proteins in seeds and roots of Le+ and Le– soybean varieties. *Plant Physiology* 81(2): 558–565.

Voelker, T.A., Staswick, P. and Chrispeels, M.J., 1986. Molecular analysis of two Phytohaemagglutinins genes and their expression in *Phaseolus vulgaris* cv. Pinto, a lectin-deficient cultivar of the bean. *The EMBO Journal* 5(12): 3075–3082.

*Walker: The Protein Protocols Handbook: Google Scholar*, n.d. Retrieved April 26, 2021, from https://scholar.google.com/scholar_lookup?title=The Protein Protocols Handbook&author=K Yamamoto&author=T Tsuji&author=T Osawa&author=JM Walker&publication_year=2002&book=The Protein Protocols Handbook

Xie, Y., Sheng, Y., Li, Q., Ju, S., Reyes, J. and Lebrilla, C.B., 2020. Determination of the glycoprotein specificity of lectins on cell membranes through oxidative proteomics. *Chemical Science* 11(35): 9501–9512.

Zhang, J., Shi, J., Ilic, S., Jun Xue, S. and Kakuda, Y., 2008. Biological properties and characterization of lectin from red kidney bean (*Phaseolus vulgaris*). *Food Reviews International* 25(1): 12–27.

CHAPTER 12

# Enzymatic Inhibitors (Protease inhibitors, Amylase inhibitors, Cholinesterase Inhibitors)

**Varun Kumar and Kanwate Balaji**

## CONTENTS



## 12.1 INTRODUCTION

Plant extracts and fractions are used for their basic health needs by 80% of the world's population. The history of mankind is described by the relationship between humans, medicinal plants, and drugs derived from medicinal plants. The phytochemicals are produced as secondary metabolites that contain several thousand compounds. Enzyme inhibitors are found in many natural products, and their discovery and production are active fields of pharmacology and biochemistry (Rauf & Jehan, 2017). As a result, inhibition of enzyme activity can obliterate a pathogen or accurate a metabolic inequity; several drug molecules are enzyme inhibitors, and often enzyme activators interact with different enzymes, raise their enzymatic actions, remove the connection, and distort the products in the enzymes' catalytic cycle (Rauf & Jehan, 2017). This chapter describes several phytoconstituents and plant species that function as α-amylase inhibitors, protease inhibitors (PIs), and acetylcholinesterase (AChE) inhibitors. The majority of research has been attracting these enzymes due to the significant modulation of a physiological disorder. Protease inhibitors (PIs), are reported from the secondary metabolites which are contributing strong beneficial agents in the regulation of disease through the inhibition of protease enzyme among them. Since 1938, the extensive circulation of protease inhibitors in the plant has been well recorded. Angiosperm seeds, including dicots and monocots, along with gymnosperm seeds, contain roughly 5–10% water-soluble protein

DOI: 10.1201/9781003178446-12

(Mutlu & Gal, 1999). Plant-derived protease inhibitors from three main families have been studied: *Fabaceae*, *Poaceae*, and *Solanaceae* (Richardson, 1991). Weder (1981) discovered that legume seed protein contains up to 6% PIs, while cereal contains about 10% PIs (Pusztai, 1972). PIs were later discovered in *Malvaceae*, *Rutaceae*, *Poaceae*, and *Moringaceae*, among other plant families (Tajini et al., 2012). Proteases are efficient executors of a common chemical event known as peptide bond hydrolysis. While most proteases cleave peptide connections between naturally occurring amino acids, other proteases have slightly altered responses. Exopeptidases (aminopeptidases and carboxypeptidases), which are directed by the NH2 and COOH termini of their corresponding substrates, target internal peptide bonds. On the other hand, the availability of structural and mechanistic information on these enzymes prompted the development of new classification schemes. Proteases are divided into six categories based on their catalytic mechanism: aspartic, glutamic, metalloproteases, cysteine, serine, and threonine proteases. Protease activity can be regulated *in vivo* via a variety of mechanisms, including gene regulation, commencement of inactive zymogens, obstruct by endogenous inhibitors, and targeting to particular compartments (Lopez & Bond, 2008).

The endoglucanase α-amylase (1,4-a-D-glucan-glucanohydrolase, EC3.2.1.1) hydrolyzes the endo α-(1,4) glycosidic linkages in starch and associated polysaccharides. The hydrolysis of starch is catalyzed first by α-amylase, which is found in human saliva, and then by pancreatic amylase, which is found in the duodenum. Human pancreatic α-amylase (HPA) is a key pharmacological mark for type 2 diabetes care. Inhibition of α-amylase, a starch, and glycogen digestion enzyme, is being investigated as a treatment for carbohydrate-absorption problems like overweight and hypertension, as well as dental caries and periodontal illnesses. Plants are a rich source of chemical constituents that can inhibit α-amylase, and they can be used as medicinal or usable food sources.

Acetylcholinesterase (AChE; E.C. 3.1.1.7) enzymes are present in all vertebrate organisms which are essential for mammalian survival, terminating cholinergic transmission at the neuromuscular junction. Since acetylcholinesterase (AChE) inhibitors are a common treatment for Alzheimer's disease, researchers are looking for new molecules with anti-AChE activity. The fact that naturally occurring compounds from plants are considered to be a potential source of new inhibitors has led to the identification of a large number of secondary metabolites and plant extracts with the ability to inhibit the enzyme AChE, which, according to the cholinergic hypothesis, increases the levels of the neurotransmitter acetylcholine in the brain, thereby improving cholinergia (Murray et al., 2013). Enzyme inhibitors are found in nature and are used and manufactured as an important part of pharmacology and biochemistry. Natural poisons are enzyme inhibitors that have evolved to protect a plant or animal from predators. The enzyme inhibitory capacity of natural compounds, medicinal plant extracts, and isolated compounds will be recorded in this book chapter.

## 12.2 CHEMISTRY

Many of the naturally occurring PIs, such as α-amylase, protease, and AChE, were further characterized by various plant species. Isookanin has been isolated from Spanish needles, *Bidens bipinnata*, and showed moderate inhibition activity on HPA (Figure 12.1) (Yang et al., 2012). Since isookanin contains two catecholic units, it is supposed to be a strong reductant, reducing iodine levels and causing false-positive results. Tiliroside is a noncompetitive inhibitor isolated from the seeds of the dog rose, *Rosa canina L.*, which inhibits porcine pancreas α-amylase (PPA) with an $IC_{50}$ of 280 mM and Ki values of 84.2 mM measured using p-nitrophenyl-alpha-D-pentaglucoside as a substrate. High-dose tiliroside is needed to reduce the postprandial plasma glucose concentration of mice treated with starch, possibly due to its poor α-amylase inhibition activity in animal models. Tiliroside can inhibit both sodium-dependent glucose transporter 1 and glucose transporter 2 mediated glucose uptake in enterocytes, resulting in anti-hyperglycemic (Figure 12.1) (Goto et al., 2012).

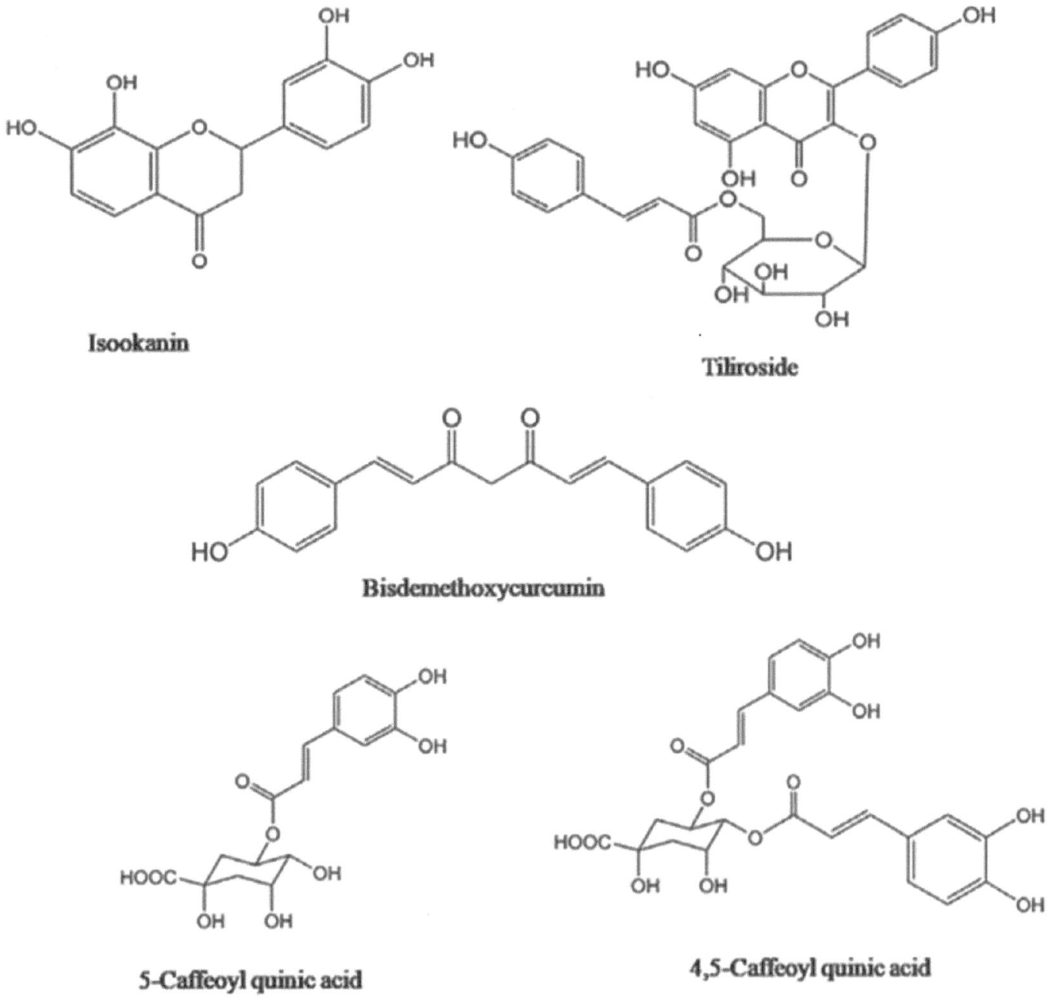


**Figure 12.1** α-amylase inhibitors: Chemical Structure of Isookanin, Tiliroside, Bisdemethoxycurcumin, and Caffeoylquinic acids (Source: Goto et al., 2012.)

Curcumin and its derivatives have been proposed as multi-targeting compounds with a wide variety of health advantages. Bisdemethoxycurcumin from the rhizome of *Curcuma longa* inhibits HPA and PPA, suggesting it may be used to reduce starch digestion rates. Kinetic study shows that it is an uncompetitive inhibitor of HPA with evident Ki of 3.0 mM (Ponnusamy et al., 2012). The major polyphenolic compounds present in green coffee beans are mono and disubstituted caffeoylquinic acids. There are three interconverting position isomers of monosubstituted caffeoylquinic acids and three dicaffeoyl quinic acids purified from green coffee beans due to the inclusion of three secondary hydroxyl groups in the quinic acid ring. The inhibition activity of these compounds on PPA-I (Narita & Inouye, 2011) was tested using p-nitrophenyl-diglucoside which, when hydrolyzed, produces p-nitrophenol and maltose. The inhibitory activity of monocaffeoyl quinic acid is highly dependent on the role of the caffeoyl groups.5-Caffeoylquinic acid (or generally known as chlorogenics acid) (see Figure 12.1) has a higher inhibition activity compared to that of 4-caffeoylquinic acid and 3-caffeoylquinic acids. Since 3,4- and 4,5-dicaffeoyl quinic acids have the same $IC_{50}$ values (20 mM), and 4,5-dicaffeoyl quinic acid has an $IC_{50}$ of 30 mM, the inhibitory activity of the three dicaffeoyl quinic acid isomers is much higher and less sensitive to the location of the ester groups (Narita & Inouye, 2011).

Anti-cholinesterase inhibitors (e.g., medications, natural toxins, pesticides, chemical warfare agents) are a wide class of chemical compounds with different physicochemical characteristics that inhibit the cholinesterase enzyme from decomposing ACh, thus increasing the amount and duration of the neurotransmitter action (Colovic et al., 2013; Pohanka, 2011). There are two types of AChE inhibitors: permanent and reversible. The majority of reversible inhibitors are used for medicinal purposes (Colovic et al., 2013). AChE is inhibited by three different types of compounds: nerve agents and tacrine are examples of compounds that bind to the active site and interact with either an esoteric or anionic site. Compounds that function in concert with the aromatic gorge, including decamethonium, as well as compounds, interact on the peripheral (β) anionic site, like huperzine and propidium *d*-tubocurarine (Pohanka, 2011). AChE inhibitory activity has been identified in several plants, suggesting that they may be useful in the management of different types of neurodegenerative disorders, including Alzheimer's disease. Ethnopharmacological methods and bioassay-guided isolation have led to the discovery of potential AChE and BuChE inhibitors in plants, including those for memory disorders (Suganthy et al., 2009). Figure 12.2 shows the structures of several essential anti-cholinesterase compounds. Alkaloids, terpenes, sterols, flavonoids, and glycosides make up the majority of these phytochemicals with possible AChE and BChE inhibitory action. The main forms of alkaloids with substantial anti-cholinesterase activity include triterpenoid alkaloids, steroidal alkaloids, indole alkaloids, isoquinoline alkaloid, and lycopodane type alkaloids, which are all capable agents for use as cholinesterase inhibitors in a clinical study.

## 12.3 DISTRIBUTION

Natural extracts obtained from plants have a broad range of pancreatic α-amylase inhibitors, that can be employed as oral medications in diabetes (Fred-Jaiyesimi, Kio, & Richard, 2009; Sudha, Zinjarde, Bhargava, & Ravi Kumar, 2011; Tundis, Loizzo, & Menichini, 2010).The chemical diversity of extract-derived molecules holds a lot of promise for new pharmacologically active compounds to be discovered. Tarling et al. (2008), for example, employed an extract from the Japanese garden plant *Crocosmia crocosmiiflora* to screen and isolate flavanols, glycosylated acyl, montbretins A, B, and C, as strong inhibitors of pancreatic α-amylase (Tarling et al., 2008). There are other flavonoids shown to be efficient inhibitors of salivary amylase, including luteolin and quercetin (Lo Piparo et al., 2008). Correspondingly, there are two potent molecules isolated from the Nepalese medicinal herb Pakhanbhed (*Bergenia ciliate*), (-)-3-O-galloylepicatechin and (-)-3-O-galloylcatechin, which were found to inhibit α-glucosidase and pancreatic α-amylase (Bhandari, Jong-Anurakkun, Hong, & Kawabata, 2008). *Curcuma longa* is a perennial *Zingiberaceae* plant found across the tropics, particularly in China, India, and Southeast Asia. For over 6,000 years, its tuber, which contains curcumin, has been utilized as a flavour and dish-colouring agent in a range of culinary uses (Kurup & Barrios, 2008). It contains a high concentration of sesquiterpenes and curcuminoids, which are responsible for a variety of biological effects Curcuminoids are anti-oxidant, anti-cancer, and anti-inflammatory compounds found in *Curcuma longa*. Bisdemethoxycurcumin (BDMC) prevents *C. longa* from inactivating human pancreaticα-amylase, a therapeutic object for type-2 diabetes oral hypoglycemic drugs. Tiliroside (kaempferol 3-O-(600-O-p-coumaroyl)-b-D-glucopy ranoside) is a glycosidic flavonoid establish in therapeutic and nutritional sources such as rose hips, linden, and strawberries (Matsuda et al., 2002; Ninomiya et al., 2007; Tsukamoto et al., 2004). In non-obese mice, tiliroside treatment substantially reduced body weight gain and visceral fat accumulation after fasting (Ninomiya et al., 2007). The researchers studied the impacts of tiliroside on carbohydrate digestion and absorption in the gastrointestinal tract and found that it reduced pancreatic-amylase-mediated carbohydrate digestion and also SGLT1- and GLUT2-mediated glucose transport in enterocytes (Goto et al., 2012).

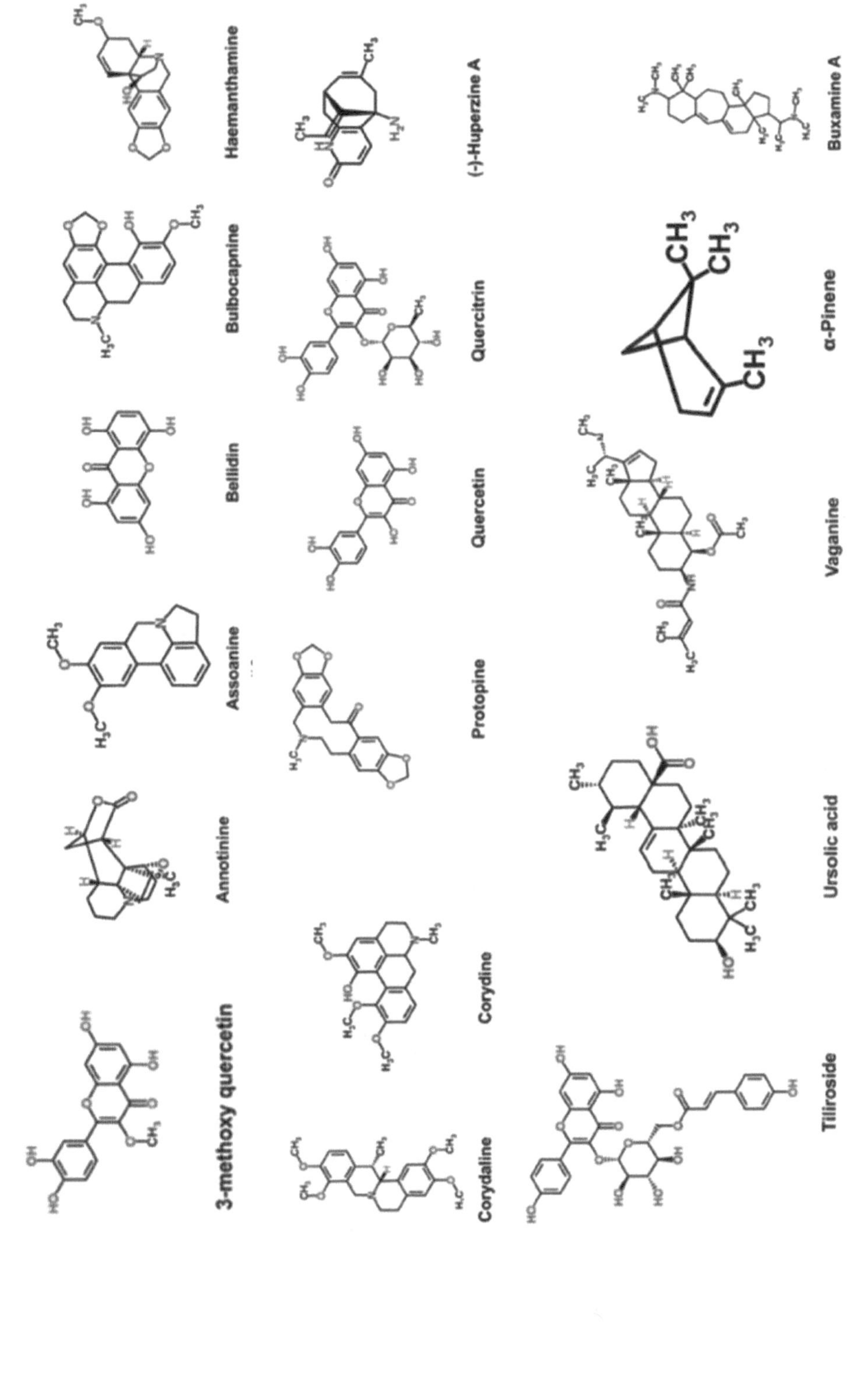


**Figure 12.2** Chemical Structure of some of important plant based AChE inhibitors. (Source: Ahmed et al., 2013.)

PIs have been isolated and characterized from a wide range of species, including animals, plants, and microbes (Christeller & Liang, 2005; Valueva & Mosolov, 2004; Haq et al., 2004; Mosolov et al., 2001; Mosolov & Valueva, 2005). PIs are needed to intend for the behaviour of their analogous proteases to be regulated, and they play an important regulatory role in a variety of biological processes. In the plant kingdom, PIs are very popular. Plant PIs (PPIs) are small proteins that have been found in the aerial parts of plants as well as in storage tissues including tubers and seeds (De Leo et al., 2002). Plants often produce them in reaction to damage or infection by pathogens or insects (Ryan, 1990). PIs function for the prevention of metabolic proteins in plants, interfering through insects' digestive processes. PIs are one of the most important defensive mechanisms used by plants to fight predators, and they are particularly effective against phytophagous insects and microorganisms. The proteins in family 13 Kunitz-type PPIs suppress serine peptidases, and they also comprise inhibitors of cysteine and aspartate proteases, according to Heibges et al. (2003). Serpin inhibitors are largely serine protease inhibitors, but they often comprise inhibitors of cysteine proteases. PIs have previously been divided into serine, cysteine, aspartate, and metallocarboxy PIs (Koiwa et al., 1997; De Leo et al., 2002; Laskowski et al., 2000). Some of the most important PIs have been illustrated in Table 12.1.

Many synthetic drugs have their origins in the plant world, and herbal medicines dominated our pharmacopoeia until around 200 years ago. In both ancient and modern cultures, medicinal plants play a significant role in health care. Many different plant sources have been used in the past to treat learning and memory problems. Furthermore, there is an increasing interest in the importance and application of natural resources in the treatment and improvement of cognitive impairments, Alzheimer's disease (AD), and its related pathologies. There are many compounds with anti-AChE activity (Table 12.2) reported. The structures of some important anti-cholinesterase compounds. Alkaloids, terpenes, sterols, flavonoids, and glycosides make up the majority of these phytochemicals with possible AChE inhibitory action. The main forms of alkaloids with substantial anti-cholinesterase activity include steroidal alkaloids, triterpenoid alkaloids, an isoquinoline alkaloid, indole alkaloids, and lycopodane-type alkaloids, making them capable agents for use as cholinesterase inhibitors in a clinical study.

## 12.4 MECHANISM OF ACTION

The α-amylase reaction mechanism involves using the retaining double displacement method to catalyze substrate hydrolysis (Van et al., 2002; Koshland, 1953). The active site contains two catalytic residues: glutamic acid and aspartic acid. The former behaves as an acid/base catalyst throughout degradation, helping to stabilize transition states, whereas the latter serves as a nucleophile throughout transition creation. Electron transfer from the glutamic acid to the glucosidic oxygen (i.e., the oxygen between two glucose molecules at subsites -1 and +1) occurs until the substrates are coupled to the active site, at which point the nucleophilic aspartate binds the glucose C (1) at subsite -1. As a result of these two events, the glycosidic bond is broken, and an oxocarbonium proton transition state is changed to a covalent intermediate. Water or a fresh glucose molecule replaces the protonated glucose molecule at the +1 subsite, attacking the glycosyl-enzyme transitional and forming an oxocarbonium proton transition state. Glutamate works by removing a proton from either water or a newly formed glucose molecule. The hydroxyl group at C1 (water) or a novel glycosidic bond between the -1 and +1 subsites is formed by oxygen from the incoming water or glucose molecule. Additional aspartic acid residues, in addition to glutamic acid and aspartic acid residues, indirectly contribute to activation by binding to the substrate's OH (2) and OH(3), causing substrate deformation (Uitdehaag et al., 1999). Apart from active site residues, homologous residues such as histidine, arginine, and tyrosine play an important role in guiding the substrate into the active site. They also control the nucleophile's correct orientation as well as the electrical

**Table 12.1 List of Protease Inhibitors Which Are Generated from the Plants Source**

| Protease Inhibitors | Origin | Role and Function | Reference |
|---|---|---|---|
| Protease inhibitor under Bowman-Brik | *Glycine max* | Degradation of immunoglobulins | Komarnytsky et al., 2006 |
| Protease inhibitor under Bowman-Brik | *Oryza sativa* | Inhibition of fungal growth | Qu et al., 2003 |
| Protease inhibitor under Bowman-Brik | *Vicia faba* | Inhibition of mycelia growth through reduction of trypsin and chymotrypsin activity | Ye et al., 2001 |
| Bowman-Brik from Soyabean inhibitor | *Glycine max* | Block the digestive protease through inhibition of aphid growth | Azzouz et al., 2005 |
| Trypsin and Chymotrypsin inhibitor | *Nicotiana alata* | Inhibition of extracellular protease | Kim et al., 2007 |
| Bowman-Brik trypsin inhibitor, Chymotrypsin/subtilisin inhibitor 2 | *Hordeum vulgare* | Blocking of subtilisin and trypsin | Pekkarinen et al., 2007 |
| Serpin1 | *Arabidopsis thaliana* | Blocking the digestive protease | Rustgi et al., 2017; Stuiver and Custers, 2011 |
| Kunitz-type protease inhibitor | *Arabidopsis thaliana* | Blocking the cysteineRD21 activity | Roberts et al., 2011; Rustgi et al., 2017 |
| Kunitz-type protease inhibitor | *Arabidopsis thaliana* | Blocking the serine and cysteine protease activity | Arnaiz et al., 2018 |
| Trypsin inhibitor from Cowpea | *Vigna unguiculata* | Inhibition of larval growth | Lingling et al., 2005; Pujol et al., 2005; Hilder et al., 1987 |
| Potato-type I inhibitor | *Solanum tuberosum*, *Nicotiana alata* | Inhibition of protease action | Dunse et al., 2010 |
| Potato-type I inhibitor | *Solanum tuberosum* | After injury and nematode infection, several expression patterns emerge | Turra et a al., 2009 |
| Potato carboxypeptidase inhibitor | *Solanum tuberosum* | Larval growth inhibition; anti-fungal activity | Quilis et al., 2007, 2014 |
| Phloem serpin-1 | *Cucurbita maxima* | Elastase inhibition | Yoo et al., 2000; Petersen et al., 2005 |
| Maize protease inhibitor | *Zea mays* | Serine protease inhibition; restricting the larval and fungal growth | Quilis et al., 2014; Vila et al., 2005 |
| Kunitz-type inhibitor from passion fruit | *Passiflora edulis Sims* | Midgut protease inhibition in lepidopteran and coleonpteran pests, as well as *Aedes aegyapti* | Botelho et al., 2014 |
| Kunitz trypsin inhibitor | *Populus Trichocarpa x p Opulus deltoides* | Midgut protease inhibition in lepidopteran and coleonpteran pests | Major and Constabel et al., 2008 |
| Kunitz inhibitor from soybean | *Glycine max* | Blocking the digestive protease in insect and parasites | Azzouz et al., 2005; Major and Constabel et al., 2008; Lee et al., 1999 |
| Serine protease inhibitor | *Arabidopsis thaliana* | Chymotrypsin inhibition; reducing the growth of larva and fungal | Laluk, 2011 |
| Serine protease inhibitor | *Beta vulgaris* | Trypsin inhibitory activity; reducing the larval growth | Smigocki et al., 2013 |
| Serine protease inhibitor | *Solanum tuberosum* | Inhibition of Trypsin and chymotrypsin | Valueva et al., 1998 |

*(Continued)*

**Table 12.1 (Continued) List of Protease Inhibitors Which Are Generated from the Plants Source**

| Protease Inhibitors | Origin | Role and Function | Reference |
|---|---|---|---|
| Serine protease inhibitor | *Fagopyrum sculentum* | Spore germination, mycelial growth, insect survival, and bacterial development are all inhibited. | Dunaevsky et al., 1997; Cheng et al., 2015 |
| Serine protease inhibitor | *Hordeum vulgare* | Inhibition of midgut protease; reducing the growth of larva and insect | Altpeter et al., 1999; Alfonso et al., 2003; Hamza et al., 2018 |
| Serine protease inhibitor | *Solanum nigrum* | Inhibit the serine protease PI-I and PI-II | Hartl et al., 2010 |
| Potato Type II protease inhibition | *Solanum americanum* | Inhibition of midgut protease | Dunse et al., 2010; Luo et al., 2012 |
| Kunitz trypsin inhibitor | *Adenanthera payonina* | Inhibition of trypsin, papain protease, midgut protease, and larval growth | Migliolo et al., 2010; da silva et la., 2014 |
| Kazal-type inhibitor | *Arabidopsis thaliana* | Reducing the conidial germination | Pariani et al., 2016 |
| Tomato catherpsin D inhibitor | *Solanum tuberosum* | Improvement of protein stability | Castilho et al., 2014; Goulet et al., 2012; Robert et al., 2013; Grosse-Holz et al., 2018 |

polarization of the substrate structure (Uitdehaag et al., 1999; Nakamura et al., 1993; Strockopytov et al., 1996; Muralikrishna & Nirmala, 2005). The mechanism of the α-amylase reaction is depicted in Figure 12.3 (Muralikrishna & Nirmala, 2005).

Two distinct protein domains make up the AChE molecule. The first is a massive catalytic domain with about 500 residues, while the second is a small C-terminal peptide with fewer than 50 residues. A membrane separates the anionic and esteratic subsites of AChE's active site. The anionic subsite attaches to the positive quaternary amine in acetylcholine, whereas the esteratic subsite hydrolyzes it into acetate and choline. Hydrolysis of the carboxyl ester yields an acyl-enzyme and free choline. A water molecule nucleophilically attacks the acyl-enzyme, generating acetic acid and renewing the liberated enzymes (Lionetto et al., 2013).The enzyme's catalytic machinery is located at the esteratic site. This is because Cholinesterases use a catalytic triad of Ser200–His440–Glu327 to increase the nucleophilicity of the catalytic serine. Gly118, Gly119, and Ala20120 make up the "oxyanion hole" (OH). The oxyanion hole containing these three peptide residues is a more useful motif for stabilizing Ach's tetrahedral intermediate than the two-pronged structures in serine proteinases (Houghton et al., 2006; Tougu, 2001). The "anionic subsite," also known as the "choline-binding subsite" or "hydrophobic subsite," is mostly aromatic residues and contains Trp84, Phe330, and Glu199. AChEs have different "peripheral anionic sites" (PAS). TcAChE is made up of aromatic and carboxylic acid residues, including Asp72, Tyr70, Tyr121, Trp279, and Phe290. Phe288 and Phe290 make up the "acyl bag," also known as the "acyl binding pocket" or "acyl-binding pocket." These are thought to play a role in controlling the size of substrates that can reach the active site20. AChE is found in three isoforms: G1 in the liver, G4 in the brain and neuromuscular endplate, and G2 in the rest of the body (Suganthy et al., 2009). Binding occurs at the active site at the bottom of the gorge in the case of alkaloids inhibitors, and positively charged nitrogen appears to be a key feature of the inhibitor. It binds to the oxyanion hole sector, primarily Trp84, as well as a lipophilic region separated from the positive charge. It inhibits AChE activity by forming hydrogen bonds with serine 200 and other catalytic residues like His 440. Some inhibitors bind to the gorge's rim as well as the peripheral anionic region (Suganthy et al., 2009). The carbonyl group of the carbamate moiety interacts with the hydroxyl group of serine 200, which is present in the catalytic triad of AchE, to form an ester in the urethane sections of the molecule. The ester is slowly hydrolyzed

**Table 12.2 AChE-Inhibitors Derived from the Plant-Based Sources**

| AChE- Inhibitors | Class Compound | Family | Plant | References |
|---|---|---|---|---|
| Lycorine, Tazettine, Crinine, 3–epi–hydroxybulbispermine, 2–demethoxy–montanine, Galanthamine | Alkaloids | *Amaryllidacae* | *Galanthus ikariae* | Ahmed et al., 2013 |
| Conypododiol | Alkaloids | *Asparagaceae* | *Asparagus adscendens* | Khan et al., 2011 |
| Bulbocapnin, corydaline | Alkaloids | *Fumariaceae* | *Corydalis cava* | Adsersen et al., 2007 |
| Gnidioidine Lycofoline, Acrifoline, Anhydrolycodolin, Annotinine, Annotine, Annotine N-oxide, Lycodoline, LycoposerramineM | Alkaloids | *Lycopodiaceae* | *Lycopodium annotinum* | Ahmed et al., 2013; Halldorsdottir et al., 2010 |
| Buxakarachiamine, Buxakashmiramin, Buxahejramine, Cyclomicrophylline-A, Cyclovirobuxeine–A, Cycloprotobuxine–C | Triterpenoid alkaloid | *Buxaceae* | *Buxus papillosa* | Ahmed et al., 2013; Parveen et al., 2001 |
| Stepharanine, cyclanoline, and *N*-methyl stepholidine | Quaternary protoberberine alkaloids | *Menispermaceae* | *Stephania venosa* | Murray et al., 2013 |
| (–)–huperzine A | Quinolizidine alkaloid | *Lycopodiaceae* | *Huperzia serrata* | Ahmed et al., 2013; Xi-can et al., 1994 |
| Uleine, Geissospermine | Indole alkaloid | *Apocynaceae* | *Himatanthus lancifolius, Geissospermum vellosii Allemao* | Murray et al., 201334, Williams et al., 2011 |
| Turbinatine and desoxycordifolie | Indole alkaloid | *Rubiaceae* | *Chimarrhis turbinata* | Suganthy et al., 2009 |
| Rutaecarpine and dehydroevodiamine | Indole alkaloid | *Rutaceae* | *Evodia rutaecarpa (Juss.) Benth* | Williams et al., 2011 |
| LegusinA, Corynoline | Indole alkaloid | *Papilionaceae* | *Desmodium pulchellum* and *D. gangeticum, Corydalis incise* | Suganthy et al., 2009 |
| Protopine, Palmatine, corynoxidine | Isoquinoline alkaloid | *Papaveraceae* | *Corydalis ternate, Corydalis speciosa* | Kim et al., 1999, 2004 |
| Berberine | | *Berberine* | *Rhizoma Coptidis* | Ji and Shen, 2011; Tang et al., 2009 |
| Hookerian H, Hookeriana I, Sarcovagine C, Homomoenjodaramine, moenjodaramine, EpipachysamineD, Dictyophlebine | steroidal alkaloid | *Buxaceae* | *Sarcococca hookeriana, Buxus hyrcana* | Johnson et al., 2013 |
| Isosarcodine, Sarcorine, Sarcodine, Sarcocine, Alkaloid–C, Sarsalignone, Vaganine, Buxamine B | Steroidal alkaloid | *Buxaceae* | *Sarcococca saligna, Buxus hyrcana, Buxus papillosa* | Ahmed et al., 2013; Choudhary, 2001; Khalid et al., 2004 |

*(Continued)*

**Table 12.2 (Continued) AChE-Inhibitors Derived from the Plant-Based Sources**

| AChE- Inhibitors | Class Compound | Family | Plant | References |
|---|---|---|---|---|
| Assoanine, 11–hydroxygalantamine, Epinorgalantamine, Sanguinine | Steroidal alkaloid | *Amaryllidaceae* | *Narcissus assoanus*, *Narcissus confuses*, *Eucharis grandiflora* | Lopez et al., 2002; Ahmed et al., 2013 |
| Α–pinene, β–pinene, Ursolic acid | Monoterpene, Pentacyclic triterpene acid | *Lamiaceae* | *Salvia potentillifolia*, *Origanum majorana* | Kivrak et al., 2009; Chung et al., 2001 |
| (+)-limonene, trans-anethole, (+)–sabinene | Terpene | *Apiaceae* | *Pimpinella anisoides* | Ahmed et al., 2013 |
| E)-β-caryophyllene, bicyclogermacrene | Sesquiterpines | *Compositae* | *Gynura bicolor DC.* | Miyazawa et al., 2016 |
| 3-Methoxy quercetin, Quercetin, Quercitrin, Quercitrin, Tiliroside | Flavonoid | *Rosaceae* | *Agrimonia pilosa* | Jung and Park, 2007 |
| quercetin-3-O- β-D-glucopyranoside, quercetin- 3-*O*-α-L-rhamnopyranosyl-(1→6)-β-D-glucopyranoside | Flavonol-*O*-glycosides | *Ginkgoaceae* | *Ginkgo biloba* | Ding et al., 2013 |
| Curcumin, bisdemethoxy curcumin, and demethoxycurcumin | Curcuminoid | *Zingiberaceae* | *Curcuma longa* L. | Ahmed and Gilani, 2009 |

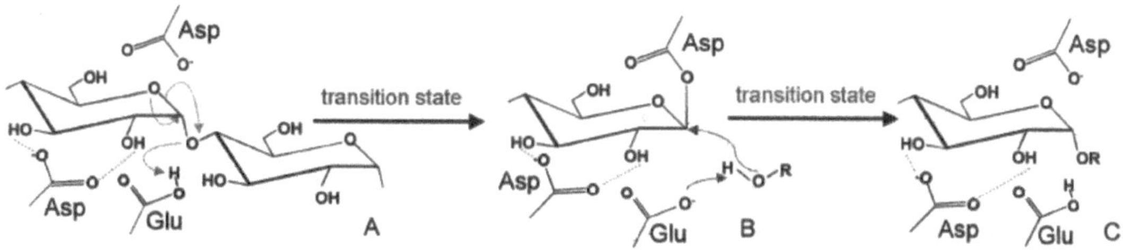


**Figure 12.3** α-amylase reaction mechanism of double displacement method. (Source: Van der Maarel et al., 2002.)

to regenerate the active parent form, interfering with the enzyme's AChE inhibitory property. As a result, the carbamate group plays a key role in AChE inhibitory action. Furthermore, the presence of an aromatic ring and a nitrogen atom promotes inhibitor binding to AChE, inhibiting its action (Suganthy et al., 2009).

Galanthamine binds to the bottom of AChE's active site gorge, interacting with both the coline-binding site and the acyl-binding pocket (Suganthy et al., 2009). The hydroxyl group at C-3 on galantamine is responsible for its successful binding to AChE, according to a structure–activity relationship analysis. Galantamine has a dual-action mechanism on the cholinergic system. It inhibits AChE and modulates nAChR activity allosterically. Galantamine binds to AChE in the brain, lowering ACh catabolism and increasing ACh levels in the synaptic cleft (Ng et al., 2015). Because of the catechol moiety in its structure, flavonoid derivatives display AChE inhibitory action, according to Ji and Zhang (2006).

Proteases are enzymes that break down polypeptide peptide linkages. Proteases are categorized according to the chemical groups involved in active catalytic. The hydroxyl group in the side chain of a serine residue in the binding site works as a nucleophile in the process that catalyzes the hydrolysis of a peptide bond in serine proteases, while the sulfhydryl group with an inside chain of a cysteine side chain does so in cysteine proteases. The nucleophile that assaults the peptide bond in aspartic acid proteases and metalloproteases is a water molecule in the binding site (arranged through binding with just an aspartyl group or a metal ion, accordingly). However, proteases can have the same catalytic mechanism but will be unrelated in amino acid sequence, as products of convergent evolution. Several authors have thoroughly reviewed the mechanisms of protease–inhibitor interaction (Chothia & Lesk, 1986; Bateman & James, 2011; Joshi et al., 2013). Inhibitors can interrelate proteases in a variety of pathways, but mainly two pathways are common for interaction (Rawlings et al., 2004). Irreversible trapping reaction is one of them which is shown by the best-known families of protease inhibitors. Irreversible trapping reaction corresponds to the serpins (I4), 2 macroglobulins, and baculovirus protein p35 inhibitors families of proteins (Rawlings et al., 2004,2010).The interaction between the protease and the inhibitor causes the hydrolysis of the peptide bond, which causes a conformational transition (see Figure 12.4A). This is a non-reversible reaction, and the inhibitor certainly does not return to its original structure. As a result, enzymes involved in trapping reactions are often referred to as suicide inhibitors. A tight-binding reaction is another often found mechanism of protease–inhibitor interaction. This mechanism is also known as a regular mechanism, and Laskowski and Qasim (2000), as well as Farady and Craik et al. (2010) have extensively identified it. This mechanism is used by all inhibitors, and it has been demonstrated for serine protease inhibitors (Rawlings et al., 2004). The standard mechanism of inhibition is used by the majority of plant serine protease inhibitors (SPIs) (Bateman and James, 2011). The inhibitors engage with the protease active site (P1) in a way similar to the enzyme-substrate interaction in strong-binding processes (see Figure 12.4B).The canonical inhibitors are also capable of inhibiting serine proteinases by various P1 specificities. The Potato II, Bowman-Birk, and Kunitz families can

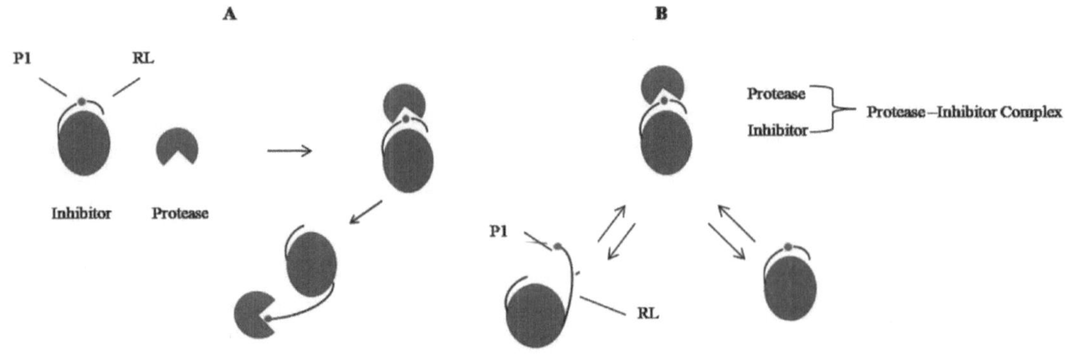


**Figure 12.4** Protease–inhibitor interaction mechanisms. (A) Trapping reactions that are irreversible. The interaction between the protease and the inhibitor causes the hydrolysis of peptide bond in the inhibitor structure, resulting in a conformational transition. (B) Tight-binding relationships which is reversible. In a similar way to the enzyme–substrate interaction, the inhibitor interacts with the protease active site. The stable form of inhibitor and changed forms of inhibitor but peptide bond of reactive site is hydrolysed coexist in a stable equilibrium in the protease-inhibitor complex. As a result, the complex's inhibitor is dissociated into its intact or modified form. RL: reactive loop; P1: PI reactive site. (Source: Clemente et al., 2019.)

all object multiple proteinases at once, with varying degrees of specificity (Chothia & Lesk, 1986). Plant SPIs that use this technique help plants prepare for unwanted proteolytic action, whether it's to monitor growth or protect against pest attack.

## 12.5 TOXICOLOGY

In the theoretical notion that natural products are safer than synthetic alternatives, plants are known to contain toxic molecules. As a result, assessing a natural product's potentially toxic effects is essential to ensure its protection and potential interest in biotechnological applications. This is accomplished by a variety of approaches, including the *in vitro* evaluation of acute toxic effects on mammalian cell lines. The inhibition of acetyl- and butyrylcholinesterase (AChE, BuChE), -glucosidase, α-amylase, and tyrosinase was studied. The extracts were non-toxic and mostly composed of flavonoids and a few compounds (roseoside and oleuropein). Natural-source molecules have a high degree of similarity and binding ability to biological structures, raising the chances of contact with a variety of biological targets (Lahlou, 2013; Placines et al., 2020). Such enzymes include AChE and BuChE, which are associated with Alzheimer's disease (AD), tyrosinase, which is connected to hyperpigmentation disorders, and glucosidase as well α-amylase, which are associated with Type 2 Diabetes Mellitus (T2DM). Several medicines have been explored in clinical studies to modify the condition reported due to their enzymatic inhibitory character (e.g., acarbose for T2DM, galantamine for AD, and kojic acid for hyperpigmentation). Nonetheless, because of the potential for unwanted effects, the pharmaceutical and cosmetic industries are increasingly interested in identifying better, more effective, and less harmful natural enzymatic inhibitors (e.g., gastrointestinal disturbances and hepatotoxicity). The extract in opioids was studied using RAW 264.7 macrophages, HEK 293 (human embryonic kidney), and HepG2 (human liver cancer). The colorimetric assay 3-(4,5-dimethylthiazol-2-yl)-2,5-diphenyltetrazolium bromide (MTT) was used to measure cellular viability (Rodrigues et al., 2014). Toxic effects of PIs from *S. aculeatissimum* (SAPI) have been assessed in an animal model until they can be used in biological applications. Fruits had the highest PI activity compared to leaves, roots, and seeds, with 54% trypsin inhibitory activity and 48% chymotrypsin inhibitory activity. All of the animals gained weight normally, with only minor differences between the control and treated classes. By the conclusion of the treatment phase, no behavioural changes or death were found. Similarly, during this period, no substantial differences in food consumption or weight gain were found between the control and treated classes. There were no major differences between the control and the serum glutamate oxaloacetate transaminase (SGOT), serum glutamate pyruvate transaminase (SGPT), alkaline phosphatase (ALP), total protein, albumin, globulin, and bilirubin levels. All of the findings were linked to the positive control, Kunitz Soy PI, which had identical haematological and biochemical patterns to the control (Krishnan & Murugan, 2016).

## 12.6 IDENTIFICATION AND QUANTIFICATION

PIs are the peptides or the proteins, have catalytic activity of enzymes/proteins, and are widely distributed in nature from viruses to all kingdoms. There are several methods to identify the PIs, caseinolytic plate assay is one of them. This is a visual method to detect the PIs. This method can be carried out using a bore well on the agar and casein plates. In the middle, well trypsin can be added and the surrounding wells were filled with the samples having PIs. After keeping for incubation, the inhibition was stopped using TCA. After that, we can identify the reduced zone which was due to the inhibition of protease trypsin. This is how one can identify the presence and absence of PIs in the given sample.

To quantify the activity of the PIs one can carry out the enzyme assay in the presence and absence of a given sample. The substrate would be casein in buffer solution (Kunitz, 1947). The protein trypsin was prepared in buffer and incubated with PI. The substrate was also prepared in the given buffer, added to the earlier mixture, and allowed to incubate. Then the reaction is terminated by adding the TCA solution. Then the following solution is subjected to centrifugation to remove the debris. Then read the supernatant against the blank in the spectrophotometer at 280 nm. In this reaction, the casein peptides were formed by the enzyme trypsin. Then these peptides were dissolved in TCA. These peptides were quantified using tyrosine as a standard. In the presence of the PI, the tyrosine activity will be reduced resulting in the formation of fewer casein peptides and vice versa. More of the casein peptides means more tyrosine activity and less PI activity. 1 U of protein activity is the amount of protein (enzyme) which releases 1 μg of tyrosine/mL of the mixture/min under a given condition. 1 U of PI activity was defined as the decrease in 1 U of OD of released casein peptides by the action of trypsin/min under given conditions (Mohan et al., 2018).

The amylase inhibitory (AIs) activity was identified and quantified by various methods. The extract having AIs mixed with amylase and buffer. Then the soluble starch was added as substrate and the reaction mixture was kept for incubation. The reaction mixture was terminated by keeping the mixture at a high temperature for 5 min. After that, one can read the absorbance of the resultant mixture. Then the AI can be quantified using maltose as standard. The HPLC-MS/MS can also be done to know the frequency of the various inhibitors within the samples. The extracts having AIs were validated with the peptide standards (Rogniaux et al., 2015). The varying amount of the AIs samples and internal standards were injected for the linear response of the specific peptides. The internal standards were used to show the matrix effect.

The sample having AI were mixed with the buffer and the enzyme solution. Then allow the mixture to incubate. Then the substrates were added in the form of starch mixed with the buffer and allowed to incubate the solution mixture. Then the reaction can be terminated using the appropriate reagent (DNS colour reagent) and kept in a boiling water bath for 10 min. Then the absorbance was measured. The acarbose was used as a standard inhibitor for the enzyme. The AIs also can be quantified using HPLC-DAD. Quantitative estimation was carried using the standard solution calibration curve.

The identification of AChEI can be carried out by using various ways: pharmacophore-based virtual screening, molecular docking, and bioassay.

## 12.7 SAFETY, PRECAUTIONS, AND REGULATION

Switching the PIs to the other forms or inhibitors may improve the reverse inhibitory effect like in the case of diseased conditions, switching the PIs to the non-nucleoside reverse transcriptase inhibitors may improve the diseased conditions (Ruiz et al., 2001;Negredo et al., 2002, Martinez et al., 1999; Moyle & Baldwin, 2000).

## 12.8 EFFECT OF PROCESSING (DRYING, FERMENTATION, BOILING, AUTOCLAVING, BAKING, BROILING, COOKING, FREEZING, FRYING, ROASTING, AND GERMINATION)

The PI shows the increased enzyme inhibitory activity in the soaked beans. The activity was dependent on the time of soaking (Shi et al., 2017; Wang et al., 2008). This activity might be due to the low leaching out effect during hydration, indicating less loss of the PI in the water. Lower heating temperature for a longer time may cleave the peptides of PIs, leading to the inactivation of the enzyme activity. When the heating was at boiling temperature the amylase inhibitors showed increased activity. The PI activity for most seeds was resistant to heating. Wati et al. (2010) stated that when the temperature increased to a higher level, the compact structure of the trypsin loosens reversibly. Furthermore, Morrison et al. (2007) suggested that the PIs might be heat stable due to their resistance against the higher heat. Vidal-Valverde et al (1997) stated that, although the PIs are from different sources, they may differ in the structure, molecule weight and composition, but have the same catalytic site. Habiba (2002), Hefnawy (2011), and Osman et al. (2002) explained that the autoclaving of raw materials like seeds (source of many PIs) resulted in the inactivation of the inhibitory activity of PIs. Slow freezing may encourage the formation of non-uniform ice crystals. This results in the breakage of the tissue (Mok et al., 2015). In dried seeds, due to the low moisture content, this loss is relatively less (Li & Sun, 2002). All these studies show the extent of enzyme inhibition inactivation by various processing methods is varied and dependent on the source of the material.

## 12.9 FUTURE SCOPE

In the last few years, new types of interesting inhibitors have been identified at a rapid rate. These inhibitors play an important role in exogenous defence in plants. Proteases play an important role in disease progression. An imbalance in proteolytic activity is responsible for a significant number of human diseases. PIs play an important role in the endogenous defence system because they help control and stabilize protease activity. Many plant-based protease inhibitors are presently in clinical trials, and several pharmaceutical firms are interested (Clemente & Arques, 2014; Clemente et al., 2010). Many plant protease inhibitors' sequences and crystal structures are accessible. Just a small number are applied in medicine as well as undergoing clinical trials (Majumdar, 2013). Plant protease inhibitors have some benefits over synthetic protease inhibitors. PPIs can also be obtained via the diet by supplementing with additional plant-based food preparations that have no harmful effects on the human body. To find potential candidates for protease inhibitors with therapeutic value derived from plants, further research is required. Given the growing population and diseases, additional PPIs for use in the management and regulation of diseases are required. This research demonstrates the enormous potential of PI derived from the plant.

There are, however, more questions that need to be answered to clear the way for functional food products containing starch hydrolase inhibitors as active ingredients. The inhibition mechanisms of the newly discovered inhibitors should be investigated further using an enzyme inhibition kinetic analysis combined with an in silico molecular docking study of the inhibitor's interaction with the enzyme. This will aid in comprehending the structural features of inhibitors that are essential for their function, as well as providing details for justification design or the quest for new types of more potent inhibitors. Different types of starch hydrolase have been shown to respond differently to inhibitors. As a result, it's important to test inhibition activity using mammalian enzymes so that the results apply to the human system.

Alzheimer's disease has a significant impact on people's personal and social lives, and cholinesterase inhibitors undoubtedly aid in the successful management and treatment of the disease. It is well established that alkaloids are the main phytoconstituents responsible for plant extracts' anti-cholinesterase function, and this knowledge could be used to develop new anti-cholinesterase drugs using alkaloids as intermediates. Even though a large number of natural plant extracts have been discovered to be effective inhibitors of AChE and BChE, only a few plants have been thoroughly researched. For optimal therapeutic use of these phytoconstituents, comprehensive studies involving amyloid and receptor-binding studies are needed. Furthermore, there is little information on the protection of both plant extracts and isolated phytoconstituents. Since there are so few animal experiments and clinical trials available, there is a need for further research in these fields. Alkaloids are the main compounds responsible for plant extracts' anti-cholinesterase activity, and these alkaloids can be used as starting materials for new types of synthetic drugs for the treatment of Alzheimer's disease. The scope of future research on the most effective plant-based inhibitors AChE, protease, and α-amylase is presented here.

## 12.10 CONCLUSION

Plants and plant-derived natural products can act as enzyme inhibitors. Researchers were led to extract bioactive compounds from plants that have excellent enzymatic activity in this book chapter. Because plant PIs have been isolated and characterized from a variety of sources, and because natural inhibitors have been made available through gene therapy and transgenic plants overexpressing particular inhibitors with therapeutic significance, the natural inhibitors' potential in medicine and agriculture is enormous, and it is still being fully explored. AchE inhibitors have therapeutic uses in Alzheimer's disease, senile dementia, ataxia, myasthenia gravis, and Parkinson's disease. The cholinergic system is the most powerful neurotransmitter system in the regulation of cognitive function. Herbal medicines are large chemical libraries that have been created for the treatment of Alzheimer's disease. Many medications currently on the market, such as plant alkaloids such as Galantamine, are aimed at treating Alzheimer's disease. Ayurveda, for example, is a traditional medicinal method that emphasizes health preservation and disease prevention over curative therapies. Diabetes mellitus is a metabolic disorder characterized by chronic hyperglycaemia and disturbances in carbohydrate, lipid, and protein metabolism caused by insulin secretion, intervention, or both. Postprandial hyperglycaemia reduction is the most important clinical method for diabetes treatment. The inhibition of enzymes that hydrolyze carbohydrates, such as alpha-amylase, is used to avoid glucose absorption.

## REFERENCES

Adsersen, A., Kjølbye, A., Dall, O., & Jäger, A. K. 2007. Acetylcholinesterase and butyrylcholinesterase inhibitory compounds from Corydalis cava Schweigg. & Kort. *Journal of Ethnopharmacology* 113(1): 179–182.

Ahmed, F., Ghalib, R. M., Sasikala, P., & Ahmed, K. M. 2013. Cholinesterase inhibitors from botanicals. *Pharmacognosy Reviews* 7(14): 121.

Ahmed, T., & Gilani, A. H. 2009. Inhibitory effect of curcuminoids on acetylcholinesterase activity and attenuation of scopolamine-induced amnesia may explain medicinal use of turmeric in Alzheimer's disease. *Pharmacology Biochemistry and Behavior* 91(4): 554–559.

Alfonso-Rubí, J., Ortego, F., Castañera, P., Carbonero, P., & Díaz, I. 2003. Transgenic expression of trypsin inhibitor CMe from barley in indica and japonica rice, confers resistance to the rice weevil Sitophilus oryzae. *Transgenic Research* 12(1): 23–31.

Altpeter, F., Diaz, I., McAuslane, H., Gaddour, K., Carbonero, P., & Vasil, I. K. 1999. Increased insect resistance in transgenic wheat stably expressing trypsin inhibitor CMe. *Molecular Breeding* 5(1): 53–63.

Arnaiz, A., Talavera-Mateo, L., Gonzalez-Melendi, P., Martinez, M., Diaz, I., & Santamaria, M. E. 2018. Arabidopsis Kunitz trypsin inhibitors in defense against spider mites. *Frontiers in Plant Science* 9: 986.

Azzouz, H., Campan, E. D. M., Cherqui, A., Saguez, J., Couty, A., Jouanin, L., & Kaiser, L. 2005. Potential effects of plant protease inhibitors, oryzacystatin I and soybean Bowman-Birk inhibitor, on the aphid parasitoid Aphidius ervi Haliday (Hymenoptera, Braconidae). *Journal of Insect Physiology* 51(8): 941–951.

Bateman, K., & NG James, M. 2011. Plant protein proteinase inhibitors: structure and mechanism of inhibition. *Current Protein and Peptide Science* 12(5): 341–347.

Bhandari, M. R., Jong-Anurakkun, N., Hong, G., & Kawabata, J. 2008. α-Glucosidase and α-amylase inhibitory activities of Nepalese medicinal herb Pakhanbhed (Bergenia ciliata, Haw.). *Food Chemistry* 106(1): 247–252.

Botelho-Júnior, S., Machado, O. L., Fernandes, K. V., Lemos, F. J., Perdizio, V. A., Oliveira, A. E., ... & Jacinto, T. 2014. Defense response in non-genomic model species: methyl jasmonate exposure reveals the passion fruit leaves' ability to assemble a cocktail of functionally diversified Kunitz-type trypsin inhibitors and recruit two of them against papain. *Planta* 240(2): 345–356.

Castilho, A., Windwarder, M., Gattinger, P., Mach, L., Strasser, R., Altmann, F., & Steinkellner, H. 2014. Proteolytic and N-glycan processing of human α1-antitrypsin expressed in Nicotiana benthamiana. *Plant Physiology* 166(4): 1839–1851.

Cheng, Z., Li, J. F., Niu, Y., Zhang, X. C., Woody, O. Z., Xiong, Y., ... & Ausubel, F. M. 2015. Pathogen-secreted proteases activate a novel plant immune pathway. *Nature* 521(7551): 213–216.

Chothia, C., & Lesk, A. M. 1986. The relation between the divergence of sequence and structure in proteins. *The EMBO Journal* 5(4): 823–826.

Choudhary, M. I. 2001. Bioactive natural products as a potential source of new pharmacophores. A theory of memory. *Pure and Applied Chemistry* 73(3): 555–560.

Christeller, J., & Liang, W. 2005. Plant serine protease inhibitors. *Protein and Peptide Letters* 12: 439–447.

Chung, Y. K., Heo, H. J., Kim, E. K., Kim, H. K., Huh, T. L., Lim, Y., ... & Shin, D. H. 2001. Inhibitory Effect of Ursolic Acid Purified from Origanum majorana L. on the Acetylcholinesterase. *Molecules & Cells* 11(2).

Clemente, A., & del Carmen Arques, M. 2014. Bowman-Birk inhibitors from legumes as colorectal chemopreventive agents. *World Journal of Gastroenterology: WJG* 20(30): 10305.

Clemente, A., Moreno, F. J., Marín-Manzano, M. D. C., Jiménez, E., & Domoney, C. 2010. The cytotoxic effect of Bowman–Birk isoinhibitors, IBB1 and IBBD2, from soybean (Glycine max) on HT29 human colorectal cancer cells is related to their intrinsic ability to inhibit serine proteases. *Molecular Nutrition & Food Research* 54(3): 396–405.

Clemente, M., Corigliano, M. G., Pariani, S. A., Sánchez-López, E. F., Sander, V. A., & Ramos-Duarte, V. A. 2019. Plant serine protease inhibitors: Biotechnology application in agriculture and molecular farming. *International Journal of Molecular Sciences* 20(6): 1345.

Colovic, M. B., Krstic, D. Z., Lazarevic-Pasti, T. D., Bondzic, A. M., & Vasic, V. M. 2013. Acetylcholinesterase inhibitors: pharmacology and toxicology. *Current Neuropharmacology* 11(3): 315–335.

da Silva, D. S., de Oliveira, C. F., Parra, J. R., Marangoni, S., & Macedo, M. L. 2014. Short and long-term antinutritional effect of the trypsin inhibitor ApTI for biological control of sugarcane borer. *Journal of Insect Physiology* 61: 1–7.

De Leo F, Volpicella M, Licciulli F, Liuni S, Gallerani R, & Ceci LR. 2002. Plant-PIs: a database for plant protease inhibitors and their genes. *Nucleic Acids Research* 30 (1): 347–348.

Ding, X., Ouyang, M. A., Liu, X., & Wang, R. Z. 2013. Acetylcholinesterase inhibitory activities of flavonoids from the leaves of Ginkgo biloba against brown planthopper. *Journal of Chemistry* 2013.

Dunaevsky, Y. E., Gladysheva, I. P., Pavlukova, E. B., Beliakova, G. A., Gladyshev, D. P., Papisova, A. I., ... & Belozersky, M. A. 1997. The anionic protease inhibitor BWI-1 from buckwheat seeds. Kinetic properties and possible biological role. *Physiologia Plantarum* 101(3): 483–488.

Dunse, K. M., Stevens, J. A., Lay, F. T., Gaspar, Y. M., Heath, R. L., & Anderson, M. A. 2010. Coexpression of potato type I and II proteinase inhibitors gives cotton plants protection against insect damage in the field. *Proceedings of the National Academy of Sciences* 107(34): 15011–15015.

Farady, C. J., & Craik, C. S. 2010. Mechanisms of macromolecular protease inhibitors. *Chembiochem* 11(17): 2341–2346.

Fred-Jaiyesimi, A., Kio, A., & Richard, W. 2009. α-Amylase inhibitory effect of 3β-olean-12-en-3-yl (9Z)-hexadec-9-enoate isolated from Spondias mombin leaf. *Food Chemistry* 116(1): 285–288.

Goto, T., Horita, M., Nagai, H., Nagatomo, A., Nishida, N., Matsuura, Y., & Nagaoka, S. 2012. Tiliroside, a glycosidic flavonoid, inhibits carbohydrate digestion and glucose absorption in the gastrointestinal tract. *Molecular Nutrition & Food Research* 56(3): 435–445.

Goulet, C., Khalf, M., Sainsbury, F., D'Aoust, M. A., & Michaud, D. 2012. A protease activity–depleted environment for heterologous proteins migrating towards the leaf cell apoplast. *Plant Biotechnology Journal* 10(1): 83–94.

Grosse-Holz, F., Madeira, L., Zahid, M. A., Songer, M., Kourelis, J., Fesenko, M., ... & van der Hoorn, R. A. 2018. Three unrelated protease inhibitors enhance accumulation of pharmaceutical recombinant proteins in Nicotiana benthamiana. *Plant Biotechnology Journal* 16(10): 1797–1810.

Habiba, R. A. 2002. Changes in anti-nutrients, protein solubility, digestibility, and HCl-extractability of ash and phosphorus in vegetable peas as affected by cooking methods. *Food Chemistry* 77(2): 187–192.

Halldorsdottir, E. S., Jaroszewski, J. W., & Olafsdottir, E. S. 2010. Acetylcholinesterase inhibitory activity of lycopodane-type alkaloids from the Icelandic Lycopodium annotinum ssp. alpestre. *Phytochemistry* 71(2–3): 149–157.

Hamza, R., Pérez-Hedo, M., Urbaneja, A., Rambla, J. L., Granell, A., Gaddour, K., ... & Cañas, L. A. 2018. Expression of two barley proteinase inhibitors in tomato promotes endogenous defensive response and enhances resistance to Tuta absoluta. *BMC Plant Biology* 18(1): 1–14.

Haq, S. K., Atif, S. M., & Khan, R. H. 2004. Protein proteinase inhibitor genes in combat against insects, pests, and pathogens: natural and engineered phytoprotection. *Archives of Biochemistry and Biophysics* 43(1): 145–159.

Hartl, M., Giri, A. P., Kaur, H., & Baldwin, I. T. 2010. Serine protease inhibitors specifically defend Solanum nigrum against generalist herbivores but do not influence plant growth and development. *The Plant Cell* 22(12): 4158–4175.

Hefnawy, T. H. 2011. Effect of processing methods on nutritional composition and anti-nutritional factors in lentils (Lens culinaris). *Annals of Agricultural Sciences* 56(2): 57–61.

Heibges, A., Salamini, F., & Gebhardt, C. 2003. Functional comparison of homologous members of three groups of Kunitz-type enzyme inhibitors from potato tubers (Solanum tuberosum L.). *Molecular Genetics and Genomics* 269(4): 535–541.

Hilder, V. A., Gatehouse, A. M., Sheerman, S. E., Barker, R. F., & Boulter, D. 1987. A novel mechanism of insect resistance engineered into tobacco. *Nature* 330(6144): 160–163.

Houghton, P. J., Ren, Y., & Howes, M. J. 2006. Acetylcholinesterase inhibitors from plants and fungi. *Natural Product Reports* 23(2): 181–199.

Ji, H. F., & Shen, L. 2011. Berberine: a potential multipotent natural product to combat Alzheimer's disease. *Molecules* 16(8): 6732–6740.

Ji, H. F., & Zhang, H. Y. 2006. Theoretical evaluation of flavonoids as multipotent agents to combat Alzheimer's disease. *Journal of Molecular Structure: Theochem* 767(1–3): 3–9.

Johnson, S., Marro, J., & Torres, J. J. 2013. Robust short-term memory without synaptic learning. *PloS One* 8(1): e50276.

Joshi, R. S., Mishra, M., Suresh, C. G., Gupta, V. S., & Giri, A. P. 2013. Complementation of intramolecular interactions for structural–functional stability of plant serine proteinase inhibitors. *Biochimica et Biophysica Acta (BBA)-General Subjects* 1830(11): 5087–5094.

Jung, M., & Park, M. 2007. Acetylcholinesterase inhibition by flavonoids from Agrimonia pilosa. *Molecules 12*(9): 2130–2139.

Khalid, A., Ghayur, M. N., Feroz, F., Gilani, A. H., & Choudhary, M. I. 2004. Cholinesterase inhibitory and spasmolytic potential of steroidal alkaloids. *The Journal of Steroid Biochemistry and Molecular Biology* 92(5): 477–484.

Khan, I., Nisar, M., Khan, N., Saeed, M., Nadeem, S., Ali, F., ... & Khan, I. A. 2011. Structural insights to investigate Conypododiol as a dual cholinesterase inhibitor from Asparagus adscendens. *Fitoterapia* 81(8): 1020–1025.

Kim, D. K., Lee, K. T., Baek, N. I., Kim, S. H., Park, H. W., Lim, J. P., ... & Eun, J. S. 2004. Acetylcholinesterase inhibitors from the aerial parts of Corydalis speciosa. *Archives of Pharmacal Research* 27(11): 1127–1131.

Kim, S. R., Hwang, S. Y., Jang, Y. P., Park, M. J., Markelonis, G. J., Oh, T. H., & Kim, Y. C. 1999. Protopine from Corydalis ternata has anticholinesterase and antiamnesic activities. *Planta Medica* 65(03): 218–221.

Kim, T. G., Kim, H. M., Lee, H. J., Shin, Y. J., Kwon, T. H., Lee, N. J., ... & Yang, M. S. 2007. Reduced protease activity in transformed rice cell suspension cultures expressing a proteinase inhibitor. *Protein Expression and Purification* 53(2): 270–274.

Kivrak, I., Duru, M. E., Öztürk, M., Mercan, N., Harmandar, M., & Topçu, G. 2009. Antioxidant, anticholinesterase and antimicrobial constituents from the essential oil and ethanol extract of Salvia potentillifolia. *Food Chemistry* 116(2): 470–479.

Koiwa, H., Bressan, R. A., & Hasegawa, P. M. 1997. Regulation of protease inhibitors and plant defense. *Trends in Plant Science* 2(10): 379–384.

Komarnytsky, S., Borisjuk, N., Yakoby, N., Garvey, A., & Raskin, I. 2006. Cosecretion of protease inhibitor stabilizes antibodies produced by plant roots. *Plant Physiology* 141(4): 1185–1193.

Koshland Jr, D. E. 1953. Stereochemistry and the mechanism of enzymatic reactions. *Biological Reviews* 28(4): 416–436.

Krishnan, V. M., & Murugan, K. 2016. Acute and subchronic toxicological evaluation of the purified protease inhibitor from the fruits of Solanum aculeatissimum Jacq. on Wistar rats. *Cogent Biology* 2(1): 1191588.

Kunitz, M. 1947. Crystalline soybean trypsin inhibitor II. General properties. *Journal of General Physiology* 30(4): 291–310.

Kurup, V. P., & Barrios, C. S. 2008. Immunomodulatory effects of curcumin in allergy. *Molecular Nutrition & Food Research* 52(9): 1031–1039.

Lahlou, M. 2013. The success of natural products in drug discovery.

Laluk, K., & Mengiste, T. 2011. The Arabidopsis extracellular unusual serine protease inhibitor functions in resistance to necrotrophic fungi and insect herbivory. *The Plant Journal* 68(3): 480–494.

Laskowski Jr, M., & Qasim, M. A. 2000. What can the structures of enzyme-inhibitor complexes tell us about the structures of enzyme substrate complexes?. *Biochimica et Biophysica Acta (BBA)-Protein Structure and Molecular Enzymology* 1477(1–2): 324–337.

Laskowski Jr, M., Qasim, M. A., & Lu, S. M. 2000. Interaction of standard mechanism, canonical protein inhibitors with serine proteinases. *Protein–Protein Recognition* 60(1): 228–279.

Lee, S. I., Lee, S. H., Koo, J. C., Chun, H. J., Lim, C. O., Mun, J. H., ... & Cho, M. J. 1999. Soybean Kunitz trypsin inhibitor (SKTI) confers resistance to the brown planthopper (Nilaparvata lugens Stål) in transgenic rice. *Molecular Breeding* 5(1): 1–9.

Li, B., & Sun, D. W. 2002. Novel methods for rapid freezing and thawing of foods–a review. *Journal of Food Engineering* 54(3): 175–182.

Lingling, L. V., Jianjun, L., Ming, S., Liyun, L., & Bihao, C. 2005. Study on transformation of cowpea trypsin inhibitor gene into cauliflower (Brassica oleracea L. var. botrytis). *African Journal of Biotechnology* 4(1): 45–49.

Lionetto, M. G., Caricato, R., Calisi, A., Giordano, M. E., & Schettino, T. 2013. Acetylcholinesterase as a biomarker in environmental and occupational medicine: new insights and future perspectives. *BioMed Research International* 2013 :1–9.

Lo Piparo, E., Scheib, H., Frei, N., Williamson, G., Grigorov, M., & Chou, C. J. 2008. Flavonoids for controlling starch digestion: structural requirements for inhibiting human α-amylase. *Journal of Medicinal Chemistry* 51(12): 3555–3561.

López, S., Bastida, J., Viladomat, F., & Codina, C. 2002. Acetylcholinesterase inhibitory activity of some Amaryllidaceae alkaloids and Narcissus extracts. *Life Sciences* 71(21): 2521–2529.

López-Otín, C., & Bond, J. S. 2008. Proteases: multifunctional enzymes in life and disease. *The Journal of Biological Chemistry* 283(45): 30433.

Luo, M., Ding, L. W., Ge, Z. J., Wang, Z. Y., Hu, B. L., Yang, X. B., ... & Xu, Z. F. 2012. The characterization of SaPIN2b, a plant trichome-localized proteinase inhibitor from Solanum americanum. *International Journal of Molecular Sciences* 13(11): 15162–15176.

Major, I. T., & Constabel, C. P. 2008. Functional analysis of the Kunitz trypsin inhibitor family in poplar reveals biochemical diversity and multiplicity in defense against herbivores. *Plant Physiology* 146(3): 888–903.

Majumdar, D. D. 2013. Recent updates on pharmaceutical potential of plant protease inhibitors. *International Journal of Medicine and Pharmaceutical Research* 3: 101–120.

Martínez, E., Conget, I., Lozano, L., Casamitjana, R., & Gatell, J. M. 1999. Reversion of metabolic abnormalities after switching from HIV-1 protease inhibitors to nevirapine. *Aids* 13(7): 805–810.

Matsuda, H., Ninomiya, K., Shimoda, H., & Yoshikawa, M. 2002. Hepatoprotective principles from the flowers of Tilia argentea (linden): structure requirements of tiliroside and mechanisms of action. *Bioorganic & Medicinal Chemistry* 10(3): 707–712.

Migliolo, L., de Oliveira, A. S., Santos, E. A., Franco, O. L., & Maurício, P. 2010. Structural and mechanistic insights into a novel non-competitive Kunitz trypsin inhibitor from Adenanthera pavonina L. seeds with double activity toward serine-and cysteine-proteinases. *Journal of Molecular Graphics and Modelling* 29(2): 148–156.

Miyazawa, M., Nakahashi, H., Usami, A., & Matsuda, N. 2016. Chemical composition, aroma evaluation, and inhibitory activity towards acetylcholinesterase of essential oils from Gynura bicolor DC. *Journal of Natural Medicines* 70(2): 282–289.

Mok, J. H., Choi, W., Park, S. H., Lee, S. H., & Jun, S. 2015. Emerging pulsed electric field (PEF) and static magnetic field (SMF) combination technology for food freezing. *International Journal of Refrigeration* 50: 137–145.

Mohan, M., Kozhithodi, S., Nayarisseri, A. and Elyas, K.K., 2018. Screening, purification and characterization of protease inhibitor from Capsicum frutescens. *Bioinformation*, 14(6): p.285.

Morrison, S. C., Savage, G. P., Morton, J. D., & Russell, A. C. 2007. Identification and stability of trypsin inhibitor isoforms in pea (Pisum sativum L.) cultivars grown in New Zealand. *Food Chemistry* 100(1): 1–7.

Mosolov, V. V., & Valueva, T. A. 2005. Proteinase inhibitors and their function in plants: a review. *Prikladnaia biokhimiia i mikrobiologiia* 41(3): 261–82.

Mosolov, V. V., Grigor'eva, L. I., & Valueva, T. A. 2001. Plant proteinase inhibitors as polyfunctional proteins (a review) *Prikladnaia biokhimiia i mikrobiologiia* 37(6): 643–50.

Moyle, G., & Baldwin, C. 2000. Switching from a PI-based to a PI-sparing regimen for management of metabolic or clinical fat redistribution. *The AIDS Reader* 10(8): 479–485.

Muralikrishna, G., & Nirmala, M. 2005. Cereal α-amylases—an overview. *Carbohydrate Polymers* 60(2): 163–173.

Murray, A. P., Faraoni, M. B., Castro, M. J., Alza, N. P., & Cavallaro, V. 2013. Natural AChE inhibitors from plants and their contribution to Alzheimer's disease therapy. *Current Neuropharmacology* 11(4): 388–413.

Mutlu, A., & Gal, S. 1999. Plant aspartic proteinases: enzymes on the way to a function. *Physiologia Plantarum* 105(3): 569–576.

Nakamura, A., Haga, K., & Yamane, K. 1993. Three histidine residues in the active center of cyclodextrin glucanotransferase from alkalophilic Bacillus sp. 1011: effects of the replacement on pH dependence and transition-state stabilization. *Biochemistry* 32(26): 6624–6631.

Narita, Y., & Inouye, K. 2011. Inhibitory effects of chlorogenic acids from green coffee beans and cinnamate derivatives on the activity of porcine pancreas α-amylase isozyme I. *Food Chemistry* 127(4): 1532–1539.

Negredo, E., Cruz, L., Paredes, R., Ruiz, L., Fumaz, C. R., Bonjoch, A., ...& Clotet, B. 2002. Virological, immunological, and clinical impact of switching from protease inhibitors to nevirapine or to efavirenz in patients with human immunodeficiency virus infection and long-lasting viral suppression. *Clinical Infectious Diseases* 34(4): 504–510.

Ng, Y. P., Or, T. C. T., & Ip, N. Y. 2015. Plant alkaloids as drug leads for Alzheimer's disease. *Neurochemistry International* 89: 260–270.

Ninomiya, K., Matsuda, H., Kubo, M., Morikawa, T., Nishida, N., & Yoshikawa, M. 2007. Potent anti-obese principle from Rosa canina: structural requirements and mode of action of trans-tiliroside. *Bioorganic & Medicinal Chemistry Letters* 17(11): 3059–3064.

Osman, M. A., Reid, P. M., & Weber, C. W. 2002. Thermal inactivation of tepary bean (Phaseolus acutifolius), soybean and lima bean protease inhibitors: effect of acidic and basic pH. *Food Chemistry* 78(4): 419–423.

Pariani, S., Contreras, M., Rossi, F. R., Sander, V., Corigliano, M. G., Simón, F., ... & Clemente, M. 2016. Characterization of a novel Kazal-type serine proteinase inhibitor of Arabidopsis thaliana. *Biochimie* 123: 85–94.

Parveen, S., Khalid, A., Farooq, A., & Choudhary, M. I. 2001. Acetyl and butyrylcholinesterase-inhibiting triterpenoid alkaloids from Buxus papillosa. *Phytochemistry* 58(6): 963–968.

Pekkarinen, A. I., Longstaff, C., & Jones, B. L. 2007. Kinetics of the inhibition of Fusarium serine proteinases by barley (Hordeum vulgare L.) inhibitors. *Journal of Agricultural and Food Chemistry* 55(7): 2736–2742.

Petersen, M. L. C., Hejgaard, J., Thompson, G. A., & Schulz, A. 2005. Cucurbit phloem serpins are graft-transmissible and appear to be resistant to turnover in the sieve element–companion cell complex. *Journal of Experimental Botany* 56(422): 3111–3120.

Placines, C., Castañeda-Loaiza, V., João Rodrigues, M., Pereira, C. G., Stefanucci, A., Mollica, A., ... & Castilho, P. C. 2020. Phenolic profile, toxicity, enzyme inhibition, in silico studies, and antioxidant properties of Cakile maritima scop.(Brassicaceae) from southern Portugal. *Plants* 9(2): 142.

Pohanka, M., 2011. Cholinesterases, a target of pharmacology and toxicology. *Biomedical Papers of the Medical Faculty of Palacky University in Olomouc*, 155(3).

Ponnusamy, S., Zinjarde, S., Bhargava, S., Rajamohanan, P. R., & RaviKumar, A. 2012. Discovering bisdemethoxycurcumin from Curcuma longa rhizome as a potent small molecule inhibitor of human pancreatic α-amylase, a target for type-2 diabetes. *Food Chemistry* 135(4): 2638–2642.

Pujol, M., Hernández, C. A., Armas, R., Coll, Y., Alfonso-Rubí, J., Pérez, M., ... & González, A. 2005. Inhibition of Heliothis virescens larvae growth in transgenic tobacco plants expressing cowpea trypsin inhibitor. *Biotecnología Aplicada* 22(2): 127–130.

Pusztai, A. 1972. Metabolism of trypsin-inhibitory proteins in the germinating seeds of kidney bean (Phaseolus vulgaris). *Planta* 107(2): 121–129.

Qu, L. J., Chen, J., Liu, M., Pan, N., Okamoto, H., Lin, Z., ... & Chen, Z. 2003. Molecular cloning and functional analysis of a novel type of Bowman-Birk inhibitor gene family in rice. *Plant Physiology* 133(2): 560–570.

Quilis, J., López-García, B., Meynard, D., Guiderdoni, E., & San Segundo, B. 2014. Inducible expression of a fusion gene encoding two proteinase inhibitors leads to insect and pathogen resistance in transgenic rice. *Plant Biotechnology Journal* 12(3): 367–377.

Quilis, J., Meynard, D., Vila, L., Avilés, F. X., Guiderdoni, E., & San Segundo, B. 2007. A potato carboxypeptidase inhibitor gene provides pathogen resistance in transgenic rice. *Plant Biotechnology Journal* 5(4): 537–553.

Rauf, A., & Jehan, N. 2017. Natural products as a potential enzyme inhibitors from medicinal plants. In *Enzyme Inhibitors and Activators.* InTech: Rijeka, Croatia, 165–177.

Rawlings, N. D. 2010. Peptidase inhibitors in the MEROPS database. *Biochimie* 92(11): 1463–1483.

Rawlings, N. D., Tolle, D. P., & Barrett, A. J. 2004. Evolutionary families of peptidase inhibitors. *Biochemical Journal* 378(3): 705–716.

Richardson, M. 1991. Seed storage proteins: the enzyme inhibitors. *Methods in Plant Biochemistry*, **5**: 259–305.

Robert, S., Khalf, M., Goulet, M. C., D'Aoust, M. A., Sainsbury, F., & Michaud, D. 2013. Protection of recombinant mammalian antibodies from development-dependent proteolysis in leaves of Nicotiana benthamiana. *PLoS One* 8(7): e70203.

Roberts, T. H., Ahn, J. W., Lampl, N., & Fluhr, R. 2011. Plants and the study of serpin biology. *Methods in Enzymology* 499: 347–366.

Rodrigues, M. J., Gangadhar, K. N., Vizetto-Duarte, C., Wubshet, S. G., Nyberg, N. T., Barreira, L., ... & Custódio, L. 2014. Maritime halophyte species from southern Portugal as sources of bioactive molecules. *Marine Drugs* 12(4): 2228–2244.

Rogniaux, H., Pavlovic, M., Lupi, R., Lollier, V., Joint, M., Mameri, H., ... & Larré, C. 2015. Allergen relative abundance in several wheat varieties as revealed via a targeted quantitative approach using MS. *Proteomics* 15(10): 1736–1745.

Ruiz, L., Negredo, E., Domingo, P., Paredes, R., Francia, E., Balagué, M., ... & Clotet, B. 2001. Antiretroviral treatment simplification with nevirapine in protease inhibitor-experienced patients with HIV-associated lipodystrophy: 1-year prospective follow-up of a multicenter, randomized, controlled study. *Journal of Acquired Immune Deficiency Syndromes* 27(3): 229–236.

Rustgi, S., Boex-Fontvieille, E., Reinbothe, C., von Wettstein, D., & Reinbothe, S. 2017. Serpin1 and WSCP differentially regulate the activity of the cysteine protease RD21 during plant development in Arabidopsis thaliana. *Proceedings of the National Academy of Sciences* 114(9): 2212–2217.

Ryan, C. A. 1990. Protease inhibitors in plants: genes for improving defenses against insects and pathogens. *Annual Review of Phytopathology* 28(1): 425–449.

Shi, L., Mu, K., Arntfield, S. D., & Nickerson, M. T. 2017. Changes in levels of enzyme inhibitors during soaking and cooking for pulses available in Canada. *Journal of Food Science and Technology* 54(4): 1014–1022.

Smigocki, A. C., Ivic-Haymes, S., Li, H., & Savić, J. 2013. Pest protection conferred by a Beta vulgaris serine proteinase inhibitor gene. *PloS One* 8(2): e57303.

Strokopytov, B., Knegtel, R. M., Penninga, D., Rozeboom, H. J., Kalk, K. H., Dijkhuizen, L., & Dijkstra, B. W. 1996. Structure of cyclodextrin glycosyltransferase complexed with a maltononaose inhibitor at 2.6 Å resolution. Implications for product specificity. *Biochemistry* 35(13): 4241–4249.

Sudha, P., Zinjarde, S. S., Bhargava, S. Y., & Kumar, A. R. 2011. Potent α-amylase inhibitory activity of Indian Ayurvedic medicinal plants. *BMC Complementary and Alternative Medicine* 11(1): 1–10.

Suganthy, N., Pandian, S. K., & Devi, K. P. 2009. Cholinesterase inhibitors from plants: possible treatment strategy for neurological disorders: A review. *International Journal of Biomedical and Pharmaceutical Sciences* 3(1): 87–103.

Tajini, F., Trabelsi, M., & Drevon, J. J. 2012. Combined inoculation with Glomus intraradices and Rhizobium tropici CIAT899 increases phosphorus use efficiency for symbiotic nitrogen fixation in common bean (Phaseolus vulgaris L.). *Saudi Journal of Biological Sciences* 19(2): 157–163.

Tang, J., Feng, Y., Tsao, S., Wang, N., Curtain, R., & Wang, Y. 2009. Berberine and Coptidis rhizoma as novel antineoplastic agents: a review of traditional use and biomedical investigations. *Journal of Ethnopharmacology* 126(1): 5–17.

Tarling, C. A., Woods, K., Zhang, R., Brastianos, H. C., Brayer, G. D., Andersen, R. J., & Withers, S. G. 2008. The search for novel human pancreatic α-amylase inhibitors: high-throughput screening of terrestrial and marine natural product extracts. *ChemBioChem* 9(3): 433–438.

Tougu, V. 2001. Acetylcholinesterase: mechanism of catalysis and inhibition. *Current Medicinal Chemistry-Central Nervous System Agents* 1(2): 155–170.

Tsukamoto, S., Tomise, K., Aburatani, M., Onuki, H., Hirorta, H., Ishiharajima, E., & Ohta, T. 2004. Isolation of cytochrome P450 inhibitors from strawberry fruit, Fragaria ananassa. *Journal of Natural Products* 67(11): 1839–1841.

Tundis, R., Loizzo, M. R., & Menichini, F. 2010. Natural products as α-amylase and α-glucosidase inhibitors and their hypoglycaemic potential in the treatment of diabetes: an update. *Mini Reviews in Medicinal Chemistry* 10(4): 315–331.

Turra, D., Bellin, D., Lorito, M., & Gebhardt, C. 2009. Genotype-dependent expression of specific members of potato protease inhibitor gene families in different tissues and in response to wounding and nematode infection. *Journal of Plant Physiology* 166(7): 762–774.

Uitdehaag, J. C., Mosi, R., Kalk, K. H., van der Veen, B. A., Dijkhuizen, L., Withers, S. G., & Dijkstra, B. W. 1999. X-ray structures along the reaction pathway of cyclodextrin glycosyltransferase elucidate catalysis in the α-amylase family. *Nature Structural Biology* 6(5): 432–436.

Valueva, T. A., & Mosolov, V. V. 2004. Role of Inhibitors of Proteolytic Enzymes in Plant Defense against Phytopathogenic Microorganisms. *Biochemistry* 69(11): 1305–1309.

Valueva, T. A., Revina, T. A., Kladnitskaya, G. V., & Mosolov, V. V. 1998. Kunitz-type proteinase inhibitors from intact and Phytophthora-infected potato tubers. *FEBS Letters* 426(1): 131–134.

Van Der Maarel, M. J., Van der Veen, B., Uitdehaag, J. C., Leemhuis, H., & Dijkhuizen, L. 2002. Properties and applications of starch-converting enzymes of the α-amylase family. *Journal of Biotechnology* 94(2): 137–155.

Vidal-Valverde, C., Frias, J., Diaz-Pollan, C., Fernandez, M., Lopez-Jurado, M., & Urbano, G. 1997. Influence of processing on trypsin inhibitor activity of faba beans and its physiological effect. *Journal of Agricultural and Food Chemistry* 45(9): 3559–3564.

Vila, L., Quilis, J., Meynard, D., Breitler, J. C., Marfà, V., Murillo, I., ... & San Segundo, B. 2005. Expression of the maize proteinase inhibitor (mpi) gene in rice plants enhances resistance against the striped stem borer (Chilo suppressalis): effects on larval growth and insect gut proteinases. *Plant Biotechnology Journal* 3(2): 187–202.

Wang, N., Hatcher, D. W., & Gawalko, E. J. 2008. Effect of variety and processing on nutrients and certain anti-nutrients in field peas (Pisum sativum). *Food Chemistry* 111(1): 132–138.

Wati, R. K., Theppakorn, T., Benjakul, S., & Rawdkuen, S. 2010. Trypsin inhibitor from 3 legume seeds: fractionation and proteolytic inhibition study. *Journal of Food Science* 75(3): C223–C228.

Weder, J. K. P., 1981. Proteinase inhibitors in the Leguminosae. pp. 533–560. In R.M. Polhill & P. H. Raven (eds.), *Advances in Legume Systematics.* Royal Botanic Gardens, England.

Williams, P., Sorribas, A., & Howes, M. J. R. 2011. Natural products as a source of Alzheimer's drug leads. *Natural Product Reports* 28(1): 48–77.

Xi-Can, T., Kindel, G. H., Kozikowski, A. P., & Hanin, I. 1994. Comparison of the effects of natural and synthetic huperzine-A on rat brain cholinergic function in vitro and in vivo. *Journal of Ethnopharmacology* 44(3): 147–155.

Yang, Z., Wang, Y., Wang, Y., & Zhang, Y. 2012. Bioassay-guided screening and isolation of α-glucosidase and tyrosinase inhibitors from leaves of Morus alba. *Food Chemistry* 131(2): 617–625.

Ye, X. Y., Ng, T. B., & Rao, P. F. 2001. A Bowman–Birk-type trypsin-chymotrypsin inhibitor from broad beans. *Biochemical and Biophysical Research Communications* 289(1): 91–96.

Yoo, B. C., Aoki, K., Xiang, Y., Campbell, L. R., Hull, R. J., Xoconostle-Cázares, B., ... & Lucas, W. J. 2000. Characterization of Cucurbita maxima phloem serpin-1 (CmPS-1): a developmentally regulated elastase inhibitor. *Journal of Biological Chemistry* 275(45): 35122–35128.

CHAPTER 13

# Glycyrrhizic Acid

**Shafiya Rafiq, Summira Rafiq, Priyanka Suthar, Gulzar Ahmad Nayik, and Harish Kumar**

## CONTENTS



## 13.1 INTRODUCTION

Glycyrrhizic acid, also called as glycyrrhizin and commonly abbreviated as GA, is a saponin found in liquorice root (Shibata et al., 1991). Liquorice, also known as licorice, regarded as the "Grandfather of Plants" is a valuable herb with both nutritional and medicinal properties (Isbrucker and Burdock, 2006). The two primary forms available in the market include root (Liquiriti radix) and the liquorice extract (*Succus liquiritiae* or *Glycyrrhizae extractum crudum*). In China, Japan, and Egypt, Glycyrrhizic acid has been known and used for decades to treat asthma, dry cough, voice hoarseness, lung diseases, mouth ulcers, and liver diseases. It has also been used to treat pectoral diseases and to quench thirst (Isbrucker and Burdock, 2006). In addition to this, it has been suggested for treatment of diseases related to bladder, kidney, body temperature, skin, nerves, and eye (Fiore et al., 2005). It is also considered as a spice due to its yellow colour, sweet flavour, and valuable pharmacological properties attributed to the presence of various types of flavonoids and terpenoids (glycyrrhizin). Owing to the non-sensitizing and whitening properties, extract and various derivatives of glycyrrhizin are used to treat various types of allergies, inflammation, and peptic ulcer, as well as in cosmetic preparations (Hayashi and Sudo, 2009).

## 13.2 OCCURRENCE, CHEMISTRY, AND BIOCHEMISTRY OF GLYCYRRHIZIC ACID

*Glycyrrhiza glabra* is a long shrub which belongs to *Leguminosae* family native to the Mediterranean region and Asia (Olukoga and Donaldson, 1998). *G. glabra var. typica* is grown in Europe's south and central parts, *var. glandulifera* is grown in central and southern Russia, and *var. violacea* is grown in Iran and Iraq, although the majority of commercial liquorice products are from *G. glabra*

DOI: 10.1201/9781003178446-13

*var. violacea*, grown in Iran and Iraq. *Licorice var. lepidota var. typica* also grows in different parts of England and the United States, but neither contributes to world production. Economically important varieties are obtained from China, Spain, Iran, Iraq, Russia, and Turkey. Even though there are no notorious prohibitions against any variety, some varieties are not sufficiently sweet to have market value. *G. uralensis* and *G. pallidifora* (Chinese licorice) is a separate Glycyrrhiza species distinguished by smaller length as compared to other varieties..

The name Glycyrrhiza itself expresses the principal characteristic of the plant, which is a combination of two Greek words, "*glykos*," which means sweet, and "*rhiza*," meaning root. This sugary taste of the root is because of glycyrrhizin, which is reported to be 50 times sweeter in comparison to refined sugar. The harvesting of the root is carried out in autumn at age 3–4 of the plant (Olukoga and Donaldson, 1998). The roots of the liquorice plant are dug out, washed, cleaned, and shifted to warehouses where other operations, including bailing, sorting, and drying are done. Millstones crush the dried roots, and the pulp is boiled to prepare the extract. Finally, this extract is cleaned and dried; usually vacuum dried to produce a paste, mould into sticks or blocks, or can be converted to powder. Liquorice paste is desired for flavouring of tobacco and cigarettes, whereas for confectionery and pharmaceuticals liquorice powder is preferred (Carmines et al., 2005). The flavonoids liquiritin, isoliquiritin, and their aglycones, which make up 1–1.5% of the water-soluble extract, give the root its bright-yellow hue. In addition to this, liquorice extract also contains essential oils, sugars, polysaccharides, salts, and low contents of nitrogenous compounds. The number and type of chemical constituents in liquorice is potentially vast and considerably influenced by a number of factors, including internal (genetic), external, and processing factors (Duke, 2000; Wang et al., 2000).

Glycyrrhizin (glycyrrhizic acid; glycyrrhizinate), a triterpenoid saponin, is the primary active ingredient of root extract and constitutes 10–25% (Fugh-Berman and Ernst, 2001). Glycyrrhizin is composed of a glycyrrhetic acid, triterpenoid aglycone, conjugated with disaccharide of glucuronic acid (Figure 13.1) (Wang et al., 2000) and exists as calcium and potassium salts of 18β-glycyrrhizic acid (also known glycyrrhizinic acid or as glycyrrhizic and a glycyrrhetinic acid glycoside) in root of liquorice plant because of its tribasic-acidic nature and ammonium salt in the market preparations (Isbrucker and Burdock, 2006). Glycyrrhizin ammoniated salt, derived from liquorice extract, is used as a flavouring agent in a variety of foods. Food Chemicals Codex has provided specifications for this salt. An analogue of glycyrrhetic acid known as Carbenoxolone (18beta-glycyrrhetinic acid hydrogen succinate) is used to treat ulcerative conditions. Glycyrrhizin gives foods an unappealing brownish hue, and the sweetness is lost in acidic conditions, limiting its use in the food and beverage industries. Liquorice and glycyrrhizin are mostly used to flavour tobacco and sweets, with

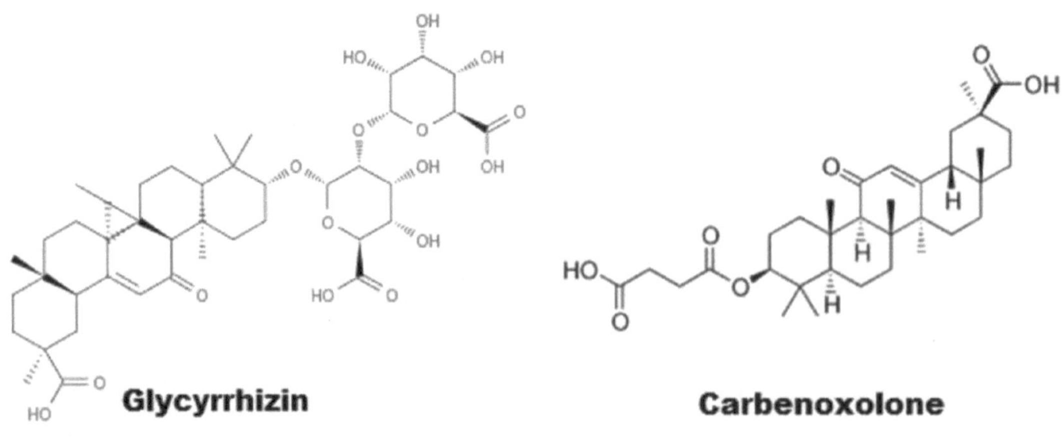


**Figure 13.1** Structure of Glycyrrhizin.

a few marginal applications in beer and ale (Fenwick et al., 1990; Reineccius, 2000). They can be used as surfactants and to reduce bitterness in drinks, saccharinated products, and pharmaceutical formulations because they have the ability to foam. Glycyrrhizin is also used as a flavour enhancer and has replaced 25% of the cocoa in products (Duke, 1985).

## 13.3 CONSUMPTION

The quantity of liquorice root and its derivatives ingested by the general public are estimated as "disappearance data," via per-person estimates of intake. This calculation is carried out by the National Academy of Sciences in annual surveys that measure the ingredients used in food (NAS, 1989). The most recent study, conducted in 1987, was based on manufacturers' voluntary reports on the amount of ingredients generated during the survey year. During the survey it was assumed that there is a limited quantity of a substance accessible and it is consumed at the retail level, irrespective of the format of consumption. This method is easy to adopt as the outcome (daily exposure) is computed by simply dividing the annual poundage by the density of population present in the survey year and the number of days per annum. Some stipulations are essential to set in the data reported in survey, since (1) amount provided is a snippet of the total volume as all manufacturers will not participate; (2) the distribution of consumption may be unequal since not everyone can consume every form of food containing the substance on a regular basis. To account for these factors, the Food and Drug Administration assumes that only a portion of the data was recorded, i.e., 60% of the actual data, and that only 10% of the population absorbs 100% of the computed number. The intake comparison was made on the basis of glycyrrhizin as a main ingredient. The total load recorded for flavouring yields a daily per capita intake of 1.6 mg per day, or 0.027 mg/kg body weight.

The values of glycyrrhizin were determined through a poll conducted by NACGM (National Association of Chewing Gum Manufacturers) members' consumption, with the help of method called PADI (Possible Average Daily Intake). Combining values of Possible Average Daily Intake and the glycyrrhizin concentration present in food provides values of high-end consumption. A total of 215 mg per day, or 3.6 mg/kg body weight, is absorbed using this process. This result was similar to the value given by FDA (246 mg/day) for intake in the United States (), with the Netherlands (4–5 g/day) being the only country to surpass it. There is a possibility of even more consumption of glycyrrhizin in individuals with craving for this flavour particularly, but it is very rare as flavour of liquorice is commonly obtained with alike-tasting substances, e.g., anise or anethole. Table 13.1 shows FDA limitations for application of liquorice root extract and its derivatives in various foods items. Approximately 90% of the liquorice obtained from the US is handed down to the tobacco

**Table 13.1 FDA Limitations for Application of Liquorice Root Extract and Its Derivatives in Various Foods Items**

| Food Category | Maximum Permissible Levels (% Glycyrrhizin) | Functioning |
|---|---|---|
| Alcoholic and non-alcoholic beverages | 0.1 and 0.15 | 1,2,3 |
| Baked goods | 0.05 | 1,2 |
| Hard and soft candy | 16.0 and 3.1 | 1,2 |
| Chewing gum | 1.1 | 1,2 |
| Herbs/seasonings | 0.15 | 1,2 |
| Plant protein-derived products | 0.15 | 1,2 |
| Vitamin/mineral | 0.5 | 1,2 |
| Other food items excluding sugar replacers | 0.1 | 1,2 |

1 – Flavouring agent; 2 – Flavour enhancer; 3 – Surface active agent (Source-Isbrucker and Burdock, 2006)

industry, and the remaining 10% is used evenly by food and pharmaceutical industries (Fenwick et al., 1990). However, intake of glycyrrhizin as a supplement is also considered noteworthy. Schulz et al. (1998) reported an intake of 200–600 mg/day of glycyrrhizin or 5–15 g of dried root for 4–6 weeks might be used for the treatment of gastrointestinal diseases. There are fair chances of acute exposures if the average amount would exceed the limit of high-end consumption because of indulgence in liquorice-flavoured products. Although such kinds of incidents may be mitigated by the presence of anise or anethole in liquorice flavours, resulting in reduction of the actual quantity of glycyrrhizin consumed. Individuals who consume tobacco flavoured with glycyrrhizin and/or liquorice or capsules as a health supplement may experience excessive intake of approximately equal likelihood but not quantitatively as high in dose.

## 13.4 ABSORPTION, METABOLISM, AND ELIMINATION

When given orally, glycyrrhizin has a low bioavailability in both humans and rats. Glycyrrhizin was detected in humans and rats after a single dose of 100–1,600 mg/kg and 50 mg/kg, respectively (Yamamura et al., 1995; Gunnarsdottir and Johannesson, 1997). However, glycyrrhetic acid was found in plasma samples of both humans and rats after consuming liquorice extract or glycyrrhizin, according to these researchers. In the majority of plasma samples, Glycyrrhizic acid concentrations were smaller and occurred later when glycyrrhizin was introduced through liquorice extract compared to when consumed as a pure compound in an equivalent dose; however, in rabbits, the opposite was reported (Cantelli-Forti et al., 1994, Hou et al., 2005). Licorice extract has also shown effects to alter pharmacokinetics in rats by increasing bile flow (Cantelli-Forti et al., 1997). The time needed to achieve the maximum concentration of glycyrrhetic acid in plasma was 10 h for glycyrrhizin consumption and 2 h extended for liquorice extract consumption. Same results were discovered in a study were eight volunteers were involved (healthy adult) conducted by Cantelli-Forti et al., 1994. They were given 800–1,600 mg glycyrrhizin in the form of ammoniated salt or liquorice extract. The lipophilic component of liquorice extract was discovered to be involved in gastric emptying and glycyrrhizin absorption (Wang et al., 1995). The main compounds, however, have not been identified. Surprisingly, neither glycyrrhetic acid nor glycyrrhizin were reported in germ-free rats' plasma, which were fed by glycyrrhizin (Takeda et al., 1996). These findings, combined with the comparably extensive lag time to reach maximal glycyrrhetic acid in plasma, point to a presystemic (first-pass) metabolic process that involves the de-glucuronidation of glycyrrhizin with the help of intestinal flora prior to glycyrrhetic acid absorption (Ploeger et al., 2001). Many researchers have discovered a number of intestinal bacterial strains involved in hydrolysis of glycyrrhizin. Examples include *Streptococcus* and *Eubacterium sp.* (Kim et al., 1999). Glycyrrhetic acid bioavailability after glycyrrhizin ingestion tends to be dose-limiting in rats. It might be because of weaknesses in either the absorption of glycyrrhetic acid or the hydrolysis mechanism (Ploeger et al., 2001). In tissues, glycyrrhizin and glycyrrhetic acid do not accumulate. Both compounds, however, bind greatly to human and rat serum albumin, and the mechanism is saturable, regardless of whether the binding sites are unique or non-specific (Ploeger et al., 2001). Glycyrrhetic acid can cross the placental barrier and be detected in rat foetuses, according to a recent report (Hundertmark et al., 2002). By extracting bile from one rat given [3H]glycyrrhetic acid and introducing it into the intestine (duodenum part) of a second rat, Iveson et al. (1971) demonstrated the enterohepatic circulation (EHC) of glycyrrhetic acid. Nearly 14% of the radioactivity was excreted in the bile of the second animal within 6 h, with totals of 29 and 31% defecated through the bile after 24 and 48 h, respectively. The presence of three glycyrrhetic acid compounds, 18-glycyrrhetyl-30-glucuronide, 18-glycyrrhetyl-3-O-glucuronide, and 18-glycyrrhetyl-3-O-sulfate, was discovered in the collected bile, indicating hepatic conjugation of glycyrrhetic acid ahead of biliary excretion. The urine excreted less than 2% of the initial dose, indicating that it is not a significant route of removal. The existence of only the parent compound as an unmodified substance in faecal extracts of rats given orally [3H]glycyrrhetic acid indicated that glucuronyl and sulphate conjugates were fully hydrolyzed by intestinal microflora prior to excretion in the faeces. It was found that 3-ketoglycyrrhetic acid was the compound after metabolization of glycyrrhetic acid in rat liver homogenates with the help of an enzyme called glycyrrhetinate dehydrogenase (Akao et al., 1990). This metabolic stage which was reversible in nature was thrice faster than the rate at which glycyrrhetic acid was oxidised. The activity of glycyrrhetinate dehydrogen was investigated further in a later study. By the twelfth week of life, enzyme activity had reached its peak. Adult male rats were given estradiol or surgical hypophysectomy, which reduced the activity of glycyrrhizinate dehydrogenase. Female rats, on the other hand, had some glycyrrhetinate dehydrogenase activity induced by hypophysectomy or testosterone administration. These results suggest that the hypothalamus–pituitary system controls the enzyme. This metabolic pathway is thought to play a minor role in glycyrrhetic acid metabolism in rats, but its existence in humans is unknown. Ploeger et al. (2001) studied the pharmacokinetics of glycyrrhizin and glycyrrhetic acid extensively. When given to rats or humans at levels that surpass the saturation of serum protein binding, glycyrrhizin and glycyrrhetic acid have a dose-dependent plasma clearance. These findings point to a bile metabolism or excretion mechanism that is restricted by hepatic ability. Owing to enterohepatic recirculation of glycyrrhetic acid and the biliary storage process of its metabolites in the gallbladder, glycyrrhetic acid in plasma display several peaks after either glycyrrhizin/glycyrrhetic acid or liquorice administration. Plasma glycyrrhetic acid concentrations peaked at 1 g/ml after 10 h for 16 healthy adults who consumed 225 mg glycyrrhizin liquorice, with second and third peaks of around 0.2 and 0.1 g/ml at 30 and 50 h, respectively (Ploeger et al., 2000). Following a fat-containing meal, these latter peaks are thought to represent a bolus re-administration of glycyrrhetic acid metabolites into the intestines via gallbladder emptying. As a consequence, complete removal from the body takes several days after a single dose, and the risk of glycyrrhetic acid accumulation increases when administered on a regular basis.

To summarise, glycyrrhizin's metabolic fate is multiplex and involves various interdependent steps. After oral administration, glycyrrhizin undergoes a foremost metabolic phase comprised of intestinal microbial metabolism to an aglycone compound and/or monoglycone. Only a small amount of glycyrrhizin is absorbed, resulting in 3MGA and glycyrrhetic acid being absorbed into the intestines. Although the hepatic metabolism and processing of 3MGA and glycyrrhetic acid in humans is unknown, it is clear that both will undergo further conjugation or reduction before being excreted through the bile. The intestinal flora most likely remetabolizes glucuronide compounds and metabolites excreted in bile, making them subject to enterohepatic recycling. Glycyrrhetic acid clearance potential is generally lower in patients with compromised hepatic function.

## 13.5 TOXICOLOGY OF GLYCYRRHIZIC ACID

Glycyrrhizic acid from Licorice (*Glycyrrhiza glabra*) is mostly utilized as a natural sweetener in food products. It is also applied in pharmaceuticals and cosmetics and generally extracted from the roots of the plant. However, broad ranges of reactions associated with glycyrrhizic acid were reported. Some cases are reported with serious illness and consumers have been admitted to the hospitals. The severity of reactions has been greatly influenced by the dose and exposure time duration. Størmer et al. (1993) described few symptoms like hypokalaemia, hypernatraemia, elevated blood pressure, oedema and reninangiotensin-aldosterone system suppression. According to Batiha et al. (2020), high dose of active compound glycyrrhizin led to pseudohyperaldosteronism, which causes the consumer hypersensitive against adrenal cortex hormones, and results in various adverse effects which includes fatigue, heart attack, water retention, high blood pressure and headache and finally leads to swellings in legs, contraindicated in pregnancy, and other health issues. Among all adverse effects, most research studies published in the field of pharmacology and biochemistry is concentrated on "hypermineralcorticosteroid" or "pseudohyperaldosteronism" effects and its respective mechanisms.

In many studies, it was reported that enzymatic processes have been affected by glycyrrhetic acid in cell culture system or tested animal models. Mainly, cytochrome P450 monooxygenase, mitochondrial oxidative phosphorylation, and N-acetyltransferase activity has been restricted in tested animals. Also, cytochrome P450 isozyme induction has been reported (Isbrucker and Burdock, 2006). Similar effect was reported by Asl and Hosseinzadeh (2008), and stated that consumption of large quantity of liquorice may led to the severe symptoms of excess mineralocorticoid like hyperkalemia and hypertension. Lowered activity of 11β-HSD2 is main reason behind hypertension. The renal conversion of cortisone from cortisol is regulated by this enzyme. Therefore, activation of renal receptors of mineralocorticoids due to liquorice intake which finally results in a state of suppressed rennin angiotensin system and excess apparent mineralocorticoid. Aforementioned, the study by Tanahashi et al. (2002) also explained that derivatives of liquorice like glycyrrhizic acid restrict the activity of 11β-HSD2 enzyme and thereby leading to the pseudoaldosteronism by its consumption. At the dose of 120 mg glycyrrhizic acid, the revealing decrease in mRNA and 11-HSD2 protein was reported. Contrasting to this, other in-vitro studies reported that treatment of glycyrrhetinic acid in mouse kidney cells M1 for 24 h didn't affect the expression level of 11-HSD2 mRNA. Thus it can be concluded that different indirect mechanism may be involved such as chronic high dose of glycyrrhizic acid suppresses the mRNA, competitive inhibitor to 11-HSD2, and protein expression of 11-HSD2. In some cases with pseudoaldosteronism, the above mentioned signs are explained by the long intake of glycyrrhizic acid. Author further discussed that adverse effect of glycyrrhizin acid was related with iron liver state. The liver iron content has been significantly reduced in feeding Sprague-Dawley (male) when 2% ammoniated glycyrrhizin was administered in diet for 14 days and faecal iron exertion was increased significantly. Also, significant weight gain in treated animal was observed, however no effect on other minerals has been reported by this diet (Nazari et al., 2017). Kwon et al. (2020) stated that increased diastolic and systolic blood pressure (DBP and SBP) and extracellular volume has been reported by intake of liquorice for 2 weeks. The elevated blood pressure via elevated extracellular fluid volume and stiffness in artery was reported due to consumption of liquorice. Author reported that meta-analysis of 18 studies (n = 337) have been reported with lowered serum potassium level and increased blood pressure by intake of licorice (3.19 mmHg for DBP and 5.45 mmHg for SBP). Furthermore, children were administered with the high-dose glycyrrhizin prenatally, i.e., above 500 mg per week showed inhibition of 11βHSD2 via liquorice confectionary maternal consumption and also showed reduced visuospatial and verbal abilities along with aggression and attention related problems. Besides this, glycyrrhizin at this dose level showed altered diurnal and stress-induced hypothalamic-pituitary-adrenocortical axis (HPAA) function in the children age group of 8.1 years with dose-dependent manner (Hosseinzadeh and Nassiri-Asl, 2015). The earlier study by Radhakrishnan et al. (2005) showed 100% mortality of Black molly was reported on day 7 when liquorice extract was given at 4 mg per litre. However, lowest experimental concentration i.e., 1 mg per litre of liqorice extract showed 17% mortality on day 25 and at 2 mg per litre liquorice extract showed increased mortality by 34% on day 15 of experiment. The effect of extract was mainly associated with inhibition of tyrosinase activity on treated animal and showed 50% inhibition in vitro in comparison with standard kojic acid inhibitor. The results were concluded that the accumulation of liquorice extract in liver tissues led to the toxicity and damaging effects.

The extract of liquorice has been recently reported as mutagenic properties at high concentration, i.e., 25 mg/mL by Abudayyak et al. (2015). The utilization of liquorice during the pregnancy has been reported with decreased gestational age significantly in human beings (Strandberg et al., 2001). According to some studies, the consumption of liquorice by pregnant ladies has led to cognitive dysfunction-related issues in children (Räikkönen et al., 2009). The results of exposure of glycyrrhizin with 0–249 mg per week dose and high exposure to above 500 mg per week groups of children has been compared and it showed significant decline in the narrative memory, visuospatial and verbal abilities, and also increase in the problems related with attention, externalizing symptoms, aggression, and rule-breaking was observed. The above effects on various cognitive functions are strongly dose related. The findings are consistent with "foetal programming" caused by glucocorticoid overexposure, and caution in consuming licorice-based foods during pregnancy is advised. HPAA functioning associated with glycyrrhizin from liquorice in children was also studied by Räikkönen et al. (2010). It is also reported by Hauksdottir et al. (2015) that consumption of liquorice may increase the risk of preeclampsia in mothers with some genetic history of the disease. Rossi et al. (1999) found that the consumption of glycyrrhizin in large quantity in the form of sweetener or drug is a susceptible subject and may lead to the symptoms similar to hypermineralcorticoidism, hypokaliaemia, hypertension, and rabdomyolysis which sometimes causes the severe arrhythmias induced due to hypokaliaemia and renal failure. Usually glycyrrhizin is isomerized into the glycyrrhetic acids 18α and 18β-. Previously, it was reported that these are principle metabolites that are responsible for hypertension and reduced diuresis, even at low doses in the tested animals (rat). Aside from its use, glycyrrhizin toxicity has been documented in many research publications, but only in rare cases, such as fatigue, potassium loss, hypertension, pseudohyperaldosterinism, and excessive acid loss. According to many studies, the ratio of cortisol and cortisone was directly associated with dose response, fluid retention, blood pressure (systolic), and fall in plasma potassium. The dose and liquorice intake directly influence the symptoms as well as the individual's susceptibility (de Putter and Donck, 2014). The study by Cartier et al. (2002) showed that the consumption of liquorice roots may be responsible for occupational asthma via and IgE-mediated mechanism, which was observed in intermediate skin reactivity reaction by using diluted liquorice root powder. Recently, Kimyon et al. (2019) reported several important potential sensitizing molecules from liquorice roots such as glycyrrhizic acid, components of flavonoids, and glycyrrhetinic acid (the breakdown product of glycyrrhizic acid). Table 13.2 shows toxicological studies of Glycyrrhizic acid or its derivatives.

The case study by Pastorino et al. (2018) reported that lethal acute intoxication was observed in a 34-year-old woman by consumption of liquorice over the period of a few months. Elinav and Chajek-Shaul (2003) stated the mechanism action of bioactive compound, glycyrrhizic acid from liquorice for hypokalemia. The author described the inhibitory action of 11 β-hydroxysteroid dehydrogenase (renal enzyme) followed by renal conversion to inactivated cortisone from cortisol. As mentioned above, this situation leads to activation of receptors of mineralocorticoids and finally results in apparent mineralocorticoids excess. Treatment of this is based on lab evidences and thorough history of hypokalemia. The complete recovery from hypokalemia can be achieved by avoiding consumption of licorice and supplementation of potassium. Oman et al. (2012) discussed the interaction of drug and liquorice with hepatic microsomal enzyme system. The study on one patient showed that the administration of liquorice led to the digoxin toxicity from hypokalemia. The extract from liquorice roots (without glycyrrhizin) causes the inhibition of cytochrome P450 3A4 (CYP3A4) and P450 systems. Authors discussed the potentiation of warfarin effects by inhibitory action on hepatic microsomal enzyme system by liquorice. The study by Abe et al. (1987) reported the effects of glycyrrhizin its derivatives (glycyrrhetinic acid and aglycon) on mouse melanoma cell (B16) culture. Cell differentiation and growth has been studied and it was reported that glycyrrhetinic acid restricts the growth of cultured cells (B16). This leads to the morphological alteration and stimulation of cells. The results showed that the glycyrrhizin also showed similar observation at much higher concentration (nearly 20 times that of glycyrrhrtinic acid).

## 13.6 CONCLUSIONS

Glycyrrhizin is the primary active component of liquorice (*Glycyrrhiza glabra*). For decades, liquorice and its extract have been used to cure many illnesses, among which are stomach ulcers, fever, bronchitis, arthritis, and many more. The FDA, European Council, and the JECFA (Joint FAO/WHO Food Additives Expert Committee) have all authorized the extract of liquorice and

**Table 13.2 Toxicological Studies of Glycyrrhizic Acid or Its Derivatives**

| Active Compound | Animals | Route of Administration | Observations | Reference |
|---|---|---|---|---|
| Ammoniated glycyrrhizin | Mice (male) | 0.4% in drinking water for consecutive 4 days before causing cold stress | During an 8-hour period of cold stress, glycyrrhizin-treated mice died more quickly than untreated mice | Kraus (1958) |
| Ammoniated glycyrrhizin | Rat (male) | 0.4% in drinking water for one week before 48-h fasting | Glycyrrhizin lowered rats' glucose mobilisation abilities. Both groups had the expected level of hypoglycemia after 24 h of fasting | Kraus (1958) |
| Ammoniated glycyrrhizin | Rat (Sprague-Dawley weanling rats) | 2% ammoniated glycyrrhizin with replacement of equivalent amount of cornstarch in the diet in chow, for 14 days | Increased in weight of body and average faecal weight, as well as increased faecal iron excretion and lower liver iron levels | West et al. (1979) |
| Glycyrrhizic acid | Rat | 0.1 and 1 mg/mL in drinking water for 12 weeks | Increased tail blood pressure and right atrial pressure due to pulmonary artery thickening and an increase in serum Na+ levels and a decrease in K+ content | Ruszymah et al. (1995) |
| Disodium glycyrrhizinate | Mice | 0.04, 0.08, 0.15, and 0.3, 0.6, or 1.25% in drinking water for 10 weeks | For females and males, the MTD (maximum tolerated dose) was 0.3 and 0.15%, respectively. In the tenth week, both animals died, with 0.6 and 1.25% of them starving to death | Kobuke et al. (1985) |
| Monoammonium glycyrrhizinate | Rat and mice | Dose level was 215, 316, and 464 mg/kg for mice. Dose for rats was 316, 464, and 681 mg/kg rats | Middle dose levels showed the slight or moderate reduction in the motility, ataxia, dyspnea, and tremor in more than 4 animals from each sex of rats and mice. The $LD_{50}$ values for mice were 325 mg/kg and 478 mg/kg for rats (24 h and 14 days) | Akasaka et al. (2008) |

glycyrrhizin. It has also been regarded as GRAS by the FEMA (Flavor and Extract Manufacturers' Association). However, some acute exposures can result if the average amount of daily consumption will be exceeded. It's fair to say that current liquorice extract and glycyrrhizinate consumption levels pose no risk.

## REFERENCES

Abe, H., Ohya, N., Yamamoto, K. F., Shibuya, T., Arichi, S., and Odashima, S. 1987. Effects of glycyrrhizin and glycyrrhetinic acid on growth and melanogenesis in cultured B16 melanoma cells. *European Journal of Cancer and Clinical Oncology*, 23(10): 1549–1555

Abudayyak, M., Nath, E. Ö., and Özhan, G. 2015. Toxic potentials of ten herbs commonly used for aphrodisiac effect in Turkey. *Turkish Journal of Medical Sciences*, 45(3): 496–506.

Akao, T., Akao, T., and Kobashi, K. 1990. Metabolism of glycyrrhetic acid by rat liver microsomes: glycyrrhetinate dehydrogenase. *Biochimica et Biophysica Acta (BBA)-Lipids and Lipid Metabolism*, 1042(2): 241–246.

Akasaka, Y., Hatta, A., Sato, T., Leuschner, J., Sasagawa, C., and Inoue, H. 2008. Acute toxicity study of monoammonium glycyrrhizinate by single intravenous administration to CD– 1 mice and CD rats. *薬理と治療*, 36(11): 1017–1023.

Asl, M. N., and Hosseinzadeh, H. 2008. Review of pharmacological effects of Glycyrrhiza sp. and its bioactive compounds. *Phytotherapy Research*, 22(6): 709–724.

Batiha, G. E. S., Beshbishy, A. M., El-Mleeh, A., Abdel-Daim, M. M., and Devkota, H. P. 2020. Traditional uses, bioactive chemical constituents, and pharmacological and toxicological activities of Glycyrrhiza glabra L.(Fabaceae). *Biomolecules*, 10(3): 352

Cantelli-Forti, G., Maffei, F., Hrelia, P., Bugamelli, F., Bernardi, M., D'Intino, P., Maranesi, M., and Raggi, M. A. 1994. Interaction of licorice on glycyrrhizin pharmacokinetics. *Environmental Health Perspectives*, 102(suppl 9): 65–68.

Cantelli-Forti, G., Raggi, M. A., Bugamelli, F., Maffei, F., Villari, A., and Trieff, N. M. 1997. Toxicological assessment of liquorice: biliary excretion in rats. *Pharmacological Research*, 35(5): 463–470.

Carmines, E. L., Lemus, R., and Gaworski, C. L. 2005. Toxicologic evaluation of licorice extract as a cigarette ingredient. *Food and Chemical Toxicology*, 43(9): 1303–1322.

Cartier, A., Malo, J. L., and Labrecque, M. 2002. Occupational asthma due to liquorice roots. *Allergy*, 57(9): 863–863.

de Putter, R., and Donck, J. 2014. Low-dose liquorice ingestion resulting in severe hypokalaemic paraparesis, rhabdomyolysis and nephrogenic diabetes insipidus. *Clinical Kidney Journal*, 7(1): 73–75.

Duke, J. A., 1985. CRC Handbook of Medicinal Herbs. CRC Press, Inc., Boca Raton, FL, pp. 215–216.

Duke, J. A., 2000. *Handbook of Phytochemical Constituents of GRAS Herbs and Other Economic Plants*. CRC Press, Inc., Boca Raton, FL, pp. 277–281.

Elinav, E., and Chajek-Shaul, T. 2003. Licorice consumption causing severe hypokalemic paralysis. *Mayo Clinic Proceedings*, 78(6): 767–768.

Fenwick, G. R., Lutomski, J., and Nieman, C. 1990. Liquorice, Glycyrrhiza glabra L.: composition, uses and analysis. *Food Chemistry*, 38(2): 119–143.

Fiore, C., Eisenhut, M., Ragazzi, E., Zanchin, G., and Armanini, D. 2005. A history of the therapeutic use of liquorice in Europe. *Journal of Ethnopharmacology*, 99(3): 317–324.

Fugh-Berman, A., and Ernst, E. 2001. Herb–drug interactions: review and assessment of report reliability. *British Journal of Clinical Pharmacology*, 52(5): 587–595.

Gunnarsdóttir, S., and Jóhannesson, T. 1997. Glycyrrhetic acid in human blood after ingestion of glycyrrhizic acid in licorice. *Pharmacology & Toxicology*, 81(6): 300–302.

Hauksdottir, D., Sigurjonsdottir, H. A., Arnadottir, M., and Geirsson, R. T. 2015. Severe, very early onset pre-eclampsia associated with liquorice consumption. *Hypertension in Pregnancy*, 34(2): 221–226.

Hayashi, H., and Sudo, H. 2009. Economic importance of licorice. *Plant Biotechnology*, 26(1): 101–104.

Hosseinzadeh, H., and Nassiri-Asl, M. 2015. Pharmacological effects of Glycyrrhiza spp. and its bioactive constituents: update and review. *Phytotherapy Research*, 29(12): 1868–1886.

Hou, Y. C., Hsiu, S. L., Ching, H., Lin, Y. T., Tsai, S. Y., Wen, K. C., and Chao, P. D. L. 2005. Profound difference of metabolic pharmacokinetics between pure glycyrrhizin and glycyrrhizin in licorice decoction. *Life Sciences*, 76(10): 1167–1176.

Hundertmark, S., Dill, A., Bühler, H., Stevens, P., Looman, K., Ragosch, V., Seckl, J. R., and Lipka, C. 2002. 11β-Hydroxysteroid dehydrogenase type 1: a new regulator of fetal lung maturation. *Hormone and Metabolic Research*, 34(10): 537–544.

Isbrucker, R. A., and Burdock, G. A. 2006. Risk and safety assessment on the consumption of Licorice root (Glycyrrhiza sp.), its extract and powder as a food ingredient, with emphasis on the pharmacology and toxicology of glycyrrhizin. *Regulatory Toxicology and Pharmacology*, 46(3): 167–192.

Iveson, P., Lindup, W. E., Parke, D. V., and Williams, R. T. 1971. The metabolism of carbenoxolone in the rat. *Xenobiotica*, 1(1): 79–95.

Kim, D. H., Lee, S. W., and Han, M. J. 1999. Biotransformation of glycyrrhizin to 18β-glycyrrhetinic acid-3-O-β-D-glucuronide by Streptococcus LJ-22, a human intestinal bacterium. *Biological and Pharmaceutical Bulletin*, 22(3): 320–322.

Kimyon, R. S., Liou, Y. L., Schlarbaum, J. P., and Warshaw, E. M. 2019. Allergic contact dermatitis to licorice root extract. *Dermatitis*, 30(3): 227–228.

Kobuke, T., Inai, K., Nambu, S., Ohe, K., Takemoto, T., Matsuki, K., Nishinal, H., Huang, I.-B., and Tokuoka, S. 1985. Tumorigenicity study of disodium glycyrrhizinate administered orally to mice. *Food and Chemical Toxicology*, 23(11): 979–983.

Kraus, S. D. 1958. Glycyrrhizin-induced Inhibition of the Pituitary-Adrenal Stress Response. *The Journal of Experimental Medicine*, 108(3): 325–328.

Kwon, Y. J., Son, D. H., Chung, T. H., and Lee, Y. J. 2020. A review of the pharmacological efficacy and safety of licorice root from corroborative clinical trial findings. *Journal of Medicinal Food*, 23(1): 12–20.

NAS. 1989. 1987 *Poundage and Technical EVects Update of Substances Added to Food*. National Academy of Sciences, Washington, DC.

Nazari, S., Rameshrad, M., and Hosseinzadeh, H. 2017. Toxicological effects of Glycyrrhiza glabra (licorice): a review. *Phytotherapy Research*, 31(11): 1635–1650.

Olukoga, A., and Donaldson, D. 1998. Historical perspectives on health The history of liquorice: the plant, its extract, cultivation, commercialisation and etymology. *The Journal of the Royal Society for the Promotion of Health*, 118(5): 300–304.

Omar, H. R., Komarova, I., El-Ghonemi, M., Fathy, A., Rashad, R., Abdelmalak, H. D., Yerramadha, M. R., Yaseen, A., Helal, E., and Camporesi, E. M. (2012). Licorice abuse: time to send a warning message. *Therapeutic Advances in Endocrinology and Metabolism*, 3(4): 125–138.

Pastorino, G., Cornara, L., Soares, S., Rodrigues, F., and Oliveira, M. B. P. 2018. Liquorice (Glycyrrhiza glabra): a phytochemical and pharmacological review. *Phytotherapy Research*, 32(12): 2323–2339.

Ploeger, B., Mensinga, T., Sips, A., Meulenbelt, J., and DeJongh, J. 2000. A human physiologically-based model for glycyrrhzic acid, a compound subject to presystemic metabolism and enterohepatic cycling. *Pharmaceutical Research*, 17(12): 1516–1525.

Ploeger, B., Mensinga, T., Sips, A., Seinen, W., Meulenbelt, J., and DeJongh, J. 2001. The pharmacokinetics of glycyrrhizic acid evaluated by physiologically based pharmacokinetic modeling. *Drug Metabolism Reviews*, 33(2): 125–147.

Radhakrishnan, N., Gnanamani, A., and Sadulla, S. 2005. Effect of licorice (Glycyhrriza glabra Linn.), a skin-whitening agent on Black molly (Poecilia latipinnaa). *Journal of Applied Cosmetology*, 23(4): 149–158.

Räikkönen, K., Pesonen, A. K., Heinonen, K., Lahti, J., Komsi, N., Eriksson, J. G., Seckl, J. R., Järvenpää, A. L., and Strandberg, T. E. 2009. Maternal licorice consumption and detrimental cognitive and psychiatric outcomes in children. *American Journal of Epidemiology*, 170(9): 1137–1146.

Räikkönen, K., Seckl, J. R., Heinonen, K., Pyhälä, R., Feldt, K., Jones, A., Pesonen, A. K., Phillips, D. I. W., Lahti, J., Järvenpää, A. L., Eriksson, J. G., Metthews, K. A., Strandberg, T. E. and Kajantie, E. 2010. Maternal prenatal licorice consumption alters hypothalamic–pituitary–adrenocortical axis function in children. *Psychoneuroendocrinology*, 35(10): 1587–1593.

Reineccius, G. A. 2000. Flavoring systems for functional foods. *Essentials of Functional Foods*. Gaithersburg, MD: Aspen Publishing, pp. 87–95.

Rossi, T., Fano, R. A., Castelli, M., Malagoli, M., Ruberto, A. I., Baggio, G., Zennaro, R., Migaldi, M., and Barbolini, G. 1999. Correlation between high intake of glycyrrhizin and myolysis of the papillary muscles: an experimental in vivo study. *Pharmacology & Toxicology*, 85: 221–229.

Ruszymah, B. H. I., Nabishah, B. M., Aminuddin, S., and Khalid, B. A. K. 1995. Effects of glycyrrhizic acid on right atrial pressure and pulmonary vasculature in rats. *Clinical and Experimental Hypertension*, 17(3): 575–591.

Schulz, V., Hänsel, R., and Tyler, V. E. 1998. Digestive system. In *Rational Phytotherapy*. Springer, Berlin, Heidelberg, pp. 167–220.

Shibata, S., Inoue, H., Iwata, S., Ma, R., Yu, L., Ueyama, H., Takayasu, J., Hasegawa, T., Tokuda, H., Nishino, A., and Iwashima, A. 1991. Inhibitory effects of licochalcone A isolated from Glycyrrhiza inflata root on inflammatory ear edema and tumour promotion in mice. *Planta Medica*, 57(3): 221–224.

Størmer, F. C., Reistad, R., and Alexander, J. 1993. Glycyrrhizic acid in liquorice: evaluation of health hazard. *Food and Chemical Toxicology*, 31(4): 303–312.

Strandberg, T. E., Järvenpää, A. L., Vanhanen, H., and McKeigue, P. M. 2001. Birth outcome in relation to licorice consumption during pregnancy. *American Journal of Epidemiology*, 153(11): 1085–1088.

Takeda, S., Ishihara, K., Wakui, Y., Amagaya, S., Maruno, M., Akao, T., and Kobashi, K. 1996. Bioavailability study of glycyrrhetic acid after oral administration of glycyrrhizin in rats; relevance to the intestinal bacterial hydrolysis. *Journal of Pharmacy and Pharmacology*, 48(9): 902–905.

Tanahashi, T., Mune, T., Morita, H., Tanahashi, H., Isomura, Y., Suwa, T., Daido, H., Gomez-Sancehz, C. E., and Yasuda, K. 2002. Glycyrrhizic acid suppresses type 2 11β-hydroxysteroid dehydrogenase expression in vivo. *The Journal of Steroid Biochemistry and Molecular Biology*, 80(4–5): 441–447.

Wang, Z., Nishioka, M., Kurosaki, Y., Nakayama, T., and Kimura, T. 1995. Gastrointestinal absorption characteristics of glycyrrhizin from glycyrrhiza extract. *Biological and Pharmaceutical Bulletin*, 18(9): 1238–1241.

Wang, Z. Y., Athar, M., and Bickers, D. R., 2000. Licorice in foods and herbal drugs: chemistry, pharmacology, toxicology and uses. In: Mazza, G., Oomah, B. D. (Eds.), *Herbs, Botanicals & Teas*. Technomic Publishing Co. Inc, Lancaster, PA, pp. 321–353.

West, L. G., Nonnamaker, B. J., and Greger, J. L. 1979. Effect of ammoniated glycyrrhizin on the mineral utilization of rats. *Journal of Food Science*, 44(5): 1558–1559.

Yamamura, Y., Santa, T., Kotaki, H., Uchino, K., Sawada, Y., and Iga, T. 1995. Administration-Route dependency of absorption of glycyrrhizin in rats: intraperitoneal administration dramatically enhanced bioavailability. *Biological and Pharmaceutical Bulletin*, 18(2): 337–341.

CHAPTER 14

# BOAA
## *A Neurotoxin*

**Sakshi Sharma, Anil Dutt Semwal, M Pal Murugan, D D Wadikar, and Ram Kumar Sharma**

## CONTENTS



DOI: 10.1201/9781003178446-14

## 14.1 INTRODUCTION

A neurotoxin, β-N-oxalyl-L-a, β-diaminopropionic acid (ODAP), or L-BOAA has been recognized to be the main cause for lathyrism or neurolathyrism disease in human. The neurotoxin ODAP was first identified in 1962 by Bell when he discovered ninhydrin-reacting substances in numerous *Lathyrus* species. Rotter et al. (1991) recommended that ODAP could have an anti-nutritive function in assimilation of food as observed in their experiments with chicks where they fed 400 g/kg (low- and medium-ODAP *L. sativus* lines) or 600 g/kg (low ODAP *L. sativus* line). Kuo et al. (1994) demonstrated the biosynthesis of BOAA from its precursor β-(isoxazolin-5-on-2-yl)-alanine (BIA) in the young seedlings.

A connection amongst the over ingestion of *L. sativus* seeds and the disease neurolathyrism, an upper motor neuron disorder depicted by a spastic paraparesis of the lower limbs, is fully acknowledged for numerous decades (Dwivedi and Prasad 1964). The neurotoxin L-BOAA, a non-protein excitatory amino acid, is observed to be present in all parts of *Lathyrus* plants (Campbell et al. 1994). However, *L. sativus* is only one of the 160 species among the *Lathyrus* genus. The other species being *L. cicera*, *L. ochrus*, *L. odoratus*, *L. roseous*, *L. pusillus*, *L. hirsutus*, *L. clymenum*, *L. latifolius*, and *L. sylvestris*, all of which are known to cause lathyrism in both humans and animals. However, the presence of BOAA toxin has reduced the consumption of this highly nutritious crop.

During recent times, incidences of neurolathyrism or lathyrism have been reported from China, Ethiopia, and India. The increased instances of lathyrism in the past led to the extensive research work being done in producing low toxin-containing varieties of grass pea through genetic and molecular approaches. Additionally, advanced food processing technologies played a significant part in reducing content of BOAA toxin from processed grass pea products. Precautions and necessary safety measures shall be adopted before giving this crop a full-fledged status for production and processing at world-wide platform.

## 14.2 CHEMISTRY OF β-ODAP

Chemically β-ODAP or BOAA or Dencichin has molecular weight of 176 and is represented by the molecular formula $C_5H_8N_2O_5$. Two forms of ODAP, viz., α- ODAP and β-ODAP isomers are available. The α- isomer of ODAP is supposed to be less toxic than the β-isomer and is not linked with neurolathyrism (Yan et al. 2006; Gresta et al. 2014). Thus, the toxicity mainly is governed by the relative proportion of β-ODAP to the total quantity of ODAP. Naturally, β:α ratio is nearly 95:5, and this ratio may vary under various circumstances. This neurotoxin BOAA is known to have a structural similarity to the neurotransmitter glutamate occurring in the *Lathyrus* species (Figure 14.1).

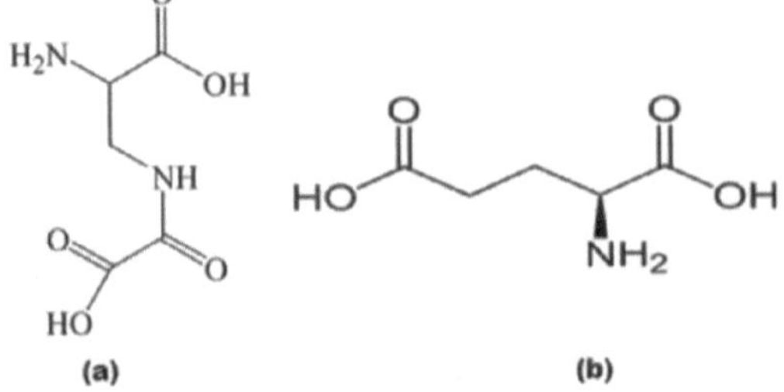


**Figure 14.1** Structure of (A) BOAA, (B) L- Glutamate.

## 14.3 LATHYRUS SATIVUS

### 14.3.1 Distribution

The grass pea plant belongs to the family *Fabaceae*, genus *Lathyrus* and species *sativus* of the *Plantae* Kingdom. It is commonly called chickling vetch, chickling pea, grass peavine, riga pea, Indian pea, Indian vetch (UK and North America), Alverjas (Venezeula), Almorta (Spain), Gilban (Sudan), Matri (Pakistan), Pisellobretonne (Italy), Guaya (Ethiopia), and Gesette (France). In India, it is popular as Khesari, Kesare, chural, Khesra, teora, karil, Karas, kasar, latri, lakhori, Lakhodi, lang, batura, santal, and chattramatur. In Nepal and Bangladesh, *L. sativus* is popular as khesari.

### 14.3.2 Botany

*L. sativus* is a sub-erect, herbaceous winter annual plant. The stems reach upto 25 to 60 cm height. The leaves of *L. sativus* plant are pinnately compound and have two leaflets; the upper ones having modified tendrils. Flower of *L. sativus* plants are generally reddish purple, pink, white, and blue in color. Pods of the plant are oblong, flat, and slightly curved. A single pod contains 3–5 seeds that may be white, yellowish, or grayish-brown in color with usual spotting or mottling (Campbell 1997).

*L. sativus* plants grow well under extreme conditions of drought, cold, and a saline environment. Grass pea plants do not even require rich and fertile soil for growth, and can grow well in low-fertility soils to heavy clays. This plant can even repel numerous pests and pathogens, and also control the growth of certain weeds (Yang and Zhang 2005, Girma and Korbu 2012). Prakash et al. (1977) observed that irrespective of the age or the variety of *L. sativus* plant, BOAA is present in all fragments of the plant. The maximum concentration was reported at vegetative stage in the leaf and at the reproductive stage in the embryo.

Grass pea plants are an ideal option for sustainable agriculture as these can fix as well as use atmospheric nitrogen thus, can be used as a good green manure for improving the quality of soil. In addition, the plant acts as ground covers reducing evaporation, and help in conserving the soil moisture.

The stem, leaf and seeds of *L. sativus* plant have potential as fine forage for animal feeding. Due to its ability to grow well under acute stress environment as well as being potential source of nutrients, this crop is an important source of food crop. *L. sativus* has a yield potential of as high as 5 tonnes/hectare under good agro-climatic environment (Briggs et al. 1983). Traditionally, *L. sativus* is regarded as a poor man's crop (Lambein et al. 2019, Khandare et al. 2020). It is cultivated as an insurance crop in drought-prone areas. Its produce was also given by the landlords as wages to the labourers.

The seeds of grass pea plants contain about 7.5 to 8.2% water, 58.2% carbohydrate (48 to 52.3% starch), 18.2 to 34.6% protein, 0.58 to 0.8% fat, 4.3 to 7.3% ash. The grains are also composed of pentose (6.8%), sucrose (1.5%), lignin (1.5%), phytin (3.6%), prolamine (1.5%), albumin (6.69%), globulin (13.3%), and glutelin (3.8%) (Campbell 1997, Bhattacharjee et al. 2018, Dilling 1919, Lisiewska et al. 2003, Rahman et al. 1974). The seeds of this crop also have been shown to consist of starch, sucrose, fixed oil, alkaloids, flavonoids, tannins, phenols, terpenes, oleo-resin, legumelin, gum resin, leguminvicilin, carbohydrates, proteins, amino acids, carotenoids, β-carotene, riboflavin, and ascorbic acid.

The seed oil of *L. sativus* possesses many medicinal benefits. It is a powerful cathartic. It can be used to treat scabies, allergy, and eczema. The kernel of grass pea is locally utilized in producing homeopathic medication. Immature pods and young vegetative parts are cooked and consumed as vegetables, or they are boiled, seasoned with salt, and eaten as a snack in Asia. In India, whole *L. sativus* seeds are boiled, or are processed into dhal and consumed in dhal form or ground into flour. In Bangladesh, roti, or flat bread made of *L. sativus* flour, is a staple food for many labourers.

In Ethiopia and Eritrea, *L. sativus* grains are mainly eaten as sauce (wot), sauce made by flour (shirowot), and sauce made from hulled split grains (kikwot). Boiled grass pea seeds, called nifro, and an unleavened bread (Kitta) made of *L. sativus* are mainly eaten at the times of food scarcity. Young plants of grass pea are also utilized as cattle fodder in many parts of the world (Campbell 1997, Ali Esmail Al-Snafi 2019). *L. sativus* has many pharmacological benefits such as anti-oxidant, anti-diabetic, analgesic, anti-pyretic, and cardio-protective effects.

Besides β-ODAP, several other neurotoxic amino acids have been found present in *L. sativus*, namely homoarginine in the seeds, and homoserine, homoserine-like compounds, and isoxazoline-like compounds in the sprouts and every part of the plant excluding the ripened seed. Homoarginine is believed to modulate BOAA toxicity (Yusuf et al. 1995). Another substance more toxic than β-ODAP and found to be present in the *Lathyrus* species is α-amino-adipinic acid (Riepe et al. 1995, Grela et al. 2001). Few other non proteinaceous and non-toxic compounds have been found in *Lathyrus* species such as β-mercaptomethylamine, β-(γ-L-glutamyl)-aminopropionitrile (BAPN), N-dimethylhydrazine, aminoacetonitrile, 2-cyanopropylamine, aminoacetichydrazide, cyanoacetic acid hydrazide, benzoic acid hydrazide, nicotinic acid hydrazide, and p-nitrobenzoic acid hydrazide (Grela et al. 2001).

## 14.4 LATHYRISM

During recent times, instances of neurolathyrism have been found in China, Ethiopia and India. Grass pea is produced in large parts of China, Burma, Nepal, India, Bangladesh, Pakistan, some parts of Europe (Italy, Portugal, Poland, and France), Africa, and South America. Various epidemics of neurolathyrism have been observed in various states of India as well as other countries in the past few decades (Sleeman et al. 1844, Cantani 1873, Bourlier 1882, Stockman 1917, Buchanan 1927, Carrot and Coulmel 1946, Kessler 1947, Rodríguez Arias 1950, Dwivedi and Prasad 1964, Barrow et al. 1974, Kulkarni and Attal 1977, Haque et al. 1996, Getahun et al. 1999, Woldemanuel et al. 2012, Giménez-Roldán and Spencer 2016). Various international symposia organized all over the world in Dhaka (1972), France (1985), London (1989), India (2012), etc. have emphasized on growing instances of neurolathyrism. Many states in India produce *L. sativus*, including Madhya Pradesh, Maharashtra, Telangana, West Bengal, Karnataka, Bihar, Gujarat, and parts of Uttar Pradesh. Khokhar and Owusu-Apenten (2003) reported that the grass pea contained high β-ODAP levels when grown in nutrient solution deficient in zinc and rich in ferrous iron. The *L. sativus* seeds from Ethiopia contained 1.25 to 25 g/kg of β-ODAP, however, β-ODAP concentration of *L. sativus* kernels from Bangladesh varied from 5 to 8 g/kg.

Sleeman et al. (1844) first gave a comprehensive description of lathyrism in India that happened in 1831 in Madhya Pradesh due to intake of *L. sativus* for long time. Soon afterwards, Irwin in 1859 reported paralysis of lower extremities due to consumption of *L. sativus* in Allahabad. The *L. sativus* grown in three districts of Chhattisgarh namely Durg, Raipur, and Bilaspur were examined for the amount of β-ODAP, which varied from 0.1 to 2.5 g/100 g by Nagarajan and Gopalan (1968). Siddique et al. (1996) examined three species of Lathyrus genus in the Mediterranean-type environments of Western Australia. The amount of ODAP in *L. ochrus* was reported to be double that of *L. sativus*. *L. cicera* was observed to contain the least content of ODAP.

Khandare et al. (2014) analysed five villages of Gondia District of Maharashtra for their *L. sativus* consumption, concentration of β-ODAP, exposure to the toxin β-ODAP, and its effect on health, and nutritional status of the people. They postulated that *L. sativus* consumption in small amounts did not lead to the crippling disease associated with the toxin.

Khandare et al. (2018) undertook a study to evaluate the present status of intake of *L. sativus* and incidences of lathyrism, with the contents of β-ODAP, protein and amino acids in three districts of Chhattisgarh state (Durg, Raipur and Bilaspur). The β-ODAP content was observed as 0.65 ±

0.13, 0.63 ± 0.14, and 0.65 ± 0.14 g/100 g from *L. sativus* grown in Durg, Bilaspur, and Raipur, respectively. In their study, they found that there was lower consumption of split *L. sativus* in these districts and thus lower occurrence of lathyrism disease.

Shiferaw and Porceddu (2018) examined 50 accessions of *L. sativus* from varied geographical locations from Ethiopia for β-ODAP concentration and potential of seed storage protein for genetic diversity. The accessions containing medium β-ODAP content on single plant basis might hold potential of favourable samples for breeding. Careful selection carried out for desired traits in genetically variable germplasm will definitely reduce the BOAA content of crop cultivar and enhance its proper utilization. Berger et al. (1999) observed ODAP content to have a positive and a negative correlation with phosphorous content of soil, and clay content and salinity, respectively.

### 14.4.1 Mechanism of Action of Toxin

Plants produce non-protein amino acid as secondary metabolites to protect them from environmental stresses (Nunn et al. 2010). These non-protein amino acids are similar in structure to the proteinogenic amino acids (Rodrigues-Correa and Fett-Neto 2019). The amount of BOAA in grass pea seeds is affected by both environmental as well as genetic factors. The amino acid β-isoxazolin-5-on-2-yl-alanine (BIA) is predominantly found in *L. sativus* during the seedling stage. This heterocyclic amino acid is also found in *Pisum sativum* and *Lens culinaris*. However, unlike in *L. sativus*, BIA does not metabolize into β-ODAP in the latter two legumes (Kuo et al. 1998).

Liu et al. (2017) carried out a study involving metabolomics for detection of metabolic processes linked with the biosynthesis of BOAA in *L. sativus*. They found an association of β-ODAP metabolism with nitrogen and sulphur metabolisms. Serine and cysteine were negatively correlated with the accumulation of β-ODAP. The amino acid serine gets converted into O-acetylserine and isoxazolin-5-one. Both these compounds are broken down into BIA by the β-cyanoalanine synthase (β-CAS) enzyme. BIA is suggested to be transformed to an intermediate 2,3,-l-diaminopropanoic acid, which gets consequently oxalylized by oxalyl-coenzyme A and forms β-ODAP. β-CAS enzyme is also included in maintaining the cysteine molecules within the β-ODAP pathway (Malathi et al. 1967; Malathi et al. 1970; Kuo et al. 1994; Kuo and Lambein 1991).

The production of isoxazolin-5-one is crucial for the biosynthesis of β-ODAP and involves metabolic activities of CAS and cysteine synthase (CS) or O-acetylserinesulfhydrylase or O-acetylserine(thiol)lyase (Ikegami et al. 1991, 1999). During biosynthesis of cysteine, CS catalyse the formation of O-acetylserine and hydrogen sulphide. The cysteine formed is then used as a substrate for CAS in detoxification of cyanide in plants (Machingura et al. 2016). The β-cyanoalanine is converted to asparagines, which further transforms to isoxazolin-5-one.

Chakraborty et al. 2018 applied a bioinformatics approach for identification and characterization of a novel *cysteine synthase* (*LsCSase*) gene from *L. sativus*. Their study lays a groundwork entailing a link between the biosynthesis of β-ODAP and *LsCSase* gene. Their study indicated that the *LsCSase* gene was up-regulated in young seedling tissues and young seeds with an enhanced level of expression under conditions of zinc-iron stress and polyethylene glycol- induced osmotic stress. Lambein et al. (2019) emphasizes on further studies incorporating genetic engineering for developing *L. sativus* lines for understanding precise activity of *CSase* gene during biosynthesis of β-ODAP.

Various *in vitro* cell culture studies have suggested BOAA to be a glutamate receptor agonist.

The excitotoxic theory is generally considered responsible for all the toxin effects of BOAA. Any interaction of BOAA with receptor has to possess considerable specific binding; however, BOAA has not shown any considerable specific binding with the glutamate receptors (Jain et al. 1998).

Some actions of the toxin BOAA are provoked through A2/A3 glutamate receptor systems that are found on chosen neurons (Ali Esmail Al-Snafi 2019). In addition, the administration of the toxin BOAA in low amounts in cerebellum exerts *in vivo* activation of glutamate receptors that are included in the management of cGMP level.

Activation of glutamate receptor and the regulation of calcium influx by means of AMPA (α-amino-3-hydroxy-5-methylisoxazole-4- propionate) receptors are critical for the neurotoxicity of BOAA (Singh et al. 2004). Roche et al. (1994) and Soderling et al. (1994) have shown that functions of glutamate receptor can be regulated by phosphorylation. The phosphorylation can regulate physiological functions from excitatory neurotransmission to the alteration of synaptic plasticity and further to neurodegenerative diseases. Phosphorylation of AMPA receptor units by Protein kinase C has been demonstrated by Roche et al. (1996). Protein kinase C regulates the calcium influx through AMPA receptors and calcium channels (Carvalho et al. 1998). BOAA is presumed to act as an agonist at AMPA type glutamate receptors (Pearson and Nunn 1981, McDonald and Morris 1984, Ross et al. 1985, Ross et al. 1989). Singh et al. (2004) suggested BOAA to be directly activating protein kinase C. The activated Protein kinase C is phosphorylating and regulating the BOAA-mediated calcium influx by means of AMPA receptors.

Toxicity of BOAA leads in inhibiting of the mitochondrial complex I restrictively in the motor cortex and lumbar spinal cord. Mitochondrial dysfunction has been proposed to be due to generation of reacting oxygen species resulting in oxidation of protein thiol groups to disulfides. The oxidation of thiol groups makes the mitochondrial complex I extremely susceptible for inactivation. Ravindranath (2002) indicated a conventional mechanism, including oxidation of protein thiol groups and the neurodegeneration caused by mitochondrial dysfunction due to the excitatory amino acid BOAA. Experimentation carried out in male mice showed that presence of BOAA leads to loss of activity of complex I and dendritic swelling of neurons in the motor cortex and lumbar cord, resulting in biochemical changes on CNS mitochondria. This further supports the observation that the oxidation of thiol groups combined with mitochondrial dysfunction as activated by BOAA are the initial consequences, further leading to neurodegeneration. The inhibition of mitochondrial complex I can be prevented through pre-treatment with the aid of inhibitor thiols such as glutathione organic compound and alpha- lipoic acid (Sriram et al. 1998). Harikiran et al. (2019) evidently pointed out that the preservation of protein thiol homeostasis through thiol delivery vehicles may provide defense against excitotoxic insults occurring due to BOAA.

Various studies have proposed generation of free radical oxygen species as a method of toxicity of BOAA after its focal hippocampal usage in rats (Van Moorhem et al. 2011). *In vitro* analysis of mouse brain slices treated by BOAA showed mitochondrial complex I (NADH dehydrogenase) inhibition (Sriram et al. 1998).

Inhibition of the enzyme TAT (tyrosine amino transferase) by BOAA in *in vitro* as well as *in vivo* studies gives a different mechanism of neurotoxicity caused by BOAA (Shashi Vardhan et al. 1997). Olney et al. (1990) proposed that the excessive manufacturing of hormone metabolites such as 6-OH amino acid, a well-known neurotoxin could possibly be the reason for neurodegeneration. Harikiran et al. (2019) suggests that the mechanism of TAT inhibition by BOAA may be used for species differentiation between black and white mice. A significant rise in the brain DOPA and other catecholamines in C57BL/6J black mice were observed by treatment with BOAA (Shashi Vardhan et al. 1997).

A centrally acting muscle relaxant named Tolperisone has been revealed to significantly lessen spasticity of patients suffering from neurolathyrism (Melka et al. 1997). Baclofen to some extent has been shown to control hypertonicity (Mukharjee and Chakravarty 2010).

Jyothi et al. (1999) studied *in vitro* metabolism of BOAA in rats, chicks, and mice. They found that BOAA up to a certain limit could be oxidized *in vivo* in mice resulting in development of $CO_2$ and oxalate. They suggested that a similar kind of pathway may be possible in humans that involves near complete oxidation of BOAA. This established the possibility of humans having a unique ability to metabolize BOAA. However, the exact biochemical procedure for metabolism of BOAA in humans is yet to be revealed. Rudra et al. (2004) postulated that certain individuals may be deficient or totally lack the ability to detoxify BOAA, and these individuals are prone to neurolathyrism. This could be the reason for only few individuals suffering from neurolathyrism.

### 14.4.2 Toxicology of Lathyrism

Two types of lathyrism, namely Neurolathyrism and Osteolathyrism, have been observed (Barone 2020). **Osteolathyrism** is a skeletal deformity of bone and is commonly associated with consumption of *L. odoratus*, *L. roseous*, *L. pusillus*, and *L. hirsutus*. The major causative agent for Osteolathyrism has been reported to be the toxin β-aminopropionitrile (BAPN). BAPN is also present in *L. sativus* and *L cicera*. **Neurolathyrism** is a spastic paraparesis associated with upper motor neuron dysfunction and occurs in variety of animals, including humans. This disease has been associated with malnutrition, poverty, scarcity due to flood, drought, conflict, etc., during which people have to rely on foods comprising a major portion of grass pea (*Lathyrus sativus* L.), purple Spanish vetchling (*Lathyrus clymenum* L.), or red chickling vetch (*Lathyrus cicera* L.). In neurolathyrism, general observed signs are weakness in hind limbs and concomitant paralysis of muscles. Initially, painful spasms are observed in lower limbs with concurrent weakness and subsequently spastic paraplegia in chronic form, thus resulting in complete and irreversible leg paralysis (Hanbury et al. 1999).

Neurolathyrism can be further divided into two types based on the ingestion of type of *Lathyrus* species. First type can be majorly associated with *L. latifolius* and *L. sylvestris*, and the causative factor being L-2, 4,-diaminobutyric acid (DABA). However, relatively few incidences have been observed and thus less clinical importance is given to DABA as compared to the second type of neurolathyrism caused by consumption of *L. sativus*, *L. cicera*, *L. clymenum*, and *L. ochrus*, and the associated causative factor is β-ODAP. The nervous system of animals confuses β-ODAP for a glutamate analogue. α-amino-3-hydroxy-5-methyl-4-isoxazole propionic acid-type glutamate receptors form strong bonds with β-ODAP, and this leads to neurons suffering excitotoxic degeneration and similar neurotoxic effects (Rao et al. 1964).

There are various risk factors involved in the development of neurolathyrism, such as heavy physical activity, gender (male), young age (about 15 to 25 years), micronutrient (Zn, Cu, Vitamin C, Vitamin A) deficiency (Rao 2001). Deficiency of zinc in the soil also leads to more BOAA toxin content in the *L. sativus* seeds (Lambein et al. 2010). A study pointed out that the blood group "O" is found to be linked with lathyrism (Getahun et al. 2002).

Molecular docking is gaining popularity and is a commonly used methodology in structure-based drug designing. Molecular docking has the advantage of being able to predict the binding interaction of small ligand entities against the targeted receptor protein active site (Harikiran et al. 2019). It can predict the most favorable three-dimensional pose of ligand to other molecules docked in a stable complex (Lengauer and Rarey 1996). Numerous studies highlighted importance of docking in understanding the binding interaction of protein–ligand interaction in drug designing (Sharma et al. 2019, 2020, 2021). For understanding the mechanism behind lathyrism, three structural analogues of BOAA were synthesized using molecular docking (Omelchenko et al. 1999). These are carbo xymethyl-alpha,beta-diaminopropanoic acid (CMDAP), N-acetyl-alpha,beta-diaminopropanoic acid (ADAP), carboxymethylcysteine (CMC) (Omelchenko et al. 1999). Inhibition for BOAA was observed to be 99. Maximum inhibition was observed for CMDAP (92), followed by CMC (65) and ADAP (61). This study by Omelchenko et al. (1999) on BOAA structural analogues established that these BOAA analogues could act with glutamate receptors without inducing any neurotoxicity. This study holds particular importance as these analogues may find their usage in the drug designing platform where they could bind with the glutamate receptors and inhibit the actions leading to neurotoxicity and thus neurolathyrism.

According to Sriram et al. (1998) sulphur amino acids possessed a protective effect against BOAA toxicity. Eguchi et al. (2011) emphasized that the deficiency of sulphur amino acids occurred by consumption of *L. sativus* diet plays a considerable role in BOAA toxicity by intensifying the oxidative stress. Based on this, Hoque et al. (2012) examined the protective effect of sulphur amino acids of cow, buffalo, sheep, and goat milk for lathyrism. They found the milk from buffalo and sheep to possess the maximum quantity of sulphur amino acids, and proposed the utilization of these animal milk sources to protect lathyrism.

Researchers have pointed out the prolonged extreme intake of grass pea to be a major factor in the development of neurolathyrism disease. According to Kislev and Hopf (1985), lathyrism appears when consumption of *L. sativus* is about 1/3rd or 1/2nd of the total diet for approximately three to six months reported that the toxicity of BOAA occurs only if the consumption of *L. sativus* pulse is more than 75% of the total diet intake, while the consumption of about 5 to 30% of total intake is considered safe. Therefore, alteration in their use or combining them with cereals for consumption has been suggested by various researchers (Lambein 2000, Getahun et al. 2005, Valamoti et al. 2011) in order to prevent getting affected by lathyrism.

Studies on animal feeds have quantified the level of β-ODAP in diet to ensure lower intake of β-ODAP. Effect of consumption of *Lathyrus* spp. as feed differs among different animal species. BOAA has been suggested to be a strong neurotoxicant and was found toxic in many animal species such as mice (Aydillo and Jiménez-Caste 1968), monkeys (Mani et al. 1971), sheep (Keeler and James 1971), young rast (La Bella et al. 1977), horses (Spencer et al. 1986), guinea pigs (Kumar et al. 2003), and chicks (Anil Kumar et al. 2018). Horses have been observed to be highly susceptible to lathyrism after feeding on *Lathyrus* spp. seeds (Steyn 1993, LoÂpez Bellido 1994). According to Stockman (1931), there is evidence for dying of pigs, horses, sheep, and cattle because of lathyrism after consumption of *Lathyrus* species seeds in their feed. Monkeys show similar effects to humans due to intake of *L. sativus*, and at times result in death (Rao et al. 1967). Many bird species were also found susceptible to lathyrism after consumption of *Lathyrus* spp. seeds (Stockman 1931).

The intermittent intake of grains of *L. cicera* or *L. sativus* is not found to cause any damage in horses and sheep. According to LoÂpez Bellido (1994), up to 50% of *L. cicera* grains could be incorporated in the feed ration of sheep with no observed symptoms of lathyrism. The grain of *L. sativus* and *L. cicera* are fed to gestating female sheep, fattening lambs, and serving male sheep (LoÂpez Bellido 1994). Franco Jubete (1991) stated a total of 350 g of *L. cicera* seed/day was consumed by lactating ewes without showing any harmful effects. Tekle-Haimanot et al. (1997) studied horses, goats, sheep, and donkeys, and found that the hind limbs developed spasticity after 1–3 years of feeding on the grains of *L. sativus*. According to them, newborn sheep and goats were found to be more prone to lathyrism, as they developed symptoms after 1–3 months.

Yadav et al. (1992) isolated bacteria from soil sludge that can utilize BOAA as their only source of carbon and nitrogen. It has been postulated that rumen microflora gets adapted to BOAA and breaks it down (Hanbury et al. 2000). According to Rasmussen et al. (1992), sheep are more tolerant to *L. sylvestris* in the food because of alteration in the rumen matter. Hanbury et al. (2000) presumed it could be due to increase in breakdown of DABA. *L. sativus* and *L. cicera* grains were incubated in the rumen fluid of sheep, and loss of more than 90% of ODAP in 4 h was observed (Farhangi 1996).

Low et al. (1990) performed an experiment where in chickens (starting at age 7 days) were fed with grains of *L. sativus* containing low ODAP content and incorporated at 82% of the diet for about 4 weeks did not get affected by lathyrism. Rotter et al. (1991) fed *L. sativus* lines, containing low (0.13%), medium (0.22%), and high (0.27%) ODAP content, at 20–80% of the diet of chickens. In young chickens, reduction in weight gain, feed intake, and feed conversion efficiency was observed when intake of *L. sativus* seeds was increased in their diet. They found no significant difference to wheat/soybean diet at 20 and 40% proportion. On the other hand, 0.27% ODAP content grain diet showed a decrease in weight gain by the chickens, feed intake by the chickens, and also the feed conversion efficiency, as compared to seed containing lower ODAP content.

Castell et al. (1994) observed similar decline in the daily weight gain and efficiency of feed conversion after intake of high ODAP content (0.30%) *L. sativus* seed by starter pigs and grower-finisher pigs. Weight of heart and spleen as a fraction of liveweight were found to decrease by increasing the amount of *L. sativus*. On the contrary, Mullan et al. (1999) observed no significant difference in ADG (Average Daily Weight Gain), VFI (Voluntary Feed Intake), and FCR (Feed Conversion Ratio) when pigs were fed with *L. cicera* grains containing 0.09% ODAP content from 15 to 110 kg liveweight at 30% of the diet. Weights of liver and kidney were also found to be undisturbed, and no symptoms of lathyrism were observed in pigs. Similarly, no reduction in average daily weight gain, voluntary feed intake, and feed conversion ratio, and also lathyrism were noticed in weaner pigs fed on *L. cicera* grains containing 0.10% ODAP contents at 15% of diet (Mullan, unpublished). When *L. cicera* was fed at 20% of the diet, ADG was observed to be 10% lower while FCR was found to increase.

Horse has been observed to develop symptoms of lathyrism after approximately 10 days of exclusive consumption, and after 2–3 months after partial consumption of *L. sativus* seeds in the diet (Ali Esmail Al-Snafi 2019). In horse, congested patches in stomach and intestines, catarrhal bronchitis, and hyperaemia of the lungs were observed. Bovines exhibit suspended rumination, constipation, small and weak pulse, paralysis of limbs, and loss of sensibility in skin. In cattle, predominant congestion of meninges with haemorrhagic patches, thick and dark blood, large quantity of bloody serum in cranium and anterior parts of spinal cord (Steyn 1933). Fikre et al. (2010) proposed that the addition of methionine to *L. sativus* as feed for chickens protected them from developing neurological symptoms.

Yerra et al. (2015) analysed *L. sativus* seeds from different Indian states, specifically Andhra Pradesh, Kerala, Bihar, Chhattisgarh, and Odisha for effect of process technologies on β-ODAP content and *in-vivo* assessment on Wistar Albino rats. The levels of β-ODAP varied among *L. sativus* grains of different states, the highest being in Bihar and the lowest in Andhra Pradesh. The soaked and boiled samples were shown to have reduced β-ODAP content significantly. Their study revealed that a better muscle co-ordination activity of Wistar Albino rats in *L. sativus* seeds from Andhra Pradesh and soaked and boiled seed, which might be attributed to lower quantity of β-ODAP content of the seed.

In an attempt to enhance our knowledge on neurolathyrism, Khandare et al. (2020) developed an animal model for studying neurolathyrism using 24 goat kids by segregating them into four groups. One group being control, the other two groups being fed with low- and high-toxin containing grass pea, and the fourth group was fed with high-toxin grass pea flour. They concluded that three goat kids were affected with neurolathyrism irrespective of the content of BOAA toxin due to consumption of *L. sativus*.

### 14.4.3 Stages of Lathyrism

The onset of lathyrism is sudden. The early symptoms of the disease are difficulty in walking, weakness in legs, and unbearable cramps. There is development of spastic paralysis in this disease which is irreversible. Pyramidal tracts are included causing motor weakness and increased tone in thigh extensors and adductors.

There are five stages of neurolathyrism (Abraham and Abay 2009):

1. **Latent Stage:** Individual appears to be healthy. However, when the individual is under physical stress, they show an ungainly gait. If *L. sativus* pulse is cut from the diet, complete reduction of the above signs is observed.
2. **No Stick Stage:** In this stage, the individual can walk with short, jerky movements without using a stick.
3. **One Stick Stage:** In the third stage, the individual can walk with a crossed gait with a general tendency to be able to walk on toes. There is stiffness in muscles perceived at this stage.
4. **Two Stick Stage:** In this stage, because of extreme bending of the knees and crossed legs, more pronounced symptoms are observed. The patient requires crutches as support. In this stage, gait is slow. The individual, after walking only a short distance, tires easily.

5. **Crowing Stages:** In this 5th stage, it becomes impossible for the individual to be in an erect posture as the knee joint is unable to support body weight. The individual has to resort to crawling by throwing his body weight on to the hands.

Commonly, 90% of cases fall under the No or One Stick Stages. The rest 10% fall under Two Stick and Crowing Stages.

## 14.5 GLIOTOXIC PROPERTIES OF BOAA

Besides neurotoxic effects, BOAA is found to possess gliotoxic properties. Exposure to BOAA induces morphological alterations in astrocytes such as vacuole formation and cellular swelling, in turn leading to cell lysis. BOAA causes a neurotoxic effect *in vitro* at 20/~M, while a relatively higher concentration is needed for lysis of astrocytes within 48 h of exposure time. However, low levels of BOAA were found to produce higher amounts of pathology when exposure time is increased (Bridges et al. 1991).

Additionally, long durations of exposure to low quantities of BOAA may compromise the functions of astrocytes, especially the EAA (Excitatory amino acid) systems where astrocytes play a significant part in both terminating the excitatory signal by high-affinity uptake and reusing the transmitter via the glutamine cycle. The overall effect of BOAA on the central nervous system results from the combined action at more than one site, owing to its gliotoxic properties (Bridges et al. 1991).

## 14.6 IDENTIFICATION AND QUANTIFICATION/ METHOD OF ESTIMATION OF β-ODAP CONTENT

Various techniques exist that either remove or reduce the amount of β-ODAP in *L. sativus* varieties by intervention of processing technologies for detoxification of grass pea seeds. For these technologies to be successful, analytical methods for detection and quantification of β-ODAP is essential. Different methods used in estimation of BOAA are given hereunder:

### 14.6.1 Ninhydrin Method

Ninhydrin method is the first known method for determination of BOAA (Cheema et al. 1971). It involves the use of electrophoresis of the *L. sativus* extract on a paper strip. It was then sprayed with 0.5% of ninhydrin in acetone, followed by heating at 80°C for 15 min before elution of ninhydrin positive band with 75% ethanol comprising copper sulphate. The absorbance was measured at 510 nm.

### 14.6.2 Colorimetric Method

Rao (1978) developed a most popular and extensively utilized method for β-ODAP estimation. It is an indirect colorimetric method involving alkaline hydrolysis of β-ODAP to oxalic acid and L-α-β-diaminopropionic acid (DAP). DAP reacts with o- phthalaldehyde (OPT) in alkaline aqueous buffer in the presence of a reducing agent mercaptoethanol. Their product is a yellow-colored substance 1- alkylthio-2-alkylisoindole, which can be analyzed at an absorbance of 420 nm. This method is, however, not selective between the isomers, as both α- and β-ODAP can hydrolyze to DAP. It is an established fact that β-ODAP isomerises to α-ODAP due to heat to an equilibrium value with a ratio of 60:40 (Bell and O'Donovan 1966). Therefore, the OPT method is disadvantageous in terms of measuring total ODAP content as it does not measure the reduction in the BOAA content in *L. sativus* products processed under different conditions of temperature, pressure and pH. This method is also considered to be non- reproducible and time consuming.

### 14.6.3 High-Performance Liquid Chromatography (HPLC) Method

The other sophisticated method involves high-performance liquid chromatography (HPLC). It includes off-line pre-column derivatization using phenyl isothiocyanate, 9-fluorenylmethyl chloroformate, dansyl chloride, and 6-aminoquinolyl-N-hydroxusuccinimyl carbamate. These methods, however, do not differentiate between the two ODAP isomers. Although the separation of the isomers can be achieved by phenyl isothiocyanate (PITC) derivatization, the experimental troublesomeness is intensified as it is challenging to segregate the derivatizing agent (Khan et al. 1994). Reversed-phase high-performance chromatography is performed with 6-aminoquinolyl-*N*hydroxysuccinimyl carbamate (AQC) derivatization (Chen et al. 2000) have also been reported, but the derivatives decompose easily at room temperature.

### 14.6.4 Enzyme-Based Detectors

Another method involves utilization of enzymes such as glutamate oxidase for their probable enzymatic action with respect to the neurotoxin β-ODAP.

Earlier, Mehta et al. (1972) described that the enzyme tryptophanase degraded the BOAA toxin to pyruvate and other products. However, monitoring the activity of tryptophanase on BOAA toxin and pyruvate formation did not prove to be successful (Moges et al. 1994). Utilization of enzyme DAP-ammonia lyase from *Pseudomonas* spp. for determining BOAA after alkaline hydrolysis of BOAA to DAP have also been reported (Rao et al. 1974).

Ammonia gets formed as an enzymatic reaction product of various nitrogen-containing compounds. Ammonia also gets released in elimination reactions of various amino acids that are catalyzed by tryptophanase. DAP is one such amino acid involved in this type of reaction (Morino and Snell 1970). DAP gets produced after hydrolysis of ODAP. An indirect estimation of β-ODAP was reported as in the presence of ketoglutarate and nicotinamide adenine dinucleotide (NADH) ammonia can be detected either in a cuvette or by flow-injection method with glutamate dehydrogenase (GIDH). Various detectors can then be utilized for measuring disappearance of NADH. Due to reaction equilibrium, glutamate formation was favoured.

Therefore, flow-injection ammonia assay system coupled with GIDH reactor was utilized to analyse the activity of tryptophanase on DAP (Moges et al. 1993). Moges et al. (1994) in their study found that glutamate oxidase acts as a catalyst in the oxidation of β-ODAP. Thereby, they utilized a reactor which contained the enzyme (in immobilized form) in the flow-injection mode. In the prereactor, the major interfering substance "glutamate" was destroyed by GluOx (glutamate oxidase) catalase. Glutamate poses a major interference as it is also present in the *L. sativus* seed extracts and undergoes oxidation much faster than the β-ODAP. One oxidation product of β-ODAP is hydrogen peroxide, which in the presence of 4-aminophenazone reacts with Trinder reagent to form quinoneimine dye in a horseradish peroxidase reactor. This dye is red in colour and can be measured at a wavelength of 512 nm spectrophotometrically. For removal of proteins and other macromolecules, whose adsorption created unreliable response, ultrafiltration technique was applied. This method has the advantage of selectivity, as glutamate oxidase specifically oxidizes only β-ODAP and does not react on α- ODAP.

### 14.6.5 Biosensors

Biosensors based on enzymes are gaining a lot of popularity these days, and proving themselves highly beneficial in food and biomedical industries, involving *in vivo* studies and regulating fermentation process after chromatographic separations. Belay et al. (1997) developed a first biosensor based on glutamate oxidase/peroxidase amperometric detection. Beyene et al. (2004) developed another amperometric biosensor involving a screen printed carbon electrode (SPCE) for detection of BOAA. In this biosensor, electrode surface was immobilized with glutamate oxidase in a Nafion-film for oxidising β-ODAP to form hydrogen peroxide that can then be detected by manganese dioxide bulk modified SPCE method.

### 14.6.6 Liquid Chromatography Employing Bio-Electrochemical Detection

Marichamy et al. (2005) analysed BOAA using liquid chromatography combined with bio-electrochemical detection system. An enzyme based amperometric biosensor, which involves oxidation of BOAA to produce hydrogen peroxide by glutamate oxidase. The hydrogen peroxide is then reduced by the enzyme horseradish peroxidase. The chromatographic separation becomes necessary as glutamate oxidase is also responsive to L- glutamate and to some extent L- aspartate, apart from BOAA. All these are capable of generating hydrogen peroxide. On contrary, the non-toxic α- isomer of the toxin is not acted upon by the glutamate oxidase. Thus, this method is β-selective and considered more accurate. The combination of both the enzymes glutamate oxidase and horseradish oxidase, at the end of a spectrographic graphite electrode, ensures the operating of biosensor at an optimum potential of -50 mV. The biosensor is designed in a way that the glutamate oxidase is immobilized as a separate layer without electrically wiring to the electrode. The mediator used for reducing hydrogen peroxide with horseradish oxidase also shows activity of glutamate oxidase. Therefore, it becomes necessary that any electrical connection does not occur between electrode and the layer of glutamate oxidase. This evades the chances of short circuit, and decreases the analytical signal, and thus the sensitivity (Marichamy et al. 2005). The glutamate oxidase has oxidised an analyte, the redox centre of the enzyme undergoes reduction simultaneously. To reoxidise glutamate oxidase, molecular oxygen reoxidises and converts to hydrogen peroxide. After hydrogen peroxide enters to the layer of the horseradish oxidase, hydrogen peroxide is reduced to hydrogen ions and water. The mediator again reoxidises the active site of horseradish oxidase enzyme, and thus is reduced by electrode to undergo catalysis again.

### 14.6.7 Modified Spectrophotometric Assay Method

Emmrich et al. (2019) developed a screening method by modifying the spectrophotometric assay method suggested by Rao in 1978. In this method, plate- based assay was developed which comprised of harvesting the plant material into 96 well plates, followed by subjecting the material to freeze-drying. Thereafter, it was pulverized and then extracted. One part of the extract obtained was hydrolysed with KOH to produce L-2, 3-diaminopropionic acid. This was reacted with Rao reagents, namely OPA and β-mercaptoethanol, to obtain a coloured dye. The absorbance of the wells in the plates can then be analysed by the help of plate-reader spectrophotometer. This method offers advantages of analysing total ODAP content in large sample numbers, and being a cost-effective method. However, this method has few disadvantages such as low sensitivity and not able to distinguish among the two ODAP isomers. These disadvantages were addressed in a yet another method described by Emmrich et al. (2019). In this method, an LCMS based method using a heavy isotope labelled internal standard (di-13C-labelled β-L- ODAP) of β-L- ODAP is developed which offers high sensitivity, β-ODAP quantification as well as authentication of new genotypes having low to zero β-ODAP content.

## 14.7 SAFETY, PRECAUTIONS, AND REGULATIONS

Various attempts have been made to develop hybrids free from β-ODAP and other toxins present in *Lathyrus* species, but none has been successful in complete removal of the toxin. β-ODAP content varies among seeds of different size, region of cultivation, and the harvesting time. Grela et al. (2000) found that the *L. sativus* cultivated in temperate regions had low lathyrogen level as compared to tropical and subtropical area. Barik et al. (2007) discovered that a polymorphism at a molecular level that is useful for genetic breeding programmes for crop improvement. Materon and Ryan (1995) have adequately quoted the significance of Zinc for crop production. De Belleroche and Clifford (1987) confirmed that the deficiency of the micronutrient Zinc has been associated with motor-neuron disease. Keeping in mind the benefit of this essential micronutrient, Abd El- Moneim et al. (2001) examined the probable effect of Zinc added to the soil in the greenhouse and the field on the amount of β-ODAP in various grass pea lines. Their study implicated that the Zinc either from the soil or by adding as a fertilizer partially reduced β-ODAP content. However, Dahiya (1976) has essentially stated that above 0.2% levels of BOAA for intake by humans are harmful. Therefore, additional technical interventions including processing methodologies and breeding approaches, at genetic and molecular level, for reducing β-ODAP content is required for this crop to gain importance in human diet and nutrition.

Public education and awareness about the dangers of lathyrism disease is very important. Prolonged consumption of *L. sativus* and in larger quantities has been known to cause irreversible paralysis.

Adulteration of legume flours such as chickpea flour and pigeon pea flour is quite frequently reported in the literature (Urga et al. 1995, 2005, Gahukar 2014). *L. sativus* seeds are utilized for the adulteration of pulses, due to their very high resemblance with the shape of pigeon pea pulse seeds. This is a common concern because of the neurotoxin BOAA being present in the *L. sativus* pulse. Majorly reported cases of grass pea adulteration are found in some Asian as well as African countries like India, Nepal, Ethiopia, etc. (Tekle-Haimanot et al. 1993, Arora et al. 1996, Gahukar 2014). Unfortunately, the presence of *L. sativus* flour in the high-quality flours of other pulses is visually undetected. Thus, various analytical techniques have been developed for the detection of the presence of neurotoxin BOAA. Large screening studies can be analysed by randomly amplified polymorphic DNA (RAPD) fingerprint technique.

FSSAI (Food Safety and Standards Authority of India) is the sole authority founded under Ministry of Health and Family Welfare, Government of India with the responsibility of security and advancement of public health through monitoring and managing of food safety. The FSS (Food Safety and Standards) Act, 2006 is the principal law for regulation of food products.

FSSAI has released a DART (Detect Adulteration with Rapid Test) booklet that includes some quick tests at household level for detecting adulterants in common food products such as milk and milk products, food grains and its products, spices, condiments, sugar, confectionary items, etc. There is, indeed, a requirement of more research work to be conducted in the future years to work out the consumption of *L. sativus* seed and flour.

Food Authority in 2016 lifted the ban on trade and storing of grass pea varieties that are having less quantity of the toxin BOAA such as Ratan, Prateek, and Mahateora. The Ministry of Agriculture requested to promote the cultivation of these low toxin-containing varieties instead of the local varieties containing higher content of the toxin BOAA in the traditional areas.

## 14.8 FOOD PROCESSING TECHNIQUES

Various food processing technologies have been recommended and evaluated for decreasing the amount of β-ODAP (Tekle-Haimont et al. 1993), however, 100% reduction could not be achieved using any processing methodology. Various thermal and non-thermal food processing treatments have been postulated. Some thermal treatments utilized for β-ODAP reduction are cooking, pressure cooking, slow cooking, roasting, and autoclaving, etc.

### 14.8.1 Effect of Soaking

Soaking is one such treatment where different soaking mediums have been examined for its effect on reduction of β-ODAP (Srivastava and Khokhar 1996). Grains are soaked in water for variable duration depending upon the type of seed. During soaking, water is absorbed by the seed. During prolonged soaking, some of nutrients also leach out with the anti-nutritional factors.

### 14.8.2 Effect of Soaking Medium

Khokhar et al. (1996) reported that soaking in different soaking media such as water, boiled water, tamarind solution, sodium chloride, lime water, sodium bicarbonate, and ascorbic acid as an effective approach in reduction of β-ODAP levels in *L. sativus* seeds. Among these, maximum reduction of about 69% β-ODAP levels were found by soaking in boiled water. Srivastava and Khokhar (1996) soaked *L. sativus* grains in different soaking media such as water, boiled water, alkaline solution, and tamarind solution. The highest reduction of β-ODAP (65 to 70%) was observed by soaking *L. sativus* in boiled water. Getahun et al. (2005) soaked grass pea seeds in water prior to cooking decreased the risk of neurolathyrism.

Srivastava et al. (2015) analysed various Indian *L. sativus* genotypes such as Ratan, Sihara local, Mahateora, Kanpur local 01, Kanpur local 02, Kanpur local 03, Nirmal, Prateek and Pusa 24 for their β-ODAP content. Genotypic differences were observed for the β-ODAP content. Among the genotypes studied Sihara local has the highest amount of β-ODAP content (1.14 mg/kg) whereas Mahateora has the lowest toxin amount (0.46 mg/kg) in the seed. *S*eeds of different varieties were subjected to processing treatments such as soaking and dehusking. The soaking treatment decreased the toxin content by 12.99%, while dehusking resulted in increase of approximately 33.77% of the toxin.

### 14.8.3 Effect of Boiling Seeds

Padmajaprasad et al. (1997) studied the effect of boiling seed of *Lathyrus* seed to reduce the content of β-ODAP. They observed that boiling of *L. sativus* seeds treatment to be effective in decreasing the concentration of β-ODAP. Boiling of *Lathyrus* seeds followed by discarding the water, β-ODAP content decreased by 90%. Tadelle et al. (2003) subjected grass pea seeds to various treatments such as soaking and cooking at 60, 75, 90°C and boiling temperatures. One-day-old Cobb broiler chicks were fed with these treated grass pea seeds. They did not observe any visible symptoms of lathyrism in the Cobb Broiler Chicks in their study.

### 14.8.4 Effect of Cooking and Roasting

Cooking has shown effective in decreasing the β-ODAP levels, depending upon cooking duration. Roasting was shown to reduce 20.61% of β-ODAP content (Tadelle et al. 2003). Grela et al. (2001) showed extrusion processing of *L. sativus* grains significantly reduced β-ODAP content. As the moisture content of *L. sativus* seeds and temperature of the extruder barrel is increased, more reduction in content of β-ODAP was observed. Yerra et al. (2016) examined different food processing methods such as roasting, soaking before roasting, soaking before boiling, tamarind water treatment germination, autoclaving, frying in oil (15, 25, and 45 min). Their study emphasized the detoxification of ODAP present in grass pea could thus progress the utilization of *L. sativus* for consumption by humans. Kebede et al. (1995) subjected *L. sativus* seeds to cooking and dry heating reduced ODAP content to about 77% and 75%, respectively. Akalu et al. (1998) studied cooking, roasting, and autoclaving of *L. sativus* seeds and flour at varying degrees of moisture content, soaking, time, temperature, and pH. The roasting treatment at 150°C for 60 min was found to effectively remove 82% of β-ODAP content.

### 14.8.5 Effect of Fermentation

Variable results were reported by different researchers on the effect of fermentation. Akalu et al. (1998) found that fermentation did not effectively reduce the content of β-ODAP in their study. Yigzaw et al. (2004), Starzyńska-Janiszewska and Stodolak (2011), and Buta et al. (2020) found significant reduction by fermentation treatment of *L. sativus*. Kuo et al. (1995) showed a reduction of 10% of β-ODAP content in *L. sativus* seeds by fermentation with *Aspergillus oryzae* NRRL 1988 for 48 h, and then subsequently fermentation with *Rhizopus oligosporus* sp T-3 for 48 h. Their study showed increased nutritional attributes such as amino acid scores for sulphur- containing as well as aromatic amino acids, protein content, and reduction in flatulence-causing factors. However, Akalu et al. (1998) reported that fermentation did not effectively reduce the content of β-ODAP in their study.

Kuo et al. (2000) carried out solid state fermentation of *L. sativus* varieties containing low toxin content with *Aspergillus oryzae* and *Rhizopus microspores* var *chinensis*, and found significant reduction in the content of β-ODAP. Also, their study reported increased amounts of amino acids such as histidine, valine, tyrosine, glutamic acid, lysine, and threonine in the fermented seeds.

### 14.8.6 Effect of Other Processing Treatment

High Hydrostatic Pressure (HHP) treatment has shown to be beneficial for reduction of β-ODAP as well as other anti-nutritional components such as oligosaccharides, phytates, and trypsin inhibitors. HHP has been shown to improve digestibility of grain proteins, higher amino acid content, and improved taste (Estrada-Girón et al. 2005, Han and Baik 2006, Boonyaratanakornkit et al. 2002, Lullien-Pellerin and Balny 2002). Recently Buta et al. (2019) in their study found that HHP treatment given to *L. sativus* seeds soaked for 6 and 12 h at 600 MPa for 25 min showed greatest decrease in the amount of toxin β-ODAP. They emphasized the importance of the combined soaking, pressure, holding time, and variety of *L. sativus* and their influence on structural changes and reduction in the β-ODAP content.

Tarade et al. (2007) evaluated the kinetic degradation of β-ODAP over the temperature range of 60 to 120°C and pH 4 and 9.2 for isothermal degradation. Non-isothermal conditions such as cooking in open pan, pressure cooker, "EcoCooker" were also studied. For prediction of β-ODAP degradation, a mathematical model was developed which worked on the basis of time and temperature of the non-isothermal process and the kinetic rate factors of the isothermal processes.

Rehman et al. (2007) carried out detoxification of *L. sativus* by various treatments such as soaking, steeping, germination, boiling in water, chemical treatments using $H_2SO_4$, $NaHCO_3$, and HCl. Steeping in water at 60 to 70°C for about 8 h, including 7 rinses, showed maximum elimination of the toxin β-ODAP. The detoxified flour obtained was added at different levels to the chapatti and about 200 g/kg of *L. sativus* flour could be added without affecting sensory attributes. It was observed that after supplementation, there was increment in the level of protein. Also, the biological value, protein efficiency ratio, net protein utilisation increased and feed quality ratio was reduced.

Dash and Ananthanarayan (2020) developed protein hydrolysates from *L. sativus* flour having reduced β-ODAP content by pre-treatments involving suspension in 70% ethanol followed by stirring at 300 rpm for 60 min and then centrifugation at 6,440 × g for approximately 30 min. The residue was vacuum dried at 40°C for 12 h and then ground and sieved to form pre-treated Kesari dhal flour. The pre-treated flour was subjected to liquid and solid state enzymatic hydrolysis using alcalase, cellulose, and amylase to produce liquid hydrolysate with improved anti-oxidant and anti-diabetic properties.

Ahmad and Nain (2020) developed a method for preparation of *L. sativus* protein free from the toxin ODAP. They reported conversion of β-ODAP to α- ODAP, and subsequent separation from protein fraction that was dependent upon pH. They emphasized that the elimination of ODAP may increase possibility of using *L. sativus* as an alternate protein source having high homoarginine content, and other health benefits such as beneficial for patients with cardiovascular diseases.

## 14.9 FUTURE PERSPECTIVE

Future line of research should focus on the following lines to exploit the wider range of benefits offered by *L. sativus* crop:

- More focus should be given to user-friendly, rapid detection methods for the common toxins such as BOAA. The research towards this aspect could play a critical role in reducing adulteration of pulses and Bengal gram flour, which is generally adulterated with *L. sativus* flour. Moreover, rapid detection techniques may prove beneficial during development of genetic and molecular techniques for improving the quality of *L. sativus* crop.
- Concerted research efforts should be made to reduce the toxic effects of BOAA through food processing techniques as an immediate or short term goal. As long term goal, efforts should be continued to develop cultivars with inherent improved nutritional quality, i.e., genotypes with low or acceptable BOAA content.
- Improved package of agronomical and protection practices should also be developed to enhance the production and productivity of this beneficial crop especially under climatic change conditions.
- Stringent actions and policies regarding prevention of adulteration of *L. sativus* in other pulses have to be given more focus.
- Animal model system and toxicology studies of the toxin BOAA should be studied in depth corresponding to the lower toxin containing varieties.

## 14.10 CONCLUSION

Grass pea plants are an ideal option for sustainable agriculture under global climate change conditions. They help diversify our food basket due to their wider adaptability and ability to grow well under harsh environments, their drought tolerance, and inherent capacity to resist different pathogen attacks. They are capable of fixing as well as using atmospheric nitrogen and help in conserving the soil moisture. The major bottleneck that prevents this is widespread consumption and cultivation is the presence of the neurotoxin BOAA. Sufficient research efforts have not yet managed to solve this problem. Therefore, focused efforts are essentially required to understand the mechanism of BOAA action, its toxicological effect, and food processing and technological interventions to reduce or remove its effect. Efforts should also develop cultivars that have an inherent capacity to produce zero or low BOAA content through conventional and biotechnological crop improvement tools.

## REFERENCES

Abd El-Moneim, A. M., Van Dorrestein, B., Baum, M., Ryan, J. and Bejiga, G. 2001. Role of ICARDA in improving the nutritional quality and yield potential of Grasspea (*Lathyrus sativus* L.) for subsistence farmers in dry areas. *Lathyrus Newsletter*, 2:55–58.

Abraham, M. and Abay, S. M. 2009. Eurolathyrism: An updated review. *Pharmacologyonline*, 1:381–388.

Ahmad, Y. and Nain, V. 2020. A convenient and robust protocol for preparation of ODAP-free Lathyrus sativus protein. *Analytical Biochemistry*, 591:113544.

Akalu, G., Johansson, G. and Nair, B. M. 1998. Effect of processing on the content of β-N-oxalyl-α, β-diaminopropionic acid (gb-ODAP) in grass pea (*Lathyrus sativus*) seeds and flour as determined by flow injection analysis. *Food Chemistry*, 62(2):233–237.

Al-Snafi, A. E. 2019. Chemical constituents and pharmacological effects of *Lathyrus sativus*: A review. *IOSR Journal of Pharmacy*, 9(6):51–58.

Arora, R. K., Mathur, P. N., Riley, K. W. and Adham, Y. 1996. *Lathyrus* genetic resources in Asia. In Proceedings of a Regional Workshop, 27-29 December 1995, Indira Gandhi Agricultural University, Raipur, India. IPGRI Office for South Asia, New Delhi.

Aydillo, N. L. and Jiménez-Caste, T. 1968. Contribution to the etiology and pathogenicity of experimental lathyrism in white mice using the exclusive digestion of fluor seeds (Lathyrus Sativus) and bland, mixed and totally and partially adjusted diets. Discussion of the deficiency and neurotoxic factors, from the clinical and histopathological viewpoints. *Trabajos del Instituto Cajal de investigaciones biologicas*, 60:157–190.

Barone, M. 2020. *Lathyrus Sativus and Nutrition: Traditional Food Products, Chemistry and Safety Issues.* Springer Nature, Cham.

Barik, D. P., Acharya, L., Mukherjee, A. K., and Chand, P. K. 2007. Analysis of genetic diversity among selected grasspea (Lathyrus sativus L.) genotypes using RAPD markers. *Zeitschrift für Naturforschung C*, 62(11–12):869–874.

Barrow M. V., Simpson, C. F. and Miller, E. J. 1974. Lathyrism: A review. *The Quarterly Review of Biology*, 49:101–128.

Belay, A., Ruzgas, T., Csöregi, E., Moges, G., Tessema, M., Solomon, T. and Gorton, L. 1997. LC– Biosensor system for the determination of the neurotoxin β-N-oxalyl-l-α, β-diaminopropionic acid. *Analytical Chemistry*, 69 (17):3471–3475.

Bell, E. A. and O'Donovan, J. P. 1966. The isolation of α-and γ-oxalyl derivatives of α, γ-diaminobutyric acid from seeds of Lathyrus latifolius, and the detection of the α-oxalyl isomer of the neurotoxin α-amino-β-oxalylaminopropionic acid which occurs together with the neurotoxin in this and other species. *Phytochemistry*, 5(6):1211–1219.

Berger, J. D., Siddique, K. H. M. and Loss, S. P. 1999. Cool season grain legumes for Mediterranean environments: The effect of environment on non-protein amino acids in Vicia and Lathyrus species. *Australian Journal of Agricultural Research*, 50(3):403–412.

Beyene, N. W., Moderegger, H., and Kalcher, K. 2004. Simple and effective procedure for immobilization of oxidases onto mno2-bulk-modified, screen-printed carbon electrodes. *South African Journal of Chemistry*, 57:1–7.

Bhattacharjee, S., Waqar, A., Barua, K., Das, A., Bhowmik, S. and Debi, S. R. 2018. Phytochemical and pharmacological evaluation of methanolic extract of Lathyrus sativus L. seeds. *Clinical Phytoscience*, 4(1):1–9.

Boonyaratanakornkit, B. B., Park, C. B. and Clark, D. S. 2002. Pressure effects on intra-and intermolecular interactions within proteins. *Biochimica et Biophysica Acta (BBA)-Protein Structure and Molecular Enzymology*, 1595(1–2):235–249.

Bourlier, A. 1882. Le lathyrisme. *Gazette Médicale de Algérie*, 17:139–141.

Bridges, R. J., Hatalski, C., Shim, S. N. and Nunn, P. B. 1991. Gliotoxic properties of the Lathyrus excitotoxin β-N-oxalyl-l-α, β-diaminopropionic acid (β-l-ODAP). *Brain Research*, 561(2):262–268.

Briggs, C. J., Parreno, N. and Campbell, C. G. 1983. Phytochemical assessment of Lathyrus species for the neurotoxic agent, β-N-oxalyl-L-α-β-diaminopropionic acid. *Planta Medica*, 47(3):188–190.

Buchanan, A. 1927. *Report on Lathyrism in the Central Province, 1896–1902*. Government Press, Nagpur, India.

Buta, M. B., Emire, S. A., Posten, C., Andrée, S. and Greiner, R. 2019. Reduction of β-ODAP and IP6 contents in *Lathyrus sativus* L. seed by high hydrostatic pressure. *Food Research International*, 120:73–82.

Buta, M. B., Posten, C., Emire, S. A., Meinhardt, A. K., Müller, A. and Greiner, R. 2020. Effects of phytase-supplemented fermentation and household processing on the nutritional quality of *Lathyrus sativus* L. seeds. *Heliyon*, 6(11):e05484.

Campbell, C. G. 1997. *Grass pea, Lathyrus sativus L. . Biodiversity International*, 18:1–91.

Campbell, C. G., Mehra, R. B., Agrawal, S. K., Chen, Y. Z., Moneim, A. A., Khawaja, H. I. T., Yadov, C. R., Tay, J. U. and Araya, W. A. 1994. Current status and future strategy in breeding grass pea (*Lathyrus sativus*). In *Expanding the Production and Use of Cool Season Food Legumes*, Springer, Dordrecht, 617–630.

Cantani, A. 1873. Latirismo (Lathyrismus) illustrata da tre casi clinici. *Il Morgagni*, 15:745–745.

Carrot, E. and Coulmel, H. 1946. Notes cliniques sur une épidémie de lathyrisme. *Revue Neurologique*, 78:572–580.

Carvalho, A. L., Duarte, C. B., Faro, C. J., Carvalho, A. P. and Pires, E. V. 1998. Calcium influx through AMPA receptors and through calcium channels is regulated by protein kinase C in cultured retina amacrine- like cells. *Journal of Neurochemistry*, 70(5):2112–2119.

Castell, A. G., Cliplef, R. L., Briggs, C. J., Campbell, C. G., and Bruni, J. E. 1994. Evaluation of Lathyrus (Lathyrus sativus L) as an ingredient in pig starter and grower diets. *Canadian Journal of Animal Science*, 74(3):529–539.

Chakraborty, S., Mitra, J., Samanta, M. K., Sikdar, N., Bhattacharyya, J., Manna, A., Pradhan, S., Chakraborty, A. and Pati, B.R. 2018. Tissue specific expression and in-silico characterization of a putative cysteine synthase gene from Lathyrus sativus L. *Gene Expression Patterns*, 27:128–134.

Cheema, P. S., Padmanaban, G. and Sarma, P. S. 1971. Mechanism of action of β-n-oxalyl-l-α, β-diaminopropionic acid, the *Lathyrus sativus* neurotoxin. *Journal of Neurochemistry*, 18(11):2137–2144.

Chen, X., Wang, F., Chen, Q., Qin, X. C. and Li, Z. 2000. Analysis of neurotoxin 3-N-oxalyl-L-2, 3-diaminopropionic acid and its α-isomer in *Lathyrus sativus* by high-performance liquid chromatography with 6-aminoquinolyl-N-hydroxysuccinimidyl carbamate (AQC) derivatization. *Journal of Agricultural and Food Chemistry*, 48(8):3383–3386.

Dahiya, B. S. 1976. Seed morphology as an indicator of low neurotoxin in *Lathyrus sativus* L. *Qualitas Plantarum*, 25(3–4):391–394.

Dash, P. and Ananthanarayan, L. 2020. Development of Kesari dal (*Lathyrus sativus*) protein hydrolysates, with reduced β-ODAP content exhibiting anti-oxidative and anti-diabetic properties. *Journal of Food Measurement and Characterization*, 14(4):2108–2125.

De Belleroche, J. S. and Clifford, F. R. (1987). Zinc, glutamate receptors and motorneurone disease. *Lancet*, 11:1082–1083.

Dilling W. J. 1919. The constituents of *Lathyrus sativus* seeds and their action. *The Journal of Pharmacology and Experimental Therapeutics*, 14(5):359–366.

Dwivedi, M. P. and Prasad, B. G. 1964. An epidemiological study of lathyrism in the district of Rewa: Madhya Pradesh. *Indian Journal of Medical Research*, 58:81–116.

Emmrich, P. M., Rejzek, M., Hill, L., Brett, P., Edwards, A., Sarkar, A., Field, R. A., Martin, C. and Wang, T. L. 2019. Linking a rapid throughput plate-assay with high-sensitivity stable-isotope label LCMS quantification permits the identification and characterisation of low β-L-ODAP grass pea lines. *BMC Plant Biology*, 19(1):1–14.

Estrada-Girón, Y., Swanson, B. G. and Barbosa-Cánovas, G. V. 2005. Advances in the use of high hydrostatic pressure for processing cereal grains and legumes. *Trends in Food Science and Technology*, 16(5):194–203.

Farhangi, M. 1996. The nutritional value of *Lathyrus cicera* grain for sheep. M.Sc. Animal Production Thesis. University of Adelaide.

Fikre, A., Yami, A., Kuo, Y. H., Ahmed, S., Gheysen, G. and Lambein, F. 2010. Effect of methionine supplement on physical responses and neurological symptoms in broiler chicks fed grass pea (*Lathyrus sativus*)-based starter ration. *Food and Chemical Toxicology*, 48(1):11–17.

Franco Jubete, F. 1991 *Los Titarros: El cultivo de Lathyrus en Castilla y LeoÂn*. Junta de Castilla y LeoÂn, Valladolid.

Gahukar, R. T. 2014. Food adulteration and contamination in India: Occurrence, implication and safety measures. *International Journal of Basic and Applied Sciences*, 3(1):47.

Getahun, H., Lambein, F., and Van der Stuyft, P. 2002. ABO blood groups, grass pea preparation, and neurolathyrism in Ethiopia. *Transactions of the Royal Society of Tropical Medicine and Hygiene*, *96*(6):700–703.

Getahun, H., Lambein, F., Vanhoorne, M., and Stuyft, P. V. D. 2005. Neurolathyrism risk depends on type of grass pea preparation and on mixing with cereals and antioxidants. *Tropical Medicine & International Health*, 10(2):169–178.

Getahun, H., Mekonnen, A., Tekle-Haimanot, R. and Lambein, F. 1999. Epidemic of neurolathyrism in Ethiopia. *The Lancet*, 354(9175):306–307.

Giménez-Roldán S. and Spencer, P. S. 2016 Azañón's disease. A 19th century epidemic of neurolathyrism in Spain. *Revue Neurologique*, 172:748–755.

Girma, D. and Korbu, L. 2012. Genetic improvement of grass pea (*Lathyrus sativus*) in Ethiopia: An unfulfilled promise. *Plant Breeding*, 131(2):231–236.

Grela, E. R., Studzinski, T., and Matras, J. 2001. Antinutritional factors in seeds of Lathyrus sativus cultivated in Poland. *Lathyrus Lathyrism Newsletter*, 2(2):101–104.

Gresta, F., Rocco, C., Lombardo, G. M., Avola, G. and Ruberto, G. 2014. Agronomic characterization and α-and β-ODAP determination through the adoption of new analytical strategies (HPLC-ELSD and NMR) of ten Sicilian accessions of grass pea. *Journal of Agricultural and Food Chemistry*, 62(11):2436–2442.

Han, I. H. and Baik, B. K. 2006. Oligosaccharide content and composition of legumes and their reduction by soaking, cooking, ultrasound, and high hydrostatic pressure. *Cereal Chemistry*, 83(4):428–433.

Hanbury, C. D., Siddique, K. H. M., Galwey, N. W. and Cocks, P. S. 1999. Genotype-environment interaction for seed yield and ODAP concentration of *Lathyrus sativus* L. and *L. cicera* L. in Mediterranean-type environments. *Euphytica*, 110(1):45–60.

Hanbury, C. D., White, C. L., Mullan, B. P. and Siddique, K. H. M. 2000. A review of the potential of *Lathyrus sativus* L. and *L. cicera* L. grain for use as animal feed. *Animal Feed Science and Technology*, 87(1–2):1–27.

Haque, A., Hossain, M., Wouters, G. and Lambein, F. 1996. Epidemiological study of lathyrism in northwestern districts of Bangladesh. *Neuroepidemiology*, 15:83–91.

Harikiran, G., Shankar, C., Kumar, V. V., Swarnalatha, C. H., Sowjanya, K. and Navya, A. 2019. A review on analogues of beta odap in treatment of neurolathyrism showing docking affinity. *Journal of Scientific Research in Pharmacy*, 8(6):62–65.

Hoque, H., Jamali, S., Akther, J. and Prodhan, S. H. 2012. Computational analysis of milk sources from different domestic animals as supplementary food source to protect Lathyrism. *International Journal of Biosciences*, 2(7):74–82.

Ikegami, F., Itakagi, S., Ishikawa, T., Ongena, G., Kuo, Y. H., Lambein, F. and Murakoshi, I. 1991. Biosynthesis of β-(isoxazolin-5-on-2-yl) alanine, the precursor of the neurotoxic amino acid β-n-oxalyl-l-α, β-diaminopropionic acid. *Chemical and Pharmaceutical Bulletin*, 39(12):3376–3377.

Ikegami, F., Yamamoto, A., Kuo, Y. H. and Lambein, F. 1999. Enzymatic formation of 2, 3-diaminopropionic acid, the direct precursor of the neurotoxin β-ODAP, in *Lathyrus sativus. Biological and Pharmaceutical Bulletin*, 22(7):770–771.

Jain, R. K., Junaid, M. A., and Rao, S. L. N. 1998. Receptor interactions of β-N-oxalyl-L-α, β-diaminopropionic acid, the Lathyrus sativus putative excitotoxin, with synaptic membranes. *Neurochemical research*, 23(9):1191–1196.

Jyothi, P., Pratap Rudra, M. P. and Rao, S. L. N. 1999. Sustained nitric oxide generation with L-homoarginine. *Research Communications in Biochemistry and Cell and Molecular Biology*, 3:223–232.

Kebede, B., Urga, K. and Nigatu, A. 1995. Effect of processing methods on the trypsin inhibitor, tannins, phytic acid and ODAP contents of grass pea seeds. *The Ethiopian Journal of Health Development*, 9(2):97–103.

Keeler, R. F. and James, L. F. 1971. Experimental teratogenic lathyrism in sheep and further comparative aspects with teratogenic locoism. *Canadian Journal of Comparative Medicine*, 35(4):332.

Kessler, A. 1947. Lathyrismus. *Monatsschrift für Psychiatrie und Neurologie* 113: 345–375.

Khan, J. K., Kuo, Y. H., Kebede, N. and Lambein, F. 1994. Determination of non-protein amino acids and toxins in Lathyrus by high-performance liquid chromatography with precolumn phenyl isothiocyanate derivatization. *Journal of Chromatography A*, 687(1):113–119.

Khandare, A. L., Babu, J. J., Ankulu, M., Aparna, N., Shirfule, A. and Rao, G. S. 2014. Grass pea consumption and present scenario of neurolathyrism in Maharashtra State of India. *The Indian Journal of Medical Research*, 140(1):96.

Khandare, A. L., Kumar, R. H., Meshram, I. I., Arlappa, N., Laxmaiah, A., Venkaiah, K., Rao, P. A., Validandi, V. and Toteja, G. S. 2018. Current scenario of consumption of *Lathyrus sativus* and lathyrism in three districts of Chhattisgarh State, India. *Toxicon*, 150:228–234.

Khandare, A. L., Kalakumar, B., Validandi, V., Qadri, S. S. Y. H., Harishankar, N., Singh, S. S. and Kodali, V. 2020. Neurolathyrism in goat (*Capra hircus*) kid: Model development. *Research in Veterinary Science*, 132:49–53.

Khokhar, S. and Apenten, R. K. O. 2003. Antinutritional factors in food legumes and effects of processing. *The Role of Food, Agriculture, Forestry and Fsheries in Human Nutrition*, 4:82–116.

Khokhar, S., Frías, J., Price, K. R., Fenwick, G. R., and Hedley, C. L. 1996. Physico-Chemical Characteristics of Khesari Dhal (Lathyrus sativus): Changes in α-Galactosides, Monosaccharides and Disaccharides during Food Processing. *Journal of the Science of Food and Agriculture*, 70(4):487–492.

Kislev, M. E. and Hopf, M. 1985. Food remains from Tell Qasille, with special reference to *Lathyrus sativus/cicera*. In A. Mazar (Ed.), *Excavations at Tell Qasille*. Institute of Archaeology, Hebrew University, Jerusalem, part 2:140–147.

Kulkarni, S. W. and Attal, H. C. 1977. An epidemiological study of lathyrism in Amgaon block, Bhandara district, Maharashtra. *Indian Journal of Medical Research*, 66:602–610.

Kumar, A., Natarajan, S., Omar, N. A. B., Singh, P., Bhimani, R., and Singh, S. S. 2018. Proteomic changes in chick brain proteome post treatment with lathyrus sativus neurotoxin, β-N-oxalyl-L-α, β-diaminopropionic acid (L-ODAP): a better insight to transient neurolathyrism. *Toxicological research*, *34*(3):267–279.

Kumar, M., Kannan, A., Upreti, R. K., Mishra, G., Khanna, S. K., and Das, M. 2003. Toxic interaction of Lathyrus sativus and manganese in guinea pig intestine. *Toxicology mechanisms and methods*, *13*(4): 295–300.

Kuo, Y. H., Bau, H. M., Rozan, P., Chowdhury, B., and Lambein, F. 2000. Reduction efficiency of the neurotoxin β-ODAP in low-toxin varieties of Lathyrus sativus seeds by solid state fermentation with Aspergillus oryzae and Rhizopus microsporus var chinensis. *Journal of the Science of Food and Agriculture*, 80(15):2209–2215.

Kumar, S., Bejiga, G., Ahmed, S., Nakkoul, H. and Sarker, A. 2011. Genetic improvement of grass pea for low neurotoxin (β-ODAP) content. *Food and Chemical Toxicology*, 49(3):589–600.

Kuo, Y. H. and Lambein, F. 1991. Biosynthesis of the neurotoxin β-N-oxalyl-α, β-diaminopropionic acid in callus tissue of *Lathyrus sativus. Phytochemistry*, 30(10):3241–3244.

Kuo, Y. H., Khan, J. K. and Lambein, F. 1994. Biosynthesis of the neurotoxin β-ODAP in developing pods of Lathyrus sativus. *Phytochemistry*, 35(4):911–913.

Kuo, Y.-H., Bau, H.-M., Quemener, B., Khan, J. K. and Lambein, F. 1995. Solid-state fermentation of *Lathyrus sativus* seeds using *Aspergillus oryzae* and *Rhizopus oligosporus* sp. T-3 to eliminate the neurotoxin ODAP without loss of nutritional value. *Journal of the Science of Food and Agriculture*, 69:81–89.

Kuo, Y. H., Ikegami, F. and Lambein, F. 1998. Metabolic routes of β-(isoxazolin-5-on-2-yl)-L-alanine (BIA), the precursor of the neurotoxin ODAP (β-n-oxalyl-l-α, β,-diaminopropionic acid), in different legume seedlings. *Phytochemistry*, 49(1):43–48.

Kusama-Eguchi, K., Yoshino, N., Minoura, A., Watanabe, K., Kusama, T., Lambein, F. and Ikegami, F. 2011. Sulfur amino acids deficiency caused by grass pea diet plays an important role in the toxicity of l-β-ODAP by increasing the oxidative stress: Studies on a motor neuron cell line. *Food and Chemical Toxicology*, 49(3):636–643.

La Bella, V., Rizza, M. L., Alfano, F. and Piccoli, F. 1997. Dietary consumption of *Lathyrus sativus* seeds induces behavioral changes in the rat. *Environmental Research*, 74(1):61–66.

Lambein, F., Diasolua Ngudi, D., and Kuo, Y. H. 2010. Progress in prevention of toxico-nutritional neurodegenerations. In *African Technology Development Forum Journal*, 6(3–4):60–65.

Lambein, F., Travella, S., Kuo, Y. H., Van Montagu, M. and Heijde, M. 2019. Grass pea (*Lathyrus sativus* L.): Orphan crop, nutraceutical or just plain food?. *Planta*, 250(3):821–838.

Lengauer, T. and Rarey, M. 1996. Computational methods for biomolecular docking. *Current Opinion in Structural Biology*, 6(3):402–406.

Lisiewska, Z., Korus, A. and Kmiecik, W. 2003. Changes in chemical composition during development of grass pea (*Lathyrus sativus* L.) seeds. *Food/Nahrung*, 47(6):391–396.

Liu, F., Jiao, C., Bi, C., Xu, Q., Chen, P., Heuberger, A. L. and Krishnan, H. B. 2017. Metabolomics approach to understand mechanisms of β-N-oxalyl-l-α, β-diaminopropionic acid (β-ODAP) biosynthesis in grass pea (*Lathyrus sativus* L.). *Journal of Agricultural and Food Chemistry*, 65(47):10206–10213.

López Bellido, L. 1994. Grain legumes for animal feed. *Neglected Crops*, 1492:273–288.

Low, R. K. C., Rotter, R. G., Marquardt, R. R. and Campbell, C. G. 1990. Use of *Lathyrus sativus* L. (var. *Seminis albi*) as a food stuff for poultry. *British Poultry Science*, 31:615–625.

Lullien-Pellerin, V. and Balny, C. 2002. High-pressure as a tool to study some proteins′ properties: Conformational modifications, activity and oligomeric dissociation. *Innovative Food Science and Emerging Technologies*, 3:209–221.

Machingura, M., Salomon, E., Jez, J. M. and Ebbs, S. D. 2016. The β-cyanoalanine synthase pathway: Beyond cyanide detoxification. *Plant, Cell and Environment*, 39(10):2329–2341.

Malathi, K., Padmanaban, G., Rao, S. L. N. and Sarma, P. S. 1967. Studies on the biosynthesis of β-N-oxalyl-l-α, β-diaminopropionic acid, the *Lathyrus sativus* neurotoxin. *Biochimica et Biophysica Acta (BBA)-General Subjects*, 141(1):71–78.

Malathi, K., Padmanaban, G. and Sarma, P. S. 1970. Biosynthesis of β-N-oxalyl-l-α, β-diaminopropionic acid, the *Lathyrus sativus* neurotoxin. *Phytochemistry*, 9(7):1603–1610.

Mani, K. S., Srlramachari, S., Rao, S. L. N. and Sarma, P. S. 1971. Experimental neurolahyrism in monkey. *Indian Journal of Medical Research*, 59(6):880–885.

Marichamy, S., Yigzaw, Y., Gorton, L. and Mattiasson, B. 2005. Isolation of obligate anaerobic rumen bacteria capable of degrading the neurotoxin β-ODAP (β-N-oxalyl-L-α, β-diaminopropionic acid) as evaluated by a liquid chromatography/biosensor analysis system. *Journal of the Science of Food and Agriculture*, 85(12):2027–2032.

Materon, L. A. and Ryan, J. 1995. Rhizobial inoculation and phosphorus and zinc nutrition for annual medics adapted to Mediterranean environments. *Agronomy Journal*, 87(4):692–698.

McDonald, B. and Morris, M. H. 1984. The statistical validity of the ratio method in financial analysis: An empirical examination. *Journal of Business Finance and Accounting*, 11(1):89–97.

Mehta, T., Hsu, A. F. and Haskell, B. E. 1972. Specificity of the neurotoxin from *Lathyrus sativus* as an amino acid antagonist. *Biochemistry*, 11(22):4053–4063.

Melka, A., Tekle-Haimanot, R. and Lambien F. 1997. Symptomatic treatment of neurolathyrism with Tolperizone HCL (Mydocalm): A randomized double blind and placebo controlled drug trial. *Ethiopian Medical Journal*, 35:77–91.

Moges, G., Solomon, T. and Johansson, G. 1993. Flow injection spectrophotometric and amperometric determinations of ammonia with glutamate dehydrogenase reactor. *Bulletin of the Chemical Society of Ethiopia*, 7(2):99–112.

Moges, G., Solomon, T. and Johansson, G. 1994. Glutamate oxidase-catalyzed oxidation of β-N-Oxalyl-L-α, β-N-diaminopropionic acid (ß-ODAP), a neurotoxin in the seeds of lathyrus sativus. *Analytical Letters*, 27(12):2207–2221.

Morino, Y. and Snell, E. E.. 1970. Tryptophanase (*Eischerichia coli* B). In: *Methods in Enzymology*, Vol. XVIIA, S. P. Colowick and N. O. Kaplan (Eds.). Academic Press, New York, 439.

Mukherjee, A. and Chakravarty, A. 2010. Spasticity mechanisms–for the clinician. *Frontiers in Neurology*, 1(149): 1–10.

Mullan, B. P., Hanbury, C. D., Hooper, J. A., Nicholls, R. R., Hagan, C. R. and Siddique, K. H. M. 1999. Lathyrus (Lathyrus cicera cv. Chalus): A potential new ingredient in pig grower diets. *Recent Advances in Animal Nutrition in Australia*, 12:12A.

Nagarajan, V. and Gopalan, C. 1968. Variation in the neurotoxin β-(N)-oxalylamino-alanine content in *Lathyrus sativus* samples from Madhya Pradesh. *Indian Journal of Medical Research*, 56(1):95–99.

Nunn, P. B., Bell, E. A., Watson, A. A. and Nash, R. J. 2010. Toxicity of non-protein amino acids to humans and domestic animals. *Natural Product Communications*, 5(3):485–504.

Olney, J. W., Zorumski, C., Price, M. T. and Labruyere, J. 1990. L-cysteine, a bicarbonate-sensitive endogenous excitotoxin. *Science*, 248(4955):596–599.

Omelchenko, I. A., Jain, R. K., Junaid, M. A., Rao, S. L. N. and Allen, C. N. 1999. Neurotoxic potential of three structural analogs of β-N-oxalyl-α, β-diaminopropanoic acid (β-ODAP). *Neurochemical Research*, 24(6):791–797.

Padmajaprasad, V., Kaladhar, M. and Bhat, R. V. 1997. Thermal isomerisation of β-N-oxalyl-L-α, β-diaminopropionic acid, the neurotoxin in *Lathyrus sativus*, during cooking. *Food Chemistry*, 59(1):77–80.

Pearson, S. and Nunn, P. B. 1981. The neurolathyrogen, β-N-oxalyl-L-α, β-diaminopropionic acid, is a potent agonist at 'glutamate preferring'receptors in the frog spinal cord. *Brain Research*, 206(1):178–182.

Prakash, S., Misra, B. K., Adsule, R. N. and Barat, G. K. 1977. Distribution of β-N-oxalyl-L-α-β diaminopropionic acid in different tissues of aging *Lathyrus sativus* plant. *Biochemie und Physiologie der Pflanzen*, 171(4):369–374.

Rahman, Q. N., Akhtar, N. I. L. O. F. A. R. and Chowdhury, A. M. 1974. Proximate composition of food-stuffs in Bangladesh. Part I. Cereals and pulses. *Journal of Scientific Industrial Research*, 9:129–133.

Rao, D. R., Hariharan, K. and Vijayalakshmi, K. R. 1974. Specific enzymic procedure for the determination of neurotoxic components (derivatives of L-. alpha.,. beta.-diaminopropionic acid) in *Lathyrus sativus*. *Journal of Agricultural and Food Chemistry*, 22(6):1146–1148.

Rao, S. L. N. 1978. A sensitive and specific colorimetric method for the determination of α, β-diaminopropionic acid and the Lathyrus sativus neurotoxin. *Analytical Biochemistry*, 86(2):386–395.

Rao, S. L. N. 2001. Do we need more research on neurolathyrism?. *Membranes*, 23:1191–1196.

Rao, S. L. N., Adiga, P. R. and Sarma, P. S. 1964. The isolation and characterization of β-N-oxalyl-L-α, β-diaminopropionic acid: A neurotoxin from the seeds of *Lathyrus sativus*. *Biochemistry*, 3(3): 432–436.

Rao, S. L. N., Sarma, P. S., Mani, K. S., Rao, T. R., and Sriramachari, S. 1967. Experimental neurolathyrism in monkeys. *Nature*, 214(5088):610–611.

Rasmussen, M. A., Foster, J. G. and Allison, M. J. 1992. *Lathyrus sylvestris* (Flat pea) toxicity in sheep and ruminal metabolism of flat pea neurolathyrogens. In James, L. F., Keeler, R. F., Bailey, E. M., Cheeke, P. R., Hegarty, M. P. (Eds.), Proceedings of the Third International Symposium on Poisonous Plants, Iowa State University Press, Ames, IA.

Ravindranath, V. 2002. Neurolathyrism: Mitochondrial dysfunction in excitotoxicity mediated by L-β-oxalyl aminoalanine. *Neurochemistry International*, 40(6):505–509.

Rehman, S. U., Paterson, A., Hussain, S., Murtaza, M. A. and Mehmood, S. 2007. Influence of partial substitution of wheat flour with vetch (*Lathyrus sativus* L) flour on quality characteristics of doughnuts. *LWT-Food Science and Technology*, 40(1):73–82.

Riepe, M., Spencer, P. S., Lambein, F., Ludolph, A. C. and Allen, C. N. 1995. *In vitro* toxicological investigations of isoxazolinone amino acids of *Lathyrus sativus*. *Natural Toxins*, 3(1):58–64.

Roche, K. W., Raymond, L. A., Blackstone, C. and Huganir, R. L. 1994. Transmembrane topology of the glutamate receptor subunit Clu-R6. *Journal of Biological Chemistry*, 269:11679–11682.

Roche, K. W., O'Brien, R. J., Mammen, A. L., Bernhardt, J. and Huganir, R. L. 1996. Characterization of multiple phosphorylation sites on the AMPA receptor GluR1 subunit. *Neuron*, 16(6):1179–1188.

Rodrigues-Corrêa, K. C. D. S. and Fett-Neto, A. G. 2019. Abiotic stresses and non-protein amino acids in plants. *Critical Reviews in Plant Sciences*, 38(5–6):411–430.

Rodríguez Arias, B. 1950. Estudio de una epidemia de latirismo en España. *Medicina Clínica* 15:370–374.

Ross, S. M., Roy, D. N. and Spencer, P. S. 1985. β-N-oxalylamino-l-alanine: Action on high-affinity transport of neurotransmitters in rat brain and spinal cord synaptosomes. *Journal of Neurochemistry*, 44(3):886–892.

Ross, S. M., Roy, D. N. and Spencer, P. S. 1989. β-N-oxalylamino-L-alanine action on glutamate receptors. *Journal of Neurochemistry*, 53(3):710–715.

Rotter, R. G., R. R. Marquardt and C. G. Campbell. 1991. The nutritional value of low lathyrogenic *Lathyrus* (*Lathyrus sativus*) for growing chicks. *British Poultry Science*. 32:1055–1067.

Rudra, M. P., Singh, M. R., Junaid, M. A., Jyothi, P. and Rao, S. L. N. 2004. Metabolism of dietary ODAP in humans may be responsible for the low incidence of neurolathyrism. *Clinical Biochemistry*, 37(4):318–322.

Sharma, S., Srivastav, S., Singh, G., Singh, S., Malik, R., Alam, M. M., Shaqiquzamman, M., Ali, S. and Akhter, M. 2020. *In silico* strategies for probing novel DPP-IV inhibitors as anti-diabetic agents. *Journal of Biomolecular Structure and Dynamics*, 39(6):2118–2132.

Sharma, S., Srivastava, S., Shrivastava, A., Malik, R., Almalki, F., Saifullah, K., Alam, M. M., Shaqiquzzaman, M., Ali, S. and Akhter, M. 2019. Mining of potential dipeptidyl peptidase-IV inhibitors as anti-diabetic agents using integrated *in silico* approaches. *Journal of Biomolecular Structure and Dynamics*, 38(18):5349–5361.

Sharma, S., Sharma, S., Pathak, V., Kaur, P. and Singh R. K. 2021. Drug repurposing using similarity-based target prediction, docking studies and scaffold hopping of lefamulin. *Letters in Drug Design and Discovery*, 18(7):733–743. https://doi.org/10.2174/1570180817999201201113712.

Shashi Vardhan K., Pratap Rudra M. P. and Rao S. L. N. 1997. Inhibition of tyrosine aminotransferase by h-N-oxalyl-L-a, h-diaminopropionic acid, the *Lathyrus sativus* neurotoxin. *Journal of Neurochemistry*, 68:2477–84.

Shiferaw, E. and Porceddu, E. 2018. Assessment of variability in grass pea germplasm using β-ODAP content and seed protein electrophoresis. *Annual Review of Food Science and Technology*, 19:316–323.

Siddique, K. H. M., Loss, S. P., Herwig, S. P. and Wilson, J. M. 1996. Growth, yield and neurotoxin (ODAP) concentration of three *Lathyrus* species in Mediterranean-type environments of Western Australia. *Australian Journal of Experimental Agriculture*, 36(2):209–218.

Singh, M. R., Rudra, M. P., Rao, S. L. N. and Singh, S. S. 2004. *In vitro* activation of protein kinase C by β-N-oxalyl-L-α, β-diaminopropionic acid, the *Lathyrus sativus* neurotoxin. *Neurochemical Research*, 29(7):1343–1348.

Sleeman, W. H. 1844. *Rambles and Recollections of an Indian Official*, Vol. I . London: J. Hatchard and Son, 478.

Soderling, T. R., Tan, S. E., McGlade-McCulloh, E., Yamamoto, H. and Fukunaga, K. 1994. Excitatory interaction between glutamate receptors and protein kinases. *Journal of Neurobiology*, 25(3):304–311.

Spencer, P., Ludolph, A., Dwivedi, M. P., Roy, D., Hugon, J. and Schaumburg, H. H. 1986. Lathyrism: Evidence for role of the neuroexcitatory amino acid BOAA. *The Lancet*, 328(8515):1066–1067.

Sriram, K., Shankar, S. K., Boyd, M. R. and Ravindranath, V. 1998. Thiol oxidation and loss of mitochondrial complex I precede excitatory amino acid-mediated neuro degeneration. *Journal of Neuroscience*, 18(24):10287–10296.

Srivastava, R. P., Singh, J., Singh, N. P. and Singh, D. 2015. Neurotoxin and other anti-nutrients of khesari (Lathyrus sativus) genotypes and their reduction by water soaking and dehusking. *Indian Journal of Agricultural Biochemistry*, 28(2):172–177.

Srivastava, S. and Khokhar, S. 1996. Effects of processing on the reduction of β-ODAP (β-N-Oxalyl-L-2, 3-diaminopropionic acid) and anti-nutrients of *Khesari Dhal, Lathyrus sativus. Journal of the Science of Food and Agriculture*, 71(1):50–58.

Starzynska-Janiszewska, A. and Stodolak, B. 2011. Effect of inoculated lactic acid fermentation on antinutritional and antiradical properties of grass pea (*Lathyrus sativus*' Krab') flour. *Polish Journal of Food and Nutrition Sciences*, 61(4): 245–249.

Steyn, D. G., 1933. *Lathyrus sativus* L. (chickling vetch khesari Indian pea) as a stock food. *Onderstepoort Journal of Veterinary Science and Animal Industry*, 1:163–171.

Stockman, R. 1917. Lathyrism. *Edinburgh Medical Journal*, 19:277–296.

Stockman, R. 1931. The poisonous principle of Lathyrus and some other leguminous seeds. *Epidemiology & Infection*, 31(4):550–562.

Tadelle, D., Alemu, Y., Nigusie, D. and Peters, K. J. 2003. Evaluation of processing methods on the feeding value of grass pea to broilers. *International Journal of Poultry Science*, 2(2):120–127.

Tekle-Haimanot, R., Abegaz, B. M., Wuhib, E., Kassina, A., Kidane, Y., Kebede, N., Alemu, T. and Spencer, P. S. 1993. Pattern of *Lathyrus sativus* (grass pea) consumption and beta-N-oxalyl-α-β-diaminoproprionic acid (β-ODAP) content of food samples in the lathyrism endemic region of northwest Ethiopia. *Nutrition Research*, 13(10):1113–1126.

Tekle-Haimanot, R., Getachew, T., Doyle, D., Kriek, N. P. J. and Spencer, P. S. 1997. Preliminary report on the development of an animal model for human neurolathyrism. In Tekle-Haimanot, R., Lambein, F. (Eds.), *Lathyrus and Lathyrism, a Decade of Progress*. University of Ghent, Belgium, 27–29.

Urga, K., Fite, A. and Kebede, B. 1995. Nutritional and antinutritional factors of grass pea (Lathyrus sativus) germplasms. *Bulletin of the Chemical Society of Ethiopia*, 9(1).

Urga, K., Fufa, H., Biratu, E. and Husain, A. 2005. Evaluation of Lathyrus sativus cultivated in Ethiopia for proximate composition, minerals, β-ODAP and anti-nutritional components. *African Journal of Food, Agriculture, Nutrition and Development*, 5(1):1–16.

Valamoti, S. M., Moniaki, A. and Karathanou, A. 2011. An investigation of processing and consumption of pulses among prehistoric societies: Archaeobotanical, experimental and ethnographic evidence from Greece. *Vegetation History and Archaeobotany*, 20(5):381–396.

Van Moorhem, M., Lambein, F. and Leybaert, L. 2011. Unraveling the mechanism of β-N-oxalyl-α, β-diaminopropionic acid (β-ODAP) induced excitotoxicity and oxidative stress, relevance for neurolathyrism prevention. *Food and Chemical Toxicology*, 49(3):550–555.

Woldeamanuel, Y. W., Hassan, A. and Zenebe, G. 2012. Neurolathyrism: Two Ethiopian case reports and review of the literature. *Journal of Neurology*, 259:1263–1268.

Yadav, V. K., Santha, I. M., Timko, M. P., and Mehta, S. L. 1992. Metabolism of the Lathyrus sativus L. neurotoxin, β-N-oxalyl-L-α, β-diaminopropionic acid, by a pure culture of a soil-borne microbe. *Journal of Plant Biochemistry and Biotechnology*, 1(2): 87–92.

Yan, Z. Y., Spencer, P. S., Li, Z. X., Liang, Y. M., Wang, Y. F., Wang, C. Y. and Li, F. M. 2006. *Lathyrus sativus* (grass pea) and its neurotoxin ODAP. *Phytochemistry*, 67(2):107–121.

Yang, H. M. and Zhang, X. Y. 2005. Considerations on the reintroduction of grass pea in China. *Lathyrus Lathyrism Newsletter*, 4:22–26.

Yerra, S., Putta, S., and Kilari, E. K. 2015. Effect of various processing methods on the mineral content of *Lathyrus sativus* seeds cultivated in different states of India. *World Journal of Pharmaceutical Research*, 4(9):1522–1530.

Yerra, S., Putta, S., and Kilari, E. K. 2016. The role of food processing the techniques in the detoxification of ODAP in Lathyrus sativus. *International Journal of Information Research and Review*, 3(8), 2818–2822.

Yigzaw, Y., Gorton, L., Solomon, T. and Akalu, G. 2004. Fermentation of seeds of Teff (*Eragrostis teff*), grass-pea (*Lathyrus sativus*), and their mixtures: Aspects of nutrition and food safety. *Journal of Agricultural and Food Chemistry*, 52(5):1163–1169.

Yusuf, H. K. M., Hoque, K., Uddin, A., Roy, B. C. and Lambein, F. 1995. Homoarginine antagonizes the toxicity of Lathyrus toxin in 1-day-old-chicks. *Bangladesh Journal of Physiology and Pharmacology*, 10(2):74–75.

CHAPTER 15

# Toxic Amino Acids and Fatty Acids

**Sanusi Shamsudeen Nassarawa, Hauwa Ladi Yusuf, and Salamatu Ahmad Sulaiman**

## CONTENTS



## 15.1 INTRODUCTION

Proteins are made up of 20 L-a-amino acids that have been coded. The availability of amino acids or crucial qualities such as chemical, thermal, and photochemical stability may influence evolutionary selection (Rodgers, Samardzic, and Main 2017). The capacity of side-chain groups to impart various functions on the synthesized protein is believed to have driven their diversity. Once peptides are linked into proteins, canonical or "protein" amino acids can undergo various post-translational changes, enhancing the protein's functional capabilities. There are around 1,000 amino acids found in nature, many of which are synthesized by plants. The 20 protein amino acids are the most

DOI: 10.1201/9781003178446-15

commonly found in the human body (Rodgers, Samardzic, and Main 2017). The toxicity of amino acids was first studied in depth in the early 1960s. Neurolathyrism, one of the earliest neurotoxic disorders known, is the most prominent example of amino acid poisoning. Some plant amino acids have gotten a lot of attention because of their toxicity (Rodgers, Samardzic, and Main 2017). This was not owing to the amino acid molecule's natural chemical reactivity but rather to its likeness to one of the "selected" 20 protein amino acids. The capacity of an amino acid to be mistaken for and substitute for a protein amino acid in a metabolic pathway or biological function determines its toxicity. This occurs most frequently during protein synthesis, although it can also happen when amino acids act as receptor agonists or enzyme substrates (Rodgers, Samardzic, and Main 2017). Protein synthesis is an essential process for all living things, and interfering with it could cause serious and widespread damage. Amino acids may have been the first plant poisons, as they might have harmed the growth of even the most rudimentary creatures that relied on protein synthesis for survival. Autotoxicity can be protected by a single host defence strategy for amino acids that target protein synthesis. The emergence of a more selective protein synthesis machinery capable of differentiating the protein amino acid from "imposters" or fast alteration of amino acids causes autotoxicity (Rodgers, Samardzic, and Main 2017).

This chapter will go over the dangers of toxic amino acids. The focus is on findings related to the chemistry and metabolism of these substances, classification, mechanism of action, toxicology, identification and quantification, safety, precautions, regulation, and future scope.

## 15.2 CHEMISTRY

The polymerization products of roughly 20 proteinogenic amino acids are peptides and polypeptides. In all 20 α-amino acids, the carboxylic acid (-COOH) and amino (-NH2) functional groups are connected to the same tetrahedral carbon atom (Tripathy et al. 2018). The R-groups connected to the -carbon distinguishes amino acids from one another, with the exception of glycine, which has a hydrogen R-group. Different structures, sizes, and electric charges (acidity/basicity) can be found in R-groups (Tripathy et al. 2018)

Amino acids (excluding glycine) are chiral and thus optically active due to the presence of four distinct substituents bonded to a carbon. Amino acids can be found in two configurations, both of which are non-superimposable mirror images of one another, albeit the L-stereoisomers are substantially more prevalent. Aromatic R-groups absorb UV radiation in certain amino acids with maximum absorption at 280 nm (Tripathy et al. 2018). In amino acids, both the acidic-COOH and basic-NH2 groups can ionize and establish ionic equilibrium in the following way:

$$R-COOH \leftrightarrow R-COO^{-}+H^{-}$$

$$R-NH\text{þ}3 \leftrightarrow R-NH2+H^{-}$$

Despite the fact that amino acids include at least two mildly acidic groups, the carboxyl group is a much more powerful acid than the amino group (Pathak and Keharia 2014). The carboxyl group is protonated at pH 7.4, whereas the amino group is not. At this pH, an amino acid with an ionizable R-group is electrically neutral, producing zwitterions.

### 15.2.1 Structural Properties

The structure, length, and non-polar hydrophobic fatty acid chains found in amino acids can vary (Tripathy et al. 2018). The structure of amino acids explains their tremendous compositional diversity and wide range of physicochemical and biological properties. Differences in the amino acid or peptide head group of Amino acids impact a surfactant's adsorption, aggregation, and biological activity. They are classified as cationic, anionic, non-ionic, or amphoteric based on the functional groups they contain. Polar amino acids were combined with a non-polar, long-chain hydrophobic moiety to generate the structure. This resulted in molecules with high surface activity, as well as chiral compounds (Pathak and Keharia 2014).

## 15.3 CLASSIFICATION

### 15.3.1 Origins

#### *15.3.1.1 Natural Class*

Specific amino acid-based molecules can reduce surface and interfacial tension, outperforming glycolipids in some cases (Nwosu, Anyaehie, and Ofoedu 2019). Lipopeptides are another name for these sorts of amino acids. Lipopeptides are low-molecular-weight molecules generated mostly by the Bacillus species. Surfactin, iturin, and Fengycins are the three subclasses of amino acids in this category.

The heptapeptide variations of the aspirin, pumilacidin, lichenin, and surfactin groups are included in the surfactin family. The peptide moiety is connected to a $C_{12}$-$C_{16}$ unsaturated linear, iso, or anteiso β-hydroxyl fatty acid chain in these types of surfactants. Surfactants are macrolactonerings in which β-hydroxyl fatty acid mediates ring closure with a C-terminal peptide (Nwosu, Anyaehie, and Ofoedu 2019).

In the iturin class, the heptapeptide is linked to multiple C14-C17 chains of fatty acids. Iturins create an amide bond with the C-terminal group, resulting in a macrolactame structure (Nwosu, Anyaehie, and Ofoedu 2019). Macrolactone rings with a Tyr side chain at the third position in the peptide sequence are known as fengycins. They have a C14-C18 linear fatty acid chain saturated or unsaturated, iso, or anteiso-hydroxylated (Nwosu, Anyaehie, and Ofoedu 2019).

#### *15.3.1.2 Synthetic Class*

The amino acids used in producing protein hydrolysates, or amino acids, can be found in many products. A surfactant family is a group of chemicals that can be easily synthesized. The most common are glucine, arginine, alanine, serine, proline, aspartic acid, glutamic acid, and leucine. N-lauroyl-L-glutamic acid and N-palmitoyl-L-glutamic acid are two common examples (Tripathy et al. 2018).

### 15.3.2 Based on Aliphatic Chain Substitution

#### *15.3.2.1 N-Substituted Amino Acids*

In N-substituted compounds, alkalinity is lost when an amino group is replaced with a lipophilic moiety or a carboxylic group. N-acyl amino acids, which are anionic, are the most basic N-substituted amino acids. An amide bond is generated between the hydrophobic and hydrophilic moieties in N-substituted amino acids. The capacity of amide linkage to create hydrogen bonds facilitates surfactant breakdown in acidic environments, making them biodegradable (Tripathy et al. 2018).

#### *15.3.2.2 C-Substituted Amino Acids*

Substitution occurs on the carboxylic group of C-substituted compounds via an amide or ester bond. C-substituted molecules, such as esters and amides, are often cationic (Tripathy et al. 2018).

#### 15.3.2.3 N- and C-Substituted Amino Acids

In the second family of surfactants, the hydrophilic moiety contains both amino and carboxylic groups. These types have an amphoteric character (Tripathy et al. 2018).

### 15.3.3 Based on the Number of the Hydrophobic Tail

The number of the hydrophobic tail and head groups divides amino acids into four categories. Amino acids include monomeric or linear amino acids, dimeric or gemini amino acids, and glycerolipid type amino acids. Linear chain surfactants are composed comprised of amino acids that have at least one hydrophobic tail. Surfactants with two polar amino acid heads connected by a single hydrophobic tail are known as bolaamphiphile amino acids. These surfactants are analogues of monoglycerides, diglycerides, and phospholipids (Tripathy et al. 2018).

## 15.4 MECHANISM OF ACTION

Amino acids are essential for protein synthesis. These are used to make methyl donor methionine. Choline, betaine, creatine, and epinephrine all require this methyl donor to be synthesized. When the amino acid methionine is not sufficiently supplied in the diet, it can be transformed into cystine. Tyrosine is the precursor to epinephrine, thyroxine, and the pigment melanin, and it can be transformed into phenylalanine. Glycine, arginine, and methionine are all involved in the synthesis of creatine. The main source of ammonia synthesis in the kidney is glutamine, which is generated from glutamate. Ammonia aids in the neutralization of excreted acid. Glycine is a medication that functions as a coupling agent, transforming benzoic and salicylic acids into hippuric and salicyclic acids. Histamine is formed when histidine is decarboxylated. In the presence of vitamin B6 and B2, tryptophan can be converted to nicotinic acid and serotonin, which can then be acetylated and methylated to form the hormone melatonin. Purine and pyrimidine synthesis uses glutamate, aspartate, and ammonia generated by amino acids (Tripathy et al. 2018).

Transamination of glutamate and aspartate produces keto acids, which are then transformed to glucose through gluconeogenesis. Pyruvic acid is formed when alanine is deaminated, an important step in glucose metabolism. Alanine, like glucose, has a similar fate. As a result, alanine is a glucose-forming amino acid. The different amino acids are utilized for energy synthesis if the food contains more proteins than is required to replace the catabolized protein. The liver and kidney have an oxidative deaminating enzyme system that can convert amino acids into keto acids, releasing ammonia in the free state. Ammonia is used in the synthesis of urea. Some amino acids are converted to glucose derivatives, whereas others are converted to acetoacetate (Tripathy et al. 2018).

## 15.5 TOXICOLOGY

Surfactants, particularly cationic surfactants, are extremely hazardous to aquatic life, including algae, fish, and molluscs. Their acute toxicity is related to their propensity for disrupting the integral membrane of the membrane. Surfactant adsorption onto interfaces is often increased when the cmc of the surfactant is reduced. Amino acids are substances that can be used as food additives, pharmaceuticals, and cosmetics. Most amino acids have low toxicity, are nontoxic, or have nontoxicity to humans and the environment due to their low toxicity levels. They are suitable for food additives because they are not harmful to humans (Morán et al. 2004). Surfactants made from amino acids are mild on the skin and do not irritate (Rodgers, Samardzic, and Main 2017). Surfactants based on arginine are recognized to be less harmful than traditional surfactants. Amino acid-based amphiphiles and their spontaneously formed cationic vesicles made of tyrosine, hydroxyproline, serine, and lysine were examined for their physicochemical and toxicological properties. (Rodgers et al. 2017). And surfactant is less ecotoxic than commonly used dodecyl trimethylammonium bromide. Researchers tested their ecotoxins and haemolytic potential. They found it was less toxic than the widely used surfactant dodecyl trimethylammonium bromide. The interaction of amino acid-based surfactants appeared harmless compared to routinely used cationic surfactants, which can be hazardous (Aralu, Chukwuemeka-Okorie, and Akpomie 2021). Sulfur-based amino acid-based surfactants have been shown to be more effective corrosion inhibitors in numerous investigations. They are simple to synthesize, inexpensive, biodegradable, and soluble in aqueous conditions (Mobin, Parveen, and Rafiquee 2017). Rhamnolipids have a better toxicological profile than synthetic surfactants. Rhamnilipids were already recognized to improve permeability (Perinelli et al. 2018).

### 15.5.1 Mechanisms of Toxicology

#### *15.5.1.1 Misincorporation into Protein*

The potential of non-protein amino acids to substitute for a protein amino acid in protein synthesis, resulting in abnormal or non-native proteins, was the first mechanism of non-protein amino acid toxicity discovered (Rodgers, Samardzic, and Main 2017). In early studies of bacteria, high quantities of non-protein amino acids were used. It was observed that if the non-protein amino acid replaced a vital component of the enzyme's active site, it might cause the enzyme to lose activity (Rodgers, Samardzic, and Main 2017). Significant structural changes to a protein caused by amino acid substitution, on the other hand, could result in a loss of function or a decrease in water solubility (Rodgers, Samardzic, and Main 2017). This was only true for a few non-protein amino acids close to protein amino acids in size, structure, and charge and was referred to as amino acid analogues, or "proteomimetic" amino acids in the case of non-protein amino acids that might be incorrectly integrated into proteins (Rodgers, Samardzic, and Main 2017).

#### *15.5.1.2 Excitotoxicity*

A new type of toxicity occurs when the ionotropic (ion-channel coupled) glutamate receptor is overstimulated. Excitotoxicity is a kind of neuronal toxicity caused by overstimulation of the glutamate receptor in the cell's excitotoxic state (Rodgers, Samardzic, and Main 2017).

#### *15.5.1.3 Nephrotoxicity*

Djenkolic acid, a powerful nephrotoxin that causes djenkolism, was discovered in the djenkol bean (*Archidendron pauciflorum*). Djenkolic acid has since been found in some Australian acacia species belonging to the *Fabaceae* subfamily *Mimosoideae*. Ingestion of djenkolic acid-containing seeds by humans can cause various symptoms such as abdominal pain, nausea, vomiting, and hematuria in as little as 2–12 h; however, susceptibility to djenkolic acid and the severity of symptoms varies greatly between people (Rodgers, Samardzic, and Main 2017). Djenkolic acid is supposed to protect against insect herbivory, but it has been discovered that the bruchid beetle, a common legume pest, prefers to feed on acacia with greater djenkolic acid concentrations (Rodgers, Samardzic, and Main 2017). This shows that bruchid beetles have evolved to detoxify djenkolic acid and may have discovered a way to exploit it.

## 15.6 IDENTIFICATION AND QUANTIFICATION

Amino acid quantification is a technique for determining the amino acid composition or content of proteins, peptides, and other pharmacological or biological preparations. The amino acid analysis is a basic biochemical technique used by scientists to determine protein composition. The method is also known as amino acid identification (Pathak and Keharia 2014). Protein complexes or protein combinations can also be tested using amino acid testing. By analyzing the concentration of free amino acids in bodily fluids such as urine, blood, or plasma, amino acid quantification can monitor or identify metabolic states. Mammals have many protein molecules, and they are a significant and required part of their diet and metabolism (Pathak and Keharia 2014). Amino acids in plant extracts have been analyzed using a variety of chromatographic methods. Some research focuses on the GC analysis of amino acids in foods (Pathak and Keharia 2014). T-butyldimethylsilyl derivatives are a moisture-stable substitute for the trimethylsilyl derivatization group. The amino acids can be quantitatively converted to the appropriate T-balyldimethylaminc derivatives (Starke, Kleinpeter, and Kamm 2001). Temperature, solvent, and reagents have all been investigated to see how they affect the efficiency of the derivatization procedure (Starke, Kleinpeter, and Kamm 2001). The EI mass spectra of T-butyldimethylsilyl amino acid derivatives are highly different. The molecular mass of the amino acid derivatives was validated using chemical ionization mass spectrometry with methane as the reagent gas (Starke, Kleinpeter, and Kamm 2001).

## 15.7 SAFETY, PRECAUTIONS, AND REGULATION

The Department of Health and Human Services has approved 18 amino acids to conventional diets as a food supplement to improve protein quality according to the Code of Federal Regulations. This review focuses solely on pre-packaged meals and dietary supplements marketed to healthy adults and analyzes the nutritional benefits of adding proteinogenic amino acids. Other uses of safe amino acids are not restricted, but they do necessitate careful consideration of the functional mix of amino acids. During the generally recognized safe determination, all important safety issues, such as production processes, dose, toxicity, and the target consumer group, should be examined. Maximum daily limits are set for each product and are dependent on the target customer group (s) (Roberts 2016). The World Health Organization has banned amino acids from food products that are not designed to increase protein quality (Smriga 2020).

Food fortification is legal in Japan and Singapore, with no direct governmental monitoring or daily limitations. Indonesia has the highest level of amino acid fortification in the world (Smriga 2020). Most countries in the region restrict amino acids to specifically formulated sports foods. Indonesia and Thailand lack a regulatory framework to regulate amino acids in food and do not authorize them in most cases. Most other countries in Asia, including China, Japan, and South Korea, restrict specific sports foods only (Smriga 2020). Amino acids are included as "other substances" in the European Commission's food fortification regulation (EC) 1925/2006. The EU food law's general horizontal regulations are the only source of advice for food formulators, according to the EC (Smriga 2020). The European Union does not allow the use of certain foodstuffs with a positive list of amino acids. The only exception is "Foods for Specific Groups" [regulation (EU) 609/2013), which includes protein-rich cereals and fish (Smriga 2020).

Amino acids are widely utilized as dietary supplements, but there is no governmental monitoring of dosage, formulation, or purity criteria. The Department of Health and Human Services says it has no plans to regulate the use of amino acids in its food supply for health reasons. Some Asian and Latin American countries do not regulate amino acid supplementation explicitly (also referred to as food supplements). Strict regulations, on the other hand, have been adopted in a few Southeast Asian countries, such as Thailand, Japan, Korea, and Singapore; it has no dietary supplement regulation at all (Pathak and Keharia 2014).

The purity level of each ingredient has an impact on a dietary supplement's overall safety rating. There have been well-documented cases of major negative consequences linked to inadvertent or commercially driven contamination (Aralu, Chukwuemeka-Okorie, and Akpomie 2021). Amino acid is a key ingredient in the diet, but it can also be found in a wide range of other dietary supplements (Aralu, Chukwuemeka-Okorie, and Akpomie 2021). There is no peer-reviewed research detailing substantial adverse reactions to an amino acid supplement overdose, even in subgroups suspected of habitually taking dietary supplements (Smriga 2020). This could be due to technological hurdles like taste and texture or other issues covered in past "Amino Acid Assessment Workshops," such as acute intestine reactions, which are the first "warning" signs of overdosing (Smriga 2020). Some countries promote amino acids to protect consumers' health from harmful side effects such as high blood pressure (Smriga 2020).

Amino acids are considered macronutrients consumed in doses of many grams per day. Amino acids are micronutrients that are ingested in big amounts. Some risk-assessment organizations employ amino acid safety factors designed for high-protein foods, while others ignore them entirely when it comes to small quantities (Smriga 2020). For example, in Brazil, the well-studied essential amino acid leucine, often used in sports supplements, is allowed in dietary supplements at a maximum of 5.6 g/d, Germany at 5.0 g/d, and Switzerland 2.4 g/d, but just 0.7 g/d in Thailand (Smriga 2020).

## 15.8 FUTURE SCOPE

Long-lived cells, such as neurons and retinal pigment epithelial cells, are more vulnerable to aggregated proteins than dividing cells because they can't distribute them among daughter cells. Neurodegenerative diseases characterize these diseases. Long-lived cell populations have been shown to increase protein misfolding. The possibility of non-protein amino acids bioaccumulating should be seriously explored, according to the researchers. Most strains of cyanobacteria produce β-N-methylamino-L-alanine, which is concentrated by cycads and flying foxes (Dunlop et al. 2013). This could be a source of bioaccumulation in the food chain since some non-protein amino acids can be misincorporated into proteins.

Non-protein amino acids can compete with protein amino acids for interactions at enzyme active sites or with receptors. Many non-protein amino acids must be present in large concentrations to have a biological effect. Some examples of situations where their toxicity is clear, such as famine and severe protein amino acid deficiency, are provided. Non-protein amino acids can cause a range of health problems, according to the Department of Health and Human Services. Parkinson's disease and amyotrophic lateral sclerosis are more than 10% hereditary. The processes that cause the disease have yet to be uncovered. Parkinson's is one of the leading causes of death in the world, according to the World Health Organization. There are no recognized causes for these diseases. Chronic exposure to proteomimetic plant non-protein amino acids may raise the burden of non-native proteins in brain cells, perhaps leading to illness in genetically sensitive people. Researchers must solve these challenges because the knowledge obtained could benefit all living beings on the planet.

## 15.9 CONCLUSION

Amino acids have been proved to have a wide range of uses in various industries, and the diversity of properties resulting from their structural variability will allow this range of applications to expand in the future. Amino acids are said to have a wide range of applications in a variety of fields. Amino acids' simple biodegradability and nontoxicity can make them superior to their synthetic equivalents when used correctly. When used correctly, amino acids can be more effective than their synthetic counterparts. When handled correctly, amino acids can make them preferable to their synthetic counterparts. High production costs and the difficulty of isolating amino acids to high purity levels are just two of the obstacles that amino acids face. Amino acids can be difficult to produce because of their structure and physiochemical capabilities. Various researchers are working to address this by identifying appropriate renewable substrates and developing cost-effective and scalable technologies.

## REFERENCES

Aralu, C.C., Chukwuemeka-Okorie, H.O. and Akpomie, K.G. 2021. Inhibition and adsorption potentials of mild steel corrosion using methanol extract of Gongronema latifoliuim. *Applied Water Science*, 11(2): 1–7.

Dunlop, R.A., Cox, P.A., Banack, S.A. and Rodgers, K.J. 2013. The non-protein amino acid BMAA is misincorporated into human proteins in place of L-serine causing protein misfolding and aggregation. *PloS One*, 8(9): 75376.

Mobin, M., Parveen, M. and Rafiquee, M.Z.A. 2017. Synergistic effect of sodium dodecyl sulfate and cetyltrimethyl ammonium bromide on the corrosion inhibition behavior of l-methionine on mild steel in acidic medium. *Arabian Journal of Chemistry*, 10: S1364–S1372.

Morán, M.C., Pinazo, A., Pérez, L., Clapés, P., Angelet, M., García, M.T., Vinardell, M.P. and Infante, M.R. 2004. Green" amino acid-based surfactants. *Green Chemistry*, 6(5): 233–240.

Nwosu, J.N., Anyaehie M.A. and Ofoedu C.E. 2019. Effect of different processing techniques on the amino acid profile of black gram. *IOSR Journal of Environmental Science, Toxicology and Food Technology*, 13(11): 79–84.

Pathak, K.V. and Keharia, H. 2014. Identification of surfactins and iturins produced by potent fungal antagonist, Bacillus subtilis K1 isolated from aerial roots of banyan (Ficus benghalensis) tree using mass spectrometry. *3 Biotech*, 4(3): 283–295.

Perinelli, D.R., Lucarini, S., Fagioli, L., Campana, R., Vllasaliu, D., Duranti, A. and Casettari, L. 2018. Lactose oleate as new biocompatible surfactant for pharmaceutical applications. *European Journal of Pharmaceutics and Biopharmaceutics*, 124: 55–62.

Roberts, A. 2016. The safety and regulatory process for amino acids in Europe and the United States. *The Journal of Nutrition*, 146(12): 2635S–2642S.

Rodgers, K.J., Samardzic, K. and Main, B.J. 2017. Toxic nonprotein amino acids. *Plant Toxins*, 2(3): 1–20.

Smriga, M. 2020. International regulations on amino acid use in foods and supplements and recommendations to control their safety based on purity and quality. *Journal of Nutrition*, 150: 2602S–2605S.

Starke, I., Kleinpeter, E. and Kamm, B. 2001. Separation, identification, and quantification of amino acids in L-lysine fermentation potato juices by gas chromatography–mass spectrometry. *Fresenius' Journal of Analytical Chemistry*, 371(3): 380–384.

Tripathy, D.B., Mishra, A., Clark, J. and Farmer, T. 2018. Synthesis, chemistry, physicochemical properties and industrial applications of amino acid surfactants: A review. *Comptes Rendus Chimie*, 21(2): 112–130.

## CHAPTER 16

# Paralytic Shellfish Toxins

**Ubaid Qayoom, Zahoor Mushtaq, and E Manimozhi**

## CONTENTS



## 16.1 INTRODUCTION

The microscopic unicellular free-floating algae (phytoplankton), the primary producers, are abundant in the world's oceans and freshwater environments. Microalgae in aquatic environments undergo explosive growth under favourable conditions producing millions of cells per liter, resulting in dense blooms (red tides), and discoloration of the water (red, reddish-brown, green, yellow-green). Additionally, anthropogenic activities contributing to climate change, increased ocean eutrophication, and commercial shipping activities are assumed to escalate these blooms' frequency and occurrence throughout the world (Campbell et al., 2011). Filter-feeding shellfish like *Mysidacea* crustaceans, oysters, clams, mussels, and scallops, and other commercially essential larvae of crustaceans and herbivorous finfish feed on microalgae rich in proteins, minerals, and vitamins. It has been reported that about 60–80 species of microalgae species often produce toxins (phycotoxins), which accumulate and concentrate in the filter-feeding shellfish and finfish, with dinoflagellates accounting for 75% of all such species (James et al., 2010). Globally, algal toxins accidents range from 50,000–5,00,000 cases annually and have a global death rate of 1.5% (Wang, 2008).

Contaminated shellfish and finfish consumption is associated with various human gastrointestinal and neurological illnesses from shellfish or fish poisoning. Algal toxins prove deadly for finfish

DOI: 10.1201/9781003178446-16

and shellfish and, in the past, have also resulted in the severe mass mortalities of marine ecosystem inhabitants, including mammals, birds, and other animals interconnected through the marine food web (Flewelling et al., 2005). Currently, five major dinoflagellate toxin poisoning syndromes have been identified that can occur from consuming contaminated shellfish, finfish, and fishery products. Toxins from diatom species causing amnesic shellfish poisoning have also been reported (Hinder et al., 2011). Among the various poisonings originating from bivalve molluscs, paralytic shellfish poisoning (PSP) is well-recognized mainly due to its well-defined neurological symptoms and high fatality (de Carvalho et al., 2019).

Paralytic shellfish toxins (PSTs) occur naturally as potent neurotoxic alkaloids, with one more familiar and well-studied saxitoxin (STX) as the reference compound. They are a family of more than 50 toxins bearing structural resemblances to one another and are causative agents of PSP. Among the family, saxitoxin (STX), neosaxitoxin (NeoSTX), gonyautoxin 1 (GTX1), and decarbamoyl-saxitoxin (dc-STX) are highly toxic (Goya et al., 2020). These toxins are mainly synthesized by certain marine dinoflagellate species affiliated with the genera *Gymnodinium*, *Alexandrium*, and *Pyrodinium* (Ben-Gigirey et al., 2020) in tropical as well as moderate climate zones. Additionally, these toxins also occur in the freshwater and brackish water habitats where several species of cyanobacteria synthesize them, e.g., *Anabaena circinalis*, *Anabaena lemmermannii*, *Aphanizomenon gracile*, *Cylindrospermopsis raciborskii*, *Lyngbya wollei*, *Aphanzomenon issatschenkoi*, *Rivularia sp., and Planktothrix sp.* (Deeds et al., 2008).

PSP incidents in humans occur worldwide due to shellfish consumption containing harmful saxitoxins and saxitoxin analogues (STXs). Moreover, humans are also exposed to saxitoxins through non-traditional vectors for PSPs such as edible crustaceans, gastropods, and finfish (Deeds et al., 2008). Recently, PSTs were reported in marine invertebrates such as starfish and ascidians in Europe, posing a PSP risk in humans through the food chain (Ben-Gigirey et al., 2020). The toxicity level for various saxitoxins profoundly affects $Na^+$ influx through voltage-gated $Na^+$ channels, therefore inhibiting the production of action potential in neurons and muscle cell membranes (Duran-Riveroll et al., 2017). More importantly, as per the 1993 Chemical Weapons Convention (CWC), saxitoxin is the sole natural marine toxin to be categorized as a Schedule 1 Chemical Warfare weapon (Cusik et al., 2013). The onset of PSP symptoms starts after 30 min or a few hours after consuming contaminated shellfish. The effect of STXs on the nervous system includes a slight tickling sensation in lips, tongue, mouth, face, headache, dizziness, nausea, numbness of extremities, difficulty in breathing, and ataxia. In extreme cases, the neurotoxin can cause paralysis, leading to cardiovascular shock, respiratory arrest, or death unless respiratory support is provided (Vilarino et al., 2018). The data over the last two decades suggests an increase in intoxications caused by PSTs. However, the actual reason behind this surge is unclear, with some researchers stating that the growth in numbers is proper and is due to increased shellfish culture and intake. Some attribute, increase in cases to the augmented and improved identification and detection of PSTs.

## 16.2 CHEMISTRY OF PSTs

Saxitoxin ($C_{10}H_{17}N_7O_4$) was the earliest PST (in 1957) extracted in a pure form from Alaska butter clam, *Saxidomus gigangteus* (Schantz et al., 1957). STX is a tetrahydropurine alkaloid having a five-membered ring and a ketone hydrate moiety stabilized by a pair of neighbouring electron-withdrawing guanidinium groups. The guanidinium groups are responsible for their high polarity, and the hydrated ketone group is vital for its toxic activity (Mons et al., 1998). The first crystalline derivative of saxitoxin was synthesized in 1975 (Bower et al., 1981), and the chemical structure of saxitoxin was later explained as a result of X-ray crystallography and nuclear magnetic resonance (Figure 16.1). Apart from STX, various STX analogues were identified by researchers in the 1970s and 1980s. STX analogues with saxitoxin as the parent compound share the typical structure of

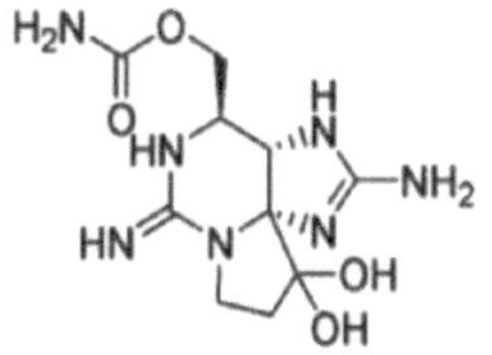

**Figure 16.1** Chemical structure of saxitoxin. (Source: Faber, 2012.)

tetrahydropurine. Based on the variations in the R4 side chain of the tetrahydropurine skeleton, PSTs are broadly classified into four subgroups: N-sulfocarbamoyl, carbamate, decarbamoyl, and deoxydecarbamoyl. The toxin analogues differentiate into more than 57 compounds based on the presence or absence of specific residues, such as the N-hydroxyl at the N1 position as well as the presence or lack of an epimeric 11-hydroxy sulfate group. The carbamate toxins may also have an N-sulfate at the N21 position and are usually referred to as N-sulfocarbamoyl analogues.

The STX analogues vary in potency from highly toxic to intermediately toxic and most minor poisonous derivatives. The Carbamate toxin, STX, NeoSTX, and Gonyautoxins 1–4 (GTX1–4) include the highly toxic analogues that act as sodium channel blockers in mammals. Decarbamoyl analogues such as dcSTX, dcGTX1–4, dcNEO, and the deoxydecarbamoyl analogues such as doGTX2, doGTX3, doSTX are believed to be of intermediate toxicity. The analogues, including *N*-sulfocarbamoyl toxins, C1-C4, B1, and B2, occur at the lowest end of the toxicity strength (Deeds et al., 2008). Interestingly, various biological factors modify PSTs, often resulting in new PSTs (called biotransformation) that microalgae cannot biosynthesize alone. Biotransformation of the PSTs may cause less toxic ones to transform or convert into analogues of more significant toxicity and *vice versa*. For instance, acidic pH combined with heat transforms C1, C2, C3, C4, GTX5, and GTX6 PSTs into more powerful toxic forms such as GTX2, GTX3, GTX1, GTX4, STX, and NeoSTX, respectively. Similarly, the transformation of the analogues such as GTX5, GTX6, C1, C2, C3, C4 into dcSTX, dcNeoSTX, dcGTX2, dcGTX3, dcGTX1, and dcGTX4, respectively, can also take place at slightly alkaline pH (WHO, 2016). Saxitoxin and STX analogues are hydrophilic and thermostable (up to 100°C) at acidic and neutral pH but are base labile and undergo rapid degradation at alkaline pH (Kodama and Sato, 2008). They are readily excreted in urine and are not able to traverse the blood-brain barrier. They do not exhibit intense ultraviolet (UV) absorbance or fluorescence. STX is highly soluble in solvents like water and methanol; sparingly soluble in acetic acid and ethanol, whereas it is practically insoluble in other organic lipid solvents and can potentially accumulate in the higher trophic levels, particularly in bivalve filter feeders (Wiese et al., 2010).

## 16.3 DISTRIBUTION

The information regarding the systemic distribution of saxitoxins in animals upon absorption is scarce. Such information is limited to a few animals (primarily mice) studies post intravenous (i.v.) or intraperitoneal (i.p.) administration of STX. These experimental studies have demonstrated that saxitoxins rapidly distribute in various tissues, including the central nervous system. Upon administering radiolabelled saxitoxin analogue in Wistar rats, maximum radioactivity was found to reach the peak level in most tissues, including the brain (Naseem, 1996). Another study in rats post a single dose (i.p.) of 5 or 10 µg STX/kg BW revealed that the saxitoxin spreads to all regions of the rat brain, with the maximum concentration of 2.36 pg/mg found in the hippocampus and a minor concentration of 0.8 pg/mg in the right and the left hemispheres. Furthermore, it was found that the concentration of STX rapidly increased in the brain with an increase in the dose, implying that a higher concentration of STX results in its faster distribution (Cervantes Cianca et al., 2007).

Distribution profiles of STX investigated by Xia and Haddad (1993) in the adult rats revealed varying levels of STX with a much higher concentration in the hippocampus, cortex, amygdala, and cerebellum compared to the brainstem and spinal cord. In adult cats, intravenously injected with STX, the distribution of STX was reported from the liver and spleen; however, STX was also found in the brain and medulla oblongata, indicating that STX can cross the blood-brain barrier (Andrinolo et al., 1999). In another study, STXs were also detected in the muscular tissue and liver of tilapia sampled in an artificial lake in Brazil (Galvao et al., 2009). The tissue distribution of STXs, as analyzed in bivalves by Garcia et al. (2015), revealed that the toxin concentration in most of the species was highest in the digestive gland, followed by the membranous mantle and adductor muscle (primary muscular system). In humans, the post-mortem analysis of tissues has revealed the presence of saxitoxins and analogues in gastric content, body fluids, and tissues like liver, kidney, and lung (Garcia et al., 2004).

## 16.4 MECHANISM OF ACTION

PSTs are inhibitory neurotoxins that trigger a weak paralysis in tissues by actively repressing the excitation of neuronal impulses. The toxins do not diffuse into the inside of the axons and act only from the outside. With its massive affinity to bind on a particular site of voltage-gated sodium ($Na^+$) ion channel, STX obstructs the short-term permeability of $Na^+$ ions by attaching firmly to a receptor position at the cell surface close to the external pore of the sodium channel. The voltage-gated sodium channels (transmembrane proteins) traverse the cell membrane of numerous excitable cells such as mammalian neurons, cardiac muscle cells, and skeletal muscle cells. The molecular targets of PSTs are voltage-gated $Na^+$ channels having a common structural motif composed of a single principal alpha ($\alpha$) subunit of a molecular weight of 220–260 kDa and 1-2 auxiliary beta ($\beta$) subunits of molecular weight 33–36 kDa (Catterall, 1984; Catterall et al., 2007). The Carbon-12hydroxyls and guanidinium groups in the saxitoxins are crucial for their attachment to the site on the $Na^+$ channel. In addition, the carbamoyl side chain is also engaged in the binding process. Overall, STX attaches to the sodium channel by aboding itself on the ion-transporting pore in the ratio of 1:1 (Satin et al., 1992; Tikhonov & Zhorov, 2005; Pearson et al., 2010). In humans or any mammal, widespread blockage of sodium channels blocks depolarization of the plasma membrane, eventually obstructing any subsequent impulse production in the peripheral nerves and skeletal fibers. This leads to an extended, relaxed state of these fibers and subsequently causes paralysis (Narahashi, 1972; Kao, 1972). STX can target specific voltage-gated sodium channels and specific membrane receptors selectively and reversibly. In a study on saxitoxin's cellular actions in de-sheathed frog sciatic nerves by Kao and Nishiyama (1965), STX was found to completely block the progression of voltage (compound action potentials). They observed a reversible impulse propagation at the dose level of 0.01 μg/mL STX in frogs and was replicable at 8 × without enduring loss. At a higher dose of 0.75 μg/mL, STX resulted in diminishing nerve-elicited spasms in the tibialis anterior devoid of the occurrence of hypotension. Doses of 0.1 μg/mL did not affect the membrane's resting potential; however, it caused total skeletal muscle impulse propagation inhibition.

During nerve impulse traversing, the escalating phase of the action potential is due to the inward sodium current. When the voltage-gated potassium ($K^+$) channels located in the plasma membrane open, they allow transit of intracellular $K^+$ towards the outside and consequential repolarization. STX and other PSTs have the ability to block the voltage-gated $Na^+$ channel highly efficiently while leaving the potassium channel unaltered. Studies of STX and analogues by Kao 1986 revealed that the 7,8,9 guanidinium functional group, which provides a cationic charge to these molecules, is involved in the strong blockade of the sodium channel. As a result, they interact with negatively charged amino acid residues in the channel. Additionally, the hydrated ketone (at C-12) is essential for this binding. Even though the carbamoyl side chain is also involved, it is not necessary for the interaction. In comparing STX to another potent neurotoxin called tetrodotoxin (TTX), many stereospecific similarities have been found (Kao and Walker, 1982), indicating that both TTX and SXT have similar functional dynamics. TTX and STX occupy receptor sites adjacent to the sodium channel's outer orifice, where the positively charged 7,8,9 guanidinium active moiety strongly interacts with negatively charged sites all around domain I and II of the channel opening. This is supplemented with many H-bonded interactions between the toxins and the channel proteins, such as those influenced by the C12 hydroxyls and the carbamoyl functional group in saxitoxin (Kao, 1993; Yang et al., 1992).

## 16.5 TOXICOLOGY

Saxitoxin and its by-products are the leading cause of PSP. PSP symptoms commence in less than 30 min after shellfish consumption and inevitably begin with a pricking or burning sensation of the lips, throat, and tongue, which proliferates to widespread numbness of the facial muscles (Llewellyn, 2006). Furthermore, symptoms may encompass diarrhoea, perspiration, and vomiting. In acute toxicity, numbness caused by STX may spread to the neck and other body extremities, resulting in muscular fragileness, deprivation of motor coordination, and eventually leads to paralysis of the affected region. In case of a fatal dose of STX, cardiovascular failure is common due to respiratory muscle paralysis. Overall, PSTs are highly potent toxins with a high mortality rate when medical support is not available. The half-life of STX varies with pH and temperature (9–28 days at 25°C and pH 7 in running water). As it enters the human body after ingestion, the half-life decreases to ~90 min, and the survival probability of affected individuals increases considerably after 12 h from ingestion or intake (Kao, 1993). As already described above, it is an effective inhibitor of the pore-forming ability of voltage-gated $Na^+$ channels in the excitable membrane of neurons (Kao & Levinson, 1986). A few studies have also established that STX can block calcium ($Ca^{2+}$) channels also (Su et al., 2004) and extend the gating of voltage-dependent potassium channels in muscle cells of the heart (Wang et al., 2003).

The intoxication levels reported in PSP cases vary greatly, ranging from a few hundred to thousands of μg STX eq./100 g of edible shellfish meat. Saxitoxin is an efficacious phycotoxin with an i.p. LD50 of 10 μg/kg BW in mice (Halstead et al., 1984). In contrast, human death has been reported after the ingestion of even 1 mg of toxin (Evans, 1969), which is due to the existence of multiple isotypes of sodium channels in mammals. These channels have differential sensitivity to saxitoxin owing to differences in the sequence of amino acid residues, particularly in the α-subunit of the channel. However, in some cases, a mutation (change in the gene's DNA sequence) may give rise to insensitivity to STX, though this is usually accompanied by a significant decrease in the gating speed of the channel (Satin et al., 1992). Also, saxitoxin and analogues show a considerable variation in their toxicity. Many reports suggest that the carbamate-derived toxins are 10–100 × potent and toxic than *N*-sulfo-carbamoyl derivatives (Llewellyn., 2006; Hall et al., 1990; Pearson et al., 2010). *N*-sulfo-carbamoyl analogues are labile and can be easily altered to the more noxious carbamate derivatives (Cembella et al., 1993; Cembella et al., 1994).

## 16.6 IDENTIFICATION AND QUANTIFICATION

Conventionally, the determination of PSTs in contaminated samples has been done by means of mouse bioassay (MBA) developed by Sommer and Mayer (1937). Due to its simplicity and reliability, the assay was later sanctioned by the Association of Official Analytical Chemists (AOAC) to detect PSTs in acidic extracts of shellfish samples (AOAC 1995). The bioassay determines a test solution's net toxicity after extraction from a 100 g shellfish sample in 100 mL of 0.1 M hydrochloric acid (HCl). 1 mL of the acid extract is then injected intraperitoneally into laboratory mice (preferably 19–21 g), and toxicity is determined in terms of a single response by correlating the time between injection to death of each mouse. Generally, the highly lethal extracts need to be diluted to lower concentrations to make certain that death happens in 5–7 min. The median death time of treated mice population is then converted into standard mouse units defined as "the minimum amount of poison that is required to kill a 20 g mouse in 15 min when 1 mL of the extract is injected intraperitoneally and is equivalent to 0.18 mg of saxitoxin" and compared with values from reference Sommer's Table for the estimate of toxicity.

The bioassay's main disadvantage is that its detection limit is approximately 40 µg saxitoxin/100 g of sample with an accuracy of ± 15–20%. Other possible penalties include the labour-intensive process, the influence of size, sex, the strain of individual mice, the non-linear relationship between toxin dose and death time, and salt interferences like NaCl, whose presence may reduce the toxicity. Additionally, the ethical concerns of using live animals for testing have led to the development of alternative analytical methods to detect marine toxins in seafood. Despite these difficulties, MBA continues to be the official screening method of PSTs in most countries that regulate PSTs in seafood.

### 16.6.1 In Vitro Tissue-Culture Assay

As discussed earlier in Section 16.4, saxitoxin and its analogues are potent neurotoxins exhibiting a high affinity for sodium channels in neurons and other cells and alter the normal function by inhibiting ion transport. The amount of interaction is proportional to toxicity.

The tissue culture assay developed in mouse neuroblastoma cells by Kogure et al. (1988) takes advantage of saxitoxin's ability to protect the cells against the combined action of two biologically active compounds: veratridine and ouabain. Mouse neuroblastoma cells enlarge and ultimately lyse upon exposure to veratridine in combination with ouabain. Veratridine is a lipid-soluble steroidal alkaloid known to stimulate uncontrolled sodium influx into nerve cells by stopping the deactivation of voltage-gated sodium ion channels after binding at receptor sites different from saxitoxin. Ouabain, also known as g-strophanthin, augments this effect by explicitly inhibiting the sodium-potassium ion pump ($Na^+/K^+$ ATPase), responsible for maintaining the membrane's resting potential by exchanging intracellular $Na^+$ ions for extracellular $K^+$ ions. When present, STX obstructs the $Na^+$ channels and ultimately inhibits the activity of the Veratridine and ouabain. Hence, the presence of STX in a contaminated sample will cause the cells to remain alive and morphologically normal. Kogure et al. (1988) recommended a mixture of 0.05 mM veratridine and 1 mM ouabain in the assay for standard analysis, which induced morphological changes in less than 1 h in the absence of saxitoxin. The proportion of cells that remain rounded, with clear and distinct cell membranes after toxin treatment, is directly proportional to the concentration of STX and its analogues.

Gallacher and Birkbeck (1992) developed a modified method for detecting and quantifying live cells after staining with Neutral Red (at 540 nm) against the tedious and subjective microscopic screening of survivor mouse neuroblastoma cells. Jellet et al. (1992) also described a similar assay using Crystal Violet dye (hexamethyl pararosaniline chloride) as a staining agent for live neuroblastoma cells. They reported a lower detection limit (LOD) of approximately 10 ng STX (eq)/mL of extract (2.0 µg STX (eq)/100 g shellfish sample). The assay results were virtually identical to that of mouse bioassay and were considerably more sensitive. This led the authors to suggest the automated tissue culture bioassay of neuroblastoma cells as a substitute to controversial live animal testing such as MBA for PSP. These studies were followed by the attempts of Manger et al. (1993), Shimojo and Iwaoka (2000), Okumura et al. (2005) to improve the cell assay.

Cell-based detection methods appear to be an excellent substitute for the MBA to screen PSTs in a variety of samples. These assays offer many advantages over the MBA as they are relatively low-cost, simple, and precise, with sensitivity similar to MBA. Additionally, the cell-based assays do not demand any highly sophisticated pieces of equipment nor specialized procedural skills.

### 16.6.2 Enzyme-Linked Immunosorbent Assay (ELISA)

ELISAs are highly sensitive analytical assays in biochemistry and are commonly used to measure antigens, proteins, etc. They involve only minimal skill to execute the assay, are cost-effective and rapid. ELISAs use the principle of pattern recognition of epitopes to detect antigens or proteins and may be designed to identify multiple toxins and their derivatives having a common recognition site. In 1964, Johnson et al. reported an immunoassay for detecting PSP involving a hemagglutination reaction; however, the sensitivity was too low for practical application. Several groups tried to develop their antigens and prepared antibodies against PSTs using various conjugated antigens using this method.

Chu and Fan (1985) developed an indirect ELISA for detecting STX by using antibodies obtained from rabbits immunized with STX-BSA mixture (saxitoxin-bovine serum albumin). The assay's detection limit lies in the range of 2–10 pg STX (0.1–0.5 ng STX/mL). However, the assay can suffer specificity issues for STX and high interference (particularly in whole mussel meat extract) in the food samples. In contrast, Kawatsu et al. (2002) reported a direct competitive ELISA to detect STX and analogues using a gonyautoxin 2/3 specific monoclonal antibody. STX was detectable at concentrations < 80 μg/100 g of shellfish sample, and the method was proposed to be convenient for qualitative screening. More sensitive, accurate, and rapid determination of STX in 0.02 to 0.8 ng/mL in human liquid blood and 0.06 to 2.0 ng/mL in dried human blood by quantitative ELISA was demonstrated by Wharton et al. (2017). They used micro-sampling devices in sample collection, allowing the uniform collection of blood samples, durable storage, and cost-effective transport.

ELISA assays could be suitable screening tools for the routine determination of saxitoxin in mussels. Micheli et al. (2002) compared two competitive ELISA formats (direct and indirect) to detect STX using the toxin-specific polyclonal antibodies raised from saxitoxin-keyhole limpet hemocyanin immunized rabbits. The LOD of STX for direct and indirect ELISA was 3 and 10 pg/mL, respectively. The major drawback of these assays is antibody cross-reaction towards some STX analogues and the lack of response towards a few others. These disadvantages, at present, prevent ELISA methods from broad acceptance for screening of PSTs in seafood. Nevertheless, their high sensitivity may render them very effective as screening tests for PSTs in some cases (Burdaspal, 1996).

### 16.6.3 Fluorometric and Colorimetric Techniques

When the saxitoxin structure was elucidated in 1971, it led to developing a new class of detection techniques based on the toxin's fluorescence measurements. The studies found that the alkaline oxidation of saxitoxin by hydrogen peroxide ($H_2O_2$) yields 8-amino-6-hydroxymethyl-2-iminopurine-3(2H)-propionic acid (AHIPA), which can be detected and quantified by fluorescence spectroscopy techniques. Bates and Rapoport (1975) developed a fluorometric assay that is reportedly 100 times more sensitive than the existing bioassay as it could detect as low as 0.003 μg STX/g meat. Further improvements in the fluorometric assay by Indrasena and Gill (1998) demonstrated an improved detection and sensitivity using hydrogen peroxide as a convenient and efficient oxidant for screening PSTs. The detection sensitivity for STX, neoSTX, GTX-1 and -4, GTX-2 and -3, C toxins and B-toxins was 0.027, 0.054, 0.023, 0.003, 0.0002, and 0.0006 pmol, respectively. The fluorescent yield in the assays can be affected by pH adjustments during extraction, before oxidation, removal of interfering co-extractants, and the presence of a variety of metals that can affect oxidation. Moreover, the toxins do not fluoresce uniformly, and for some of the carbamate toxins, fluorescence is very weak. The latter problem can be resolved by utilizing multiple fluorescences and colorimetric assays on the same samples. Taking this into account, Gershey et al. (1977) described a simple calorimetric method (at 555 nm wavelength) coupled to the ion exchange chromatographic column to detect and quantify saxitoxin based upon the oxidation reaction of 2,3-butanedione with guanidine or other compounds containing the guanidino group. The minimum detectable concentration in the actual analytical solution was 40 μg/100 g of shellfish meat. However, such methods consume more time per sample and need pH adjustments for fluorometric techniques.

Fluorimetric and colorimetric techniques could also be paired to design a single procedure, allowing the determination of PSTs from crude extracts of STX, GTX1-4, and NeoSTX. Mosley et al. (1985) applied this idea to develop a method that used fluorimetric and the Folin-Ciocalteu reagent assays separating PSTs in a linear gradient elution from a cation-exchange solid column. They reported the process to be superior to the MBA for specific purposes like research (Mosley et al., 1985).

### 16.6.4 Chromatographic and Mass Spectrometry Techniques

High-performance liquid chromatography (HPLC) is undeniably, from a practical standpoint, one of the most potent techniques existing today to screen and quantify PSTs. PSTs only possess a weak innate chromophore that requires modification and conversion to a more substantial derivative through an oxidation (or derivatization) reaction before fluorescence detection. Most of the HPLC methods for PST screening and identification are based on the preparation or extraction of samples with hydrochloric acid (HCl), pre-or post-column oxidation of the PSTs, separation of oxidized derivatives and the natural toxins by liquid chromatographic (LC), and finally, detection of the oxidation products of PSTs by measuring fluorescence. Generally, the oxidation of PSTs in basic solution ($pH > 7$) leads to the formation of purine products that are fluorescent in acidic solution, are examined with a fluorescence sensor, and eventually, the specific toxin intensities are calculated. Two standard chromatographic techniques, known as post-column and pre-column oxidation methods, are principally based on this acidification of sample extracts and the oxidation products' fluorescence intensity in the solution.

The first reports of the HPLC procedure for screening of PSPs were published in 1984 (Sullivan et al., 1984, Oshima et al., 1984), which reached a certain degree of popularity and success after several changes. Sullivan's group successfully separated underivatized PSP toxins using ion-pair chromatography. Sullivan et al. (1985) comparatively evaluated their own developed HPLC method and the mouse bioassay (AOAC OMA959.08 MBA) to determine its applicability to shellfish toxicity monitoring. A good correlation ($r = 0.92$) was determined for the 40 samples exhibiting toxicity in the bioassay (i.e., > 35 pg STX/100 g). The main drawbacks of this procedure were the instability of the cyano columns and the low sensitivity shown to N-l-hydroxy toxins. Additionally, the coelution of STX and dc-STX (de-carbamoyl saxitoxin) constituted an unnecessary drawback given that STX is 2 × toxic than that of dc-STX, thus gives an inaccurate estimate of total PSP toxicity.

Simultaneously, Oshima et al. (1984) attempted to improvise by modifying the initial oxidation reaction from the technique of Bates and Rapoport (1975), which was observed to be inadequate and unsuccessful for N-1-hydroxylated toxins. Following trials with different oxidizing agents, Oshima et al. found that ten-butyl hydroperoxide yielded exceedingly fluorescent derivatives upon oxidation by hydrogen peroxide ($H_2O_2$), even in the case of previously non-fluorescing ones, including GTX1, GTX4, and neoSTX following. The technique separated the epimers like GTX2 and GTX3, but this was not the case for GTX3 and GTX5, GTX1, and GTX4. The LOD was within the range of 0.04 to 2.2 nmol for GTX1-4, neoSTX, and STX. Later in the same decade, Oshima's group described an entire identification method based on ion-pair chromatography of 15 naturally occurring PSTs in mussels contaminated by *Gymnodiniumcatenatum* (Oshima 1989). However, the process consists of three separate isocratic runs on a $C_8$ bonded silica gel column to analyze all the PSTs in every sample and is slow and labour-intensive. These initial attempts led to the development of more accurate and reliable methodologies, principally the variations of the ion pair and the column (Franco and Fernandez-Vila 1993; Diener et al., 2006; Rourke et al., 2008).

HPLC combined with a post-column electrochemical oxidation system (ECOS) has potential application for the analysis of PSTs in the dinoflagellate, cyanobacteria, and shellfish samples (Boyer and Goddard, 1999). PSTs are oxidized into fluorescent derivatives by a coulometric electrochemical cell positioned in-line between the column outlet and the fluorescence sensor. The system is more advantageous than the previous ones as it has a more straightforward instrumental setup and avoids the reagent instability problems. However, the system has certain disadvantages linked to the upkeep and endurance of the oxidizing probe. Efforts by Jaime et al. (2001), employing the electrochemical post-column oxidation technique (PCOX) combined with chromatography, led to the successful single step separation of various PSTs, demonstrating the suitability of this method for the analysis in biological samples. Later on, another variant method of using a single ion-exchange chromatography step with sodium acetate ($C_2H_3NaO_2$) as mobile phase successfully determined and detected PSTs by FLD (Papageorgiou et al., 2005). The toxins C1, C2, GTX1-4, NeoSTX, and STX were separated with significantly less resolution of dcSTX/ STX.

In a collaborative study, Riet et al. (2011) developed a reversed-phase liquid chromatography method with PCOX and FLD (AOAC Official Method, 2011.02) for analysis for PSTs, including STX neoSTX, GTX1-5, dcGTX2-3, dcSTX, and N-sulfocarbamoyl GTX2-3. The method was developed to replace the AOAC reference biological method (AOAC *Official Method* SM 959.08) and serve as a substitute for the pre-column oxidation LC scheme (AOAC *Official Method* SM, 2005.06). 5 g shellfish samples, post homogenization, were mixed with 5 mL of 0.1 M HCl and incubated in a boiling water bath for 5 min, cooled down. pH was set to the range of 2–4 (preferably 3). The mixture was centrifuged, and an appropriate amount of supernatant was pipetted out and deproteinated with trichloroacetic acid ($C_2HCl_3O_2$). For the analysis of GTXs and STXs, the chromatography of the filtered extract was done on a $C_{18}$ silica column with a gradient step utilizing 11 mM heptane sulfonic acid ($C_7H_{16}O_3S$)/5.5 mM phosphoric acid buffer system (pH 7.1). The extract was also chromatographed on a $C_8$ silica column using a 2 mM tetra-butyl-ammonium phosphate isocratic buffer system (pH 5.8) to determine the *N*-sulfocarbamoyl gonyautoxins (C1–4). PCOX derivatized the toxins at 85°C in a phosphoric acid ($H_3PO_4$) or a periodic acid ($H_5IO_6$) buffer system using strong 0.75 M nitric acid ($HNO_3$). Final detection of the products was done by measuring fluorescence (excitation λ: 330 nm, emission λ: 390 nm).

Rey et al. (2016) proposed the new single run method using a porous graphitic carbon column in HPLC-FLD simultaneously determined 13 PSTs in approximately 30 min with improved detection limits. High-performance liquid chromatography-tandem mass spectrometry (HPLC-MS/MS) was used to evaluate the natural incidence of eight PSTs, including STX, neoSTX, GTXs, C1, and C2 in shellfish. The LODs (limits of detection) and LOQs (limit of quantification) were established in the range of 1.32–11.29 μg/kg and 0.33–5.52 μg/kg (Yang et al., 2017).

There has been tremendous progress, in recent years, in the use of liquid chromatography (LC) with electrospray ionization-mass spectrometry (ESI-MS) to detect and quantitate PSTs in a variety of samples. ESI-MS is a reliable and robust screening method for PSTs, attributed to the structural characteristics of the saxitoxins, whereby they give rise to the group of powerful ions in both the positive and negative ion modes.

In 1989, Quilliam et al. developed a method for detecting STX using liquid chromatography-mass spectrometry (LC-MS) ion-spray ionization. For 1 μL sample injection in single ion recording (Selected Ion Monitoring) and focussing on positive ions, they defined a concentration detection limit (LOD) of 0.1 μM from flow injection analysis, which is ~5 × sensitive than the AOAC MBA technique. While utilizing LC-MS, Quilliam et al. (1993) attained mass spectra (typically $MS^1$-spectra) of several oxidation products to distinguish periodate oxidation derivatives of PSTs. However, the technique had a downside due to significantly reduced sensitivity for the parent toxins. The authors deduced that "The overall sensitivity is such that pre-column oxidation combined with LC/MS will not be a competitive method for the trace level analysis of PSP toxins." In conclusion, it is safe to say that using ESI-MS paired with conventional LC methodologies has its advantages. However, the direct replacement of fluorescence detection in these methodologies provides analytical challenges because of ion-pair reagents such as heptafluorobutyric acid ($C_4HF_7O_2$) as mobile phases in the column. These reagents are generally regarded as unfitting for interconnecting and interfacing with MS to screen and detect PSTs (Quilliam, 2003a; Dell'Aversano et al., 2005), even though specific evidence of successful reverse-phase ESI-MS methods has been reported (Dahlmann et al., 2003).

A distinct methodology using HILIC (Hydrophilic interaction chromatography) in tandem with ESI-MS was first reported by Quilliam (2003b), and Dell'Aversano et al. (2005). Due to suitability, the technique has become the choice method for separating small polar molecules. The principle of this technique is based on the fact that the double-charged toxins, including STX, NeoSTX, dcNEO, and dcSTX, exhibit longer retention periods due to their higher interaction with the stationary phase matrix. Similarly, shorter retention times are observed for the singly charged GTXs and the neutral C toxins. In this method, epimeric pairs are separated by earlier elution of specific epimers due to the reduction in positively charged molecular substrates in specific a-forms attributed to the interaction between the C8 guanidinium group and the 11-hydroxy sulfate group. Following these reports, attempts were made for utilization of HILIC-ESI-MS for determination of various PSTs in a range of samples, including zooplankton, namely *Calanus finmarchicus* (Durbin et al., 2002), octopus (Robertson et al., 2004), phytoplankton (Dahlmann et al., 2003; Collins et al., 2009), purified toxin preparations (Munday et al., 2013), and snails (Jen et al., 2014). One of the effective methods involving HILIC with ESI and SRM in positive ion mode was developed by Zhuo et al. (2013), using what they referred to as QuEChERS (quick, easy, cheap, effective, rugged, and safe). The method could be validated for ten PST analogues. It was used with precision in oyster, clam, and mackerel species, and the studies reported good toxin recoveries. The only major problem with the technique was the prolonged sample processing and analysis periods, reducing the sample throughput.

A new Hydrophilic interaction liquid chromatography method (fusion HILIC-UHPLC-MS/MS) was developed by Boundy et al. (2015) that retains polar moieties by various retention mechanisms. The technique consists of a speedy and uncomplicated sample preparation protocol by a one-step dispersive extraction in 1% Acetic acid ($CH_3COOH$), followed by a feasible clean-up step employing solid-phase extraction cartridges of amorphous graphitized carbon polymer. HILIC was performed and attained complete separation of all interfering related products within a period of 11 min. Both positive and negative ion mode SRMs were incorporated ESI-MS/MS. Consequently, the method successfully overcame the major issues with previously defined methods by allowing accurate, rapid, and efficient analysis of PSTs from different samples. The technique was later subjected to a full-scale validation by Turner et al. (2015). The validation process involved detecting and quantifying STX, neoSTX, dcNEO, dcSTX, doSTX, GTX1–6, dcGTX1,-2,-4, C1–4, and M toxins. Overall, the validation process vouched for the acceptable performance characteristics of the method concerning its specificity, strength, recovery, linearity, accuracy, and duplicability. Most of all, the sensitivity of the process (54 mg STX di-HCl eq/kg ) proved to be outstanding in contrast to LC-FLD-based techniques. In contrast, the LOQs for AOAC 2005.06 and AOAC 2011.02 were 784 and 358 mg STX di-HCl eq/kg, respectively (Turner et al., 2015). It also proved better with LC-FLD AOAC 2005.06 following an extensive study of comparative analysis of over 1,100 contaminated shellfish samples. Consequently, the technique may be regarded fit for the aim of swift, precise, and reproducible detection and screening of a large number of PSTs in a broad range of shellfish species.

## 16.7 SAFETY AND REGULATION

PSP is a severe toxicity condition caused by toxins present in seafood and poses a significant danger to seafood and human well-being. A review of regulatory limitations of PSTs and other toxins for several countries can be found in FAO (2004). Humans can develop PSP owing to the consumption of contaminated raw or cooked shellfish containing high concentrations of STX. Classically, 80 μg STX equivalents (eq)/100 g tissue is regarded as the action level (AL) or regulatory limit (RL) (generally half of the permissible exposure limit) of the STX (e.g., as in the USA). ALs for various marine toxins of public health importance in the US can be found in the FDA's Fish and Fisheries Products Hazards and Controls Guidance draft available at FDA's website. Wekell et al. (2004) first established the action plan based on detecting PSTs using MBA. However, long before, Sommer and Meyer (1937) had standardized and defined a mouse unit (MU) of toxin as "the amount of toxin that killed a 20 g mouse within 10–20 min (using an extract of 100 g sample tissue boiled in HCl)." The value was estimated to be 200 MU/100 g shellfish extract based on preparation and extractions. By employing a conversion factor of 0.2 μg STX (eq) equivalent to 1 MU, the LOD was defined as 40 μg STX (eq)/100 g sample. The limit of 80 μg was set as a compromise between the MBA and LOD, and the minimum quantity of 200 μg STX (eq)/100 g was described for causing toxicity and illness at that time. Eventually, this action level was adopted as a standard, and to date, this action level seems adequate. In the USA, the data suggest that infections in recent times primarily result from recreational and subsistence fisheries in closed or untested waters.

FAO (2004) reviewed the 500 reported cases of human PSP and established a provisional LOAEL (lowest observed adverse effect level) of 2.0 μg STX (eq)/kg BW. A 3 × UF (Uncertainty Factor) applied to the LOAEL resulted in an Acute Reference Dose (ARfD) of 0.7 μg STX (eq)/kg BW. Based on the same data, EFSA (2009) identified a LOAEL of 1.5 μg STX (eq)/kg BW and applied a 3 × UF, establishing an ARfD of 0.5 μg STX (eq)/kg BW. An uncertainty factor for intra-species variation was not used as a minor sickness is easily reversible, and the recognized human toxicity cases included a broad spectrum of individuals.

There is no medically authorized remedy or antidote for saxitoxin poisoning, and the management for poisoned individuals is only supportive and symptom-driven. Decontamination and removal of toxins from the stomach and intestines using activated charcoal is suggested for patients who present within 4 h of ingestion. If a patient reports within 1 h of ingestion of toxins, a nasogastric or orogastric lavage is generally performed, and toxicants are flushed out.

## 16.8 EFFECT OF PROCESSING ON THE REMOVAL OF PSTs

Many edible shellfish species have been associated with the illness caused by PSTs, such as clams, oysters, and mussels. Thermal processing is one of the widely used tools for effective removal or reduction of toxins in many kinds of seafood and has been used for a long time. To test the reduction of PST levels in bivalve molluscs, Medcof et al. (1947) determined the effects of domestic cooking, shucking, and commercial canning on removing or reducing PSTs from clams. Cooking raw material for 15–20 min in a covered pot, boiling in water for 20 min, and pan-frying for 15 min reduced the PST content of bivalve meat by approximately 70%. Shucking demonstrated no reduction of PST content. However, canning (as practised commercially) had a good effect on the decrease of PST content. Noguchi et al. (1980) examined the impact of sterilization on quantitative aspects of PSTs in canned scallops (*Patinopecten yessoensis*) and reported a good reduction in toxicity levels. The content of PSTs continued to decrease post canning procedures throughout the storage period. Similar results were earlier obtained by Prakash (1971) by demonstrating around 90% decontamination during the sterilization procedure.

In another attempt to reduce the toxicity level of PSTs in seafood, Lawrence et al. (1994) attempted the use of hot steam and boiling on a commercial lobster species (*Homarus americanus*) from the Canadian coast. The results demonstrated that such processing techniques lower the PSP content by an average of 54% in hepatopancreases, with an overall reduction of approximately 70% PSTs per hepatopancreas. They analyzed the hepatopancreases of 45 lobsters (divided into three groups) individually for total PSP toxicity using the standard MBA. Individual toxins determination was also done using HPLC employing a pre-oxidation procedure of the toxins. Overall, boiling or steaming decreased the total toxicity (eqSTX/ hepatopancreas) by ~65% against the toxicity values of fresh/raw lobster samples.

Vieites et al. (1999) monitored the basic canning process of brine-stored and -pickled mussels (*Mytilus galloprovincialis*) to investigate fluctuations in quantitative toxin profiles and overall toxicity values of PSTs. The process involved cooking, steaming, and sterilization and lead to a substantial and reproducible drop in PST levels in mussel meat ( > 50% of initial toxicity level of samples) as estimated by MBA and HPLC methods. Additionally, they observed maximum destruction of PSTs during the sterilization phase of the process of mussel samples in brine.

## 16.9 CONCLUSION AND FUTURE SCOPE

PSP is a severe set of symptoms, and the toxins (PSTs) accountable for this sickness carry a significant seafood safety concern, as well as risks to human health and welfare. The growing knowledge and understanding of the toxin dynamics, toxicity profiles, and effective management have reduced the PSP cases and associated mortality rates over the last few decades. While the earliest and most extensively used mouse bioassay technique has offered a helpful tool for assessing the toxicity of paralytic shellfish poisoning for a long time, efforts have been directed to establish more appropriate and reliable regulatory methods and seek alternatives to the controversial MBA. All the methodologies and techniques reported for screening of PSTs to date have their benefits and drawbacks. In addition, serious global efforts are being made towards the increased use of analytical methods that do not involve live animals (e.g., MBA) for toxicity testing. Current chemical testing techniques are effective but complex and time-consuming. The development of biomarkers like genes and proteins associated with PSP as an alternate method for screening PSTs has good potential, as is evident from recent research. Advanced and pioneering supervision policies, including the on-board dockside examination infrastructure, should be followed to improve and maintain vigilance to ensure that the public consumes only toxin-free seafood harvests.

## REFERENCES


Andrinolo, D., Michea, L.F., and Lagos, N. 1999. Toxic effects, pharmacokinetics and clearance of saxitoxin, a component of paralytic shellfish poison (PSP), in cats. *Toxicon*, 37(3): 447–464.

Association of Official Analytical Chemists (AOAC). 1995. *Paralytic shellfish poison, biological method. Official methods of analysis*, 16th edition. AOAC, Washington, DC, method 959.08.

Bates, H.A., and Rapoport, H. 1975. Chemical assay for saxitoxin, the paralytic shellfish poison. *Journal of Agricultural and Food Chemistry*, 23(2): 237–239.

Ben-Gigirey, B., Rossignoli, A.E., Riobó, P., and Rodríguez, F. 2020. First report of paralytic shellfish toxins in marine invertebrates and fish in Spain. *Toxins*, 12(11): 723.

Boundy, M.J., Selwood, A.I., Harwood, D.T., McNabb, P.S., and Turner, A.D. 2015. Development of a sensitive and selective liquid chromatography–mass spectrometry method for high throughput analysis of paralytic shellfish toxins using graphitised carbon solid phase extraction. *Journal of Chromatography A*, 1387: 1–12.

Bower, D.J., Hart, R.J., Matthews, P.A., and Howden, M.E. 1981. Nonprotein neurotoxins. *Clinical Toxicology*, 18(7): 813–863.

Boyer, G.L., and Goddard, G.D. 1999. High performance liquid chromatography coupled with post-column electrochemical oxidation for the detection of PSP toxins. *Natural Toxins*, 7(6): 353–359.

Burdaspal, P.A. 1996. Bioassay and chemical methods for analysis of paralytic shellfish poison. In *Progress in Food Contaminant Analysis*, ed. J. Gilbert, 219–253. Springer, Boston, MA.

Campbell, K., Rawn, D.F., Niedzwiadek, B., and Elliott, C.T. 2011. Paralytic shellfish poisoning (PSP) toxin binders for optical biosensor technology: problems and possibilities for the future: a review. *Food Additives and Contaminants*, 28(6): 711–725.

Catterall, W.A. 1984. The molecular basis of neuronal excitability. *Science*, 223(4637): 653–661.
Catterall, W.A., Cestèle, S., Yarov-Yarovoy, V., Frank, H.Y., Konoki, K., and Scheuer, T. 2007. Voltage-gated ion channels and gating modifier toxins. *Toxicon*, 49(2): 124–141.
Cembella, A., Shumway, S.E., and Lewis, N. 1993. A comparison of anatomical distribution and spatio-temporal variation of paralytic shellfish toxin composition in two bivalve species from the Gulf of Maine. *Journal of Shellfish Research*, 12: 389–403.
Cembella, A.D., Shumway, S.E., and Larocque, R. 1994. Sequestering and putative biotransformation of paralytic shellfish toxins by the sea scallop Placopecten magellanicus: seasonal and spatial scales in natural populations. *Journal of Experimental Marine Biology and Ecology*, 180(1): 1–22.
Chu, F.S., and Fan, T.S. 1985. Indirect enzyme-linked immunosorbent assay for saxitoxin in shellfish. *Journal of the Association of Official Analytical Chemists*, 68(1): 13–16.
Cianca, R.C.C., Pallares, M.A., Barbosa, R.D., Adan, L.V., Martins, J.M.L., and Gago-Martínez, A. 2007. Application of precolumn oxidation HPLC method with fluorescence detection to evaluate saxitoxin levels in discrete brain regions of rats. *Toxicon*, 49(1): 89–99.
Collins, C., Graham, J., Brown, L., Bresnan, E., Lacaze, J.P., and Turrell, E.A. 2009. Identification and toxicity of Alexandrium tamarense (Dinophyceae) in Scottish waters. *Journal of Phycology*, 45(3): 692–703.
Cusick, K.D., and Sayler, G.S. 2013. An overview on the marine neurotoxin, saxitoxin: genetics, molecular targets, methods of detection and ecological functions. *Marine Drugs*, 11(4): 991–1018.
Dahlmann, J., Budakowski, W.R., and Luckas, B. 2003. Liquid chromatography–electrospray ionisation-mass spectrometry based method for the simultaneous determination of algal and cyanobacterial toxins in phytoplankton from marine waters and lakes followed by tentative structural elucidation of microcystins. *Journal of Chromatography A*, 994(1–2): 45–57.
de Carvalho, I.L., Pelerito, A., Ribeiro, I., Cordeiro, R., Núncio, M.S., and Vale, P. 2019. Paralytic shellfish poisoning due to ingestion of contaminated mussels: a 2018 case report in Caparica (Portugal). *Toxicon: X*, 4: 100017.
Deeds, J.R., Landsberg, J.H., Etheridge, S.M., Pitcher, G.C., and Longan, S.W. 2008. Non-traditional vectors for paralytic shellfish poisoning. *Marine Drugs*, 6(2): 308–348.
Dell'Aversano, C., Hess, P., and Quilliam, M.A. 2005. Hydrophilic interaction liquid chromatography–mass spectrometry for the analysis of paralytic shellfish poisoning (PSP) toxins. *Journal of Chromatography A*, 1081(2): 190–201.
Diener, M., Erler, K., Hiller, S., Christian, B., and Luckas, B. 2006. Determination of paralytic shellfish poisoning (PSP) toxins in dietary supplements by application of a new HPLC/FD method. *European Food Research and Technology*, 224(2): 147–151.
Durán-Riveroll, L.M., and Cembella, A.D. 2017. Guanidinium toxins and their interactions with voltage-gated sodium ion channels. *Marine Drugs*, 15(10): 303.
Durbin, E., Teegarden, G., Campbell, R., Cembella, A., Baumgartner, M.F., and Mate, B.R. 2002. North Atlantic right whales, Eubalaena glacialis, exposed to paralytic shellfish poisoning (PSP) toxins via a zooplankton vector, Calanus finmarchicus. *Harmful Algae*, 1(3): 243–251.
European Food Safety Authority (EFSA). 2009. Scientific opinion of the panel on contaminants in the food chain on a request from the European Commission on marine biotoxins in shellfish – summary on regulated marine biotoxins. *The EFSA Journal*, 1306: 1–23.
Evans, M.H. 1969. Mechanism of saxitoxin and tetrodotoxin poisoning. *British Medical Bulletin*, 25(3): 263–267.
Faber, S. 2012. Saxitoxin and the induction of paralytic shellfish poisoning. *Journal of Young Investigators*, 23(1): 1–7.
Flewelling, L.J., Naar, J.P., Abbott, J.P., Baden, D.G., Barros, N.B., Bossart, G.D., Bottein, M.Y.D., Hammond, D.G., Haubold, E.M., Heil, C.A., and Henry, M.S. 2005. Red tides and marine mammal mortalities. *Nature*, 435(7043): 755–756.
Food and Agriculture Organization of the United Nations (FAO). 2004. *Marine Biotoxins*. Paper 80. FAO Food and Nutrition, Rome.
Franco, J.M., and Fernández-Vila, P. 1993. Separation of paralytic shellfish toxins by reversed phase high performance liquid chromatography, with post-column reaction and fluorimetric detection. *Chromatographia*, 35(9–12): 613–620.
Gallacher, S., and Birkbeck, T.H. 1992. A tissue culture assay for direct detection of sodium channel blocking toxins in bacterial culture supernates. *FEMS Microbiology Letters*, 92: 101–107.

Galvao, J.A., Oetterer, M., do Carmo Bittencourt-Oliveira, M., Gouvêa-Barros, S., Hiller, S., Erler, K., Luckas, B., Pinto, E., and Kujbida, P. 2009. Saxitoxins accumulation by freshwater tilapia (Oreochromis niloticus) for human consumption. *Toxicon*, 54(6): 891–894.

Garcıa, C., del Carmen Bravo, M., Lagos, M., and Lagos, N. 2004. Paralytic shellfish poisoning: post-mortem analysis of tissue and body fluid samples from human victims in the Patagonia fjords. *Toxicon*, 43(2): 149–158.

García, C., Pérez, F., Contreras, C., Figueroa, D., Barriga, A., López-Rivera, A., Araneda, O.F., and Contreras, H.R. 2015. Saxitoxins and okadaic acid group: accumulation and distribution in invertebrate marine vectors from Southern Chile. *Food Additives & Contaminants: Part A*, 32(6): 984–1002.

Gershey, R.M., Neve, R.A., Musgrave, D.L., and Reichardt, P.B. 1977. A colorimetric method for determination of saxitoxin. *Journal of the Fisheries Board of Canada*, 34(4): 559–563.

Goya, A.B., Tarnovius, S., Hatfield, R.G., Coates, L., Lewis, A.M., and Turner, A.D. 2020. Paralytic shellfish toxins and associated toxin profiles in bivalve mollusc shellfish from Argentina. *Harmful Algae*, 99: 101910.

Hall, S., Strichartz, G., Moczydlowski, E., Ravindran, A., and Reichardt, P.B. 1990. *The saxitoxins: sources, chemistry, and pharmacology*. ACS Publications.

Halstead, B.W., Schantz, E.J., and World Health Organization. 1984. *Paralytic shellfish poisoning*. World Health Organization, Geneva, Switzerland.

Hinder, S.L., Hays, G.C., Brooks, C.J., Davies, A.P., Edwards, M., Walne, A.W., and Gravenor, M.B. 2011. Toxic marine microalgae and shellfish poisoning in the British isles: history, review of epidemiology, and future implications. *Environmental Health*, 10(1): 1–12.

Indrasena, W.M., and Gill, T.A. 1998. Fluorometric detection of paralytic shellfish poisoning toxins. *Analytical Biochemistry*, 264(2): 230–236.

Jaime, E., Hummert, C., Hess, P., and Luckas, B. 2001. Determination of paralytic shellfish poisoning toxins by high-performance ion-exchange chromatography. *Journal of Chromatography A*, 929(1–2): 43–49.

James, K.J., Carey, B., O'halloran, J., and Škrabáková, Z. 2010. Shellfish toxicity: human health implications of marine algal toxins. *Epidemiology & Infection*, 138(7): 927–940.

Jellett, J.F., Marks, L.J., Stewart, J.E., Dorey, M.L., Watson-Wright, W., and Lawrence, J.F. 1992. Paralytic shellfish poison (saxitoxin family) bioassays: automated endpoint determination and standardization of the in vitro tissue culture bioassay, and comparison with the standard mouse bioassay. *Toxicon*, 30(10): 1143–1156.

Jen, H.C., Nguyen, T.A.T., Wu, Y.J., Hoang, T., Arakawa, O., Lin, W.F., and Hwang, D.F. 2014. Tetrodotoxin and paralytic shellfish poisons in gastropod species from Vietnam analyzed by high-performance liquid chromatography and liquid chromatography–tandem mass spectrometry. *Journal of Food and Drug Analysis*, 22(2): 178–188.

Johnson, H.M., Frey, P.A., Angelotti, R., Campbell, J.E., and Lewis, K.H. 1964. Haptenic properties of paralytic shellfish poison conjugated to proteins by formaldehyde treatment. *Proceedings of the Society for Experimental Biology and Medicine*, 117(2): 425–430.

Kao, C.Y. 1972. Pharmacology of tetrodotoxin and saxitoxin. *Federation Proceedings*, 31(3): 1117–1123.

Kao, C.Y. 1993. Paralytic shellfish poisoning. *Algal Toxins in Seafood and Drinking Water*, 75: 86.

Kao, C.Y., and Levinson, S.R. 1986. *Tetrodotoxin, saxitoxin, and the molecular biology of the sodium channel*. New York Academy of Sciences.

Kao, C.Y., and Nishiyama, A.N.D.A. 1965. Actions of saxitoxin on peripheral neuromuscular systems. *The Journal of Physiology*, 180(1): 50.

Kao, C.Y., and Walker, S.E. 1982. Active groups of saxitoxin and tetrodotoxin as deduced from actions of saxitoxin analogues on frog muscle and squid axon. *The Journal of Physiology*, 323(1): 619–637.

Kawatsu, K., Hamano, Y., Sugiyama, A., Hashizume, K., and Noguchi, T. 2002. Development and application of an enzyme immunoassay based on a monoclonal antibody against gonyautoxin components of paralytic shellfish poisoning toxins. *Journal of Food Protection*, 65(8): 1304–1308.

Kodama, M., and Sato, S. 2008. Metabolism of paralytic shellfish toxins incorporated into bivalves. *Food Science and Technology-New York-Marcel Dekker*, 173: 165.

Kogure, K., Tamplin, M.L., Simidu, U., and Colwell, R.R. 1988. A tissue culture assay for tetrodotoxin, saxitoxin and related toxins. *Toxicon*, 26(2): 191–197.

Lawrence, J.F., Maher, M., and Watson-Wright, W. 1994. Effect of cooking on the concentration of toxins associated with paralytic shellfish poison in lobster hepatopancreas. *Toxicon*, 32(1): 57–64.

Llewellyn, L.E. 2006. Saxitoxin, a toxic marine natural product that targets a multitude of receptors. *Natural Product Reports*, 23(2): 200–222.

Manger, R.L., Leja, L.S., Lee, S.Y., Hungerford, J.M., and Wekell, M.M. 1993. Tetrazolium-based cell bioassay for neurotoxins active on voltage-sensitive sodium channels: semiautomated assay for saxitoxins, brevetoxins, and ciguatoxins. *Analytical Biochemistry*, 214(1): 190–194.

Medcof, J.C., Leim, A.H., Needler, A.B., Needler, A.W.H., Gibbard, J., and Naubert, J. 1947. Paralytic shellfish poisoning on the Canadian Atlantic coast. *Bulletin: Fisheries Research Board of Canada*, 75: 1–32.

Micheli, L., Di Stefano, S., Moscone, D., Palleschi, G., Marini, S., Coletta, M., Draisci, R., and Delli Quadri, F. 2002. Production of antibodies and development of highly sensitive formats of enzyme immunoassay for saxitoxin analysis. *Analytical and Bioanalytical Chemistry*, 373(8): 678–684.

Mons, M.P., Van Egmond, H.P., and Speijers, G.J.A. 1998. *Paralytic shellfish poisoning: A review*. National Institute of Public Health and the Environment, Bilthoven, The Netherlands.

Mosley, S., Ikawa, M., and Sasner Jr, J.J. 1985. A combination fluorescence assay and Folin-Ciocalteu phenol reagent assay for the detection of paralytic shellfish poisons. *Toxicon*, 23(3): 375–381.

Munday, R., Thomas, K., Gibbs, R., Murphy, C., and Quilliam, M.A. 2013. Acute toxicities of saxitoxin, neosaxitoxin, decarbamoyl saxitoxin and gonyautoxins 1&4 and 2&3 to mice by various routes of administration. *Toxicon*, 76: 77–83.

Narahashi, T.O.S.H.I.O. 1972. Mechanism of action of tetrodotoxin and saxitoxin on excitable membranes. *Federation Proceedings*, 31(3): 1124–1132.

Naseem, S.M. 1996. Toxicokinetics of [3H] saxitoxinol in peripheraland central nervous system of rats. *Toxicology and Applied Pharmacology*, 141(1): 49–58.

Noguchi, T., Ueda, Y., Onoue, Y., Kono, M., Koyama, K., Hashimoto, K., Takeuchi, T., Seno, Y., and Mishima, S. 1980. Reduction in toxicity of highly PSP [paralytic shellfish poison]-infested scallops [Patinopecten yesoensis] during canning process and storage. *Bulletin of the Japanese Society of Scientific Fisheries*, 46(11): 1339–1344.

Okumura, M., Tsuzuki, H., and Tomita, B.I. 2005. A rapid detection method for paralytic shellfish poisoning toxins by cell bioassay. *Toxicon*, 46(1): 93–98.

Oshima, Y. 1989. Latest advance in HPLC analysis of paralytic shellfish toxin. *Mycotoxins and Phycotoxins*, 88: 319–326.

Oshima, Y., Machida, M., Sasaki, K., Tamaoki, Y., and Yasumoto, T. 1984. Liquid chromatographic-fluorometric analysis of paralytic shellfish toxins. *Agricultural and Biological Chemistry*, 48(7): 1707–1711.

Papageorgiou, J., Nicholson, B.C., Linke, T.A., and Kapralos, C. 2005. Analysis of cyanobacterial-derived saxitoxins using high-performance ion exchange chromatography with chemical oxidation/fluorescence detection. *Environmental Toxicology: An International Journal*, 20(6): 549–559.

Pearson, L., Mihali, T., Moffitt, M., Kellmann, R., and Neilan, B. 2010. On the chemistry, toxicology and genetics of the cyanobacterial toxins, microcystin, nodularin, saxitoxin and cylindrospermopsin. *Marine Drugs*, 8(5): 1650–1680.

Prakash, A. 1971. Paralytic shellfish poisoning in eastern Canada. *Bulletin: Fisheries Research Board of Canada*, 177: 22–27.

Quilliam, M.A. 2003a. Chemical methods for lipophilic shellfish toxins. In *Manual on Harmful Marine Microalgae*, Intergovernmental Oceanographic Commission (UNESCO), Paris. 211–246.

Quilliam, M.A. 2003b. The role of chromatography in the hunt for red tide toxins. *Journal of Chromatography A*, 1000(1–2): 527–548.

Quilliam, M.A., Thomson, B.A., Scott, G.J., and Siu, K.M. 1989. Ion-spray mass spectrometry of marine neurotoxins. *Rapid Communications in Mass Spectrometry*, 3(5): 145–150.

Quilliam, M.A., Janeček, M., and Lawrence, J.F. 1993. Characterization of the oxidation products of paralytic shellfish poisoning toxins by liquid chromatography/mass spectrometry. *Rapid Communications in Mass Spectrometry*, 7(6): 482–487.

Rey, V., Botana, A.M., Alvarez, M., Antelo, A., and Botana, L.M. 2016. Liquid chromatography with a fluorimetric detection method for analysis of paralytic shellfish toxins and tetrodotoxin based on a porous graphitic carbon column. *Toxins*, 8(7): 196.

Robertson, A., Stirling, D., Robillot, C., Llewellyn, L., and Negri, A. 2004. First report of saxitoxin in octopi. *Toxicon*, 44(7): 765–771.

Rourke, W.A., Murphy, C.J., Pitcher, G., van de Riet, J.M., Burns, B.G., Thomas, K.M., and Quilliam, M.A. 2008. Rapid post-column methodology for determination of paralytic shellfish toxins in shellfish tissue. *Journal of AOAC International*, 91(3): 589–597.

Satin, J., Kyle, J.W., Chen, M., Bell, P., Cribbs, L.L., Fozzard, H.A., and Rogart, R.B. 1992. A mutant of TTX-resistant cardiac sodium channels with TTX-sensitive properties. *Science*, 256(5060): 1202–1205.

Schantz, E.J., Mold, J.D., Stanger, D.W., Shavel, J., Riel, F.J., Bowden, J.P., Lynch, J.M., Wyler, R.S., Riegel, B., and Sommer, H. 1957. Paralytic shellfish poison. VI. A procedure for the isolation and purification of the poison from toxic clam and mussel tissues. *Journal of the American Chemical Society*, 79(19): 5230–5235.

Shimojo, R.Y., and Iwaoka, W.T. 2000. A rapid hemolysis assay for the detection of sodium channel-specific marine toxins. *Toxicology*, 154(1–3): 1–7.

Sommer, H., and Meyer, K.F. 1937. Paralytic shellfish poison. *Archives of Pathology*, 24: 560–598.

Su, Z., Sheets, M., Ishida, H., Li, F., and Barry, W.H. 2004. Saxitoxin blocks L-type ICa. *Journal of Pharmacology and Experimental Therapeutics*, 308(1): 324–329.

Sullivan, J.J., and Wekell, M.M. 1984. *Determination of paralytic shellfish poisoning toxins by high pressure liquid chromatography*. ACS Publications, Washington, USA.

Sullivan, J.J., Wekell, M.M., and Kentala, L.L. 1985. Application of HPLC for the determination of PSP toxins in shellfish. *Journal of Food Science*, 50(1): 26–29.

Tikhonov, D.B., and Zhorov, B.S. 2005. Modeling P-loops domain of sodium channel: homology with potassium channels and interaction with ligands. *Biophysical Journal*, 88(1): 184–197.

Turner, A.D., McNabb, P.S., Harwood, D.T., Selwood, A.I., and Boundy, M.J. 2015. Single-laboratory validation of a multitoxin ultra-performance LC-hydrophilic interaction LC-MS/MS method for quantitation of paralytic shellfish toxins in bivalve shellfish. *Journal of AOAC International*, 98(3): 609–621.

Van De Riet, J., Gibbs, R.S., Muggah, P.M., Rourke, W.A., MacNeil, J.D., and Quilliam, M.A. 2011. Liquid chromatography post-column oxidation (PCOX) method for the determination of paralytic shellfish toxins in mussels, clams, oysters, and scallops: collaborative study. *Journal of AOAC International*, 94(4): 1154–1176.

Vieites, J.M., Botana, L.M., Vieytes, M.R., and Leira, F.J. 1999. Canning process that diminishes paralytic shellfish poison in naturally contaminated mussels (Mytilus galloprovincialis). *Journal of Food Protection*, 62(5): 515–519.

Vilariño, N., Louzao, M.C., Abal, P., Cagide, E., Carrera, C., Vieytes, M.R., and Botana, L.M. 2018. Human poisoning from marine toxins: unknowns for optimal consumer protection. *Toxins*, 10(8): 324.

Wang, D.Z. 2008. Neurotoxins from marine dinoflagellates: a brief review. *Marine Drugs*, 6(2): 349–371.

Wang, J., Salata, J.J., and Bennett, P.B. 2003. Saxitoxin is a gating modifier of HERG K+ channels. *The Journal of General Physiology*, 121(6): 583–598.

Wekell, J.C., Hurst, J., and Lefebvre, K.A. 2004. The origin of the regulatory limits for PSP and ASP toxins in shellfish. *Journal of Shellfish Research*, 23(3): 927–930.

Wharton, R.E., Feyereisen, M.C., Gonzalez, A.L., Abbott, N.L., Hamelin, E.I., and Johnson, R.C. 2017. Quantification of saxitoxin in human blood by ELISA. *Toxicon*, 133: 110–115.

WHO (World Health Organization). 2016. *FAO/WHO technical paper on toxicity equivalence factors for marine biotoxins associated with bivalve molluscs*. WHO, Geneva, Switzerland.

Wiese, M., D'agostino, P.M., Mihali, T.K., Moffitt, M.C., and Neilan, B.A. 2010. Neurotoxic alkaloids: saxitoxin and its analogs. *Marine Drugs*, 8(7): 2185–2211.

Xia, Y., and Haddad, G.G. 1993. Neuroanatomical distribution and binding properties of saxitoxin sites in the rat and turtle CNS. *Journal of Comparative Neurology*, 330(3): 363–380.

Yang, L., Kao, C.Y., and Oshima, Y. 1992. Actions of decarbamoyloxysaxitoxin and decarbamoylneosaxitoxin on the frog skeletal muscle fiber. *Toxicon*, 30(5–6): 645–652.

Yang, X., Zhou, L., Tan, Y., Shi, X., Zhao, Z., Nie, D., Zhou, C., and Liu, H. 2017. Development and validation of a liquid chromatography-tandem mass spectrometry method coupled with dispersive solid-phase extraction for simultaneous quantification of eight paralytic shellfish poisoning toxins in shellfish. *Toxins*, 9(7): 206.

Zhuo, L., Yin, Y., Fu, W., Qiu, B., Lin, Z., Yang, Y., Zheng, L., Li, J., and Chen, G. 2013. Determination of paralytic shellfish poisoning toxins by HILIC–MS/MS coupled with dispersive solid phase extraction. *Food Chemistry*, 137(1–4): 115–121.

CHAPTER 17

# Maitotoxin

## *The Marine Toxin*

**Harpreet Kaur, Sukriti Singh, and Arashdeep Singh**

### CONTENTS



## 17.1 INTRODUCTION

Numerous marine creatures produce powerful poisons, turning themselves noxious as a protection technique against predators. Interestingly, different creatures can get noxious by collecting poisons among their own targets. Some species of dinoflagellates, which are marine and microbial photosynthetic eukaryotes, create profoundly poisonous metabolites. The toxins of dinoflagellate contaminate the food hierarchy and affect the various consumers. The accumulation of such toxins by various filter-feeding organisms, particularly bivalves, have no detrimental consequences on themselves (Plakes and Dickey, 2010), but when consumed by their predators, such as marine mammals and fish, and eventually humans, who consume toxic seafood (Fusetani and Kem, 2009). The natural marine products such as maitotoxin, brevetoxins, okadaic acid, palytoxin, and ciguatoxin consist of complicated structures and, due to their effective biological actions, they attract the interest of biochemists, natural product scientists, as well as synthetic chemists and pharmacological scientists. All of these compounds are metabolites of polyketide represented by polyhydroxy groups and polycyclic ethers. These compounds derived their names from the tremendous fish fatalities and food intoxication in which they were found to be connected; for instance, maitotoxin and ciguatoxin deduced their names from ciguatera (Plakes and Dickey, 2010; Fusetani and Kem, 2009), Florida coastal fish mortality gave rise to brevetoxins (Hashimoto, 1979) and shellfish poisoning to okadaic acid (Yasumoto, 2001; Reyes et al., 2014). These toxins are produced by multicellular marine eukaryotic algae, mainly dinoflagellates. The raphidophytes and hapophytes are other microalgae phyla also believed to be associated with fish fatality and toxicity. In the last few decades, the

DOI: 10.1201/9781003178446-17

isolation and characterization of toxic metabolic substances with higher molecular mass from these phytoflagellates have been accomplished. Among those, the well-known example is maitotoxin (MTX-1), the structure of maitotoxin was first described by Murata and Yasumoto in 1993 (Rey, 2007). Subsequently, palytoxin (Yasumoto, 1971), zooxanthellatoxins (Yasumoto et al., 1976) and prymnesins (Friedman et al., 2008) were promulgated from microalgae.

Maitotoxin (MTX-1) and its analogues (MTX-2 and MTX-3) are polyether compounds that are water-soluble and created by the starins of dinoflagellate G. *toxicus*. The predecessor of maitotoxin is also created by *Ostereopsis spp.*, *Prorocentrum spp.*, *Amphidinium carterae, Coolia monotis*, and *cadinium* species. The ciguateric fish "*Ctenochaetus stiatus*" also known as "*Maito*" in Tahiti was the fish from which the maitotoxins was isolated first time and therefore named "Maitotoxin" from that fish. After that, the herbivorous fishes and creatures that feed on G. Toxicus were biotransformed this toxin to ciguatoxins. Maitotoxin bioaccumulates just like ciguatoxins; when they move up the food hierarchy into elevated vital levels. Although, maitotoxin is different toxin; but supposed to give rise to ciguatera, however, with distinct symptoms as compared to those brought about by ciguatoxins. Maitotoxin developed the contraction dependent on calcium ions, in skeleton muscle and smooth muscle. The influx of calcium ions increased by maitotoxins through excitable membranes, and thereby causing neurotransmitter and hormone secretion, cell depolarization, and disintegration of phosphoinositides (essential in maintaining the role of fundamental proteins of cell membrane). The actions of maitotoxins dependent on calcium take place due to the existence of tetrodotoxin and absenteeism of sodium ions, prohibiting the functioning of sodium channels. MTX is found to be one of the powerful toxins known to inhibit the mouse at the rate of LD50, i.e., 0.13 mg/kg IP, i.e., 1 mg of maitotoxin is sufficient to kill 1,000,000 mice (Hambright et al., 2014). However, the oral potency of maitotoxin is quite lower (Kelley et al., 1986), which may be attributed to the less intestinal absorption resulting from the hydrophilicity and its high molecular weight. Accordingly, maitotoxin is principally located in the analogues tissues linked to the fish alimentary tract and is supposed to take part in the poisoning of ciguatera fish, when liver tissues and gut are ingested (Pisapia et al., 2017).

## 17.2 HISTORY OF MAITOTOXIN

In 1976, the maitotoxin was primarily reported inside the gut of the bristletooth surgeonfish known as "*Ctenochaetus striatus*" ("*Maito*" in Tahitian, hence its name) accumulated in French Polynesia "Tahiti" and in the beginning, believed to causing the multiple symptoms of ciguatera (Yasumoto et al., 1976). Subsequently, after 11 years, the toxin recovered from the strains of dinoflagellate Gambier (Yasumoto et al., 1987) confirmed about the toxin source segregated from the contaminated fish. The purified maitotoxin can solubilize in hydrophillic solvents, i.e., methanol, water, and dimethylsulphoxide and is available as a clear amorphous solid but it is moderately reliable in alkaline and has no stability in acidic environment. The pure maitotoxin has tendency to adhere both plastic and glass surfaces in aqueous solution (Murata and Yasumoto, 2000). At the same time, when maitotoxin dissolved in extract of methanol-water, it showed the maximum absorbance of UV (single) at 230 nm (Yaokoyama et al., 1988) owing to the existence of a conjugated diene within the molecule (C2-C3-C4-C144) as shown in Figure 17.1. The investigations utilizing purified maitotoxin revealed that the abrupt rise of intracellular $Ca^{2+}$ ($iCa^{2+}$) and instant influx of external $Ca^{2+}$ concentrations in various cells may be the caused by maitotoxin (Reyes et al., 2014). The $Ca^{2+}$ ion influx brought about by maitotoxin accelerates various secondary events, such as, breakdown of phosphoinositide (Gusovsky et al., 1990), neuronal cells depolarization (Ogura et al., 1984), reaction of acrosome in sperm (Trevino et al., 2006; Amano et al., 1993), contraction of smooth muscle (Ohizumi and Yasumoto, 1983a; Ohizumi et al., 1983a), noradrenaline (Ohizumi et al., 1983a; Takahashi et al., 1983), neurotransmitters secretion, e.g., dopamine (Taglialatela et al., 1986), hormones secretion,

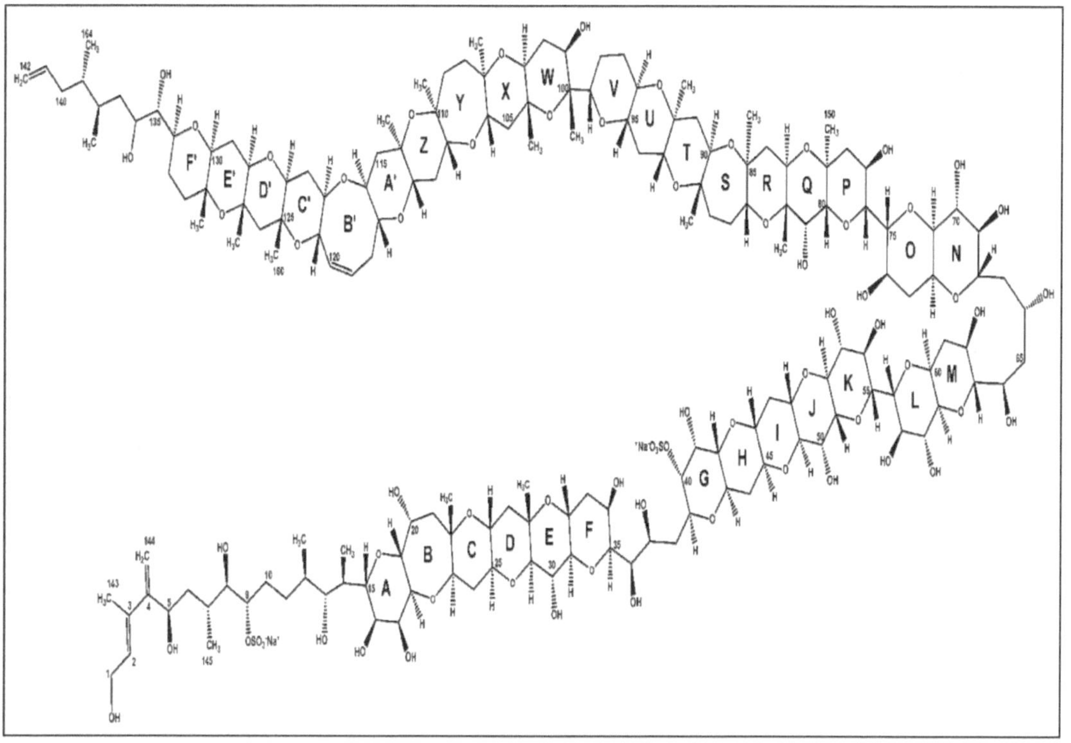

**Figure 17.1** Complete stereochemistry of Maitotoxin as obtained by Sasaki et al. (1996) and Nonomura et al. (1996).

e.g., insulin (Soergel et al., 1990), GABA (Pin et al., 1988), activation, or formation large oncotic/ cytolytic poes (Schilling et al., 1999), and inflammatory intermediates (histamine (Columbo et al., 1992), and arachidonic acid (Choi et al., 1990).

## 17.3 ORIGIN OF MAITOTOXIN

As we know, the aquatic single celled dinoflagellate G. *toxicus* is a phytoplanktonic creature, and can also located worldwide in tropical waters on the surface of algae. The ciguatera and maitotoxin produced by it which multiply through food chains as contaminated herbivorous fish consumed by carnivorous fish. The maitotoxin mainly found in the gut and liver of fishes rather than in their flesh (Yasumoto, 1971). The huge predatory fish including grouper, barracuda, snapper, amberjack, and shark contain higher concentrations of toxins. The ciguatera fish contamination can take place almost worldwide because there are no boundaries for the fish industry, and therefore marine products are transported to various nations. The dwellers or travellers of endemic regions should avoid taking moray eel or barracuda, being careful with red snapper and grouper, and recommend finding out about regional fish analogous to ciguatera. Subsequently, there is no standardized procedure for decontamination of fish or to differentiate the poisoned fish due to its appearance or smell, it is recommended to prevent consuming the gut of fish and to avoid eating huge predacious reef fish (Friedman et al., 2008; Skinner et al., 2011). It has been predicted during the upcoming years, the climate of the southeastern Gulf of Mexico and northern Caribbean will increase to 2.5°C–3.5°C (Sheppard and Rioja-Nieto, 2005). The hot weather supports the growth of G. *toxicus* (Chateau-Degat et al., 2005) and probably changes the migration patterns of fish. The outbreaks of ciguatera have been associated with the increase in temperature of sea surface in the South Pacific Ocean (Hale et al., 1999). In 1977, Yasumoto concluded that the maitotoxin was produced by dinoflagellate G. *toxicus*, he used to take 10 years to cultivate this microorganism so as to collect sufficient medium to recover this toxin and therefore to characterize its structural integrity (Yokoyama et al., 1988; Murata and Yasumoto, 2000). The maitotoxin was available commercially for some years, for research purposes and was utilize to analyse the $Ca^{2+}$ dynamics in different cell types.

## 17.4 TOXICITY OF MAITOTOXIN

A number of diseases can occur due to the human consumption of seafood poisoned with toxins caused by aquatic phytoplankton (Skinner et al., 2011; Falkoner, 1993; Baden et al., 1995). Hence, these toxins can be attributed to various chronic and acute health hazards not only in human beings but also in a wide range of animal species. According to scientific reports, these toxic compounds are often odourless, tasteless, acid, and heat liable, the standard methods of food testing cease to determine and terminate these toxins in poisoned seafood. The ciguatera symptoms may be mild to severe and can last from a few days to many years. About 400 varieties of fishes are classified as ciguateric and carry definite combinations of toxins. The main symptom of ciguateric varies from abdominal cramps, vomiting, nausea, itching, reversal of temperature, and neurological and gastrointestinal disorders. These toxins can be transmitted to a foetus or infant through the placenta or breast milk, respectively (Friedman et al., 2008; Skinner et al., 2011). Ciguatera is mainly responsible for primarily neurological symptoms as compared to maitotoxin, which is supposed to be not significant for causing ciguatera symptoms due to its lower concentration in fish. Nevertheless, it must be noteworthy that the distinguished differences in toxicity might be attributed to the consequences of chemical modifications of the toxins likely to be occurred as they move throughout the food chain, and consequently, it is difficult for them to make an immediate association among the particular toxin and diverse symptoms. The identification of ciguatera is entirely dependent on the existence of common symptoms associated with patients who had a recent history of fish consumption. Ciguatera is fat-soluble while maitotoxin is soluble in water; however, it would accumulate in the organ, such as the liver, rather than in the flesh of fish (Lewis, 2006). The oral potency of maitotoxin is very low in contrast to their elevated lethality rate when introduced intraperitoneally (i.p.); however, purified maitotoxin is considerably more poisonous than ciguatera. For instance, in mice, the lethality rate of ciguatera is 0.45 μg/kg IP and for maitotoxin it is about 0.13 μg/kg IP. The specific lethal dose is correlated to the source of sample, strain of mouse, procedure of sample preparation, because the maitotioxin binds to plastic and glass and therefore its standard concentration are not well known. The infusion of maitotoxin to mice can develop dyspnea, piloerection, low body temperature, mild convulsions or tremors, advanced paralysis, and longer death times. The increased dosage of maitotoxin can develop similar symptoms to ciguatera toxin, including convulsions with gasping and shorter death durations. The diverse strains of G. *toxicus* give rise to three different molecules of maitotoxin. There are similar symptoms of injecting MTX-1 and MTX-2 in mice, excluding the shorter death duration exhibited by MTX-2. The additional symptoms induced by MTX-3 include severe gasping that enhance the death rates; in spite of this, HPLC extra purification of MTX-3 lowers the symptoms of gasping, recommending that the another bioactive compounds may be available in crude preparation (Holmes and Lewis, 1994). The MTX-1 and MTX-3 are quite similar in producing duration of death. The toxicity of the 3 different forms can be reduced 200-fold by desulfonation of Maitotoxin (solvolysis) (Holmes and Lewis, 1994). The ELISA (enzyme-linked immunosorbent assay) or RIA (radioimmunoassay) have been recognized over the last few years to analyse ciguatera toxin, for instance, the Hokama enzyme immunoassay stick test (Hokama, 1985). The Cigua-Check® is a commercially available kit to detect toxin and is utilized by restaurants or fishermen to avoid consumption of poisoned fish. But this kit can only analyze the presence of ciguatera toxin. The mass spectrometry and HPLC (high-performance liquid chromatography) can be used to detect the contaminated fish samples by MTX and CTX; however, this method is expensive, and lack of availability is a problem in high-risk zones like small islands. To date, the antidote for ciguatera is not available but symptoms of chronic ciguatera such as paresthesias and fatigue can be diminished by some medications like amitriptyline. There are also palliative cures such as medicinal teas, consumed in both the West Indies and Indo-Pacific regions. Unfortunately, none of these remedies have been appropriately regulated to come up with effective treatment (Friedman et al., 2008; Skinner et al., 2011). The infected individuals are recommended to avoid consumption of nut oils, nuts, and alcohol for about six months after the contamination so as to prevent the reoccurrence of symptoms.

## 17.5 STRUCTURE OF MAITOTOXIN

Maitotoxin (MTX) is a distinctive and larger, naturally available product having a molecular weight of 3422 Da. The size and lethality rate of maitotoxin is much larger than palytoxin. However, the lower availability of samples has hindered the appropriate evaluation at pharmacological level. The complete maitotoxin structure was discovered in 1993. MTX was recovered from cultured strain GII-1, i.e., dinoflagellates *Gambierdiscus toxicus*. Following purification, this observation stated that MTX is considered to be the largest marine toxin which is non-polymeric, and contained a ladder-shaped cyclic polyether, particularly composed of 28 hydroxyl groups, 32 fused cyclic ether, 2 sulfates, 21 methyl groups, and 98 chiral centres (For di-sodium salt, the mono-isotopic mass = 3423.5811 Da, and molecular formula: C164H256O68S2Na2). The stereochemistry of complete molecule of maitotoxin was described in 1996 (Figure 17.1). The stereochemistry among J and K rings was opposed by Gallimore and Spencer (2006) due to repetitious concept for the biosynthesis of aquatic polyethers of ladder shaped. Later on, the observations by Nicolaou et al. (2007) and Nicolaou and Frederick (2007) encouraged the initially allocated structure derived from data of NMR spectroscopy, computational analysis, specifying the chemical synthesis and GHIJK ring analysis by NMR technique. This controversy can be resolved by X-ray studies of crystal structure of MTX. The other two analogues of maitotoxin, i.e., MTX-2 and MTX-3, were revealed by Holmes and Lewis (1994) and Holmes et al. (1990). A single strain known as "Australian *Gambierdiscus*" from Queensland (NQ1) produces Maitotoxin-2 (MTX-2) (Holmes et al., 1990). The lethality dose of this strain is LD50 in mice of about 0.080 $\mu g/kg^{-1}$ IP, i.e., less toxic (1.6-fold) as compared to MTX [1]. The MTX-2 molecular structure has not been studied yet. The LC-LRMS analysis of sample isolated from NQI strain was performed by Lewis, et al. (1994) and revealed that MTX-2 is mono-sulfate in nature and its molecular weight (MW) as mono-sodium salt is about 3298 Da. The isolation of Maitotoxin-3 (MTX-3) was carried out from WC1/1 strain, i.e., Australian *Gambierdiscus* (Holmes and Lewis, 1994). The similar symptoms as that of MTX and MTX-2 was detected for Maitotoxin-3, and found to be poisonous in mice, but deficiency of pure extract of compound hindered to detect its potency limits (i.p. LD50 in mice) (Holmes and Lewis, 1994). MTX-3 elutes prior to MTX-2 more slowly than the MTX on a reversed-phase column, while utilizing the linear gradient to come across with nitrile/water (Holmes and Lewis, 1994). However, during the usage of acetonitrile-water, the UV-spectrum of MTX-3 consists of two peaks, at wavelength of 200 nm (a minor peak) and at wavelength of 235 nm (major peak), moderately higher as compared to MTX and MTX-2) (Holmes and Lewis, 1994). The LC-LRMS analysis of WC1/1 strain in IS+ acquisition mode was performed by Lewis et al. (1994) and concluded that the di-sulfated nature of MTX-3 (as disodium salt) and its molecular weight (MW) is 1060.5 Da. The original molecular structure of MTX-3 has remained to be study. However, the complete study of MTX-2 and MTX-3 and their molecular structures are not well defined; the common structural characteristic of the MTX class of toxins that is well known is the availability of a single group of sulfate ester. The analysis based on desulfatation of MTX and its analogues carried out by Holmes and Lewis (1994) observed that at minimum one of the groups of sulfate ester is crucial for functionality.

## 17.6 SYNTHESIS OF MAITOTOXIN

Since the extraction of maitotoxins, extensive study on the synthesis of maitotoxin has been done. By using computational chemistry, Nicolaou and co-workers synthesized the maitotoxins by using domain systems as it is a large molecule. In this chapter, a number of mechanisms are summarized that were analyzed during the past three decades and are redefined, extrapolated, and implemented by researchers required by the various groups associated with the developing genre of marine bio toxins. These methods were used in fragments by various researchers and for maitotoxins all these methods were used to synthesize the various given domains.

1. In this method substrate carries a vinyl moiety which is strategically being placed adjoining the epoxide groups to the extremity that helps the stereo and region selective hydroxyl epoxide openings by six-membered creating cyclic ethers (Nicolaou et al., 1985, 1989a, b). This method changes the way in which completely five-exo ring formation is observed with no olefinic bond in pyran system. This method has been found reliable and has been continuously used for the complete mechanism of polyether marine toxins.
2. A subsequent procedure was developed to analyze the synthesis of cyclic ethers of six-membered category that revolves around the inclusion of $\alpha$ and $\beta$ ester of unsaturation moiety and also pendant hydroxyl group (Nicolaou et al., 1989c)
3. During 1990, the metathesis was the valuable appliance for organic synthesis (Sasaki et al., 1996) contributed to creativity relevant for the reaction required in the formation of cyclic ether (Clark, 2006). In this method, olefinic esters as substrates utilized the Tebbe reagent to form the polyether fragments (Tebbe et al., 1978). Later, the use of Takai–Utimoto type reagents was done in the reaction (Takai et al., 1994).

Nowadays, the emerging synthetic techniques have authorized the significant advancement for the mechanism of marine polyether bio toxins. Carbohydrates have been used as a starting material (Chirality) and therefore such procedures contributed the various sources to create the varying rings/domains of neurotoxin (Nicolaou and Aversa, 2011).

The confront of maitotoxin and latest development has been implemented in asymmetrical catalysis used to develop the alternative techniques required for the chemical synthesis of ether rings begin with prochiral building units. In this method, acyl furans undergoes an asymmetric phase transfer hydrogenation where ruthenium is used as a catalyst to afford furanyl alcoholsin, resulting in better productivity with increased enantiomeric purity. Further, hydroxy furfurans are oxidized with N-bromosuccinimide, and produce the large cyclic groups by acquiring Achmatowicz rearrangement. However, this approach has been already implemented for the creation of various cyclic groups involved in maitotoxin, containing the building units.

Gallimore and Spencer (2006) studied the stereochemical uniformity in various marine toxins and found that all the earlier proposed models such as Cane-Celmer-Westley (1974) and other proposed models (Shimizu, 1986; Nakanishi, 1985) reveal only fragments of biosynthesis of the marine toxins and these have been restricted to the brevetoxins. Nicolaou and team workers first synthesized the maitotoxin domain (Figure 17.2, Figure 17.3, and Figure 17.4). The Achmatowicz rearrangement or Noyori reduction were the principal reactions involved in ring formation required in this mechanism (Fujii et al., 1996). The emergence of the latest methodologies has been designed by the venture of chemical synthesis that permits the formation of relative portion of such molecules by primarily developing the structural disintegration of ladder-shaped polyether toxins. The substantial advancement in the formation of various polycyclic marine ethers has been emphasized since 2000 (Nicolaou et al., 2008; Nakata, 2010)

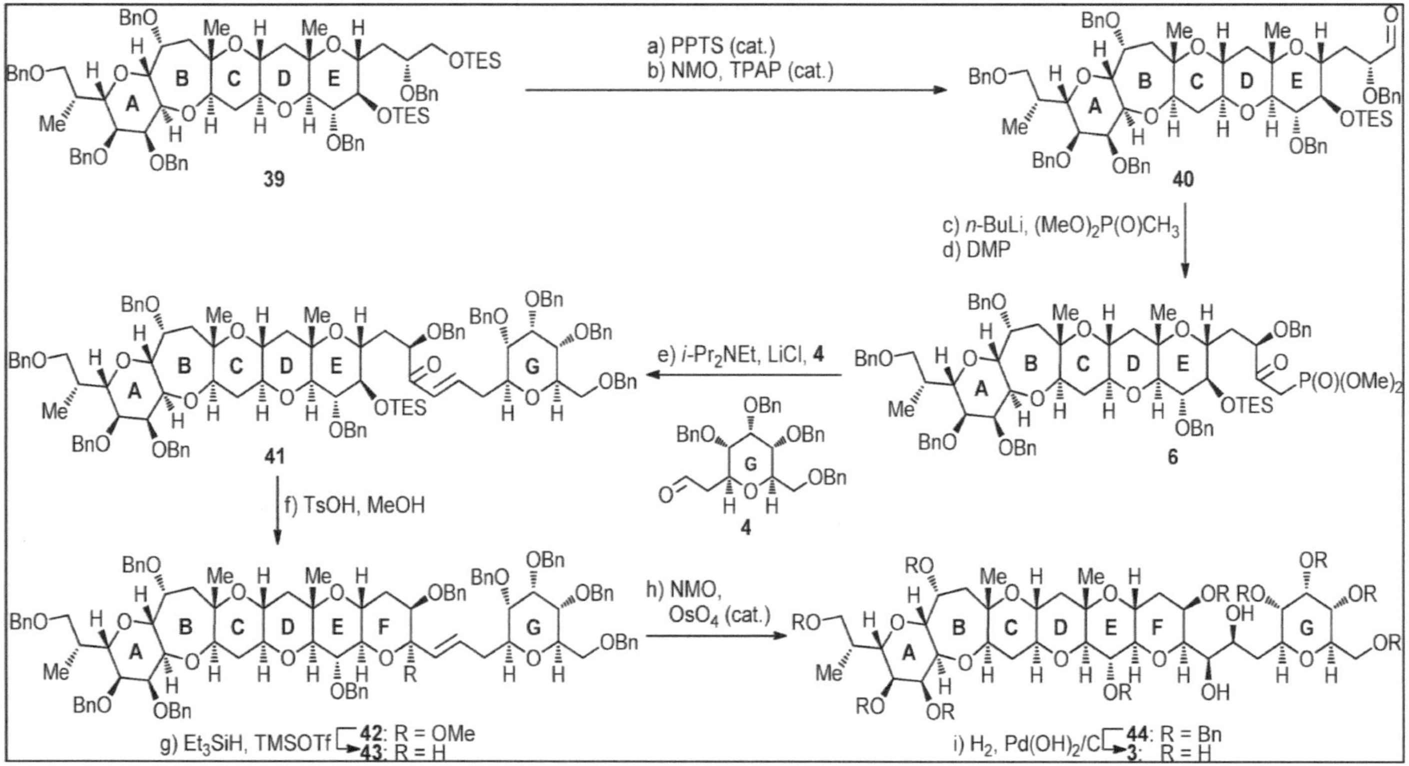


**Figure 17.2** Complete synthesis of maitotoxins ABCDEF ring system (Nicolaou et al., 2010) (reprinted with permission) **Reagents/Conditions** (a) **8** (1.5 equiv), 9-BBN (0.5 M in THF, 4.5 equiv), THF, 25°C, 4 h; then $KHCO_3$ (0.5 M aq., 13.5 equiv), 25°C, 20 min; then **7**, SPhos (0.3 equiv), $Pd(OAc)_2$ (0.15 equiv), 25°C, 72 h, 90%; (b) $BH_3$•THF (1.0 M in THF, 10.0 equiv), THF, 0°C, 18 h; then $H_2O_2$ (35% aq., 100 equiv), NaOH (1.0 M aq., 200 equiv), 25°C, 6 h, 70% (R-diastereomer) plus 15% (§-diastereomer); (c) DMP (4.0 equiv), $CH_2Cl_2$, 0 f 25°C, 2 h, 97% for **37**, 84% for $C_{23}$-*epi*-**37**; (d) imid. (200 equiv), PhMe, 105°C, 120 h, 65% plus 26% recovered starting material ($C_{23}$-*epi*-**37**); (e) **37** (1.0 equiv), $Zn(OTf)_2$ (5.0 equiv), EtSH:$CH_2Cl_2$ (1:5), 25°C, 20 h; (f) TESCl (10.0 equiv), imid. (20 equiv), $CH_2Cl_2$, 25°C, 1 h, 91% over the two steps; (g) *m*-CPBA (2.5 equiv), $CH_2Cl_2$, 0°C, 30 min; then $AlMe_3$ (2.0 M in hexanes, 5.0 equiv), 0°C, 30 min, 94%.

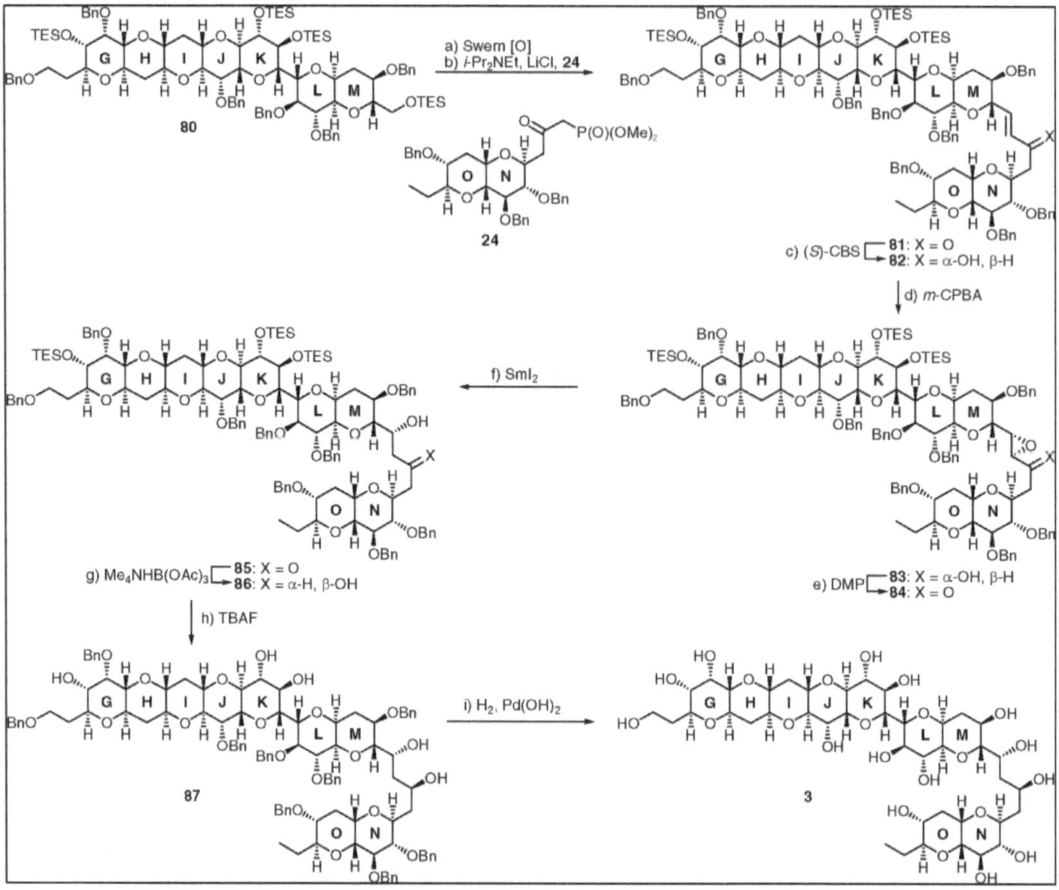


**Figure 17.3** Complete synthesis of maitotoxins GHFJKLMNO ring system (reprinted with permission) **Reagents and conditions**: (a) **6** (3.0 equiv), 9-BBN (0.5 M in THF, 8.0 equiv), THF, 60°C, 3 h; then KHCO3 (1.0 M in H2O, 20 equiv), 25°C, 30 min; then SPHOS (0.2 equiv), $Pd(OAc)_2$ (0.1 equiv), **76** (1.0 equiv), 25°C, 48 h, 72%; (b) $BH_3$•THF (1.0 M in THF, 10 equiv), THF, 0°C, 18 h; then $H_2O_2$ (35% aq., 100 equiv), NaOH (1.0 M aq., 200 equiv), 25°C, 5 h, 85%; (c) DMP (2.0 equiv), $CH_2Cl_2$, 25°C, 2 h, 93%; (d) TsOH (2.0 equiv), MeOH, 50°C, 18 h; (e) TMSOTf (5.0 equiv), $Et_3SiH$ (10 equiv), $CH_3CN$, 0°C, 30 min, 95% over the two steps; (f) TESCl (20 equiv), imid. (25 equiv), $CH_2Cl_2$, 25°C, 3 h, 96%.

## 17.7 PHYSIOLOGICAL ACTIVITY AND MODE OF ACTION OF MAITOTOXIN

The most poisonous marine compounds found till date are maitotoxins and up to now four toxin and its analogues are found namely MTX-1, MTX-2, MTX-3, and MTX-4 from variant dinoflagellate strains (Murray et al., 2018; Pisapia et al., 2017; Holmes and Lewis, 1994). The studies so far on effects of maitotoxins are at cellular level and actual mode of action has not been completely elucidated. Earlier the activation of voltage-gated calcium channel was found to be the mode of action for maitotoxin (Takashi et al., 1982; Cataldi et al., 1999). Researchers observed that maitotoxin increases calcium in plasma membrane by initiating the calcium access mechanism independent of voltage. However, the activation of non-selected ion channels possibly associated with transient receptor potential canonical 1 (TRPC1) have been exhibited by MTX (Morales-Tlalpan and Vaca, 2002; Meunier et al., 2009). $Ca^{2+}$, an important secondary intracellular messenger, is responsible for secretion, contraction, development, fertilization, and proliferation in cells. It creates a wide range

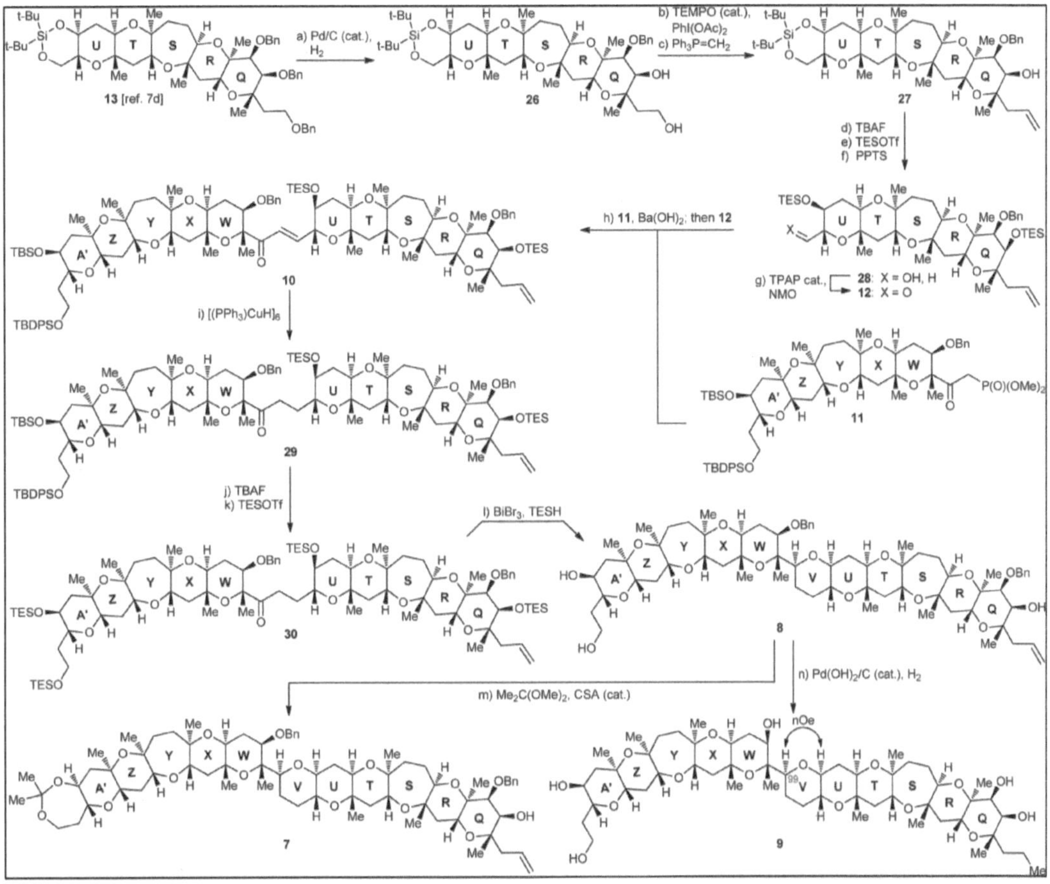

**Figure 17.4** Complete synthesis of maitotoxins QRSTVWXYZ ring system (reprinted with permission) **Reagents and conditions**: (a) 10% Pd/C (0.2 equiv), $H_2$, EtOH, 25 °C, 4 h, 80%; (b) TEMPO (0.3 equiv), $PhI(OAc)_2$ (2.0 equiv), $CH_2Cl_2$, 40 °C 2.5 h; then additional TEMPO (0.5 equiv), 40 °C, 1 h; (c) $CH_3PPh_3Br$ (10 equiv), NaHMDS (0.6 M in PhMe, 9.0 equiv), THF, 0 °C, 10 min; then crude aldehyde, 0 °C, 1 h, 77% over two steps; (d) TBAF (1.0 M in THF, 4.0 equiv), THF, 25 → 45 °C, 4 h; (e) TESOTf (6.0 equiv), 2,6-lutidine (8.0 equiv), 25 °C, 1 h, quant. over two steps; (f) PPTS (0.07 equiv), MeOH, −10 °C, 1 h, 76%; (g) NMO•$H_2O$ (3.0 equiv), TPAP (0.05 equiv), 4 Å MS, $CH_2Cl_2$, 0 → 25 °C, 1 h; (h) 11 (1.0 equiv), $Ba(OH)_2$•$8H_2O$ (1.5 equiv), THF:$H_2O$ (6:1); then 12, 25 °C, 4.5 h, 78% over two steps;(i) $[(PPh_3)CuH]_6$ (1.5 equiv), PhMe, 25 °C, 3 h, 97%; (j) TBAF (1.0 M in THF, 6.0 equiv), THF, 25 °C, 5 h; (k) TESOTf (8.0 equiv), 2,6-lutidine (10 equiv), $CH_2Cl_2$, 0 °C, 1 h, 88% over two steps; (l) $BiBr_3$ (0.5 M in MeCN, 3.0 equiv), TESH (50 equiv), MeCN:$CH_2Cl_2$ (4:1), −10 °C, 2 h, 81%; (m) 2,2-dimethoXypropane (50 equiv), CSA (0.2 equiv), $CH_2Cl_2$, 25 °C, 1 h, 83%; (n) 20% $Pd(OH)_2$/C (0.6 equiv), $H_2$, EtOH, 25 °C, 28 h, quant.

of spatial and temporal signals. Maitotoxins have been found to have effect on $Ca^{2+}$ homeostasis by elevating the $Ca^{2+}$ concentration and can be prove as an important tool in understanding the changes in intracellular $Ca^{2+}$ level as it is of specific interest, involving secretion of hormones, activated cell death, and fertilization (Reyes et al., 2014).

In various cells, like in fibroblasts of skin, large conducting channels get activated which causes lysis in cell, but this action has been found to be maitotoxin concentration-dependant. Murata et al. (1994) studied the change in activity of maitotoxin after removing sulfate ester group or hydrogenation of molecules and found that it reduces the activity of maitotoxin by several degrees as the potential of maitotoxin to cause the influx of $Ca^{2+}$ ions or breakdown of phosphoinositide in glioma cells or insulinoma decreases. Maitotoxin has been observed, for example, to causes achrosome reaction in sperm (Treviño et al., 2006), release of arachidonic acid (Choi et al., 1990), secretion of dopamine and insulin (Taglialatela et al., 1986).

Pharmacological analysis revealed that ion channels with controlled voltage are mainly responsible for pore gating, ion conductance, and pore regulation. These channels have been found to be target of potent neurotoxins such as polypeptide, alkaloids, and hydrophilic low molecular mass toxins. Once these toxins bind themselves at a particular receptor site, they have ability to change the channel functionality. These days, the receptor sites beside the protein channel of six variant neurotoxins have been recognized on ion channels with controlled voltage utilizing different neurotoxins. It is hypothesized that maitotoxins show the switching of gating dependent on voltage which opens the calcium channels voltage-gated at resting potential of membrane. This activation of voltage-gated calcium channels occurs as a consequence of activating a nonselective cation current (Estacion, 2000). Studies done by Kakizaki *et al. (2006) showed that the influx of* $Ca^{2+}$ *accumulates into cells of* cultured brainstem following a lag phase of maitotoxin which specified the permeability of $Ca^{2+}$ ions by reacting in an open state on calcium channel and avoiding its closing.

## 17.8 CONCLUSION

Maitotoxin is an effective polyether toxin extracted from the strain of dinoflagellate *Gambierdiscus toxicus*, while ciguatoxin is considered as one of the general toxins responsible for the poisoning of ciguatera fish (CFP). It is a polycyclic ether derived from polyketide which contains four fused enlarged cyclic compounds (MW-3422 Da). Maitotoxins' mechanism involves the uptake of $Ca^{2+}$ and its activated processes in a large number of various types of cells. The varied biological activity of maitotoxins facilitate it to gain attraction as a pharmacological tool so as to elucidate the cellular processes dependent on $Ca^{2+}$, comprising secretion of hormones, activated cell death, and fertilization. The extensive analysis by biological and organic scientists has been inspired by maitotoxins due to its complex structure and complex mechanism process. Among them, the understanding of both its biochemical and organic synthesis, moreover, their biological target stays incomplete. The present inadequacy of generally available maitotoxin underestimates the significance for acquiring its organic synthesis, with the intention that it again becomes readily accessible for analysis on dynamics of $Ca^{2+}$ in various methods and therefore assist to associate with its putative receptors. This may be open to good knowledge of the way the molecular mechanisms take part in the action of maitotoxins, which may assist in describing the distinct discrepancies in its practical modes. Understanding of this section may also assist in required medication or an antidote of ciguatera.

## REFERENCES

Amano, T., Okita, Y., Yasumoto, T. and Hoshi, M. 1993. Maitotoxin induce sacrosome reaction and histone degradation of starfish A sterinapectinifera sperm. *Zoological Science*, 10: 307–312.

Baden, D., Fleming, L. E. and Bean, J. A. 1995. Marine toxins. In *Handbook of Clinical Neurology: Intoxications of the Nervous System Part II. Natural Toxins and Drugs*, F. A. de Wolff (Ed.). Elsevier Press, Amsterdam, the Netherlands, pp. 141–175.

Cataldi, M., Secondo, A., D'Alessio, A., Taglialatela, M., Hofmann, F., Klugbauer, N. Di Renzo, G. and Annunziato, L. 1999. Studies on maitotoxin-induced intracellular Ca2+ elevation in Chinese hamster ovary cells stably transfected with cDNAs encoding for L-type $Ca^{2+}$ channel subunits. *Journal of Pharmacology and Experimental Therapeutics*, 290: 725–730.

Chateau-Degat, M., Chinain, M., Cerf, N., Gingras, S., Hubert, B. and Dewailly, E. 2005. Seawater temperature, Gambierdiscus spp. variability and incidence of ciguatera poisoning in French Polynesia. *Harmful Algae*, 4: 1053–1062.

Choi, O. H., Padgett, W. L., Nishizawa, Y. U. K. I. O., Gusovsky, F. A. B. I. A. N., Yasumoto, T. A. K. E. S. H. I. and Daly, J. W. 1990. Maitotoxin: Effects on calcium channels, phosphoinositide breakdown, and arachidonate release in pheochromocytoma PC12 cells. *Molecular Pharmacology*, 37(2): 222–230.

Clark, S. 2006. Construction of fused polycyclic ethers by strategies involving ring-closing metathesis. *Chemical Communication*, 34: 3571–3581.

Columbo, M., Taglialatela, M., Warner, J. A., Macglashan, D. W., Yasumoto, T., Annunziato, L. and Marone, G. 1992. Maitotoxin, a novel activator of mediator release from human basophils, induces large increase in cytosolic calcium resulting in histamine, but not leukotriene-Crelease. *Journal of Pharmacology and Experimental Therapeutics*, 263: 979–986.

Estacion, M. 2000. Ciguatera toxins: Mechanism of action and pharmacology of maitotoxin. In *Seafood and Freshwater Toxins: Pharmacology, Physiology and Detection*, L. Botana (Ed.). Marcel Dekker, Inc., New York, pp. 473–504.

Falkoner, I. 1993. *Algal Toxins in Seafood and Drinking Water.* Academic Press, San Diego, CA, pp. 224.

Friedman, M. A., Fleming, L. E., Fernandez, M., Bienfang, P., Schrank, K., Dickey, R., Bottein, M.-Y. et al. 2008. Ciguatera fish poisoning: Treatment, prevention and management. *Marine Drugs*, 6: 456–479.

Fujii, A. Hashiguchi, S. Uematsu, N., Ikariya, T. and Noyori, R. 1996. Ruthenium(II)-Catalyzed asymmetric transfer hydrogenation of ketones using a formic acid–triethylamine mixture. *Journal of Americann Chemical Society*, 118: 2521–2522.

Fusetani, N. and Kem, W 2009. Marine toxins: An overview. *Progress in Molecular and Subcellular Biology*, 46: 1–44.

Gallimore, A. R. and Spencer, J. B. 2006. Stereochemical uniformity in marine polyether ladders—implications for the biosynthesis and structure of maitotoxin. *AngewandteChemie International Edition*, 45: 4406–4413.

Gusovsky, F., Bitran, J. A., Yasumoto, T. and Daly, J. W 1990. Mechanism of maitotoxin-stimulated phosphoinositide breakdown in HL-60 cells. *Journal of Pharmacology and Experimental Therapeutics*, 252: 466–473.

Hale, S., Weinstein, P. and Woodward, A. 1999. Ciguatera (fish poisoning), elniño and the pacific sea surface temperatures. *Ecosystem Health*, 5: 20–25.

Hambright, K. D., Zamor, R. M., Easton, J. D., and Allison, B. 2014. Algae. In: Wexler, P. (Ed.), *Encyclopedia of Toxicology*, 3rd edition vol 1. Elsevier Inc., Academic Press, pp. 130–141.

Hashimoto, Y. 1979. Marine organisms which cause food poisoning. In *Marine Toxins and Other Bioactive Marine Metabolites*. Japan Scientific Society Press, Tokyo, Japan, pp. 91–105.

Hokama, Y. 1985. A rapid, simplified enzyme immunoassay stick test for the detection of ciguatoxin and related polyethers from fish tissues. *Toxicon*, 23: 939–946.

Holmes, M. and Lewis, R. 1994. Purification and characterization of large and small maitotoxins from cultured Gambierdiscustoxicus. *Natural Toxins*, 2: 64–72.

Holmes, M. J., Lewis, R. J. and Gillespie, N. C. 1990. Toxicity of Australian and French Polynesian strains of *Gambierdiscustoxicus* (Dinophyceae) grown in culture: Characterization of a new type of maitotoxin. *Toxicon*, 28: 1159–1172.

Kakizaki, A., Takahashi, M., Akagi, H., Tachikawa, E., Yamamoto, T., Taira, E., Yamakuni, T. and Ohizumi, Y. 2006. $Ca^{2+}$ channel activating action of maitotoxin in cultured brainstem neurons. *European Journal of Pharmacology*, 536: 223–231.

Kelley, B. A., Jollow, D. J., Felton, E. T., Voegtline, M. S. and Higerd, T. B. 1986. Response of mice to *Gambierdiscustoxicus* toxin. *Marine Fisheries Review*, 48: 35–37.

Lewis, R. 2006. Ciguatera: Australian perspectives on a global problem. *Toxicon*, 48: 799–809.

Lewis, R. J., Holmes, M. J., Alewood, P. F. and Jones, A. 1994. Ionspray mass spectrometry of ciguatoxin-1, maitotoxin-2 and -3, and related marine polyether toxins. *Natural Toxins*, 2: 56–63.

Meunier, F. A., Mattei, C. and Molgo, J. 2009. Marine toxins potently affecting neurotransmitter release. *Progress in Molecular and Sub-cellular Biology*, 46: 159–186.

Morales-Tlalpan, V. and Vaca, L. 2002. Modulation of the maitotoxin response by intracellular and extracellular cations. *Toxicon*, 40: 493–500.

Murata, M. and Yasumoto, T. 2000. The structure elucidation and biological activities of high molecular weight algal toxins: Maitotoxin, prymnesins and zooxanthellatoxins. *Natural Product Reports*, 17(3): 293–314.

Murata, M., Naoki, H., Matsunaga, S., Satake, M. and Yasumoto, T. 1994. Structure and partial stereochemical assignments for maitotoxin, the most toxic and largest natural non-biopolymer. *Journal of the American Chemical Society*, 116(16): 7098–7107.

Murray, J. S. Boundy, M. J. Selwood, A. I. and Harwood, D. T. 2018. Development of an LC–MS/MS method to simultaneously monitor maitotoxins and selected ciguatoxins in algal cultures and P-CTX-1B in fish. *Harmful Algae*, 80: 80–87.

Nakanishi, K. 1985. The chemistry of brevetoxins: A review. *Toxicon*, 23: 473–479.

Nakata, T. 2010. SmI2-induced cyclizations and their applications in natural product synthesis. *Chemical Record*, 10: 159–172.

Nicolaou, K. C., Aversa, R. J., Jin, J., and Rivas, F. 2010. Synthesis of the ABCDEFG ring system of maitotoxin. *Journal of the American Chemical Society*, 132: 6855–6861.

Nicolaou, K. C., and Aversa, R. J. 2011. Maitotoxin: an inspiration for synthesis. *Israel Journal of Chemistry*, 51: 359–377.

Nicolaou, K. C. and Frederick, M. O. 2007. On the structure of maitotoxin. *AngewandteChemie International Edition*, 46: 5278–5282.

Nicolaou K. C, Duggan, M. E., Hwang, C. K. and Somers, P. K. 1985. Activation of 6-endo over 5-exo epoxide openings. Ring-selective formation of tetrahydropyran systems and stereocontrolled synthesis of the ABC ring framework of brevetoxin B. *Journal of Chemical Society, Chemical Communication*, 19: 1359–1362.

Nicolaou, K. C, Prasad, C. V. C., Somers, P. K. and Hwang, C. K. 1989a. Activation of 6-endo over 5-exo hydroxy epoxide openings. Stereoselective and ring selective synthesis of tetrahydrofuran and tetrahydropyran systems. *Journal of the American Chemical Society*, 111: 5330–5334.

Nicolaou, K. C, Prasad, C. V. C, Somers, P. K. and Hwang, C. K. 1989b. Activation of 7-endo over 6-exo epoxide openings. Synthesis of oxepane and tetrahydropyran systems. *Journal of the American Chemical Society*, 111: 5335–5340.

Nicolaou, K. C., Hwang, C. K. and Duggan, M. E. 1989c. Synthesis of the FG ring system of brevetoxin B. *Journal of the American Chemical Society*, 111: 6682–6690.

Nicolaou, K. C., Cole, K. P., Frederick, M. O., Aversa, R. J. and Denton, R. M 2007. Chemical synthesis of the GHIJK ring system and further experimental support for the originally assigned structure of maitotoxin. *AngewandteChemie International Edition*, 46: 8875–8879.

Nicolaou, K. C., Frederick, M. O., Burtoloso, A. C., Denton, R. M., Rivas, F., Cole, K. P., Aversa, R. J., Gibe, R., Umezawa, T. and Suzuki, T. 2008. Chemical synthesis of the GHIJKLMNO ring system of Maitotoxin. *Journal of the American Chemical Society*, 130: 7466–7476.

Nonomura, T., Sasaki, M., Matsumori, N., Murata, M., Tachibana, K. and Yasumoto, T. 1996. The complete structure of maitotoxin, part II: Configuration of the C135-C142 side chain and absolute configuration of the entire molecule. *AngewandteChemie International Edition*, 35: 1675–1678.

Ogura, A., Ohizumi, Y. and Yasumoto, T. 1984. Calcium-dependent depolarization induced by a marine toxin, maitotoxin, in a neuronal cell. *The Japanese Journal of Pharmacology*, 36: 315.

Ohizumi, Y. and Yasumoto, T. 1983a. Contractile response of the rabbit aorta to maitotoxin, the most potent marine toxin. *The Journal of Physiology*, 337: 711–721.

Ohizumi, Y., Kajiwara, A. and Yasumoto, T. 1983a. Excitatory effect of the most potent marine toxin, maitotoxin, on the guinea-pig vas deferens. *Journal of Pharmacology and Experimental Therapeutics*, 227: 199–204.

Pin, J. P., Yasumoto, T. and Bockaert, J. 1988. γ-aminobutyric acid release is due not only to the aminobutyric acid release is due not only to the opening of calcium channels. *Journal of Neurochemistry*, 50: 1227–1232.

Pisapia, F., Sibat, M., Herrenknecht, C., Lhaute, K., Gaiani, G., Ferron, P. J., Fessard, V., Fraga, S., Nascimento, S. M., Litaker, R. W., Holland, W. C., Roullier, C. and Hess, P. 2017. Maitotoxin-4, a Novel MTX analog produced by Gambierdiscusexcentricus. *Marine Drugs*, 15(7): 220–222.

Plakas, S. M., and Dickey, R. W. 2010. Advances in monitoring and toxicity assessment of brevetoxins in molluscan shellfish. *Toxicon*, 56: 137–149.

Rey, J. 2007. *Ciguatera*. University of Florida, IFSA Extension, Gainesville, FL, 741, pp. 1–5.

Reyes, J. G., Sánchez-Cárdenas, C., Acevedo-Castillo, W., Leyton, P., López-González, I., Felix, R., Gandini, M. A., Treviño, M. B. and Treviño, C. L. 2014. Maitotoxin: Anenigmatic toxic molecule with useful applications in the biomedical sciences. In *Seafood and Freshwater Toxins: Pharmacology, Physiology and Detection*, Botana, L. M. (Ed.). CRC Press, Boca Raton, FL, 2014, pp. 677–694.

Sasaki, M., Matsumori, N., Maruyama, T., Nonomura, T., Murata, M, Tachibana, K. and Yasumoto T. 1996. The complete structure of maitotoxin, part I: Configuration of the C1-C14 side chain. *Angewandte Chemie International Edition in English*, 35: 1672–1675.

Schilling, W. P., Wasylyna, T., Dubyak, G. R., Humphreys, B. D. and Sinkins, W. G 1999. Maitotoxin and P2Z/P2X(7) purinergic receptor stimulation activate a common cytolytic pore. *American Journal of Physiology-Cell Physiology*, 277: C766–C776.

Sheppard, C. and Rioja-Nieto, R. 2005. Sea surface temperature 1871–2099 in 38 cells in the Caribbean region. *Marine Environmental Research*, 60: 389–396.

Shimizu, Y. 1986. *Natural Toxins: Animal, Plant and Microbial*, J. B. Harris (Ed.). Clarendon, Oxford, pp.123.

Skinner, M. P., Brewer, T. D., Johnstone, R., Fleming, L. E. and Lewis, R. J. 2011. Ciguatera fish poisoning in the Pacific Islands (1998 to 2008). *PLoS Neglected Tropical Diseases*, 5: 1416.

Soergel, D. G, Gusovsky, F., Yasumoto, T. and Daly J. W. 1990. Stimulatory effects of maitotoxin on insulin release in insulinoma HIT cells: Role of calcium uptake and phosphoinositide breakdown (1990) *Journal of Pharmacology and Experimental Therapeutics*, 255: 1360–1365.

Taglialatela, M., Amoroso, S., Yasumoto, T., Di Renzo, G. and Annunziato, L. 1986. Maitotoxin and Bay-K-8644: Two putative calcium channel activators with different effects on endogenous dopamine release from tuberoinfundibular neurons. *Brain Research*, 381: 356–358.

Takahashi, M. Ohizumi, Y. and Yasumoto, T. 1982. Maitotoxin, a $Ca^{2+}$ channel activator candidate. *Journal of Biological Chemistry*, 257: 7287–7289.

Takahashi, M., Tatsumi, M., Ohizumi, Y. and Yasumoto, T. 1983. $Ca^{2+}$ channel activating function of maitotoxin, the most potent marine toxin known, in clonal rat pheochromocytoma cells. *Journal of Biological Chemistry*, 258: 944–949.

Takai, T., Li, M., Sylvestre, D., Clynes, R., and Ravetch, J. V. 1994. FcR $\gamma$ chain deletion results in pleiotrophic effector cell defects. *Cell*, 76: 519–529.

Tebbe, F. N., Parshall, G. W., and Reddy, G. D. 1978. Olefin homologation with titanium methylene compounds. *Journal of the American chemical society*, 100: 3611–3613.

Treviño, C. L., De la Vega-Beltrán, J. L., Nishigaki, T., Felix, R. and Darszon, A. 2006. Maitotoxin potently promotes $Ca^{2+}$ influx in mouse spermatogenic cells and sperm, and induces the acrosome reaction. *Journal of Cellular Physiology*, 206: 449–456.

Yasumoto, T. 1971. Toxicity of the surgeonfishes. *Bulletin of the Japanese Society of Scientific Fisheries*, 37: 724–734.

Yasumoto, T. 2001. The chemistry and biological function of natural marine toxins. *The Chemical Record*, 1(3): 228–242.

Yasumoto, T., Bagnis, R. and Vernoux, J. 1976. Toxicity of the surgeonfishes-II properties of the principal water soluble toxin. *Bulletin of the Japanese Society of Scientific Fisheries*, 42: 359–366.

Yasumoto, T., Seino, N., Murakami, Y. and Murata, M. 1987. Toxins produced by benthic dinoflagellates. *Biology Bulletin*, 172: 128–131.

Yokoyama, A., Murata, M., Oshima, Y., Iwashita, T. and Yasumoto, T. 1988. Some chemical properties of maitotoxin, a putative calcium channel agonist isolated from a marine dinoflagellate. *The Journal of Biochemistry*, 104: 184–187.

CHAPTER 18

# Palytoxin

**Tanu Malik, Ramandeep Kaur, Ajay Singh, and Rakesh Gehlot**

## CONTENTS



## 18.1 INTRODUCTION

Due to seafood's delectable taste and nutritional value, it is immensely popular both at home and abroad. Many developed and large geography-bounded countries have seashores at their outskirts. This is the reason why those inhabitants adapted to Western-style food habits through the consumption of seafood. We have a lot of options available among sea produce, viz.: fish, lobsters, algae, crab, and corals which vary from sea to sea and region to region. Seafood consumption has risen throughout time as people's living conditions have improved and the fishing and aquaculture businesses have expanded dramatically. However, incidences of seafood poisoning have become increasingly common, posing a serious threat to people's health and welfare as well as major financial losses to the fish sector (Ciminiello et al., 2012). The marine toxin is one of the most common causes of seafood poisoning (Dowsett et al., 2011). Palytoxin and related compounds are nonproteinaceous natural molecules with super-carbon chains ranging from 2659 to 2680 Da and 127 to 131 carbons (Ciminiello et al., 2012a). The composition reveals that there is a family of palytoxins, each with a different molecular weight, depending on the organisms from which they are derived. Palytoxins have been detected in sea anemones, polychaete worms, crabs, and herbivorous fishes, in addition to zoanthids, showing that the toxin was accumulated through the food chain in animals living near zoanthid colonies (Mebs, 1998).

These sophisticated polyketides were generated by the genus *Ostreopsis*, which is mainly found in tropical and temperate oceans (Gleibs and Mebs, 1999; Lenoir et al., 2004). *Dinoflagellates* of

DOI: 10.1201/9781003178446-18

the genus *Ostreopsis* have been identified as the most likely source of palytoxin (Usami et al., 1995; Taniyama et al., 2003). In reality, many toxins with palytoxin-like properties have been identified and named based on the organisms that produced them (Vale and Ares, 2007). Five of the nine different *Ostreopsis* species have been identified as toxic material producers (Vale and Ares, 2007), but only four of them have been named: Ostreocin-D, a potent palytoxin analogue produced by *Ostreopsis siamensis* with an $LD_{50}$ value of 0.75 μg/kg when given intraperitoneally (Usami et al., 1995), *Ostreopsis lenticularis* produces neurotoxic ostreotoxins, *Ostreopsis mascarenensis* produces mascarenotoxins, and *Ostreopsis ovata* has recently been described as ovatoxin-a producer (Ciminiello et al., 2008). Palytoxin is a toxin produced by a number of marine organisms that may be transferred to humans by contaminated seafood, skin contact, or inhalation (Deeds and Schwartz, 2010).

Habermann (1989) validated the presence of the proposed palytoxin-induced ion channel as the target. In tropical and subtropical latitudes, serious sickness, and even death have been reported after eating seafood contaminated with palytoxin analogues since the 1970s (Tubaro et al., 2011). The presence of direct palytoxin analogues in seafood leftovers was only confirmed in a few occasions (Pelin et al., 2016a). Screening examinations on seafood samples purchased during the poisoning event, together with clinical findings and symptoms, revealed that palytoxin-contaminated seafood was the source of the health issues in numerous other instances. Palytoxin poisoning causes symptoms such as nausea, fatigue, diarrhoea, vomiting, dizziness, numbness of the extremities, muscle cramps, paresthesia, restlessness, respiratory discomfort, angina-like chest pains, abnormal blood pressure and heart rate, hemolysis, and electrocardiogram alterations such as an elevated T wave and bradycardia. Patients died in spectacular circumstances 15 hours to 4 days after seafood poisonings, typically after being taken to the hospital. A peculiar metallic taste in seafood is one of the most obvious indicators of probable palytoxin exposure (Pavaux et al., 2020). Symptoms do not emerge at the same time as big cell *Ostreopsis* densities or during flowering, but only at certain times. According to Vila et al. (2016), who conducted a relevant epidemiological and ecological study in a Mediterranean hotspot in 2013, symptoms developed near the conclusion of the exponential stage and the beginning of the stationary phase of the bloom. In the following years, this trend was approximately reproduced in that hotspot (Abós-Herràndiz et al., unpublished). Why pollutants and/or pieces of *Ostreopsis* may be aerosolized, and if these toxins constitute the disease's causal agent, are yet unknown. Palytoxin has an average $LD_{50}$ of 25 ng/kg for rabbits (the most susceptible species) and 50 ng/kg for mice following intraperitoneal injection, making it one of the most active aquatic toxins (Ares et al., 2005; Riobó and Franco, 2011). Palytoxin induces a wide range of pharmacological effects in all animal cells that have been observed.

## 18.2 STRUCTURE

Palytoxin (CAS Registry Number 77734-91-9) is a large non-proteinaceous molecule (C129H223N3O54) with a molecular weight of 2680.13 Da (Figure 18.1) that was discovered in *Palythoa toxica* in 1981 by 2 distinct research groups (Moore and Bartolini, 1981; Uemura et al., 1981). Palytoxin is a super-carbon-chain molecule that has the longest continuous carbon-atom chain of any natural molecule. There are lipophilic and hydrophilic zones in it. Palytoxin is a polyalcohol having a lengthy, partly unsaturated aliphatic chain interleaved with five sugar moieties, beginning with an OH group and finishing with an $NH_2$ group, and a total of 64 chiral centres (Munday, 2011). Palytoxin can have over $10^{21}$ stereoisomers because of this activity and the presence of eight double bonds susceptible of cis/trans isomerization (Katikou, 2007). It is second only to maitotoxin in the category of natural toxins with long continuous carbon atom chains (Kita and Uemura, 2010). It has many hydroxyl groups and two diene motifs along its backbone. Because of its vast scale and lack of repeated units, determining the complete composition, including stereochemistry, is genuinely

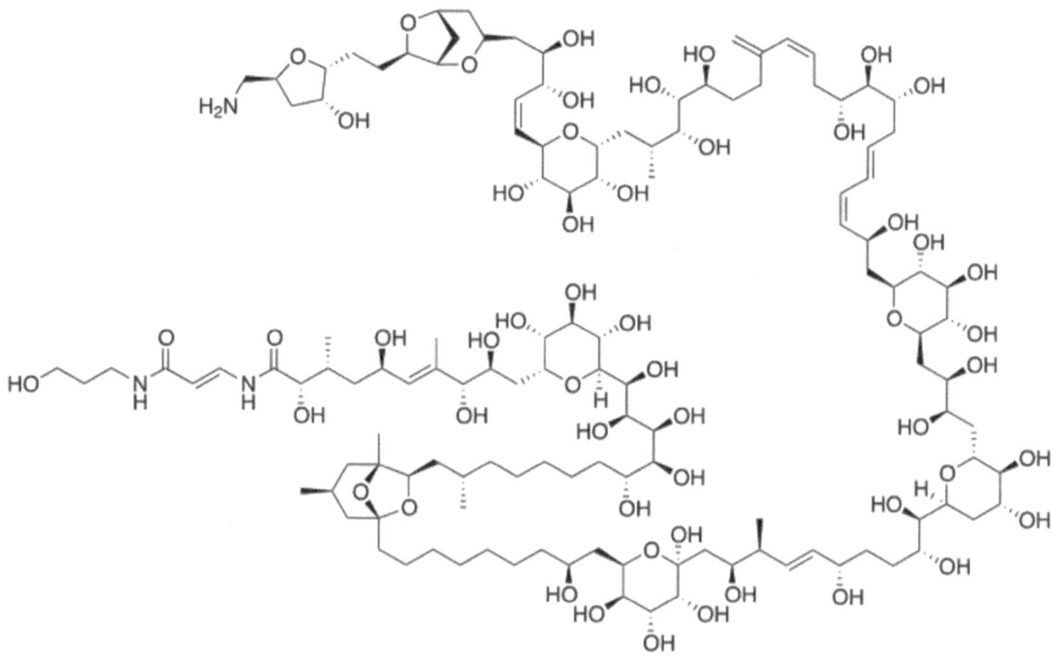


**Figure 18.1** Chemical structure of marine toxin palytoxin.

a "tour de force" (Ares et al., 2005). It is heat-stable, not inactivated by heat, and stable in neutral aqueous solutions for long periods of time; but, fast breakdown occurs in acid or alkaline conditions, resulting in loss of toxicity (Katikou, 2007).

In an aqueous solution, palytoxin forms a dimeric structure, and the interaction of the two palytoxin molecules is most likely aided by the terminal amino group. Acetylation has been demonstrated to limit the formation of dimers and reduce palytoxin's in vitro biological activity by roughly 100 times. In addition to palytoxin, a number of its congeners have been found so far. They differ from palytoxin in that they contain more or fewer hydroxyl and/or methyl groups, as well as chiralities, which may influence their poisonous efficacy (Tartaglione et al., 2016). Only a few palytoxin analogues have been chemically and/or physiologically studied. Soft corals have yielded two isomers of 42-hydroxy-palytoxin (42S-OH-50S-palytoxin) generated from *Palythoa toxica*, as well as its stereoisomer with a conformational inversion at C50 (42S-OH-50R-palytoxin) produced from *Palythoa tuberculosa* (Ciminiello et al., 2014). Other palytoxin congeners found in *Okinawan P. tuberculosa* include homopalytoxin, bishomopalytoxin, neopalytoxin, and deopalytoxin (Silva et al., 2015).

## 18.3 DISTRIBUTION

Palytoxin is a very poisonous non-peptide chemical that has biological action even at low doses. There have been several palytoxin congeners discovered, all of which derive from the dinoflagellate genus *Ostreopsis. Dinoflagellates* may be found in both tropical and temperate settings, making them a versatile species. The fact that they have a wide geographic range and may be utilised in a number of seafood dishes has further contributed to the concern. Palytoxin was initially found in *Palythoa toxica*, a Hawaiian zoantharian (Moore and Scheuer, 1971). Palytoxin and its structural congeners have now been discovered in other *Palythoa* species including Hawaiian *Palythoa vestitus*, Australian *Palythoa mammilosa*, West Indian *Palythoa caribaeorum*, and Japanese *Palythoa tuberculosa*, and *Palythoa aff. margaritae*. Palytoxin has been detected in a wide range of marine organisms, including xanthid crabs, other crustaceans, gastropods, cephalopods, echinoderms, and fish, as well as marine invertebrates of the *Palythoa* genus (Bire et al., 2013). Two systematic tests on the transmission of Palytoxin in coral reefs populated with Palytoxin-producing *Palythoa* were carried out in the Caribbean Sea (Gleibs and Mebs, 1999). Palytoxin was commonly spread in the areas studied, according to these reports, which used a delayed hemolysis assay and HPLC analysis to detect it.

Palytoxin has been found in mussels, sponges, soft corals, and gorgonians, as well as two zoantharian species and polychaete worms (Gleibs and Mebs, 1999). Palytoxin can build up in aquatic food systems, causing food poisoning in people who consume seafood (Aligizaki et al., 2011). As a result, Palytoxin is a major public health concern. Palytoxin and analogue toxins have been found in vector animals, including seafood, produced by a variety of marine organisms. As a result, ecosystems should be considered when attempting to comprehend Palytoxin distribution. After being extracted from the marine zoanthid *Palythoa toxica*, palytoxin was identified in numerous soft corals of the genus *Palythoa* (Moore and Scheuer, 1971). *Palytoxin*'s source is unclear in *Palythoa* zooxanthids, though it is likely to be bacteria or symbiotic microbes. There was also an instance of palytoxin poisoning produced by skin contact with zoanthid corals (Hoffmann et al., 2008). Although additional species in the group have subsequently been revealed to possess Palytoxin analogues, *Ostreopsis siamensis* was the first dinoflagellate to be associated to the production of dangerous compounds linked to Palytoxin (Taniyama et al., 2003). Over time, the number of dangerous Ostreopsis species has grown, and new palytoxin-like compounds have been discovered. Ostreocins were the first reported analogues in the bloom of Ostreopsis mascarenensis in the southwest Indian Ocean, followed by mascarenotoxins (further Palytoxin analogues) (Lenoir et al., 2004).

When it comes to Palytoxin, it's important to know the difference between seafood species that can only adsorb and integrate toxins in the digestive system (perhaps owing to the existence of toxin-producing microalgae that aren't further adsorbed) and those that can adsorb and integrate the poison in numerous tissues. Palytoxin presence may be "circumstantial" in the first scenario due to feeding behaviour prior to the catch of the seafood species, but toxins may be distributed, digested, stored, or expelled in the second scenario. Toxins may be located in more tissues, are more stable, and may be identified at higher quantities as a consequence of bioaccumulation, whereas metabolism may result in a greater number of Palytoxin derivatives, each with a different hazard potential.

## 18.4 MECHANISM OF ACTION

Palytoxin and its congeners have been extensively researched for their pharmacological pathways and toxicological effects over the last few decades. Much of the empirical evidence comes from in vitro and in vivo experiments on experimental animals. Palytoxin and its congeners have a wide range of deleterious effects on people and animals due to a number of mechanisms. Palytoxin and its congeners impair ion homeostasis pathways in both excitable and non-excitable tissues, according to several investigations. Palytoxin causes $K^+$ efflux, $Ca^{2+}$ inflow, and membrane depolarization by binding to the $Na^+/K^+$ ATPase pump and transforming it to a non-selective ionic pore (Tubaro et al., 2011). Palytoxin is a sort of secondary metabolite with no recognised physiological role in cells.

Temperature, saltiness, lighting or nutrition, depth or macroalgal substrate, and strain characteristics (isolation location, culture length, culture development phase) can all influence toxin production (Gémin et al., 2020). Palytoxin's mode of action has been thoroughly researched (Figure 18.2).

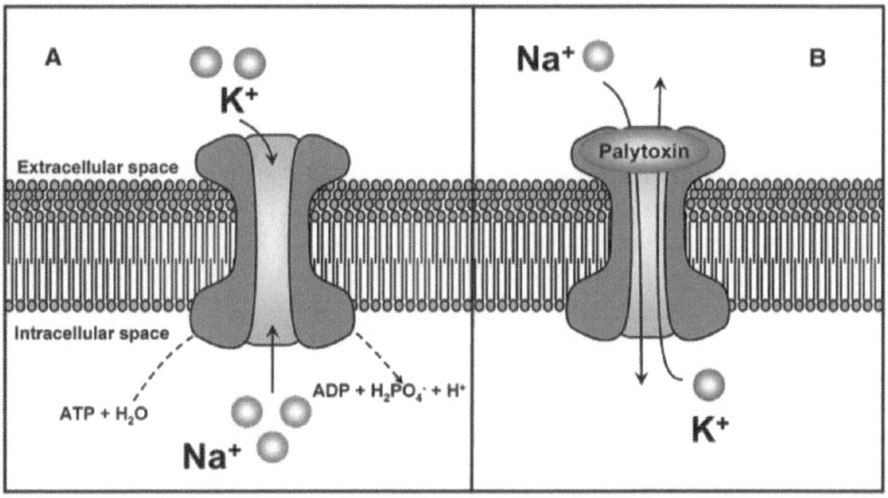


**Figure 18.2** Palytoxin's molecular mechanism of action. A. The Na+ K+-ATPase's normal function in cells entails the energy-dependent transport of Na+ and K+ ions across the plasma membrane against concentration gradients, with three Na+ ions transferred from intracellular to extracellular and two K+ ions imported into the cell per one ATP molecule hydrolyzed by the enzyme. B. Binding one palytoxin molecule to the enzyme's external side turns it into a cation channel, allowing Na+ and K+ ions to flow across the plasma membrane along concentration gradients, with Na+ inflow into and K+ efflux from the cell's interior. (Adapted from Rossini and Bigiani, 2011, Order Number:5061250719379.)

The Na+/K+ ATPase channel (Rodrigues et al., 2008) is a transmembrane protein (commonly referred to as a sodium pump) that transports three Na+ and two K+ out of the cell via ATP hydrolysis. The sodium pump generates an electrochemical gradient that is required for cell homeostasis to be maintained (Wu, 2009). Palytoxin binds to the extracellular portion of the Na+/K+ ATPase, turning it into a non-specific, permanently open ion channel that prevents active Na+ and K+ passage through the cell membrane. The ensuing membrane depolarization and substantial increase in $Ca^{2+}$ in the cytosol (Satoh et al., 2003) obstruct several of the cell's most crucial activities. Cell death is frequently associated with a shift in intracellular cation content, particularly an increase in calcium (Valverde et al., 2008).

In addition to inducing the release of K+ from numerous cell types and depolarizing every excitable tissue studied, palytoxin has a wide range of secondary pharmacological effects (Wu, 2009). Only a few of these include cardiovascular symptoms, hemolysis, histamine, prostaglandin, and norepinephrine production, platelet aggregation, bone resorption, and sperm motility inhibition (Pelin et al., 2016b). Other studies have linked palytoxin and its analogue ostreocin-D to the cytoskeleton in intestinal and neuroblastoma cells (Ares et al., 2009). As per the research, Palytoxin and ostreocin-D signalling cascades deform the actin filament system; however, factors other than Ca 2+ influx may be involved in how these toxins change the cellular actin cytoskeleton. According to the findings, ostreocin-D works in the same way as Palytoxin, indicating that the two toxins have similar targets. Despite this, minor structural changes between Palytoxin and ostreocin-D result in a substantial reduction in ostreocin-cytotoxicity D's and hemolytic potency. Palytoxin, like 12-O-tetradecanoylphorbol-13-acetate (TPA), is a powerful tumour promoter, but it does not activate protein kinase C, which is the receptor for the prototype skin tumour promoter. As a result, a better understanding of palytoxin activity would disclose unique elements of tumour promotion that may be used for anticancer purposes—a idea that was proposed in the 1990s but has since been forgotten (Munday, 2008).

## 18.5 TOXICITY

Human health effects from exposure to Palytoxin, a toxin produced by Ostreopsis, are indicative of its chemical ecology. Health effects may occur as a result of eating potentially Palytoxin-contaminated fish, or as a result of close exposure to seawater and/or aerosol during Ostreopsis blooms. Tubaro et al. (2011) looked into the characterization of human poisonings that may have been caused by Palytoxin toxicity. Since the 1970s, severe illness and even death have been recorded in tropical and subtropical latitudes after eating seafood that may have been polluted with palytoxin. Just a few cases were verified by direct Palytoxin identification in seafood leftovers among them. Screening investigations on seafood samples collected or purchased during or before the poisoning event, in conjunction or not with clinical findings and symptoms, indicated that Palytoxin-contaminated seafood was the source of the health issues in numerous additional cases. Palytoxin is a very poisonous non-peptide chemical that has biological action even at low doses. Because of the poison's effects on animals, notably humans, this toxin and its equivalents have become a global concern. The fact that they may be used in a variety of seafood recipes and have a wide geographic range has added to the issue (Chang et al., 2020).

Food poisoning (clupeotoxism) and respiratory intoxications have been linked to palytoxin toxicity in humans. Palytoxin enters the food chain and accumulates in tropical marine fish like sardines, herrings, and anchovies, producing clupeotoxism-related neurological and gastrointestinal problems. In recent years, palytoxin poisoning in humans has taken on novel forms. Patients in Germany and the United States were poisoned via dermal absorption after touching zoanthid corals in their home aquariums. In addition, a patient who attempted to remove a *Palythoa* coral was found to have inhaled human Palytoxin. There are numerous more anecdotal pieces of evidence of intoxications connected to aquarium zoanthids on internet marine aquarium sites. After being exposed to Ostreopsis ovata bloom aerosols during leisure or professional activities, people in Italy developed respiratory illnesses. Fever with considerable respiratory disturbances such as bronchoconstriction, moderate dyspnea, and wheezes is one of the symptoms produced by ovatoxin-a from aerosols, while conjunctivitis has also been observed in certain cases (Ramos and Vasconcelos, 2010). The prevalence of novel pathways of Palytoxin and its analogues toxicity has been highlighted in studies, as well as the concerns that aquarium hobbyists confront while keeping zoanthid in these aquaria.

## 18.6 IDENTIFICATION AND QUANTIFICATION

Palytoxins are identified and quantified in various ways such as *in vitro* and *in vivo* assays, analytical chemical assays, and immunological assays (Table 18.1). It is vital for human safety to identify the species that generate palytoxin. The hazardous impact of receptor binding or a cell line is used in the in vitro procedures. The impact of receptor binding on the $Na^+/K^+$ ATPase pump, which is tagged with a fluorescent dye, is detected. Fluorescence polarisation can also be used to determine it (Alfonso et al., 2012). The other approaches are based on the neuro2a cell line, 3-(4,5-dimethyl thiazol-2-yl)-2,5-diphenyltetrazolium bromide, and palytoxin's hemolytic activity against erythrocytes (Nicolas et al., 2015; Brovedani et al., 2016). In vivo approaches, on the other hand, such as the mouse bioassay, rely on the injection of a shellfish extract. Stretching of the lower back and rear limbs, spasms, restricted movement, ataxia, deterioration of the forelimbs, gasping for air, and eventually death have all been reported.

Immunological tests are based on an antibody recognising a specific portion of the palytoxin molecule (Fraga et al., 2016). High-performance liquid chromatography (HPLC), electrospray ionisation mass spectrometry (EI-MS), and liquid chromatography linked to mass spectrometry (LC-MS) are the most often utilised analytical procedures. Methods based on other ionisation technique have been found to be effective in detecting palytoxin. In both positive and negative ion modes, fast-atom bombardment (FAB) has been employed to detect palytoxin and ostreocin-D.

**Table 18.1 Methods of Quantification of Palytoxin**

| Species | Method of Quantification | Reference |
|---|---|---|
| Shellfish | Use of lithium iodine and formic acid as additives in liquid chromatography-mass spectrometry (LC-MS/MS) | Klijnstra and Gerssen, (2018) |
| *Palythoa Canariensis* | A microsphere-based immunoassay and ultrahigh-pressure liquid chromatography | Fraga et al. (2017) |
| Mussel, dinoflagellates, and soft coral | Microsphere based flow cytometry method | Fraga et al. (2016) |
| Scallops and clams | Enzyme-linked aptamer-based biosensor | Gao et al. (2017) |
| Marine and freshwater microorganisms | Dual-phase liquid chromatography coupled to triple quadrupole and quadrupole time-of-flight MS/MS platform | Wunschel et al. (2018) |
| Inland and coastal waters | High-Performance Liquid Chromatography- Heated Electro Spray Ionisation Tandem Mass Spectrometry | Merlo et al. (2020) |
| Marine water | Electro-chemical-luminescence-based sensor | Zamolo et al. (2012) |
| Shellfish | Fluorescence polarization | Alfonso et al. (2012) |
| *M. galloprovincialis* | Cytotoxicity assay (neuroblastoma cells) | Espiña et al. (2009) |
| Mussels | Novel Sensitive Cell-Based Immunoenzymatic Assay | Pelin et al. (2018) |

(Ciminiello et al., 2011). Using a hypersyl ODS C18 column eluted with a combination of water and acidified with pure acetonitrile and trifluoroacetic acid to pH 2.5, Lenoir et al. (2004) developed an LC-MS technique for measurement of palytoxin. However, no quantitative findings were presented for the mascarenensis extract. Every approach has advantages and disadvantages. The disadvantage of the in vivo approach is that the administration route is unethical. Furthermore, the approach has a low selectivity for the molecule that causes the observed effect. The use of in vitro procedures is a viable option. There is no need for a pricey conventional solution. An observed reaction, on the other hand, will still need confirmation via a confirmatory procedure. Immunological techniques are both sensitive and quick. In contrast, if an antibody only recognises a portion of the palytoxin, cross-reactivity with the molecule may be poor, resulting in an over- or under-estimate of palytoxin concentration. Analytical chemistry based on analysis can be used for confirmation. The drawback of analytical chemical procedures is that they want specific toxicity standards for each analogue (Riobó and Franco, 2011).

While the methods described above are more routinely used and assessed for seafood safety, alternative technologies, such as the Surface plasmon resonance (SPR) biosensor, may prove to be effective detection techniques in the future. It has mostly been employed in business and scientific research to evaluate molecular interactions, especially for drug analysis (Taylor et al., 2008). An inhibition-type antibody binding technique is utilised to discover toxins using an SPR biosensor technique. This capacity to detect toxins in the 15–400 mg/100g range; nevertheless, the antibody challenge outlined before also applied here. High detection capabilities, label-free, real-time, and minimal sample size are key advantages of SPR biosensors. This technique, predictably, will play an essential role for regulatory reasons in the future (Etheridge, 2009).

Aside from the type of identification utilised, sample extraction is critical. Boiling hydrochloric acid extraction is the most typical method (AOAC, 2000). This approach can turn less effective poisons into high-toxicity congeners. While there's a potential that linked diseases might arise during human digestion, the extraction is deemed safe. In contrast, fewer abrasive methods are necessary for the investigation of the innate toxin profile (Etheridge, 2010).

## 18.7 SAFETY, PRECAUTIONS, AND REGULATION

The major concern for human health is palytoxin entry into the human food chain. There is increasing evidence of adverse effects linked with ocular, cutaneous, inhalational, or exposure to aquarium soft corals polluted by palytoxin. The several cases reported described that the risk of human poisonings with these species is constantly rising. The signs and symptoms include commonly the nervous (tremors, ataxia, and paresthesia), gastrointestinal (nausea), cardiovascular (electrocardiogram alterations), skeletomuscular (spasms, weakness, and myalgia), and respiratory (coughing and rhinorrhea). Well-known method, corals as aquaria decorative elements lead to concern of this poisoning as a rising sanitary issue (Pelin et al., 2016a). Palytoxin and its congeners are highly complex toxic, which are common in all seafood. Various studies reported that palytoxins are lethal for humans. Inhalation or skin exposure following contact with aerosolized seawater during Ostreopsis blooms and during seafood handling has the most devastating repercussions (Nordt et al., 2011). The European Food Safety Authority used 200 ng palytoxin/kg as a reference point, an ARfD of 0.2 g/kg for the sum of palytoxin and ostreocin-D, and a tolerance limit of 30 g/kg for clam meat due to a lack of accurate quantitative evidence on palytoxin toxicity in humans due to a lack of accurate quantitative evidence on palytoxin toxicity in humans (EFSA, 2009).

## 18.8 EFFECT OF PROCESSING ON PALYTOXIN

Presence of toxins in seafood is a serious health concern worldwide. The various treatments are given to seafood to make the food toxin-free. Canned seafood is common in many parts of the world as it is rich in omega-3 fatty acids, proteins, and vitamins, and has low trans-fat. Heat sterilization is most frequently used for the destruction of toxins (Rodríguez et al., 2016). The various treatment used for the destruction of toxins is summarized in Table 18.2.

Other methods used for this purpose such as ozonation, irradiation, supercritical $CO_2$ extraction by way of acetic acid, evisceration, and freezing (Reboreda et al., 2010). Food irradiation has been known as an effective technology worldwide, which is capable of reducing or destroying ubiquitous pathogens that infect raw foods. However, studies on the utilization of irradiation in the mussel tissue for detoxification are limited (McCarron et al., 2007). According to European Union authorizations, the maximum allowable radiation dose for shellfish is 3 kGy, whereas the maximum allowed radiation dose for frozen peeled shrimp is 5 kGy (European Union Parliament, 2009). Ozone has mostly been utilised to purify drinking water. Previous research by Gacutan et al. (1985) on the use of ozone for shellfish detoxification demonstrated that ozone gas may effectively inactivate the toxins of *Perna viridis* infected with *Pyrodinium bahamense*.

**Table 18.2 Effect of Processing on Seafood Toxins**

| Species | Processing Type | Effect on Toxins | Reference |
|---|---|---|---|
| Mussels | • Steaming at 100°C for 5 min<br>• Autoclaving (121°C for 20 min) | • No increase or decrease in toxicity after steaming<br>• 50% reduction in total toxicity after treatment with an autoclave | Rodríguez et al. (2016) |
| Shellfish | • Gamma radiations | • Highest dose of gamma radiations resulted in the decrease in concentration of toxins | McCarron et al. (2007) |
| Shellfish | • Ozonation (15 $mg/kg^{-1}$ for 6 h)<br>• γ-irradiation (6 kGy) | • Reduction was more in ozone-treated samples as compared to irradiated samples | Louppis et al. (2011) |
| Mussels | • Ozonation (for 90 min) | • Shelf-life of 12 days was observed for vacuum-packaged ozonated mussels as compared to control sample (9 days) | Manousaridis et al. (2005) |
| Shellfish | • Supercritical atmosphere with acetic acid | • Up to 90% toxin is eliminated | González et al. (2002) |

There are numerous methods for industrial detoxification. The toxicity of *Acanthocardia tuberculatum* can be reduced by using hydrosolubility of saxitoxin and derivatives, followed by cooking, washing, and sterilising. Other writers have confirmed the lowering of toxin levels by using alkaline solutions followed by cooking and washing (Lagos et al., 2001). The utilisation of bacteria from quick detoxifying species (blue mussel—*Mytilus edulis*) has been studied, and the findings have been positive (Donovan et al., 2008). Even if the end product is not economically viable, it is possible to reduce toxic levels using supercritical $CO_2$ (Gonzalez et al., 2002). The use of amphoteric chemicals as a feed to "wash" the poison has been explored due to the lipophilic nature of the toxin. The addition of N-acetylcysteine, a glutathione precursor, to mussel metabolism, which would increase the speed of natural detoxifying processes, is a third option (Lagos et al., 2001).

## 18.9 FUTURE PERSPECTIVE

With the discovery of palytoxin chemicals in mussels, *Ostreopsis Dinoflagellates*, and cyanobacteria, it is now thought that vectors such as shellfish might pose a concern to human health in areas where these species are widespread. However, a major stumbling block is the lack of pure standards for palytoxin analogues. Characterizing the effects, activity, and contribution of these chemicals to intracellular signalling is critical. Palytoxin is a well-known toxin that may cause biochemical and biophysical reactions such as cytoskeleton reorganisation and ion channel gating. As a result, more research into palytoxin's interactions with all cytoskeletal substances such as cellular proteins, microtubules, and microfilaments is required. Although further in vitro research is needed to confirm this, the entire study leads to the conclusion that palytoxin alters the cytoskeleton, but that the cytoskeleton is also implicated in the toxin action and is required for palytoxin activity. These have vital uses in the chemical industry, aquaculture, and medicinal research, with a special focus on the discovery and development of cytotoxic chemicals that can be used to treat cancer. Because there is no comprehensive knowledge on palytoxin's hazardous potential and no particular therapy for palytoxin poisoning, medication is useful (Louzao et al., 2011).

## 18.10 CONCLUSION

Palytoxin and its analogues are one of the most potent seafood toxins. These are not generally detected by appearance, smell, and taste of contaminated food, and also cannot be removed by smoking, brining, marinating, freezing, and cooking. Palytoxin poisoning is a devastating illness, and the toxins that cause it pose a significant threat to seafood safety and human health. The neurological system, gastrointestinal, cardiovascular, skeletomuscular, and respiratory systems are all affected. Over the course of the year, knowledge of the origins, vectors, viable toxin testing procedures, and monitoring strategies has reduced illnesses and fatalities. Various sensitive, quick, and proven procedures were applied due to human health threats. A systematic strategy to identifying and measuring palytoxin in seafood will lead to a better understanding of the risks posed by palytoxin's presence and risk assessment.

## REFERENCES

Alfonso, A., Fernández-Araujo, A., Alfonso, C., Caramés, B., Tobio, A., Louzao, M. C., and Botana, L. M. 2012. Palytoxin detection and quantification using the fluorescence polarization technique. *Analytical Biochemistry*, *424*(1), 64–70.

Aligizaki, K., Katikou, P., Milandri, A., and Diogène, J. 2011. Occurrence of palytoxin-group toxins in seafood and future strategies to complement the present state of the art. *Toxicon*, *57*(3), 390–399.

Horwitz, W. 2000. Protein (crude) in nuts and nut products. Improved Kjeldahl method (AOAC Official Method 950.48). *Officials Methods of Analysis of AOAC International*, 17th ed. AOAC International: Gaithersburg, MD, USA.

Ares, I. R., Cagide, E., Louzao, M. C., Espina, B., Vieytes, M. R., Yasumoto, T., and Botana, L. M. 2009. Ostreocin-D impact on globular actin of intact cells. *Chemical Research in Toxicology*, *22*(2), 374–381.

Ares, I. R., Louzao, M. C., Vieytes, M. R., Yasumoto, T., and Botana, L. M. 2005. Actin cytoskeleton of rabbit intestinal cells is a target for potent marine phycotoxins. *Journal of Experimental Biology*, *208*(22), 4345–4354.

Biré, R., Trotereau, S., Lemée, R., Delpont, C., Chabot, B., Aumond, Y., and Krys, S. 2013. Occurrence of palytoxins in marine organisms from different trophic levels of the French Mediterranean coast harvested in 2009. *Harmful Algae*, *28*, 10–22.

Brovedani, V., Sosa, S., Poli, M., Forino, M., Varello, K., Tubaro, A., and Pelin, M. A. 2016. Revisited hemolytic assay for palytoxin detection: Limitations for its quantitation in mussels. *Toxicon*, *119*, 225–233.

Chang, E., Deeds, J., and Spaeth, K. 2020. A case of long-term neurological and respiratory sequelae of inhalational exposure to palytoxin. *Toxicon*, *186*, 1–3.

Ciminiello, P., Dell'Aversano, C., Dello Iacovo, E., Fattorusso, E., Forino, M., Grauso, L., Tartaglione, L., Guerrini, F., Pezzolesi, L., Pistocchi, R., and Vanucci, S., 2012a. Isolation and structure elucidation of ovatoxin-a, the major toxin produced by *Ostreopsis ovata*. *Journal of the American Chemical Society*, *134*(3), 1869–1875. https://doi.org/10.1021/ja210784u.

Ciminiello, P., Dell'Aversano, C., Fattorusso, E., Forino, M., Tartaglione, L., Grillo, C., and Melchiorre, N. 2008. Putative palytoxin and its new analogue, ovatoxin-a, in Ostreopsis ovata collected along the Ligurian coasts during the 2006 toxic outbreak. *Journal of the American Society for Mass Spectrometry*, *19*(1), 111–120.

Ciminiello, P., Dell'Aversano, C., Iacovo, E. D., Fattorusso, E., Forino, M., and Tartaglione, L. 2011. LC-MS of palytoxin and its analogues: State of the art and future perspectives. *Toxicon*, *57*(3), 376–389.

Ciminiello, P., Dell'Aversano, C., Iacovo, E. D., Fattorusso, E., Forino, M., Tartaglione, L., and Penna, A. 2014. First finding of Ostreopsis cf. ovata toxins in marine aerosols. *Environmental Science and Technology*, *48*(6), 3532–3540.

Ciminiello, P., Forino, M. and Dell'Aversano, C. 2012. Seafood Toxins: Classes. In Sources, and Toxicology. Handbook of Marine Natural Products, 1345–1387.

Deeds, J. R., and Schwartz, M. D. 2010. Human risk associated with palytoxin exposure. *Toxicon*, *56*(2), 150–162.

Donovan, C. J., Ku, J. C., Quilliam, M. A., and Gill, T. A. 2008. Bacterial degradation of paralytic shellfish toxins. *Toxicon*, *52*(1), 91–100.

Dowsett, N., Hallegraeff, G., van Ruth, P., van Ginkel, R., McNabb, P., Hay, B., and McLeod, C. 2011. Uptake, distribution and depuration of paralytic shellfish toxins from Alexandrium minutum in Australian greenlip abalone, Haliotis laevigata. *Toxicon*, *58*(1), 101–111.

EFSA Panel on Contaminants in the Food Chain (CONTAM). 2009. Scientific Opinion on marine biotoxins in shellfish–Palytoxin group. *EFSA Journal*, *7*(12), 1393.

Espiña, B., Cagide, E., Louzao, M. C., Fernandez, M. M., Vieytes, M. R., Katikou, P., and Botana, L. M. 2009. Specific and dynamic detection of palytoxins by in vitro microplate assay with human neuroblastoma cells. *Bioscience Reports*, *29*(1), 13–23.

Etheridge, S. M. 2010. Paralytic shellfish poisoning: Seafood safety and human health perspectives. *Toxicon*, *56*(2), 108–122.

European Union Parliament. 2009. List of Member States' authorizations of food and food ingredients which may be treated with ionising radiation. *Official Journal of European Union C*, *283*(52), 5.

Fraga, M., Vilariño, N., Louzao, M. C., Fernández, D. A., Poli, M., and Botana, L. M. 2016. Detection of palytoxin-like compounds by a flow cytometry-based immunoassay supported by functional and analytical methods. *Analytica Chimica Acta*, *903*, 1–12.

Fraga, M., Vilariño, N., Louzao, M. C., Molina, L., López, Y., Poli, M., and Botana, L. M. 2017. First identification of palytoxin-like molecules in the atlantic coral species palythoa canariensis. *Analytical Chemistry*, *89*(14), 7438–7446.

Gacutan, R. Q., Tabbu, M. Y., Aujero, E. J., and Icatlo, F. 1985. Paralytic shellfish poisoning due to Pyrodinium bahamense var. compressa in Mati, Davao Oriental, Philippines. *Marine Biology*, *87*(3), 223–227.

Gao, S., Zheng, X., Hu, B., Sun, M., Wu, J., Jiao, B., and Wang, L. 2017. Enzyme-linked, aptamer-based, competitive biolayer interferometry biosensor for palytoxin. *Biosensors and Bioelectronics*, *89*, 952–958.

Gémin, M. P., Réveillon, D., Hervé, F., Pavaux, A. S., Tharaud, M., Séchet, V., and Amzil, Z. 2020. Toxin content of Ostreopsis cf. ovata depends on bloom phases, depth and macroalgal substrate in the NW Mediterranean Sea. *Harmful Algae*, *92*, 101727.

Gleibs, S., and Mebs, D. 1999. Distribution and sequestration of palytoxin in coral reef animals. *Toxicon*, *37*(11), 1521–1527.

González, J. C., Fontal, O. I., Vieytes, M. R., Vieites, J. M., and Botana, L. M. 2002. Basis for a new procedure to eliminate diarrheic shellfish toxins from a contaminated matrix. *Journal of Agricultural and Food Chemistry*, *50*(2), 400–405.

Habermann, E. 1989. Palytoxin acts through Na+, K+-ATPase. *Toxicon*, *27*(11), 1171–1187.

Hoffmann, K., Hermanns-Clausen, M., Buhl, C., Büchler, M. W., Schemmer, P., Mebs, D., and Kauferstein, S. Q. 2008. A case of palytoxin poisoning due to contact with zoanthid corals through a skin injury. *Toxicon*, *51*(8), 1535–1537.

Katikou, P. 2007. Chemistry of palytoxins and ostreocins. In Phycotoxins: chemistry and biochemistry (pp. 75–93). Blackwell Publishing.

Kita, M., and Uemura, D. 2010. Marine huge molecules: The longest carbon chains in natural products. *The Chemical Record*, *10*(1), 48–52.

Klijnstra, M. D., and Gerssen, A. 2018. A sensitive lc-ms/ms method for palytoxin using lithium cationization. *Toxins*, *10*(12), 537.

Lagos, N., Rutman, M., Blamey, J., Ocaranza, M. P., Chiong, M., Hinrichsen, J. P., and Lopez, C. 2001. U.S. Patent No. 6,171,626. Washington, DC: U.S. Patent and Trademark Office.

Lenoir, S., TenHage, L., Turquet, J., Quod, J. P., Bernard, C., and Hennion, M. C. 2004. First evidence of palytoxin analogues from an Ostreopsis mascarenensis (dinophyceae) benthic bloom in southwestern indian Ocean 1. *Journal of Phycology*, *40*(6), 1042–1051.

Louppis, A. P., Katikou, P., Georgantelis, D., Badeka, A. V., and Kontominas, M. G. 2011. Effect of ozonation and γ-irradiation on post-harvest decontamination of mussels (Mytillus galloprovincialis) containing diarrhetic shellfish toxins. *Food Additives and Contaminants: Part A*, *28*(12), 1735–1744.

Louzao, M. C., Ares, I. R., Cagide, E., Espiña, B., Vilariño, N., Alfonso, A., and Botana, L. M. 2011. Palytoxins and cytoskeleton: An overview. *Toxicon*, *57*(3), 460–469.

Manousaridis, G., Nerantzaki, A., Paleologos, E. K., Tsiotsias, A., Savvaidis, I. N., and Kontominas, M. G. 2005. Effect of ozone on microbial, chemical and sensory attributes of shucked mussels. *Food Microbiology*, *22*(1), 1–9.

McCarron, P., Kotterman, M., de Boer, J., Rehmann, N., and Hess, P. 2007. Feasibility of gamma irradiation as a stabilisation technique in the preparation of tissue reference materials for a range of shellfish toxins. *Analytical and Bioanalytical Chemistry*, *387*(7), 2487–2493.

Mebs, D. 1998. Occurrence and sequestration of toxins in food chains. *Toxicon*, *36*(11), 1519–1522.

Moore, R. E., and Bartolini, G. 1981. Structure of palytoxin. *Journal of the American Chemical Society*, *103*(9), 2491–2494.

Moore, R. E., and Scheuer, P. J. 1971. Palytoxin: A new marine toxin from a coelenterate. *Science*, *172*(3982), 495–498.

Munday, R. 2008. Occurrence and toxicology of palytoxins. *Food Science and Technology-New York-Marcel Dekker*, *173*, 693.

Munday, R. 2011. Palytoxin toxicology: Animal studies. *Toxicon*, *57*(3), 470–477.

Nicolas, J., Bovee, T. F. H., Kamelia, L., Rietjens, I. M. C. M., and Hendriksen, P. J. M. 2015. Exploration of new functional endpoints in neuro-2a cells for the detection of the marine biotoxins saxitoxin, palytoxin and tetrodotoxin. *Toxicology in Vitro*, *30*, 341–347.

Nordt, S. P., Wu, J., Zahller, S., Clark, R. F., and Cantrell, F. L. 2011. Palytoxin poisoning after dermal contact with zoanthid coral. *The Journal of Emergency Medicine*, *40*(4), 397–399.

Pavaux, A. S., Berdalet, E., and Lemée, R. 2020. Chemical ecology of the benthic dinoflagellate genus ostreopsis: Review of progress and future directions. *Frontiers in Marine Science*, *7*, 498.

Pelin, M., Brovedani, V., Sosa, S., and Tubaro, A. 2016a. Palytoxin-containing aquarium soft corals as an emerging sanitary problem. *Marine Drugs*, *14*(2), 33.

Pelin, M., Florio, C., Ponti, C., Lucafò, M., Gibellini, D., Tubaro, A., and Sosa, S. 2016b. Pro-inflammatory effects of palytoxin: An in vitro study on human keratinocytes and inflammatory cells. *Toxicology Research*, *5*(4), 1172–1181.

Pelin, M., Sosa, S., Brovedani, V., Fusco, L., Poli, M., and Tubaro, A. 2018. A novel sensitive cell-based immunoenzymatic assay for palytoxin quantitation in mussels. *Toxins*, *10*(8), 329.

Ramos, V., and Vasconcelos, V. 2010. Palytoxin and analogs: Biological and ecological effects. *Marine Drugs*, *8*(7), 2021–2037.

Reboreda, A., Lago, J., Chapela, M. J., Vieites, J. M., Botana, L. M., Alfonso, A., and Cabado, A. G. 2010. Decrease of marine toxin content in bivalves by industrial processes. *Toxicon*, *55*(2–3), 235–243.

Riobó, P., and Franco, J. M. 2011. Palytoxins: Biological and chemical determination. *Toxicon*, 57(3): 368–375.

Rodrigues, A. M., Almeida, A. C. G., Infantosi, A. F., Teixeira, H. Z., and Duarte, M. A. 2008. Model and simulation of Na+/K+ pump phosphorylation in the presence of palytoxin. *Computational Biology and Chemistry*, *32*(1), 5–16.

Rodríguez, I., Alfonso, A., Antelo, A., Alvarez, M., and Botana, L. M. 2016. Evaluation of the impact of mild steaming and heat treatment on the concentration of okadaic acid, dinophysistoxin-2 and dinophysistoxin-3 in mussels. *Toxins*, *8*(6), 175.

Rossini, G. P., and Bigiani, A. 2011. Palytoxin action on the Na+, K+-ATPase and the disruption of ion equilibria in biological systems. *Toxicon*, *57*(3), 429–439.

Satoh, E., Ishii, T., and Nishimura, M. 2003. Palytoxin-induced increase in cytosolic-free Ca2+ in mouse spleen cells. *European Journal of Pharmacology*, *465*(1–2), 9–13.

Silva, M., Pratheepa, V. K., Botana, L. M., and Vasconcelos, V. 2015. Emergent toxins in North Atlantic temperate waters: A challenge for monitoring programs and legislation. *Toxins*, *7*(3), 859–885.

Taniyama, S., Arakawa, O., Terada, M., Nishio, S., Takatani, T., Mahmud, Y., and Noguchi, T. 2003. Ostreopsis sp., a possible origin of palytoxin (PTX) in parrotfish Scarus ovifrons. *Toxicon*, *42*(1), 29–33.

Tartaglione, L., Pelin, M., Morpurgo, M., Dell'Aversano, C., Montenegro, J., Sacco, G., ... and Tubaro, A. 2016. An aquarium hobbyist poisoning: Identification of new palytoxins in Palythoa cf. toxica and complete detoxification of the aquarium water by activated carbon. *Toxicon*, *121*, 41–50.

Taylor, A. D., Ladd, J., Etheridge, S., Deeds, J., Hall, S., and Jiang, S. 2008. Quantitative detection of tetrodotoxin (TTX) by a surface plasmon resonance (SPR) sensor. *Sensors and Actuators B: Chemical*, *130*(1), 120–128.

Tubaro, A., Durando, P., Del Favero, G., Ansaldi, F., Icardi, G., Deeds, J. R., and Sosa, S. 2011. Case definitions for human poisonings postulated to palytoxins exposure. *Toxicon*, *57*(3), 478–495.

Uemura, D., Ueda, K., Hirata, Y et al. 1981. Structure of palytoxin. Tetrahedron, *22*, 2781–2784.

Usami, M., Satake, M., Ishida, S., Inoue, A., Kan, Y., and Yasumoto, T. 1995. Palytoxin analogs from the dinoflagellate Ostreopsis siamensis. *Journal of the American Chemical Society*, *117*(19), 5389–5390.

Vale, C., and Ares, I. R. 2007. Biochemistry of palytoxins and ostreocins. *Phycotoxins: Chemistry and Biochemistry*, 95–118.

Valverde, I., Lago, J., Vieites, J. M., and Cabado, A. G. 2008. In vitro approaches to evaluate palytoxin-induced toxicity and cell death in intestinal cells. *Journal of Applied Toxicology: An International Journal*, *28*(3), 294–302.

Vila, M., Abós-Herràndiz, R., Isern-Fontanet, J., Àlvarez, J., and Berdalet, E. 2016. Establishing the link between Ostreopsis cf. ovata blooms and human health impacts using ecology and epidemiology. *Scientia Marina*, *80*, 107–115. doi: 10.3989/ scimar.04395.08A

Wu, C. H. 2009. Palytoxin: Membrane mechanisms of action. *Toxicon*, *54*(8), 1183–1189.

Wunschel, D. S., Valenzuela, B. R., Kaiser, B. L. D., Victry, K., and Woodruff, D. 2018. Method development for comprehensive extraction and analysis of marine toxins: Liquid-liquid extraction and tandem liquid chromatography separations coupled to electrospray tandem mass spectrometry. *Talanta*, *187*, 302–307.

Zamolo, V. A., Valenti, G., Venturelli, E., Chaloin, O., Marcaccio, M., Boscolo, S., and Prato, M. 2012. Highly sensitive electrochemiluminescent nanobiosensor for the detection of palytoxin. *ACS Nano*, *6*(9), 7989–7997.

CHAPTER 19

# Gonyautoxin

**Gifty Sawhney, Parveen Kumar, and Suraj P Parihar**

## CONTENTS



## 19.1 INTRODUCTION

**Gonyautoxins (GTX)** are a group of poisonous chemicals generated naturally by algae. They belong to the Saxitoxins family of neurotoxins, which also includes a group of molecule known as Decarbamoylsaxitoxin (dcSTX), Neosaxitoxin (NSTX), and Saxitoxin (STX). These Gonyautoxins are all analogues of Saxitoxin, the most well-known and researched toxin in this category, and they are all part of the shellfish poison (SP) family of Phycotoxins. Gonyautoxin-1 (GTX-1) to Gonyautoxin-8 (GTX-8) are the eight compounds currently classified to the Gonyautoxins group (Figure 19.1). The intake of Gonyautoxins by molluscs infected with poisonous algae can induce an illness condition termed Paralytic Shellfish Poisoning (PSP).

DOI: 10.1201/9781003178446-19

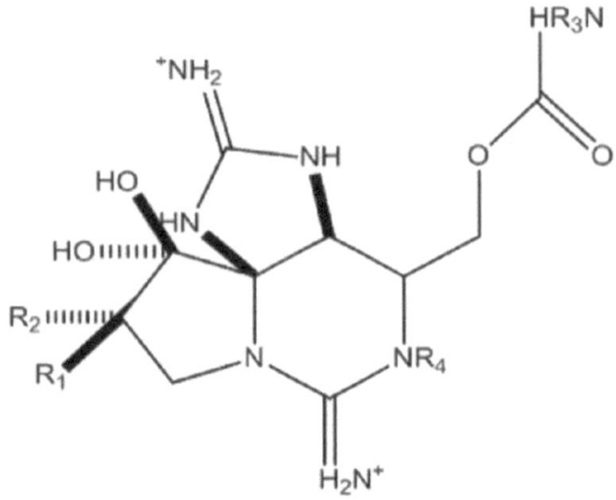


| | R1 | R2 | R3 | R4 |
|---|---|---|---|---|
| STX | H | H | H | H |
| GTX1 | $OSO_3^-$ | H | H | OH |
| GTX2 | $OSO_3^-$ | H | H | H |
| GTX3 | H | $OSO_3^-$ | H | H |
| GTX4 | H | $OSO_3^-$ | H | OH |
| GTX5 | H | H | $SO_3^-$ | H |
| GTX6 | H | H | $SO_3^-$ | OH |
| 11,11-dhSTX | OH | OH | H | H |

**Figure 19.1** Some naturally occurring Paralytic Shellfish Poisons.

PSPs are generated by a variety of marine dinoflagellates, including *Alexandrium tamarense* and *Alexandrium catenella*, and subsequently accumulate in shellfish that eat the dinoflagellates (Asakawa et al., 1995, Hall et al., 1990). Consumption of toxin-contaminated shellfish can result in paralysis and, in rare cases, mortality in humans. PSP is mostly induced by eating molluscan shellfish that have acquired PSP toxins. When filter-feeding shellfish consume poisonous phytoplankton, namely the dinoflagellate *Alexandrium* (formerly called Protogonyaulax or earlier), Gonyaulax, and many species of freshwater cyanobacteria, the PSP group of water-soluble, non-protein toxins is enriched (Anderson et al., 2012, Pearson et al., 2010). Different species and strains of shellfish and dinoflagellates influence the number and duration of the toxin combination maintained in the soft tissues of shellfish, as well as other variables such as ecological parameters (Bricelj et al., 1990) (Álvarez et al., 2019). The Gonyautoxins are the most common toxins found in shellfish along the eastern shore of North America belong to the PSP group (GTX), GTX-2, and GTX-3 (Locke and Thibault, 1994) (Hallegraeff, 1993). Because bivalve molluscs filter-feed on sea algae, PSPs tend to accumulate in their digestive organs primarily, but not entirely (Cembella and Shumway, 1995, Chen and Chou, 2001, Choi et al., 2003). PSPs pose a major concern to the food supply since they are unaffected by commercial disinfection or cooking (Gill et al., 1985, Indrasena and Gill, 1999), especially during seasons of hazardous algal blooms. There are no practical techniques for PSP detoxification of living shellfish (Bricelj and Shumway, 1998).

## 19.2 COMPONENTS

There are at a minimum 18 distinct toxin components in PSP toxins, including Gonyautoxin (GTX), Neosaxitoxin (neoSTX), and Saxitoxin (STX) (Figure 19.1) (Garthwaite, 2000, Garthwaite et al., 2001). A comprehensive ELISA screening method for detecting DSP, ASP, PSP, and NSP toxins (including Yessotoxin) in extracts has been developed. Only suspicious shellfish samples may be identified using this approach, which can then be examined using procedures that have been certified by international regulatory bodies. A Saxitoxin-horseradish peroxidase and a Gonyautoxin 2/3 (GNTX2/3)-specific monoclonal antibody-based direct competitive enzyme immunoassay combination was developed by Kawatsu (Kawatsu et al., 2002). At concentrations below the regulatory limit, dc-GNTX2/3, GNTX2/3, GNTX1/4, C1/2 neoSTX, and STX were detected. Some diatoms produce a non-dinoflagellate toxin Domoic acid (Figure 19.2), which is a marine toxin linked to Amnesic Shellfish Poisoning (ASP).

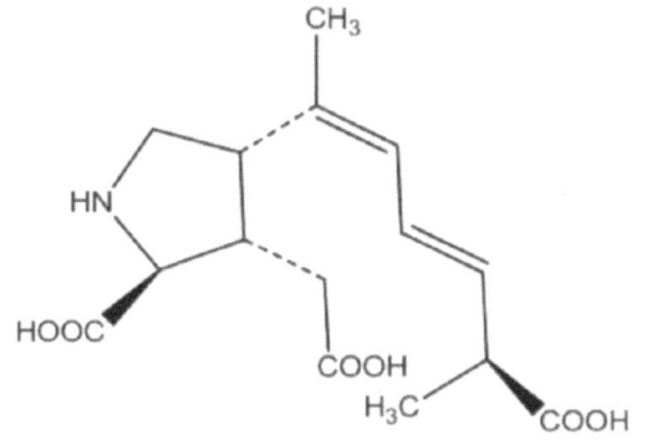


**Figure 19.2** Structure of Domoic acid.

## 19.3 GEOGRAPHICAL DISTRIBUTION, INCIDENCE, AND PREVALENCE

PSP-inducing organisms are becoming more widely distributed, and each year these have been reported in about 2,000 instances throughout the world, with a 15% death rate (Hallegraeff, 1993). Blooms of the poisonous dinoflagellate *Gonyaulax tamerensis* have been causing significant health and economic issues along Canada's, the United States', and the United Kingdom's North Atlantic beaches. It is a common issue that happens often, and in some circumstances persistently, along North America's Pacific and Atlantic coastlines, as well as Japan, South Africa, New Zealand, and Australia, Southeast Asia, as well as Central and South America (Shimizu, 1987) (Tu, 1988). In 1974, yearly global incidences were estimated to number over 1,600 cases per year, with over 300 fatalities (Mills and Passmore, 1988). Although the shell poisoning caused by the flora is similar to that caused by *Gonyaulax catenella* on the west coast by Paralytic Shellfish Poisoning (PSP), PSP's toxic components on the eastern coast are not the same as PSP (Saxitoxin, STX [LoCicero, 1975]), which had recently been determined by x-ray crystallography (Schantz et al., 1975, Bordner et al., 1975) and was later approved. As a very hygroscopic amorphous material, GTX-2, the main component of the novel toxins, was acquired. Although it was hard to accurately determine the toxicity due to its high hygroscopicity, the toxicity achieved was extremely high in both GTX-2 and -3 in very small quantities.

## 19.4 TOXICITY

More than 50 Saxitoxin analogues were reported as of 2010 (Wiese et al., 2010). Procedures that allow for its detection are now available for measuring Saxitoxin and a large number of its seafood congeners. Such a method enables the assessment of individual toxin concentrations in the sample of seafood, allowing for the determination of the sample's overall toxicity, as well as the relative toxicity of the various components and enables an evaluation of a potential menace to human wellbeing.

The "Toxicity Equivalence Factors" (TEFs) in which the toxic nature of Saxitoxin congeners is defined are the relative toxicity of saxitoxin congeners, which is a quotient of the Saxitoxin itself. An MBA for Saxitoxin congeners TEF estimates was once again utilized. In the 1930s, Sommer and Meyer devised a test for Saxitoxin itself on the basis of the connection between the pure Saxitoxin injected into mice and animal mortality (Sommer and Meyer, 1937). The quantity of Saxitoxin in the injected sample, given in "Mouse Units," was calculated using the authors' table of death times. However, this MBA has only been verified for Saxitoxin, it has successfully been developed to congeners of Saxitoxin, and TEFs for such congeners have been calculated using this data (Chain, 2010).

Due to a mice bioassay (MBA), which includes death as an endpoint intraperitoneal inoculation of the extract of seafood, the assessment has been made over the course of many years for the safety of seafood for human use. The Association of Official Analytical Chemists has certified this test as a reference technique for paralytic shellfish toxins. Many people consider such an experiment to be unethical, and its veracity is questioned because it is administered intraperitoneally rather than orally, through which individuals are exposed to PSP poisons.

## 19.5 CHEMISTRY

Toxins isolated from Alexandrium cats cells taken during a blooming episode at Opua Bay, Marlborough Sounds, New Zealand, in 2013 were used in this study. Toxins were gathered and purified using preparation columns before being chemically converted to other analogues if necessary, with beforehand reported procedures (Kochn et al., 1981, Laycock et al., 1994). For reasons of efficiency, hot diluted acetic acid was extracted for toxin extraction from bulk cultures of *A. catenella*. By centrifugation and filtering, cell debris was eliminated. The toxins were recuperated by chromatography of the activated carbon column. Further processing and processing employed filtration gel and chromatography of ion exchange.

To provide concentrated stock solutions, the cleansed toxins were dissolved with 10 mm acetic acid. The dilution of these solutions was precisely synthesized volumetrically, measured with purity, and dosage was determined using fluorescence detection, fluid chromatography, and mass spectrometry (Boundy et al., 2015). All toxins produced were calibrated using certified reference materials (CRMs), with the exception of C-3 and -4 and GTX-6, for which no CRM were available certified by Canadian National Research Council (NRC). Instead, C-3 and -4 were measured using the C-1 and -2 to GTX-2 and -3 conversion as a control for GTX-1 and -4 synthesized by hydrolysis (Costa et al., 2014, Oshima, 1995).

With the non-certified C-3 and -4 reference materials from the NRC and National Research Institute for Fisheries Sciences located in Japan, the concentration given from this technique was in good accord. GTX-6 has directly been measured using non-certified NRC referencing material and validated by acid hydrolysis quantification of neoSTX. As pairs of epimers, there are C-1 and -2, C-3 and -4, and dcGTX-2 and -3. These combinations were balanced to provide a proportion of roughly 3:1 before toxicological analysis (Figure 19.3). This is the same frequency in molluscs infected with these toxins. A technique of enhanced carbs and three types of chromatography were isolated, Bio Gel P-2, Amberslitis CG-50, and Bio-Rex 70, from the poisonous digestive gland of *Patinopecten Yessoensis* (GTX1), one of the main paralytic crustacean toxins. The GTX1 scallop was thus achieved in TLC and also in the electrophoresis of cellulose acetate membrane. The

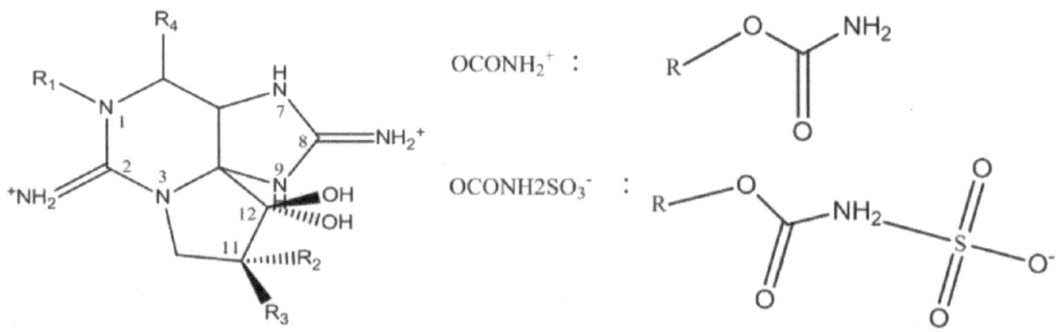


**Figure 19.3** Different groups in the structure of PSPs.

existence of a mole of $-OSO_3^-$ for each mole of poison was indicated by the elemental analysis and IR spectroscopy.

The main components of paralytic shellfish poison (PSP) in the scallop *Patinopecten yessoensis* collected from Ofunato Bay in 1976 through 1979, as well as Funka Bay in 1979 and 1980 (Hwang et al., 1987), were Gonyautoxin-1 (GTX1) and Gonyautoxin-2 (GTX2). The bivalve *Mya arenaria* and the causal plankton *Gonyaulax tamarensis* were also affected by the presence of these two toxins.

1) We previously described a method for isolating GTX2 from poisonous scallops, along with its characteristics.
2) In the case of GTX1, however, the structure and characteristics, including toxicity, have yet to be determined. These circumstances motivated us to conduct the current research. We developed a method for isolating GTX1 from the poisonous scallop digestive gland and analyzing it for structure, specific toxicity, and other characteristics.

### 19.5.1 Isolation of GTX1

Following early tests, it was discovered that the technique indicated in Figure 19.4 was the most effective for separating GTX1 from the poisonous scallop. Two volumes of 80% ethanol, whose pH was adjusted to 2.0 with conc. HCI, were given to the digestive gland (e.g., 3.6 kg; total toxicity, 760,000 MU). The mixture was homogenized for 5 minutes before being centrifuged for 30 minutes at 3,000 rpm. The residue was extracted many times more in the same way. The extracts were mixed, distilled under decreased pressure, and defatted using chloroform in an equal volume. The extract was then batch-treated with activated charcoal (Wako), and the toxin precipitated was collected with 1% acetic acid in 20% ethanol and evaporated to dryness in a vacuum (Figure 19.5). The

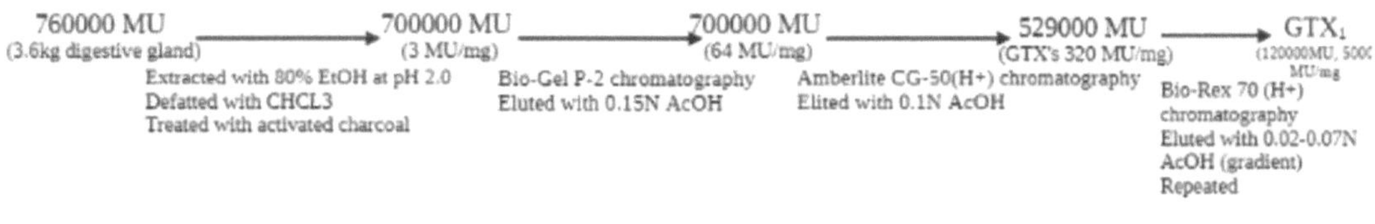


**Figure 19.4** An outline of isolation procedure of $GTX_1$ from toxic scallop digestive gland.

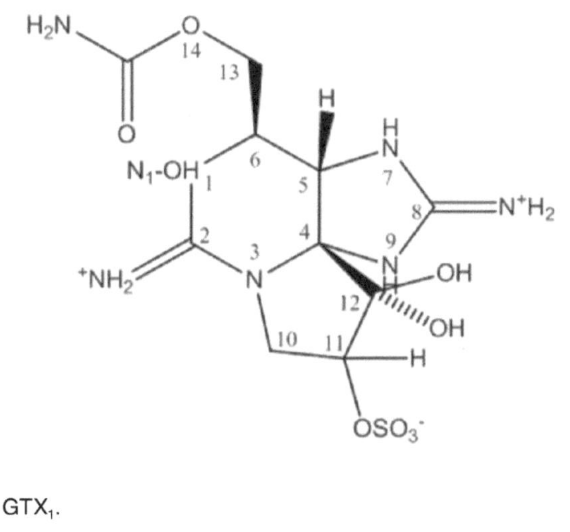


**Figure 19.5** Structure of $GTX_1$.

material was dissolved in a tiny quantity of water and a pH of 5.5 was achieved using 1 N NaOH. A Bio-Gel P-2 (Bio-Rad Lab.) column was used to apply the solution (6.5 x 50 cm). After washing the column with water, 0.15 N acetic acid was used to enhance it. The hazardous portions were mixed and put to an Amberlite CG-50 (H+, Rohm and Haas) column (2.5 x 35 cm). 0.1 N acetic acid was used to elute the TXs at a flow rate of 1.0 ml/min. The GTX fractions were mixed and chromatographed on a Bio-Rex 70 (H+, Bio-Rad Lab.) column (0.8 x 90 cm) using a linear gradient of 0.02 and 0.07 N acetic acid at 1.0 ml/min. Following the aforementioned method, GTX1-rich fractions were mixed, concentrated, and chromatographed several times. Finally, the fractions containing GTX were mixed and freeze-dried.

As previously reported, GTX2 was isolated from the scallop and utilized as a positive control, along with a genuine specimen of Saxitoxin (STX) graciously provided by Dr. Campbell of the United States Public Health Service.

#### *19.5.1.1 Separation by Thin-Layer Chromatography and Electrophoresis*

With a solvent system of pyridine-ethylacetate-acetic acid-water, thin-layer chromatography (TLC) was conducted on silica gel pre-coated plates (5 x 20 cm, Merck) (75: 25: 15: 30). Electrophoresis was performed for 30 minutes at 0.8 mA/cm width on a 5 x 18 or 12 × 12 cm cellulose acetate strip (Chemetron) in 0.08 M Tris-HCI buffer pH 8.7. Following a thin-layer chromatographic or electrophoretic run, the plate or strip was sprayed with 1% hydrogen peroxide, heated at 110°C for 10 minutes, and a fluorescent spot caused by GTX1 or other PSPs was identified under UV illumination at 365 nM.

In a research study, attempts were undertaken to isolate GTX1 from the scallop digestive gland using the SHIMIZU, S technique (Oshima et al., 1977), but no satisfactory results were achieved. After a number of experiments, the authors determined that the technique described above (Figure 19.4) was the most effective (it is essentially the same as the procedure described earlier for GTX2). Separating the hazardous component from the extract using activated charcoal proved successful. GTX group was extracted selectively using chromatography on the Amberlite CG-50 column. It was subsequently treated to Bio-Rex 70 column chromatography, which resulted in partial separation of the various GTX contents. The GTX1-rich fractions were mixed, rechromatographed on a Bio-Rex 70 column many times, and ultimately freeze-dried. When a digestive gland sample corresponding to 760,000 MU was utilized as the starting material, the yield was 24 mg and the overall toxicity was 120,000 MU.

### 19.5.2 Total Synthesis of (+)-Decarbamoylsaxitoxin and (+)-Gonyautoxin 3

The primary agents of PSP, Saxitoxin (STX 1) and its equivalents (Figure 19.1; Table 19.1), are powerful neurotoxins synthesized by dinoflagellates (Llewellyn, 2006, Lim et al., 2007). STXs have high affinity for voltage-gated sodium channels (NaChs), where binding limits sodium ion intake and delays depolarization mechanisms neuronal cell, are thought to be the cause of PSP. STXs have been utilized as a pharmacological tool to explore the characteristics of NaChs due to their distinct pharmacological characteristics. STXs have a quaternary C4 N, N-aminal carbon in their tricyclic bis-guanidine structure. STXs contain two guanidium ions that act as sodium cation mimics. Both the C5 and C6 substituents are orientated in an anti-diaxial configuration, according to X-ray crystallographic study of STXs (Dell'Aversano et al., 2008). Because of their distinctive, highly polar, and heteroatom-rich structural features, STXs have attracted the curiosity of synthetic groups, which have produced four thorough syntheses of members of this alkaloid family. In 1977 and 1992, Kishi and colleagues were the first to describe complete syntheses of ((+)-STX (1) and (-)-Decarbamoylsaxitoxin (dcSTX) (ent-3) (Fleming and Du Bois, 2006).

**Table 19.1 Different Groups in the Structure of PSPs**

| Group | Analogue | R1 | R2 | R3 | R4 |
|---|---|---|---|---|---|
| C toxins | C1 | H | H | $OSO_3^-$ | $OCONHSO_3^-$ |
| | C2 | H | $OSO_3^-$ | H | $OCONHSO_3^-$ |
| | C3 | OH | H | $OSO_3^-$ | $OCONHSO_3^-$ |
| | C4 | OH | $OSO_3^-$ | H | $OCONHSO_3^-$ |
| GTXs | dcGTX-2 | H | H | $OSO_3^-$ | OH |
| | dcGTX-2 | H | $OSO_3^-$ | H | OH |
| | dcGTX-1 | OH | H | $OSO_3^-$ | OH |
| | dcGTX-4 | OH | $OSO_3^-$ | H | OH |
| | GTX-2 | H | H | $OSO_3^-$ | $OCONH_2$ |
| | GTX-3 | H | $OSO_3^-$ | H | $OCONH_2$ |
| | GTX-1 | OH | H | $OSO_3^-$ | $OCONH_2$ |
| | GTX-4 | OH | $OSO_3^-$ | H | $OCONH_2$ |
| | GTX-5 (B1) | H | H | H | $OCONHSO_3^-$ |
| | GTX-6 (B2) | OH | H | H | $OCONHSO_3^-$ |
| STXs | dcSTX | H | H | H | H |
| | dcSTX | H | H | H | OH |
| | dcNEO | OH | H | H | OH |
| | STX | H | H | H | $OCONH_2$ |
| | NEO | OH | H | H | $OCONH_2$ |

Jacobi and colleagues have developed an azomethine imine cycloaddition technique for synthesizing ((+)-STX (1) (Fleming and Du Bois, 2006). Du Bois and colleagues developed Rh-catalyzed amination techniques (Fleming and Du Bois, 2006) for the production of (+)-STX (1) and (+)-Gonyautoxin-3 (GTX 3). The efficacy of this strategy is still debatable. The test relies on injection intraperitoneally, which eliminates the function of the digestive system in either detoxifying or enhancing the toxicological impact of certain chemicals. Furthermore, the MBA is a bioassay rather than a toxicological test, and TEFs generated from this approach have been demonstrated to be unrelated to TEFs derived from median fatal doses calculated by authorized toxicological procedures (Munday et al., 2013). The MBA also assumes that the dose–death time correlations for Saxitoxin congeners are the same as those for Saxitoxin. This has also been demonstrated to be incorrect (Munday et al., 2013). The scientific opinion of the European Food Safety Authority (EFSP), which emphasized the necessity to develop strong TEFs based on the relative oral toxicity of the Saxitoxin congener, noted the insufficiency of the existing TEFs for assessment of risk (Chain, 2010). In the recent review by the Expert Panel of TEFs, the most important parameter was the relative toxicity by oral administration and revisions to currently used TEFs in certain Saxitoxin congeners were recommended by the expert panel (Organization, 2016). The continuation of these studies was carried out using two methods of oral administration and comparing this data with the acute toxicities of Gonyautoxin-5 (GTX-5), Gonyautoxin-6 (GTX-6), Gonyautoxin-2 and -3 decarbamoyl (dcGTX-2 and -3), decarbamoyl Neosaxitoxin (dcNeoSTX), gonyautosulfocarbamoyl-2 and -3 (C-1 and -2) and N-sulfocarbamoyl Gonyautoxin-1 and -4 (C-3 and -4).

Biosynthesized paralytically by prokaryotic and eukaryotic marine organisms, paralytic shellfish toxins bind and block Na+ ion canal isoforms of human voltage at doses from 10–5 m to 10–1. The de-novo synthesis of three poisons, Gonyautoxin-2, Gonyautoxin-3, 11-Dihydroxysaxitoxin, are described. Key measures include a Pictet–Spengler diastereoselective reaction and a sulfonyl guanidine intramolecular amination of N-guanidyl pyrrol. In terms of rat NaV1.4; IC50s from GTX-2, GTX-3 and -11, 11-dhSTX are 22 nM, 15 nM and 2.2 μM correspondingly.

The voltage-gated Na+ ion channels (NaVs), which are the fundamental biochemical components of neuronal cell electrical transmission, are responsible for increased stage of action potentials (MacKenzie et al., 2021). These channel outer pores are obscured by paralytic shellfish (PSP) toxins which impede Na+ ion flow (Kao and Levinson, 1986). These substances provide detailed details of human poisoning in the 18th century. University of California researchers connected the appearance in San Francisco in 1927 of some poisonous moules with the blooms of *Alexandrium catenella*, the dinoflagellate algae species (Trainer et al., 2003, Evans, 1964). Since this groundbreaking paper, more than 50 small molecules which are structurally similar toxins have been identified with a range of dinoflagellate and cyanobacterial origins (Figure 19.1) (Mulcahy et al., 2016, Cusick and Sayler, 2013).

In 1975, the molecular architecture of a single-toxin (+) Saxitoxin was discovered by Clardy and Rapoport (STX) (Schuett and Rapoport, 1962, Bordner et al., 1975). Two deadly substances from Hepatopancreases of infected clams, first designated as epimeric forms of C11-hydroxylated STX, were discovered in a finding by Simizu (Bordner et al., 1975, Shimizu et al., 1976). The diastereomerics were designated after the dinoflagellate from which the two chemicals were obtained, as Gonyautoxin-2 (GTX 2) and Gonyautoxin-3 (GTX-3). Schantz changed the structures of the GTX-2 and GTX-3 to the appropriate 11α and 11β-sulfate esters subsequently (Boyer and Schantz, 1978).

Several PSPs have been discovered, all of which have a tricyclic bis-guanidinium core in common (Mulcahy et al., 2016, Llewellyn, 2006). STX and GTX bind to the receptor extracellularly of voltage-gated Na+ ion channels, establishing contact with the loops that constitute the filter for Na+ ion selectivity, and sterically inhibiting the penetration route of ion, according to electrophysiological and biochemical observations (Thomas-Tran and Du Bois, 2016, Choudhary et al., 2002). Chemical alteration of natural products has proved particularly difficult due to the difficulties of separation and the extremely polar nature of these molecules (Thottumkara et al., 2014, Robillot et al., 2009). The synthesis of three naturally occurring PSPs, 11, 11-dihydroxysaxitoxin (11, 11-dhSTX), Gonyautoxin-2 (GTX 2), Gonyautoxin-3 (GTX-3) and has been made possible by elaboration of this structure (Figure 19.6).

After prolonged treatment with aqueous NaOAc, using reversed phase HPLC; synthetic GTX-3 was purified and could be epimerized to a 3:1 combination of GTX-2/GTX-3. (0.3 M) (Shimizu et al., 1976). RP-HPLC was used to separate the diastereomeric guanidinium toxins, and the IC50 values for each compound against heterologously produced rNaV1.4 (CHO cell) were obtained independently. The IC50 values of GTX-2 and GTX-3 were measured to be 1.7 nM and 2.1 nM, respectively, which accord with published descriptions of their relative potency (Figure 19.7 and 19.8) (Mulcahy et al., 2016). These investigations are the first de novo synthesis of any of the sulfated GTXs that we are aware of. Nagasawa's GTX-3 preparation is perhaps the only reporting of this nature (Iwamoto et al., 2009, Iwamoto et al., 2007).

Saxitoxin, Neosaxitoxin, and the Gonyautoxins are small molecules with bis-guanidinium structures that are distinctive in both structure and shape. They are the main components of PSPs (Mulcahy and Du Bois, 2008). These extremely polar, heteroatom-rich compounds work as corks, preventing ion flow through voltage-gated Na+ channels (NaV) and therefore limiting electrical impulse in cells (Kao and Levinson, 1986). The toxins' complex molecular structure, along with their value as pharmacological tools for ion channel research, has sparked efforts to assemble them from scratch. Saxitoxin (STX) preparations and one decarbamoyloxy form have been reported in three previous investigations (Tanino et al., 1977, Kishi, 1980, Iwamoto et al., 2007). This study outlines the first approach to synthesize synthetic toxins to any of the more than 20 known sulfated toxins, Gonyautoxin-3 (GTX-3) (Figure 19.8) (Louzao et al., 2003, Fleming, 2006).

The 5-member cyclic guanidine in GTX-3 has become the focus of our synthetic investigation following our recent disclosures of an oxidative technique for the production of 2-aminoimidazoline (Kim et al., 2006). A Rh-bound guanidine nitrene, a reactive molecule capable of altering both C-H and -bonds, is considered to be involved in this transition. Amination of a pyrrole nucleus by

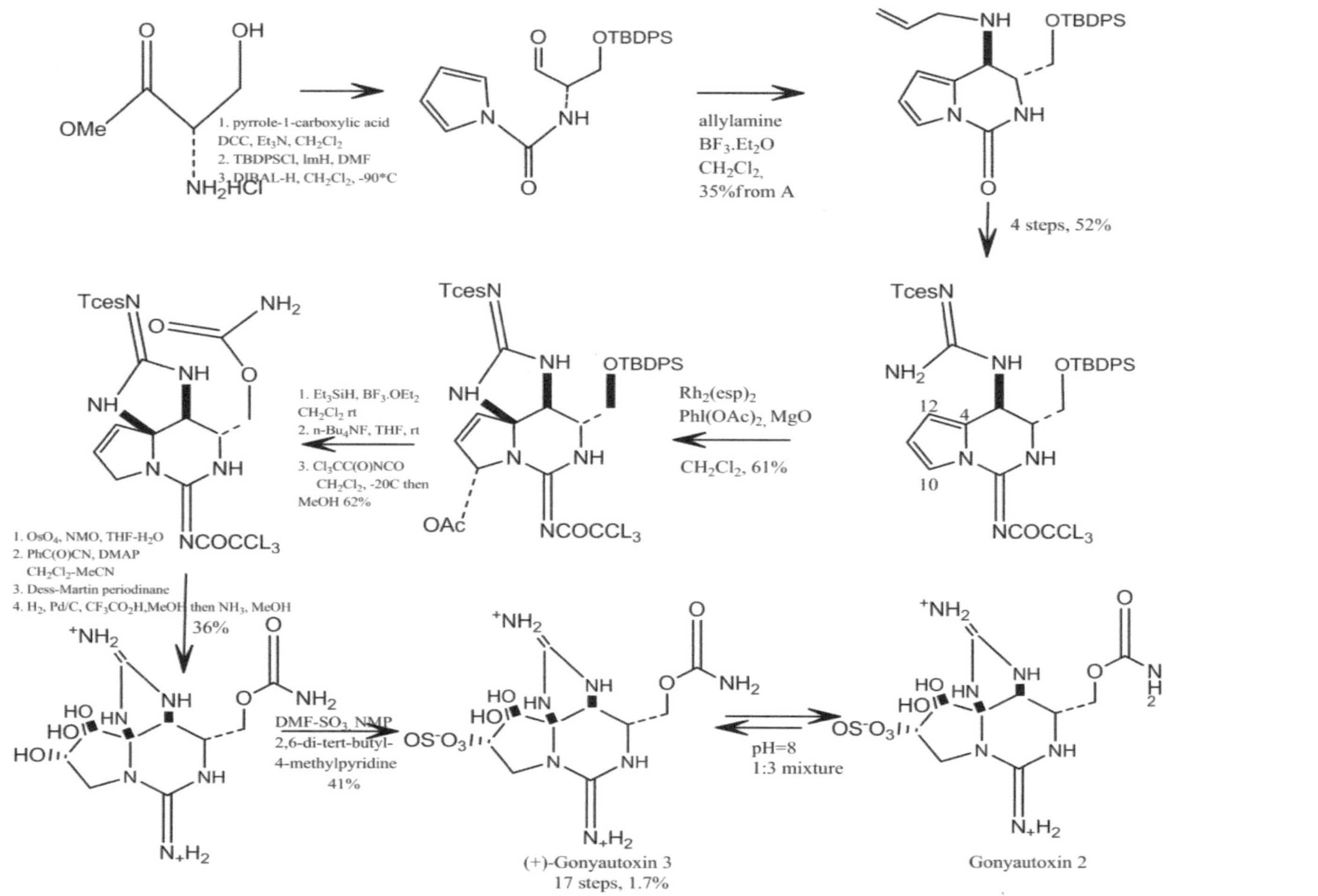


**Figure 19.6** Synthesis of (+)-Gonyautoxin-3. A Rhodium Catalyzed Amination Reaction (D Title E) is the first asymmetric synthesis of Gonyautoxin-3 (GTX-3) to access the tricyclic core of the toxins present in over thirty natural products. It is proposed that the amination process (D → E) be performed by aziridination of C4 and C12, followed by the nucleophilic attack of C10 with by the acetic acid produced in the reaction as a by-product. In aqueous acidic solution, GTX-3 epimerizes to GTX-2. Tces = trichloroethoxysulfonyl (Cl3CCH2OSO2)Rh2(esp)2 = bis[rhodium(α,α,α',α'-tetramethyl-1,3-benzenedipropionic acid).

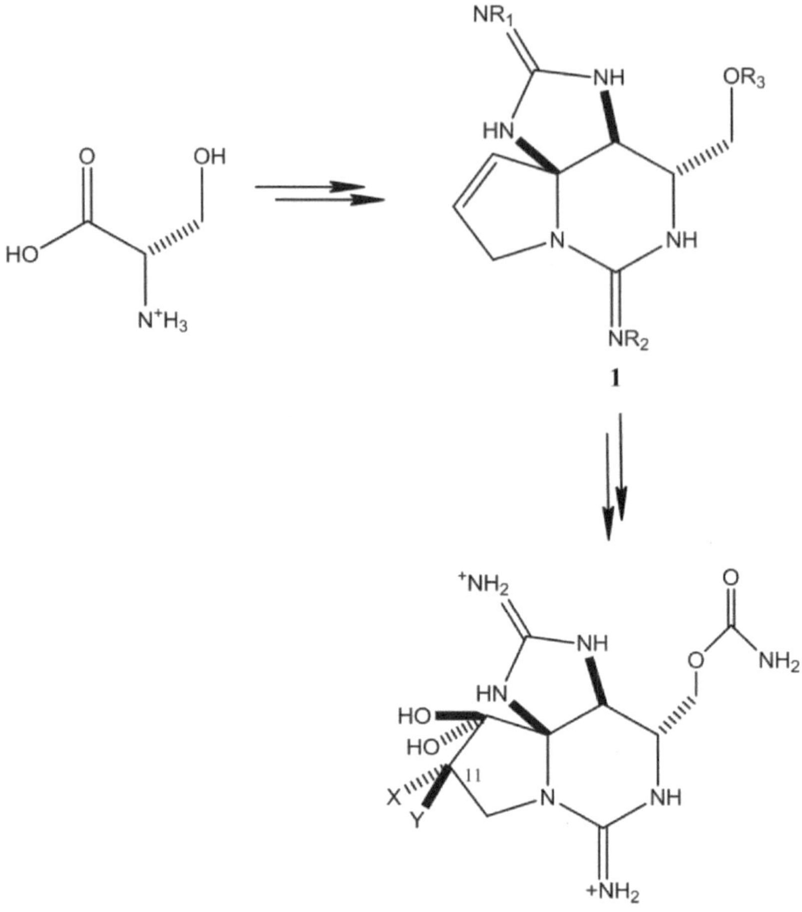


natural and designed
paralytic shellfish toxins

**Figure 19.7** Divergent pathway to C11-derived guanidinium toxins from intermediate-1.

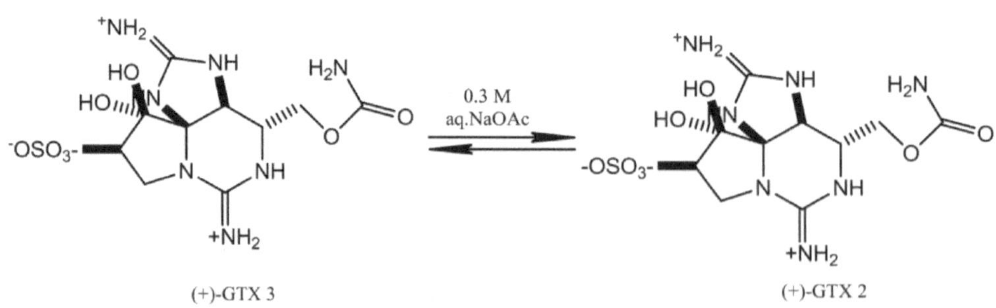


Epimerization of GTX 3 affords GTX 2 as a ~1:3 mixture
at equilibrium. The two diastereomers are separable by RP-HPLC

**Figure 19.8** Divergent pathway to C11-derived guanidinium toxins from intermediate-1.

the guanidine nitrenoid revealed a unique use of this technique for making GTX-3 (Figure 19.8). A stretched aziridine or dipolar molecule might be used in this reaction, with a nucleophile attacking either C10 or C12 to produce the required tricyclic core.

Regardless of the region-chemical hindrance, such a method reduces the GTX problem to a simple bicyclic intermediate 1. A route to bis-guanidine 1 was devised using this method, which involved the intramolecular addition of a pyrrole to an activated imine. Despite the lack of precedence, this Pictet–Spengler reaction may be promptly examined since the required precursor 2 is readily available from serine. The conversion of L-serine methyl ester to aldehyde 5 is the first step in the production of GTX-3 (Scheme 1) (Boger and Patel, 1987). The trans-substituted urea 6 with > 20:1 diastereoselectivity is obtained by condensation of this aldehyde with allylamine followed by treatment with BF3•OEt2, which causes the required ring closure (Collum et al., 1984). If the C5/C6 stereochemistry (GTX numbering) in this product is produced under kinetic control, the observed feeling of induction might be explained by a confirmation that minimizes allylic strain between the substituents on C6 and N7. A four-step process for sequential allyl deprotection and isothiourea formation (cf., step e, 6–7, Tces) (SO3CH2CC13) was developed to efficiently forward 6 to the required amination precursor 7. Of note is the development of a single-step process for sequential allyl deprotection and isothiourea formation (cf., step e, 6-7, Tces) (SO3CH2CC13).

## 19.5.3 GTX5

Gonyautoxin-5 (GTX5) was extracted from poisonous oyster *Crassostrea gigas* specimens obtained in Yamaguchi Prefecture's Senzaki Bay. The digestive glands were extracted with acidic ethanol, then subjected to activated charcoal treatment and three different forms of chromatography: Bio-GelP-2, Amberlite CG-50, and Bio-Rex 70. In both thin-layer chromatography and cellulose acetate membrane electrophoresis, the GTX-5 preparation produced was homogenous. The specific mortality was determined to be 280 MU/mg, which is significantly lower than the Gonyautoxin-1, Gonyautoxin-2, or Saxitoxin values (STX). Mild acid hydrolysis, on the other hand, enhanced the toxicity of the product by five times. STX was discovered in the hydrolyzate along with two unidentified components. The GTX-5 had a PMR spectrum that was quite similar to that of STX and included around one mole of sulphate per mole.

These findings show that GTX-5 has the carbamoyl-N-sulfo-saxitoxin structure. Depending on the species of causative plankton, the species of infected bivalves, and their habitats, the chromatographic or electrophoretic patterns of paralytic shellfish poison (PSP) varies. 1) PSP has a variety of Gonyautoxin (GTX) and Saxitoxin (STX) components, as is widely known. Gonyautoxin-5 (GTX-5) was discovered in 1975 in *Protogonyaulax catenella*, which flowered in Owase Bay, Mie Prefecture, and was given the name JGX1. 2) The same toxin was discovered in the infected bivalves. 2) GTX-5 was later found in the *P. tamarensis* culture, 3) the mussel *Mytilussp*, collected in Oda Bay, Kagawa Prefecture, and 4) the scallop *Placopecten magellanicus*, collected in the Bay of Fun, 5) and the oyster *Crassostrea gigas* from Yamaguchi Prefecture's Senzaki Bay. 6) Based on studies in Japan, GTX-5 appears to be generated exclusively by *P. catenella*, which is found in the western portion of the country. This, along with a few other factors, leads us to believe that GTX-5 is a forerunner to later PSP components. One of the authors 4) preliminarily reported on the isolation and characterization of GTX-5, revealing its low toxicity. The following technique deals with the isolation of GTX-5 from Senzaki Bay's poisonous oysters, as well as the structure and certain characteristics of the toxin.

### *19.5.3.1 Material*

In January 1980, culturally farmed specimens of the oyster *Crassostrea gigas* were collected from Senzaki Bay in Yamaguchi Prefecture. Nearly 10 kg of the edible portion was promptly frozen, transported to the University of Tokyo's Laboratory of Marine Biochemistry, and maintained frozen for about a year at - 20°C. The digestive glands (1.8 kg) were taken from the slightly thawed frozen oysters and utilized to isolate GTX-5.

#### *19.5.3.2 Isolation of GTX-5*

The digestive glands were homogenized in an Ultra-Turrax homogenizer with about the same volume of 1% acetic acid in 80% ethanol and centrifuged at 5,000 rpm for 10 minutes. The aforementioned processes were performed four more times for the residual. The supernatants were mixed together, concentrated under decreased pressure, and chloroform defatted. 1N NaOH was used to adjust the pH of the aqueous solution to 5, and 21 g of water-washed activated charcoal was added to it. The charcoal was produced using 1% acetic acid in 20% ethanol after being repeatedly rinsed with water. The eluted toxic fractions were mixed, concentrated, and adjusted to pH 5.5 before being put on a Bio-Gel P-2 column (535 cm). The column was regularly cleaned with water at a rate of 41 gallons per minute. The hazardous fractions were freeze-dried after the toxin was eluted with 0.15 N acetic acid. The resulting yellow powder was diluted in a little amount of water and applied to an Amberlite CG-50 (H+ form, 1.5, 95 cm) column. The column was cleaned with water first, then with 0.1 and 0.5 N acetic acid, and finally with 0.1 N HCI. The majority of the toxin was eluted using 300 ml water and 330 ml 0.5 N acetic acid. Three toxin peaks were identified: CG-A, -B, and -C. Unbound toxins made up the majority of the peak CG-A eluted with water. The GTX group was represented by peaks CG-B and -C, which were eluted with 0.5 N acetic acid. Peak CG-B (GTX group) was chromatographed many times on a Bio-Rex 70 (H+ form, 0.8 95 cm) column. GTX-5 was eluted using 0.1 N acetic acid in the first run, and a linear gradient of acetic acid from 0 to 0.02 N and 0 to 0.01 N in the second and third runs, respectively.

#### *19.5.3.3 Identification of GTX-5*

The Rf value in thin-layer chromatography (TLC) and the Rm value in electrophoresis were used to identify GTX-5. TLC was performed with two solvent systems [pyridine: ethylacetate: water: acetic acid (75: 25: 30: 15) and tert-butanol: acetic acid: water (2: 1: 1)] on 5 × 20 cm silica gel precoated plates (Merck). Electrophoresis was carried out on 5 × 18 cm cellulose acetate strips (Chemetron) for 30 minutes at 0.8 mA/cm in 0.08 M Tris-HCI buffer pH 8.7. Toxins were discovered under UV light at 365 nM after the plates or strips were sprayed with 1% hydrogen peroxide and heated at 110°C for 10 minutes.

#### *19.5.3.4 Degradation of GTX-5*

4 ml of 0.01 N HC1 was added to the purified GTX-5 (0.5 mg), and the solution was divided into two equal parts. One part was evaporated to dryness under decreased pressure at 40°C, while the other was exposed to four cycles of evaporation-dissolution. After those procedures were completed, each sample was evaluated using TLC, electrophoresis, or a mouse assay. These findings clearly imply that GTX-5 is STX sulphate, with the sulphate positioned at the carbamate amino group next to carbon-13 in Figure 19.9, rather than at carbon-11 as in GTX-18) or GTX-2. During the course of the research, we noticed that the GTX-5 did not produce its epimer.

GTX-5 was isolated in a highly pure form for the first time, and its structure was proposed as stated above. The specific toxicity of 280 MU/mg is significantly lower than STX, GTX-1, and GTX-2, when treated with dilute HCl, however, it dramatically enhanced its toxicity. The hydrolyzate was subjected to electrophoretic and chromatographic tests, which revealed the presence of some STX. This might mean that GTX-5 is a precursor of STX in infected *Protogonyaulax* plankton or bivalves, and that it is transformed to STX in the cell by enzymatic or nonenzymic activity.

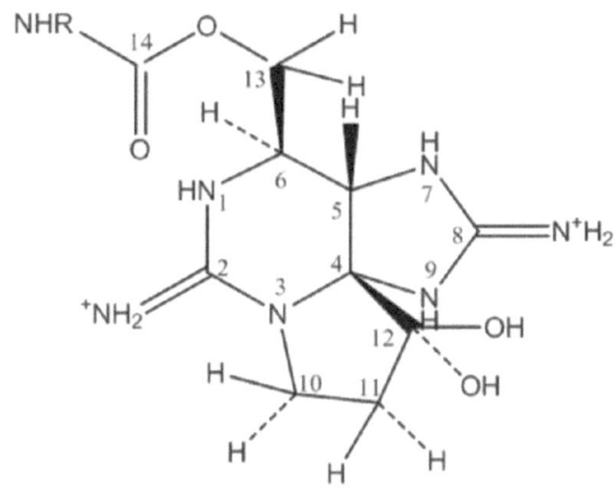

GTX$_5$: R= $SO_3^-$
STX: R=H

**Figure 19.9** Structure of GTX-5.

## 19.6 MECHANISM OF ACTION

Saxitoxin and Gonyautoxin, two toxic metabolites of those algae, block nervous communication, inflammation of the fingertips and lips, giddiness and stunning, confusing talk and breathing immobilization. Saxitoxin is an extremely toxic chemical that has a lethal dosage of 0.2 g for mice since it was isolated directly from the Alaskan butter clam. Before it was revealed to be a dinoflagellate metabolite.

In the membranes of neurons and most electrically excitable cells, voltage-gated sodium channels are responsible for the rising phase of the action potential. PSP toxins are chemicals that have a high affinity for sodium channels that reversibly obstruct neural transmission by adhering to enough sodium ion channels inside an axon, limiting depolarization, and therefore action potential propagation and neuronal transmission (Catterall, 1993) (Catterall, 2000, Lagos and Andrinolo, 2000, Goldin, 2001). The topical administration of tiny amounts of PSP toxins causes flaccid paralysis of striated muscle for dose-dependent durations, according to the molecular mechanism and physiological impact of these toxins. Despite this, the therapeutic usefulness of Saxitoxin and its analogues has been limited due to its systemic toxicity (Lagos and Andrinolo, 2000, Andrinolo et al., 1999, Andrinolo et al., 2002).

The neurological system is influenced by Gonyautoxins, which are neurotoxins. They can bind to site 1 of the α-subunit of voltage-dependent sodium channels in the postsynaptic membrane with a high affinity. After the synapse, these channels are in charge of starting action potentials. PSP toxins attach to synaptic membranes, preventing the production and propagation of action potentials and therefore blocking synaptic activity (Andrinolo et al., 1999).

## 19.7 TOXICOLOGICAL EVALUATION OF SAXITOXIN, NEOSAXITOXIN, GONYAUTOXIN-2, GONYAUTOXIN-2 PLUS -3 AND DECARBAMOYLSAXITOXIN WITH THE MOUSE NEUROBLASTOMA CELL BIOASSAY

Saxitoxin (SIX) and other PSP toxin family members are potent neurotoxins; quantities greater than 80 pg STX equivalents (eq.)/l00 g organic tissue are regarded as seriously hazardous to human beings, and the legal limit for shellfish selling in Canada and many other nations has been established in that proportion. PSP symptoms have been recorded in Canada after ingestion of 40 and 500 ug STX eq. of toxin; one case included a person who ate shellfish and was later found to have toxin levels as low as 200 pg STX eq./100 g tissue (Jellett et al., 1995). Toxin levels in shellfish vary greatly; in some cases, exceptionally high levels have been observed [for example, 150,000 pg STX eq./100 g scallop digestive gland] (Jamieson and Chandler, 1983).

Individual toxin peaks are identified using HPLC based on retention durations. As a result, this technique is very reliant on the availability of particular toxin standards. Serological methods are highly selective for the particular toxin with variable cross reactivity, but not for the full PSP family, with a number of closely related toxins. The bioassay on mice and tissue culture both measure toxicity altogether, but not particular toxin levels. These two bioassays showed statistically similar findings throughout the series of PSP toxin concentrations assessed by both techniques in a test of 50 shellfish extracts and 10 dinoflagellate extracts (Jellett et al., 1992).

In establishing techniques covering the whole 24-member toxin group PSP, including a number of widely reported significant PSPs, the absence of individual pure poisons as standard, antigens and co-chromatography, or to assess the particular toxicity of each individual toxin was a big hurdle (Hall et al., 1990). Until recently, STX was only commercially accessible in limited, costly amounts. The gracious distribution, without of charge, of the limited amounts of STX accessible from Sherwood Hall of the United States Food and Drug Administration has been as the basis for much of the shellfish screening programme and numerous scientific investigations over the years (US FDA; Washington, DC, USA).

The extension of the supply of purified individual PSP members would be highly useful for the development of new approaches, improved procedures, and the availability of confirmed reference material and assistance in the structural and toxicity of compounds. To this end, a significant effort encompassing numerous organizations, including the National Research Council of Canada (NRC), Fisheries and Oceans Canada, National Health and Welfare Canada, and Dalhousie University, was organized to produce sufficient quantities of the toxigenic dinoflagellate *Alexandrium excauatum* to allow separation of STX, Neosaxitoxin (NEO), and a mixture of GTX-2 and -3, as well as Decarbamoylsaxitoxin (dcSTX) preparation in a large amount. (Locke and Thibault, 1994). These concentrated chemicals were mass-produced and chemically described in considerable detail by Laycock et al. (1994) (Locke and Thibault, 1994).

The permanence of each of these toxin formulations was investigated by Laycock et al. in 1994, utilizing particular treatment and storage environments, which are commonly used as cell biological toxicity reference solutions. The absence of pure toxins to be used for co-chromatographic usage as standards, antigens, and the particular toxicity of each toxin has been a major stumbling block in evolving methods to cover the full range of the 24-member PSP toxin group (Hall et al., 1990) maybe perhaps a few of the main PSP toxins most often detected. Until recently, STX was only commercially accessible in limited, costly amounts.

Over the years several Shellfish screening initiatives, as well as other research programmes, have been founded by the liberal distribution of the modest STX available from the Sherwood Hall, the United States Food and Drug Administration (US FDA; Washington, DC, USA). Over the years several Shellfish screening initiatives, as well as other research programmes, have been founded by the liberal distribution of the modest STX available from the Sherwood Hall, the United States Food and Drug Administration (US FDA; Washington, DC, USA). Because GTX-2 in the solution isomerizes over the period to form combinations of all GTX-2 and GTX-2/3. GTX-2/3 determinations (chemical and bioassays) were performed at the same time after the solutions were prepared. The GTX-2/3 combination was available in two molar proportions of GTX-2 to GTX-3: I: 2.5 for Preparation 1 (GTX-2/3-l) and 4: I for Preparation 2 (GTX 2/3-2) (Figure 19.10). Decarbamoylsaxitoxin was refined by ion-exchange column chromatography on a 2.6 x 20-cm column of BioRex 70 (Bio-Rad) H+ eluted with a linear gradient of acetic acid to 3 M after acid hydrolysis of STX in 6 M HCI in a sealed evacuated tube at 100°C for 4 hours. Until otherwise specified,

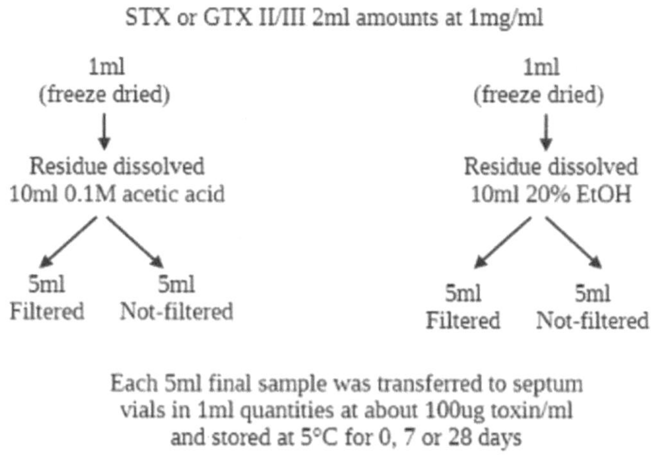


**Figure 19.10** STX and GTX-2/3-1 preparation method for stability assessment over time and filtration effectiveness.

all toxin solutions were freeze-dried or kept in 0.1 M acetic acid at 2°C, unless otherwise stated. STX, 99 pg/ml; NEO, 160 pg/ml; dcSTX, 110 pg/ml; GTX-2, 98.4 pg/ml; GTX-2/3-1, 96.7 pg/ml; GTX-2/3-2, 149.0 pg/ml were the toxin concentrations determined by capillary electrophoresis (CE) against NRC PSP-I. The US FDA provided pure Saxitoxin dihydrochloride (FDA STX).

## 19.8 PHARMACOLOGICAL PROPERTIES

The fact that all of the patients' anal sphincters relaxed immediately after infiltration indicates that this toxin induces paresis in the internal sphincters and lowers anal tone when injected locally. The fact that all patients kept their anorectal inhibitory and anocortical reflexes fully functioning was a significant result in this study, suggesting that the infiltration prevents the muscle from contracting excessively while allowing normal performance. The paralysis of the injected sphincter reduces anal tone while the other muscles remain unaffected. The local dosage reinjections went off without a hitch or adverse effects. The injected sphincter is paralysed, decreasing anal tone, while the other muscles are unaffected. The paretic effect might continue up to a week. During a 14-month follow-up, no adverse effects were found in the patients, indicating that this therapy strategy is safe.

Since 1993, botulinum toxin has been used to treat idiopathic anal fissure, with healing rates ranging from 60% to 96% in two to six months (Jost and Schimrigk, 1993) (Jost, 1997, Jost and Schimrigk, 1994, Gui et al., 1994, Brisinda et al., 1999, Maria et al., 1998). The healing rate is linked to the regimen dosage, which in long-term treatments (6–12 months) with two doses of toxin permitted recovery in 96% of patients. From the fifth day following injection, that this toxin decreased anal tone in all patients Botulinum toxin (Maria et al., 1998, Mínguez et al., 1999), in all of its therapeutic applications, is well documented for starting to produce its relaxing effect in around five days (Jost and Schimrigk, 1993).

For the pace and time of anal fissure healing, the instantaneous sphincter relaxation caused by Gonyautoxin, as well as the volume injection in which the toxin is administered (0.5 ml each side), are critical. Both of these characteristics distinguish these toxins from other pharmaceutical therapies. Because of its tiny thickness, even when the poison is penetrated into the internal anal sphincter, 1-ml volume of toxin should travel to the surrounding area and reach the exterior anal sphincter.

Gonyautoxin periarticular infiltration, on the other hand, has a powerful analgesic impact, with 100% of patients experiencing great pain relief and functional recovery following total knee arthroplasty (TKA). Periarticular injections of Gonyautoxin have been found to be safe and effective in the treatment of TKA discomfort, allowing patients to return to work sooner. All patients were given a conventional painkiller regimen after surgery: 100 mg of intravenous ketoprofen and 1,000 mg of oral acetaminophen every 8 hours for 3 days. The pain score on the Visual Analog Scale (VAS) and range of motion were measured at 12, 36, and 60 hours after surgery. At all times, all of the patients were able to fully extend their knees. During the follow-up period, no side effects or adverse responses to Gonyautoxin were observed. Patients obtained pain alleviation without the usage of opioids because of the Gonyautoxin infiltration, which was both safe and efficient.

## ABBREVIATIONS USED

**CRMs** Certified reference materials
**dcSTX** Decarbamoylsaxitoxin
**EFSP** European Food Safety Authority
**GTX** Gonyautoxin
**MBA** Mice Bioassay
**neoSTX** Neosaxitoxin
**PSP** Paralytic Shellfish Poisoning
**STX** Saxitoxin
**TEFs** Toxicity Equivalence Factors

## ACKNOWLEDGEMENT

The authors would like to express their utmost gratitude and appreciation to Director, CSIR-Indian Institute of Integrative Medicine. We also thank the Department of Science and Technology-India for providing research fellowship to Gifty Sawhney via fellowship code no. DST/INSPIRE Fellowship/2017/IF170212.

## REFERENCES

Álvarez, G., Díaz, P. A., Godoy, M., Araya, M., Ganuza, I., Pino, R., Álvarez, F., Rengel, J., Hernández, C. and Uribe, E. 2019. Paralytic shellfish toxins in surf clams mesodesma donacium during a large bloom of alexandrium catenella dinoflagellates associated to an intense shellfish mass mortality. *Toxins*, 11: 188.

Anderson, D. M., Alpermann, T. J., Cembella, A. D., Collos, Y., Masseret, E. and Montresor, M. 2012. The globally distributed genus alexandrium: multifaceted roles in marine ecosystems and impacts on human health. *Harmful Algae*, 14: 10–35.

Andrinolo, D. O., Iglesias, V., García, C. and Lagos, N. 2002. Toxicokinetics and toxicodynamics of gonyautoxins after an oral toxin dose in cats. *Toxicon*, 40: 699–709.

Andrinolo, D. O., Michea, L. F. and Lagos, N. 1999. Toxic effects, pharmacokinetics and clearance of saxitoxin, a component of paralytic shellfish poison (psp), in cats. *Toxicon*, 37: 447–464.

Asakawa, M., Miyazawa, K., Takayama, H. and Noguchi, T. 1995. Dinoflagellate alexandrium tamarense as the source of paralytic shellfish poison (psp) contained in bivalves from hiroshima bay, hiroshima prefecture, japan. *Toxicon*, 33: 691–697.

Boger, D. L. and Patel, M. 1987. Activation and coupling of pyrrole-1-carboxylic acid in the formation of pyrrole n-carbonyl compounds: pyrrole-1-carboxylic acid anhydride. *The Journal of Organic Chemistry*, 52: 2319–2323.

Bordner, J., Thiessen, W. E., Bates, H. A. and Rapoport, H. 1975. Structure of a crystalline derivative of saxitoxin. Structure of saxitoxin. *Journal of the American Chemical Society*, 97: 6008–6012.

Boundy, M. J., Selwood, A. I., Harwood, D. T., Mcnabb, P. S. and Turner, A. D. 2015. Development of a sensitive and selective liquid chromatography–mass spectrometry method for high throughput analysis of paralytic shellfish toxins using graphitised carbon solid phase extraction. *Journal of Chromatography A*, 1387: 1–12.

Boyer, G., Schantz, E. and Schnoes, H. K. 1978. Journal of the *Chemical Society: Chemical Communications*, 52: 889–890.

Bricelj, V., Lee, J., Cembella, A. and Anderson, D. 1990. Uptake kinetics of paralytic shellfish toxins from the dinoflagellate alexandrium fundyense in the mussel mytilus edulis. *Marine Ecology Progress Series*, 63: 177–188.

Bricelj, V. M. and Shumway, S. E. 1998. Paralytic shellfish toxins in bivalve molluscs: occurrence, transfer kinetics, and biotransformation. *Reviews in Fisheries Science*, 6: 315–383.

Brisinda, G., Maria, G., Bentivoglio, A. R., Cassetta, E., Gui, D. and Albanese, A. 1999. A comparison of injections of botulinum toxin and topical nitroglycerin ointment for the treatment of chronic anal fissure. *New England Journal of Medicine*, 341: 65–69.

Catterall, W. A. 1993. Structure and function of voltage-gated ion channels. *Trends in Neurosciences*, 16: 500–506.

Catterall, W. A. 2000. From ionic currents to molecular mechanisms: the structure and function of voltage-gated sodium channels. *Neuron*, 26: 13–25.

Cembella, A. and Shumway, S. 1995. Anatomical and spatio-temporal variation in psp toxin composition in natural populations of the surfclam spisula solidissima in the gulf of maine. *Harmful Marine Algal Blooms*, Lavoisier Science Publishers, Paris, Lassus, P., Arzul, G., Erard-Le Denn, E., Gentien, P., Marcaillou-Le Baut, C. (Eds.): 421–426.

Chain, E. P. O. C. I. T. F. 2010. Scientific opinion on marine biotoxins in shellfish–cyclic imines (spirolides, gymnodimines, pinnatoxins and pteriatoxins). *Efsa Journal*, 8: 1628.

Chen, C. Y. and Chou, H. N. 2001. Accumulation and depuration of paralytic shellfish poisoning toxins by purple clam hiatula rostrata lighttoot. *Toxicon*, 39: 1029–1034.

Choi, M.-C., Hsieh, D. P. H., Lam, P. K. and Wang, W.-X. 2003. Field depuration and biotransformation of paralytic shellfish toxins in scallop chlamys nobilis and green-lipped mussel perna viridis. *Marine Biology*, 143: 927–934.

Choudhary, G., Shang, L., Li, X. and Dudley Jr, S. C. 2002. Energetic localization of saxitoxin in its channel binding site. *Biophysical Journal*, 83: 912–919.

Collum, D. B., Kahne, D., Gut, S. A., Depue, R. T., Mohamadi, F., Wanat, R. A., Clardy, J. and Van Duyne, G. 1984. Substituent effects on the stereochemistry of substituted cyclohexanone dimethylhydrazone alkylations. An x-ray crystal structure of lithiated cyclohexanone dimethylhydrazone. *Journal of the American Chemical Society*, 106: 4865–4869.

Costa, P. R., Moita, T. and Rodrigues, S. M. 2014. Estimating the contribution of n-sulfocarbamoyl paralytic shellfish toxin analogs gtx6 and c3+ 4 to the toxicity of mussels (mytilus galloprovincialis) over a bloom of gymnodinium catenatum. *Harmful Algae*, 3: 35–40.

Cusick, K. D. and Sayler, G. S. 2013. An overview on the marine neurotoxin, saxitoxin: genetics, molecular targets, methods of detection and ecological functions. *Marine Drugs*, 11: 991–1018.

Dell'aversano, C., Walter, J. A., Burton, I. W., Stirling, D. J., Fattorusso, E. and Quilliam, M. A. 2008. Isolation and structure elucidation of new and unusual saxitoxin analogues from mussels. *Journal of Natural Products*, 71: 1518–1523.

Evans, M. 1964. Paralytic effects of "paralytic shellfish poison" on frog nerve and muscle. *British Journal of Pharmacology and Chemotherapy*, 22: 478–485.

Fleming, J. J. 2006. *Using Small Molecules To Investigate The Voltage-Gated Sodium Channel: A Total Synthesis Of (+)-Saxitoxin*, Stanford University, Stanford, CA.

Fleming, J. J. and Du Bois, J. 2006. A Synthesis Of (+)-Saxitoxin. *Journal Of The American Chemical Society*, 128: 3926–3927.

Garthwaite, I. 2000. Keeping shellfish safe to eat: a brief review of shellfish toxins, and methods for their detection. *Trends In Food Science and Technology*, 11: 235–244.

Garthwaite, I., Ross, K. M., Miles, C. O., Briggs, L. R., Towers, N. R., Borrell, T. and Busby, P. 2001. Integrated enzyme-linked immunosorbent assay screening system for amnesic, neurotoxic, diarrhetic, and paralytic shellfish poisoning toxins found in new zealand. *Journal Of Aoac International*, 84: 1643–1648.

Gill, T., Thompson, J. and Gould, S. 1985. Thermal resistance of paralytic shellfish poison in soft-shell clams. *Journal Of Food Protection*, 48: 659–662.

Goldin, A. L. 2001. Resurgence of sodium channel research. *Annual Review Of Physiology*, 63: 871–894.

Gui, D., Anastasio, G., Maria, G., Cassetta, E., Bentivoglio, A. and Albanese, A. 1994. Botulinum toxin for chronic anal fissure. *The Lancet*, 344: 1127–1128.

Hall, S., Strichartz, G., Moczydlowski, E., Ravindran, A. and Reichardt, P. 1990. The saxitoxins: sources, chemistry, and pharmacology, 418: 29–65.

Hallegraeff, G. M. 1993. A review of harmful algal blooms and their apparent global increase. *Phycologia*, 32: 79–99.

Hwang, D.-F., Noguchi, T., Nagashima, Y., Liao, I.-C. and Hashimoto, K. 1987. Assay of anatomical distribution of toxicity in purple clam ten frozen clam specimens were arbitrarily taken, partially thawed, shucked, and were in-dividually dissected into digestive gland, siphon. *Nippon Suisan Gakkaishi*, 53: 623–626.

Indrasena, W. and Gill, T. 1999. Thermal degradation of paralytic shellfish poisoning toxins in scallop digestive glands. *Food Research International*, 32: 49–57.

Iwamoto, O., Koshino, H., Hashizume, D. and Nagasawa, K. 2007. Total synthesis of (–)-decarbamoyloxysaxitoxin. *Angewandte Chemie*, 119: 8779–8782.

Iwamoto, O., Shinohara, R. and Nagasawa, K. 2009. Total synthesis of (–)-and (+)-decarbamoyloxysaxitoxin and (+)-saxitoxin. *Chemistry–An Asian Journal*, 4: 277–285.

Jamieson, G. and Chandler, R. 1983. Paralytic shellfish poison in sea scallops (placopecten magellanicus) in the west atlantic. *Canadian Journal Of Fisheries And Aquatic Sciences*, 40: 313–318.

Jellett, J., Stewart, J. and Laycock, M. 1995. Toxicological evaluation of saxitoxin, neosaxitoxin, gonyautoxin ii, gonyautoxin ii plus iii and decarbamoylsaxitoxin with the mouse neuroblastoma cell bioassay. *Toxicology In Vitro*, 9: 57–65.

Jellett, J. F., Marks, L. J., Stewart, J. E., Dorey, M. L., Watson-Wright, W. and Lawrence, J. F. 1992. Paralytic shellfish poison (saxitoxin family) bioassays: automated endpoint determination and standardization of the in vitro tissue culture bioassay, and comparison with the standard mouse bioassay. *Toxicon*, 30: 1143–1156.

Jost, W. 1997. One hundred cases of anal fissure treated with botulin toxin. *Diseases Of The Colon and Rectum*, 40: 1029–1032.

Jost, W. H. and Schimrigk, K. 1993. Use of botulinum toxin in anal fissure. *Diseases Of The Colon and Rectum*, 36: 974.

Jost, W. H. and Schimrigk, K. 1994. Therapy of anal fissure using botulin toxin. *Diseases Of The Colon and Rectum*, 37: 1321–1324.

Kao, C. and Levinson, S. 1986. *Tetrodotoxin, Saxitoxin, And The Molecular Biology Of The Sodium Channel*, New York Academy Of Sciences, 479:1–445.

Kawatsu, K., Hamano, Y., Sugiyama, A., Hashizume, K. and Noguchi, T. 2002. Development and application of an enzyme immunoassay based on a monoclonal antibody against gonyautoxin components of paralytic shellfish poisoning toxins. *Journal Of Food Protection*, 65: 1304–1308.

Kim, M., Mulcahy, J. V., Espino, C. G. and Du Bois, J. 2006. Expanding the substrate scope for c– h amination reactions: oxidative cyclization of urea and guanidine derivatives. *Organic Letters*, 8: 1073–1076.

Kishi, Y. 1980. Total Synthesis Of D, 1-Saxitoxin. *Heterocycles*, 14: 1477–1495.

Koehn, F. E., Ghazarossian, V. E., Schantz, E., Schnoes, H. and Strong, F. 1981. Derivatives of saxitoxin. *Bioorganic Chemistry*, 10: 412–428.

Lagos, N. W. and Andrinolo, D. 2000. Paralytic Shellfish Poisoning (Psp): toxicology and kinetics. *Food Science And Technology-New York-Marcel* Dekker, 28(6):203–216.

Laycock, M. V., Thibault, P., Ayer, S. W. and Walter, J. A. 1994. Isolation and purification procedures for the preparation of paralytic shellfish poisoning toxin standards. *Natural Toxins*, 2: 175–183.

Lim, P.-T., Sato, S., Van Thuoc, C., Tu, P. T., Huyen, N. T. M., Takata, Y., Yoshida, M., Kobiyama, A., Koike, K. and Ogata, T. 2007. Toxic alexandrium minutum (dinophyceae) from vietnam with new gonyautoxin analogue. *Harmful Algae*, 6: 321–331.

Llewellyn, L. E. 2006. Saxitoxin, a toxic marine natural product that targets a multitude of receptors. *Natural Product Reports*, 23: 200–222.

Locicero, V. R. 1975. *Proceedings Of The* First *International Conference On Toxic Dinoflagellate Blooms*, The Massachusetts Science And Technology Foundation, 8: 279–293.

Locke, S. and Thibault, P. 1994. Improvement in detection limits for the determination of paralytic shellfish poisoning toxins in shellfish tissues using capillary electrophoresis/electrospray mass spectrometry and discontinuous buffer systems. *Analytical Chemistry*, 66: 3436–3446.

Louzao, M. C., Vieytes, M. R., Cabado, A. G., Vieites Baptista De Sousa, J. M. and Botana, L. M. 2003. A fluorimetric microplate assay for detection and quantitation of toxins causing paralytic shellfish poisoning. *Chemical Research In Toxicology*, 16: 433–438.

Mackenzie, T. M., Abderemane-Ali, F., Garrison, C. E., Minor Jr, D. L. and Du Bois, J. 2021. Differential effects of modified batrachotoxins on voltage-gated sodium channel fast and slow inactivation.

Maria, G., Brisinda, G., Bentivoglio, A. R., Cassetta, E., Gui, D. and Albanese, A. 1998. Botulinum toxin injections in the internal anal sphincter for the treatment of chronic anal fissure: long-term results after two different dosage regimens. *Annals Of Surgery*, 228(5): 664.

Mills, A. and Passmore, R. 1988. Pelagic Paralysis. *The Lancet*, 331: 161–164.

Mínguez, M., Melo, F., Espí, A., García-Granero, E., Mora, F., Lledó, S. and Benages, A. 1999. Therapeutic effects of different doses of botulinum toxin in chronic anal fissure. *Diseases Of The Colon and Rectum*, 42: 1016–1021.

Mulcahy, J. V. and Du Bois, J. 2008. A stereoselective synthesis of (+)-gonyautoxin 3. *Journal Of The American Chemical Society*, 130: 12630–12631.

Mulcahy, J. V., Walker, J. R., Merit, J. E., Whitehead, A. and Du Bois, J. 2016. Synthesis of the paralytic shellfish poisons (+)-gonyautoxin 2,(+)-gonyautoxin 3, and (+)-11, 11-dihydroxysaxitoxin. *Journal Of The American Chemical Society*, 138: 5994–6001.

Munday, R., Thomas, K., Gibbs, R., Murphy, C. and Quilliam, M. A. 2013. Acute toxicities of saxitoxin, neosaxitoxin, decarbamoyl saxitoxin and gonyautoxins 1and4 and 2and3 to mice by various routes of administration. *Toxicon*, 76: 77–83.

Organization, W. H. 2016. Toxicity equivalence factors for marine biotoxins associated with bivalve molluscs, 59: 15–24

Oshima, Y. 1995. Postcolumn derivatization liquid chromatographic method for paralytic shellfish toxins. *Journal Of Aoac International*, 78: 528–532.

Oshima, Y., Buckley, L. J., Alam, M. and Shimizu, Y. 1977. Heterogeneity of paralytic shellfish poisons. Three new toxins from cultured gony aulax tamarensis cells, mya arenaria and saxidomus giganteus. *Comparative Biochemistry And Physiology Part C: Comparative Pharmacology*, 57: 31–34.

Pearson, L., Mihali, T., Moffitt, M., Kellmann, R. and Neilan, B. 2010. On the chemistry, toxicology and genetics of the cyanobacterial toxins, microcystin, nodularin, saxitoxin and cylindrospermopsin. *Marine Drugs*, 8: 1650–1680.

Robillot, C., Kineavy, D., Burnell, J. and Llewellyn, L. E. 2009. Synthesis of bifunctional saxitoxin analogues by biotinylation. *Toxicon*, 53: 460–465.

Schantz, E. J., Ghazarossian, V., Schnoes, H. K., Strong, F., Springer, J., Pezzanite, J. O. and Clardy, J. 1975. Structure of saxitoxin. *Journal Of The American Chemical Society*, 97: 1238–1239.

Schuett, W. and Rapoport, H. 1962. Saxitoxin, the paralytic shellfish poison. Degradation to a pyrrolopyrimidine. *Journal Of The American Chemical Society*, 84: 2266–2267.

Shimizu, Y. 1987. Dinoflagellate toxins. In, the biology qfdinof7agellutes. Edited by fjr taylor. Blackwell scientific press, oxford, uk, 15: 282–289.

Shimizu, Y., Buckley, L. J., Alam, M., Oshima, Y., Fallon, W. E., Kasai, H., Miura, I., Gullo, V. P. and Nakanishi, K. 1976. Structures of gonyautoxin II and III from the east coast toxic dinoflagellate gonyaulax tamarensis. *Journal Of The American Chemical Society*, 98: 5414–5416.

Sommer, H. and Meyer, K. 1937. Paralytic Shell-Fish Poisoning. *Arch. Pathol.*, 24: 560–98.

Tanino, H., Nakata, T., Kaneko, T. and Kishi, Y. 1977. A stereospecific total synthesis of dl-saxitoxin. *Journal Of The American Chemical Society*, 99: 2818–2819.

Thomas-Tran, R. and Du Bois, J. 2016. Mutant cycle analysis with modified saxitoxins reveals specific interactions critical to attaining high-affinity inhibition of Hnavl. 7. *Proceedings Of The National Academy Of Sciences*, 113: 5856–5861.

Thottumkara, A. P., Parsons, W. H. and Du Bois, J. 2014. Saxitoxin. *Angewandte Chemie International Edition*, 53: 5760–5784.

Trainer, V. L., Eberhart, B.-T. L., Wekell, J. C., Adams, N. G., Hanson, L., Cox, F. and Dowell, J. 2003. Paralytic shellfish toxins in puget sound, washington state. *Journal Of Shellfish Research*, 22: 213–223.

Tu, A. T. 1988. *Marine Toxins And Venoms*, M. Dekker, 18: 587.

Wiese, M., D'agostino, P. M., Mihali, T. K., Moffitt, M. C. and Neilan, B. A. 2010. Neurotoxic alkaloids: saxitoxin and its analogs. *Marine Drugs*, 8: 2185–2211.

CHAPTER 20

# Dendrotoxin

**Younis Ahmad Hajam, Javid Ahmad Malik, Raksha Rani, and Rajesh Kumar**

## CONTENTS



## 20.1 INTRODUCTION

*Dendroaspis angusticeps* is a green mamba snake found in the eastern part of the world and its venom has various strange types of pharmacological actions, such as the stimulation of "nerve-muscle preparations" (Barrett and Harvey, 1979). A prejunctional action is only due to these pharmacological actions that makes the easy release of acetylcholine. It was reported that this action is due to the presence of a protein present in the venom named as dendrotoxin (Harvey and Karlsson, 1980). It was shown that dendrotoxin has the potential to block the potassium current of neural cells (Dolly et al., 1984; Benoit and Dubois, 1986; Halliwell et al., 1986; Penner et al., 1986; Stansfeld et al., 1986; Anderson and Harvey, 1988).

In the venom of *Dendroaspis angusticeps*, the protein dendrotoxin or α-dendrotoxin is the "major facilitatory protein (MFS)". Fifty-nine amino acids are present in a single chain in the protein dendrotoxin which are cross-linked with each other by three disulfide bonds (Joubert and Taljaard, 1980). The other similar types such as β, γ, and δ-dendrotoxins were also found in the

DOI: 10.1201/9781003178446-20

venom of *Dendroaspis angusticeps* (Benishin et al., 1988). Other types of dendrotoxin are also present in the green mamba snake found in the western parts of the world, i.e., "*Dendroaspis viridis*" (Mehraban et al., 1986), and the black mamba snake, "*Dendroaspis polylepis*" (Strydom, 1973; Harvey and Karlsson, 1982). These dendrotoxins show similarity to "Kunitz serine protease inhibitors", for instance "aprotinin", or "bovine pancreatic trypsin inhibitor", though it was reported that dendrotoxins weakly inhibit trypsin and also that inhibitors of protein do not block potassium channels (Harvey and Karlsson, 1982; Marshall and Harvey, 1992). It was reported in the previous studies that to isolate the proteins of potassium channels dendrotoxins are used as probes (Black et al., 1988, Rehm and Lazdunski, 1988; Parcej and Dolly, 1989). It was also reported that dendrotoxins are also used to show the potassium channel distribution in the nervous system (Bidard et al., 1989; Pelchen-Matthews and Dolly, 1989; Awan and Dolly, 1991). The increase in the interest in pharmacological roles of dendrotoxins is due to the increase in the study of different potassium channels and their physiological roles. In the body cells there is presence of $K^+$ channels and these $K^+$ channels contribute to the regulation of membrane potential. There are various types of potassium channels which are expressed by individual cells. These cells play an important role for $K^+$ ions and can open and close a pore for $K^+$ ions and give response to voltage change, change in intracellular $Ca^+$ level or specific ligands; though the most common channels are voltage-gated channels. The modulation of $K^+$ channel function can be done by the use of a number of toxins isolated from bee venom, scorpion venom, sea anemones, and snake venom (Dreyer, 1990). A single molecule of dendrotoxin binds in the external vestibule of the potassium channel and obstructs the entry of $K^+$ ion from outside, and therefore plays a role in the blocking of ionic current. The $\alpha_4\beta_4$ complexes are there which act as "voltage-gated potassium channels" (MacKinnon, 1991) in which integral membrane proteins are α-subunits which contain the ion pore, and at the same time the peripheral proteins are β-subunits, which modulate the inactivation rate of the "α-subunits" (Rettig et al., 1994; Morales et al., 1995; Majumder et al., 1995). Each α-subunit consists of six membranes which are spanning alpha helices, S1–S6, and a P region which is a pore-forming domain, present between S5 and S6, in this region the toxins come and bind. The three residues of amino acid, such as A352, E353, and Y379 are dangerous for the binding of toxins as revealed by site-directed mutagenesis of the pore-forming sequence (Hurst et al., 1991). There is a dramatic reduction that occurred 26 times due to the E353 mutation into serine in the affinity of the binding of toxin. There was also a reduction in the affinity when there is a substitution of A352 or Y379, but there the substitution is less effective than E353. The higher effect of these residues was shown when the substitution occurs cooperatively. Dendrotoxin (DTXs) is one of the classes of $K^+$ channel blockers. This class I potassium channel blockers, i.e., dendrotoxins, have been studied in extensive detail, and these are small proteins isolated from the *Dendroaspis angusticeps* venom (Dufton, 1985; Harvey and Anderson, 1985). The voltage-gated $K^+$ channels like "Shaker-related Kv1 channels" are blocked by these dendrotoxins. About 60 types of residues of amino acids are present in the dendrotoxins and these also have three intramolecular disulfide bonds. The structure of dendrotoxins is very similar to the "Kunitz-type protease inhibitors" like "bovine pancreatic trypsin inhibitor (BPTI)", although dendrotoxins do not have any activity to inhibit proteases. The different types of dendrotoxins are isolated from the venom of various snakes coming under various species of *Dendroaspis genus*, such as from the "*Dendroaspis polylepis polylepis*" (black mamba snake) venom, three types of dendrotoxins-I, (Strydom, 1973), from the *Dendroaspis angusticeps* (green mamba snake venom), the α-dendrotoxin (Dolly, 1992) and from the venom of "*Dendroaspis polylepis*", dendrotoxin-K (Strydom, 1973). It has been reported that dendrotoxins are of special interest because these have the potential to target voltage-sensitive $K^+$ channel of neurons with high affinities. The $K^+$ channel Kv1.1, $K^+$ channel Kv1.2, and $K^+$ channel Kv1.6 are blocked by dendrotoxin-I expressed in the oocytes of *Xenopus* and the dendrotoxin-K only block Kv1.1 potassium channel, although both of these dendrotoxins have 60% sequence homology (Robertson et al., 1996). Moreover, $K^+$ channels Kv1.1 and Kv1.2 are blocked by α-DTX with almost equal affinity (IC50; 20 nM), but for other cloned channels it has more than 10 times less affinity (Grissmer et al., 1994) (Figure 20.1).

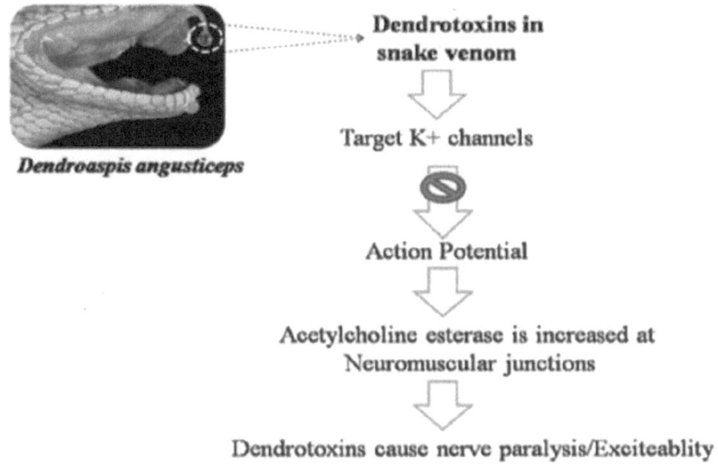


**Figure 20.1** Shows the effect of dendrotoxins on neuro-muscular nerve impulse conduction.

## 20.2 CHEMISTRY

The "major facilitatory protein" found in the venom of *Dendroaspis angusticeps* is "dendrotoxin or α-dendrotoxin". The dendrotoxin has 59 amino acids present in a single chain and cross-linked to each other by 3 disulfide bonds (Joubert and Taljaard, 1980). Dendrotoxins are similar in position and structure to "Kunitz serine proteinase inhibitors", for instance, "aprotinin or bovine pancreatic trypsin inhibitor (BPTI)", and other related proteins have also been isolated from the venom of "*Dendroaspis polylepis polylepis*" (Strydom, 1973, 1976), though their activity was not known. Two toxins named "toxin I" and "toxin K" or Dp1 or DpK were found to be active when the effect of homologues were tested on the release of acetylcholine (Harvey and Karlsson, 1982). In the venom of black mamba snakes, numerous type of "homologues of α-dendrotoxin" named β-, γ-, and δ-dendrotoxins were found (Benishin et al., 1988), and in the venom of *Dendroaspis viridis*, which is a western green mamba snake, other types of DTXs were found (Mehraban et al., 1986), additionally to those were found in *Dendroaspis polylepis*. On the other hand, the fourth species of mamba snake, which is *Dendroaspis jamesoni*, has no dendrotoxins present. Furthermore, several homologues of dendrotoxins, which are "kalicludines", were also isolated from *Anemonia sulcafa* (Schweitz et al., 1995). It should be noted that of the green mamba snakes that are coming from Kenya, dendrotoxin has only been isolated from them, no dendrotoxins were present in the venom of green mamba snakes that originated from South Africa (Lauridsen et al., 2016), and for this reason they may represent a subspecies. There are 59 types of amino acid residues present in dendrotoxin, which includes 6 half Cys. Earlier, the molecules of same size and composition are isolated from the *Dendroaspis polylepis* venom, i.e., black mamba snake (Laustsen et al., 2015), and *Dendroaspis viridis*, i.e., western green mamba snake. The sequences of several components that are separated from black mamba venom were determined and these highly resemble each other. These also resemble "Kunitz-type protease inhibitors", like "bovine pancreatic trypsin inhibitor (BPTI)". The 3D structure of "bovine pancreatic trypsin inhibitor" has been well established by "X-ray crystallography" (Huber et al., 1972; Deisenhofer and Steigemann, 1975), "nuclear magnetic resonance" (Wagner and Wüthrich, 1982), and by "neutron diffraction" (Wlodawer et al., 1984). Though the crystal structure of "dendrotoxin" is unknown and the solution structure of homologues components isolated from the "*Dendroaspis polylepis*" venom has been homologues to "bovine pancreatic trypsin inhibitors" (Arseniev et al., 1982; Keller et al., 1983; Pardi et al., 1983). The "circular dichroism spectra" of protein that are similar to dendrotoxin from the mamba snake venom are homologues to that of bovine pancreatic trypsin inhibitors (Hollecker et al., 1982; Hollecker and Creighton, 1983). A model which is based on the structure of bovine pancreatic trypsin inhibitors and E and K components of black mamba snake is helpful to determine the 3D structure of dendrotoxins. Between Cystein-7 and Cystein-57, Cystein-16 and Cystein-40, and Cystein-32 and Cystein-53 there is a formation of the 3 disulphide bonds of bovine pancreatic trypsin inhibitors which finally form a highly stable and globular structure. The formed structure is pear-shaped; its length is about 3 nM with a diameter about 2 nM. There are two loops (residues 11–23 and 34–35) on the top of the molecule which is linked by 16–40 disulphide bonds. There is a twisted anti-parallel double stranded β-sheet structure formed by the main sequence and at the "N-terminus" and towards the "C-terminus" there is a presence of two short α-helical regions (Huber et al., 1972). Moreover, though dendrotoxin and its similar structure will most likely be conventional to the general shape described for bovine pancreatic trypsin inhibitors, there may be some major differences. Certainly, it was revealed from the circular dichroism spectra for bovine pancreatic trypsin inhibitors, "toxin I" and "toxin K" that the conformation of "toxin K" is similar with the conformation of bovine pancreatic trypsin inhibitors in some regions than toxin I. The refolding studies showed that the toxins stability, particularly in the region around 16–40 disulphide bond, is different from that of bovine pancreatic trypsin inhibitors.

## 20.3 STRUCTURE–ACTIVITY RELATIONSHIPS

Though the protease inhibitors and the toxins that block the $K^+$ channel have a similar 3D structure and their amino acid sequences are highly similar, there must be some distinctness to explain for their various pharmacological activities (Harvey et al., 1984a; Swaminathan et al., 1996; Dufton and Harvey, 1998; Nishio et al., 1999). Chemical changes of local toxins and genetic engineering are involved in experiments to produce mutated toxins have been performed so as to identify the residues which are highly significant for the dendrotoxins' interaction with the protein of $K^+$ channel. The understanding about the interaction of toxins with their target cells is in a growing phase, and the dissimilarity among the toxins like "α-dendrotoxin" and "toxin K", which shows different preferences for various $K^+$ channel subtypes. Danse et al. (1994) reported that there is a synthetic gene which encodes for α-dendrotoxin and it has been expressed in *Escherichia coli*, and some mutants were prepared of it, and it was found that when Lysine triplet 28 ± 30 mutated into Ala± Ala ± Gly then the binding affinity is reduced to synaptosomal membranes up to four-fold. It indicated that the residues of lysine are present in the dendrotoxins but these are not present in protease inhibitors, so these are not the main determinant of the binding affinity of the toxins for the channels of $K^+$. Comparable results were also obtained with toxin I when there was acetylation of individual residues of lysine. It was observed that when there is a modification of Lysine 28 and Lysine 30, the binding affinity of toxin I was unaffected; on the other hand, a clear loss in the activity was observed when there is acetylation of Lysine 5 in α-dendrotoxin, and signifying that in the binding of potassium channel this residue was involved (Harvey et al., 1997). A study has been carried out on an extensive mutational analysis in which there was mutation of 26 residues out of 59 into Ala (Gasparini et al., 1998). The profound loss of affinity for the binding of $K^+$ channel was produced when there were substitutions of Lysine 5 and Leucine 9. The residues which affect the affinity for binding were present in the N-terminal region of the toxin. It seems that a common structural characteristic of toxin to block voltage-gated potassium channel is the association of a main lysine residue in association with residues of leucine, tyrosine, and phenyl alanine (Dauplais et al., 1997; Gasparini et al., 1998; Alessandri-Haber et al., 1999). Smith et al. (1995) has been successfully cloned and expressed Toxin K and Smith et al. (1997) and Wang et al. (1999a) studied some mutant toxins. There were implications in the interactions of two regions of the toxin with binding sites for radiolabelled toxin K and α-dendrotoxin: "the β-turn region (residues 24 ± 28 in toxin K)" and "Lys

3 (the equivalent to α-dendrotoxin's Lys 5)" (Smith et al., 1997). These regions are important for the capability of toxin K to block K+ current in oocytes which expresses $K^+$ channels Kv1.1 (Wang et al. 1999a). Moreover, by using site-directed mutagenesis, δ-dendrotoxin has been studied widely (Imredy and MacKinnon, 2000). For the study of interaction of toxins with cloned channels Kv1.1, there is a presence of seven residues such as Lysine 3, Tyrosine 4, Lysine 6, Leucine 7, Proline 8, Arginine 10, and Lysine 26, which were found to be very important. The residue which is important for α-dendrotoxin, δ-dendrotoxin, and toxin K is present near the N-terminus is lysine residue and the various additional residues present in each toxin are important for the binding of the individual toxin to their sites of target. It might have been predicted that Leu-7 residue of δ-dendrotoxin is critical following the work on "α-dendrotoxin", "sea anemone toxins", and "scorpion toxins" (Dauplais et al., 1997; Gasparini et al., 1998; Alessandri-Haber et al., 1999). Furthermore, in δ-dendrotoxin, mutation of Leucine 7 to alanine has no effect on its blocking potency. The obvious needs for a neighbouring hydrophobic residue which is present near the Lys is fulfilled in δ-dendrotoxin by Tyrosine 4, it leads to a sixteen-fold affinity loss when there is mutation of Lys to alanine (Imredy and MacKinnon, 2000). Though there is a general assumption that the lysine residues present at the side chain in the dendrotoxins plugs into the pore of the ion channel, in the Kv1.1 potassium channel there is mutation of residues of amino acids near the pore led. It was concluded that binding of δ-dendrotoxin takes place near the pore entrance but does not act as a physical plug (Imredy and MacKinnon, 2000).

## 20.4 MECHANISM OF ACTION

### 20.4.1 Binding to $K^+$ Channel Proteins

It was reported by most of the authors that the radiolabelled dendrotoxins shows strong and particular binding to membranes from the brain (Black et al., 1988; Rehm and Lazdunski, 1988; Parcej and Dolly, 1989; Sorensen and Blaustein, 1989; Harvey and Anderson (1985) and Dolly and Parcej (1996). It has been assumed that, for the attachment of the toxin, the binding site is on a potassium channel protein. It was reported that the sequence of "rat cortex potassium channel" also called as "rKv1.2" is mostly similar with the N-terminal sequence of an isolated protein that binds to the dendrotoxin. From the cDNA that was cloned from the brain of a rat, the rKv1.2 is deduced (Scott et al., 1990; Newitt et al., 1991). There was a reconstruction of proteins in lipid bilayers which were isolated on a dendrotoxin affinity column and it was found that dendrotoxin blocks the activity of potassium channels (Rehm et al., 1989b). Moreover, antibodies which are against parts of the mouse brain sequence cross-react with the protein which binds the dendrotoxins (Rehm et al., 1989a). Various studies were conducted on the proteins which bind to α-dendrotoxin isolated from "bovine cerebral cortex" showed that there was association of α-subunits of four large transmembrane proteins with four small accessory beta subunits (Parcej et al., 1992). Various evidences were provided that there were hetero-oligomeric combinations of various α-subunits within the Kv1 family present in the brain when precipitation experiments with subtype-specific antibodies were done (Scott et al., 1994; Wang et al., 1999b). On the synaptic membranes from the brains of rats there is attachment of radiolabelled toxin K to channels; the solublization and immunoprecipitation of these radiolabelled toxins K was done with antibodies specific for "Kv1.1 subunits", "Kv1.2 subunits", or "Kv1.4 subunits". Affinity chromatography was used for the further separation by using toxin I columns. Evidences was obtained for native channels that contains combinations like "1:1 ‡ 1:2, 1:1 ‡ 1:4, 1:1 ‡ 1:2 ‡ 1:6, and possibly 1:1 ‡ 1:4 ‡ 1:6" (Wang et al., 1999b). It was indicated by such types of findings that the behaviour of native channels will not reflect directly by the cloned channels that were expressed in mammalian cells. Though, to produce the suitable oligomere in vitro, like "β-accessory subunits" attempts are starting to have success (Shamotienko et al., 1999). Another

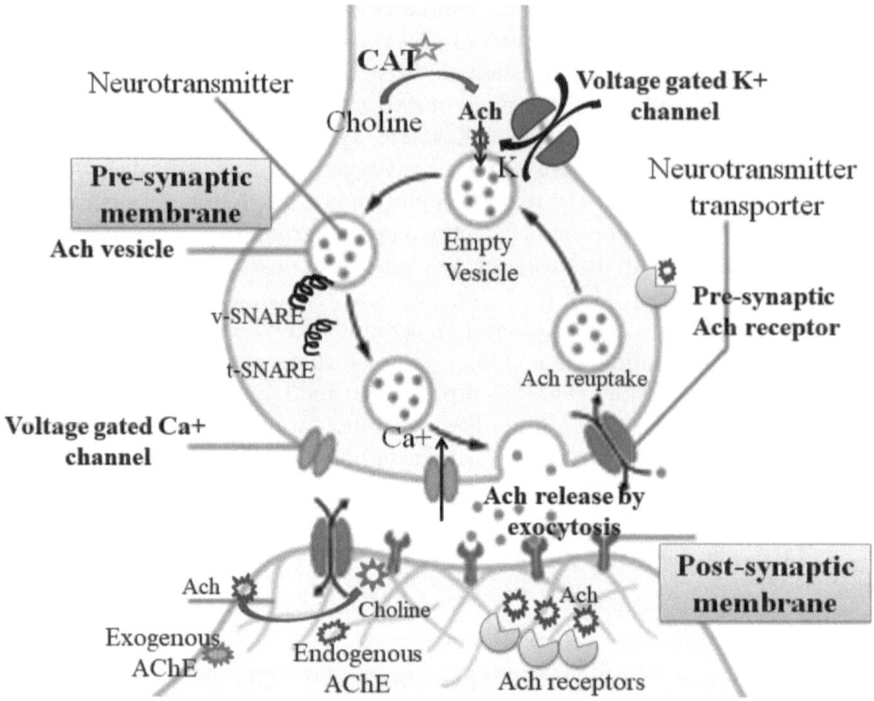


**Figure 20.2** Action mechanism of dendrotoxins on synaptic transmission.

time, for suitable native behaviour dendrotoxins have been used as tools to probe the expressed channels (Figure 20.2).

### 20.4.2 Distribution of Dendrotoxin Binding Sites

The dendrotoxins labelled as 123I have been used to study the distribution of binding sites present in the brain (Bidard et al., 1989; Pelchen-Matthews and Dolly, 1989; Awan and Dolly, 1991). Synapses rich areas have mainly dense labelling. The areas in the rat's brain are "thalamus, midbrain, and neocortex", which have high densities of binding sites for "125I-toxin I" (Bidard et al., 1989). δ-dendrotoxin does not block all the binding sites of "125I- α-dendrotoxin" (Awan and Dolly, 1991). It indicates that various subtypes of dendrotoxins binding sites are there maybe various hetero-oligomeric combinations of subunits of potassium channels. In the brain sections of monkey and human beings binding sites for "125I-α-dendrotoxin" have also been found (Kumar and Gupta, 2018). It has been found in cynomolgus monkey and human that 125I-α-dendrotoxin binds in hippocampal tissue (Schechter et al., 1994). It has also been found in the post-mortem samples from the patients having "multiple sclerosis" that dendrotoxin binds higher than normal in demyelinated plaques (Keighley et al., 1994). It has been found in the samples of hippocampus from the patient who had died from "Alzheimer's disease" there were loss of "α-dendrotoxin" and "toxin K" binding sites, with aging-related changes have also seen in the brains of rats (Cochran and Pratt, 1997).

### 20.4.3 Block of Cloned Potassium Channels

For most of the potassium channels the circular DNA has been cloned or expressed in the oocytes of *Xenopus* or in cell lines of mammals and the channels derived from neurons are sensitive to dendrotoxin. The potassium currents like "Kv1.1, Kv1.2, Kv1.6, Kd < 20 nM" that are derived from circular DNA have been blocked by α-dendrotoxin and toxin I while other potassium channels like "Kv1.3, Kv1.4, Kv1.5, Kv3.1, Kv3.4, Kv4.1" shows insensitiveness to high concentration of dendrotoxin (Grissmer et al., 1994). The relation of some differences may be depends upon the expression system such as oocyte or mammalian cells, but other may be related to the microRNA amount which is injected into the oocyte (Guillemare et al., 1992). It was reported that toxin K is active on "homo-oligomeric Kv1.1 channels" as compared to other channels when studies on cloned channels was done (Robertson et al., 1996). On the Kv1.1 channels that were expressed in Chinese hamster cells of ovary the IC50 for toxin K was 30 pM, while for greatly similar δ-dendrotoxin, it was 1.8 (Owen et al., 1997). Though, it has been reported that for δ-dendrotoxin, an IC50 of 30 pM on potassium channel Kv1.1 was expressed in the oocytes of *Xenopus* (Hopkins, 1998). The sequences of clones that are sensitive or insensitive to dendrotoxin can be compared or mutated for the localization of binding site for dendrotoxin on the polypeptide of potassium channel (Hurst et al., 1991; Tytgat et al., 1995). The reduction in the binding affinity of dendrotoxins is due to the mutation between the H5 loop of Kv1.1 channels and S5 or S6 transmembrane domains. Alanine 352, glutamic acid 353, and Tyrosine 379 are the amino acids which are involved. All the four subunits that are present in the potassium channel are work together with a dendrotoxin, and to block the potassium channels only a single toxin molecule is enough. The effect of toxin I and delta dendrotoxin was examined in a study on various heteromultimers of "Kv1.1, Kv1.2, and Kv1.4 subunits" that has been co-expressed in pairs in the oocytes of *Xenopus*. It has been found that for toxin block of potassium current, there is requirement of a single toxin sensitive site, and suggests that different subtypes of dendrotoxin may interact differently with various multimers of potassium channels (Hopkins, 1998). The majority of the electrophysiological results with dendrotoxins and cloned channels are related with the toxins which causes a pore block of potassium channel. Though, it has been shown that channel kinetics that are present in oocytes expression system are slow down by toxin I (Robertson et al., 1996), and it has also been shown in some studies that all the current even in the "homo-oligomeric toxin-sensitive channel" cells do not eliminate by the toxins.

Though, it is generally observed that dendrotoxins are specific for "voltage-activated potassium channels" of the Shaker family, an inward rectifier K+ channel is blocked by "δ-dendrotoxin", renal outer medullary potassium1 channel (ROMK1), with low affinity (Kd of 150 nM) after that with this it ultimately blocks potassium channel Kv1.1 or Kv1.6 (Imredy et al., 1998). Moreover, on the inward rectifying potassium channel1, δ-dendrotoxin showed no effect and it has been concluded by comparing sequences and renal outer medullary potassium1 channel protein that binding of the toxin occurring at the mouth of pore of renal outer medullary potassium1 channel, although current is not completely blocked through the pore. Interestingly, "α-dendrotoxin" showed no effect on the renal outer medullary potassium1 channel.

## 20.5 TOXICOLOGY

### 20.5.1 Block of Potassium Currents in Central Nervous System

It has been reported that a part of the transient potassium current in "hippocampal pyramidal cells" inhibited by dendrotoxin (Dolly et al., 1984; Halliwell et al., 1986). It has been indicated in various studies conducted in tissue culture of hippocampal cells that fast-activating current is blocked by dendrotoxin, as compared to slowly inactivating D current or fast-transient A current (Storm, 1988; Wu and Barish, 1992). The experiments that have been conducted on neurons separated from sensorimotor cortex of rats showed similar results (Foehring and Surmeier, 1993). By measuring the "$^{86}Rb^+$ efflux" from synaptosomes and by extracellular recording from the nerve terminals in "rat olfactory cortex" a comparable effect has been confirmed (Benishin et al., 1988; McGivern et al.,

1993). The channels that are sensitive or insensitive to dendrotoxins might be expressed by the same neuron in the various locations of cell. The potassium current is present in cerebellar basket cells in their terminals and dendrotoxins block the potassium current while the $K^+$ current which have concentration up to 200 nM in the cell bodies, dendrotoxin did not block them (Southan and Robertson, 1998a, Southan and Robertson, 2000). In addition to this, various kinds of dendrotoxins can have different selectivities. Based on the effects on various "$^{86}Rb^+$ efflux from synaptosome" components, dendrotoxins may be divided into two subgroups (Benishin et al., 1988): the inactivating portion of $^{86}$Rb+ efflux is blocked by α- and δ-dendrotoxin, and on the other hand, the non-inactivating flux is selectively blocked by the β- and γ-dendrotoxin.

### 20.5.2 Motor Neurons

The period of action potential is extended by the dendrotoxin I in "nodes of Ranvier" of the sciatic nerves of frogs, by blocking a portion of potassium current (Weller et al., 1985), and there is a particular block of f1 components of potassium current (Benoit and Dubois, 1986; Brau et al., 1990). The single channel recording experiments on "*Xenopus* axons" have been performed to confirm the above statement (Jonas et al., 1989), where the single channel conductance was 23 pS which was blocked by dendrotoxin. The same kind of fast-activating potassium currents are present in "the paranomodal regions" of "rat motor nerve fibres" and these regions are highly sensitive to dendrotoxin "(IC50 of 8 nM)" (Corrette et al., 1991). After the "demyelination of motor nerves" there can be detection of "high affinity binding sites" for $^{123}$I-dendrotoxin. From the sciatic nerves of rats, the recording of single channel $K^+$ currents can also be done after demyelination (Safronov et al., 1993). In the axons of rats (Safronov et al., 1993) and *Xenopus* (Koh and Vogel, 1996), three types of channels were differentiated. The first one is "fast inactivating F channels" which have 30 pS conductance in isotonic solution of $K^+$, the second one is "intermediate I channels" with 18 pS conductance, and the third one is "slowly inactivating S channels" with 10 pS conductance. Intermediate I current with IC50 of 2.8 nM in rats and 6.8 nM in *Xenopus* is selectively blocked by α-dendrotoxin. This reduces the active channel numbers and showed no effect on "single channel amplitude". Furthermore, it was reported that two types of channels having 25 and 45 pS conductance are present in human axons (Reid et al., 1999) and these two channels were blocked by "1 mM α-dendrotoxin".

### 20.5.3 Peripheral Nervous System

It has been demonstrated that dendrotoxins have the potential to block potassium channels of peripheral sensory neurons. In the "dorsal root ganglion cells" of guinea pigs, a portion of "non-inactivating potassium current" is blocked by α-dendrotoxin (Penner et al., 1986). The repetitive firing action potential in the nodose ganglion of rats and guinea pigs is produced in the presence of dendrotoxin by some cells (Stansfeld et al., 1986, 1987, 1991; McAlexander and Undem, 2000). In a tissue culture of dorsal root ganglion neurons of rat, dendrotoxin blocks the $K^+$ channels, it was confirmed in an experiment by patch clamping in which the "single channel conductance" of sensitive channels was 5–10 pS (Stansfeld and Feltz, 1988). Potassium currents are also present in the adult rat's sensory neurons, and these are very sensitive to dendrotoxins "(IC50 about 20 nM)" (Akins and McCleskey, 1993). In the sensory neuron of rats, the slowly inactivating and non-inactivating voltage-dependent potassium currents are blocked by many homologues of dendrotoxins, such as α-dendrotoxin, β-dendrotoxin, γ-dendrotoxin, and δ-dendrotoxin, toxins I and K, but with dissimilar potencies (Hall et al., 1994). The "non-inactivating voltage-dependent potassium currents" are selectively blocked by δ-dendrotoxin (IC50 of 0.24 nM), and "slowly inactivating voltage-dependent $K^+$ currents (IC50 of 1 nM)" are more actively blocked α-dendrotoxin as compared to δ-dendrotoxin. In the Schwann cells of rabbit, a "voltage-dependent $K^+$ current" is also blocked by α-dendrotoxin "(Kd of 1.3 nM)" (Baker et al., 1993), though the channel is not completely obstructed by the toxin, but induces openings with a smaller conductance (Baker and Ritchie, 1996). A delayed rectifier potassium current in "C6 astrocytoma cells" shows sensitivity towards dendrotoxin I (IC50 of 9 nM) and this current are there because of the potassium channels Kv1.1 (Wang et al., 1992). However, the expression of Kv1.1 appears to be quite low in "oligodendrocyte progenitor cells" from the brains of mice, where "Kv1.4, Kv1.5, and Kv1.6" are more abundant (Schmidt et al., 1999). $K^+$ currents in the microglia are not blocked by dendrotoxins (Eder et al., 1995).

### 20.5.4 Autonomic Nervous System (ANS)

In the sympathetic and parasympathetic branches of ANS the release of transmitter is facilitated by dendrotoxin and toxin I (Harvey et al., 1984b; Anderson, 1985). The origin of facilitatory action is found to be presynaptic at "the neuromuscular junction" in "the somatic nervous system". It seems that the beginning of the action is faster in ANS; this is the major difference and washing helps to reverse the effect of the toxin more readily. In the preparation of vas deferens of mice, a detailed study was done about the action of toxin I (Anderson, 1985). The responses of dendrotoxin elevates to indirect stimulation. The postsynaptic sensitivity towards norepinephrine, acetylcholine, or KCl does not change at the time of utmost increase of the responses to nerve stimulation, it indicates a presynaptic action site. No evidence is available regarding the action of toxin I that it interferes with any of hypothesized presynaptic feedback mechanisms and the transmitter release in the preparation might be influenced by it. For instance, various effects have been excluded on "presynaptic α- and β-adrenoceptors", "prostanoid receptors", "muscarinic and nicotinic cholinoceptors", and "angiotensin receptors". It has been concluded that toxin has direct action on the nerve and affects transmitter release (Anderson, 1985). "Voltage-sensitive calcium channels" is not affected by this action, though the $K^+$-evoked release of norepinephrine from the "clonal rat phaeochromocytoma cell line PC12" is not affected by dendrotoxin. In the cell bodies of sympathetic ganglion of rats, $K^+$ current is blocked by dendrotoxin (Halliwell et al., 1986). Neuronal excitability might be enhanced by such actions and *in vivo* these actions facilitate the release of transmitter. However, few ganglia are present in the isolated "vas deferens preparation". Therefore, the action of toxin I is directly on the axons of nerves or terminals of nerves. On the chick oesophagus preparation, a related conclusion regarding the action of dendrotoxin was found, which receives "parasympathetic innervation" (Anderson, 1985). However, from action on "ganglionic cell bodies" there may be large contribution from this kind of action in this preparation. However, current of $K^+$ in sympathetic nerve cell bodies may be blocked by dendrotoxins. The $K^+$ current in "adrenal chromaffin cells" in a tissue culture is not blocked by dendrotoxins.

### 20.5.5 Sensory Nervous System

There are two reports in which action of dendrotoxin on peripheral sensory neurons has been described (Penner et al., 1986; Stansfeld et al., 1986). A portion of "non-inactivating $K^+$ currents" is selectively and irreversibly blocked by dendrotoxin in the cells of dorsal root ganglion from guinea pigs (Penner et al., 1986). The recurring firing of action potential is produced by the A-cells when stimulated in the presence of "3–10 nM dendrotoxin" or "1–30 μm 4-aminopyridine" in rat's nodose ganglia (Stansfeld et al., 1986). The presence of slowly inactivating K+ currents was revealed in studies that were done by using voltage clamps; however, dendrotoxin blocked them reversibly. Contrary to the findings at "the neuromuscular junction" (Harvey, 1982), the actions of dendrotoxin and 4-aminopyridine were equally selective on the "nodose ganglion cells" (Stansfeld et al., 1986).

### 20.5.6 Effects on the Release of Transmitter: Skeletal-Muscle Neuromuscular Junctions

Following the observation of the effect of venom of green mamba snake (Barrett and Harvey, 1979), the first effect of dendrotoxins which has to be characterized is the facilitation of release of transmitter (Harvey and Karlsson, 1980; Harvey and Karlsson, 1982; Anderson, 1985; Anderson and Harvey, 1988). Afterward, obstruction of some potassium channels of neurons explained the facilitatory effects of the dendrotoxins. At the neuromuscular junctions of mice and frogs, the effect of dendrotoxins elevates the "quantal content" and induces the "single nerve action potential" to cause small bursts of recurring activity. It has been suggested that a fast-activating potassium channel should be blocked by dendrotoxin which helps to control the nerve-terminal excitability (Anderson and Harvey, 1988; Harvey and Anderson, 1987). It has been reported that dendrotoxins also block the "slow kinetics potassium channels" in the presence of tetraethyl ammonium, which is a "non-selective $K^+$ channel blocker" (Dreyer and Penner, 1987). In the motor and sensory neurons of the spinal cord of frogs, recurring firing of action potential is induced by α-dendrotoxin (Poulter et al., 1989), and in the hippocampal slices long-term potentiation is induced by toxin I (Kondo et al., 1992). Epileptiform activity is induced by dendrotoxin when injected into the central nervous system (Velluti et al., 1987; Silveira et al., 1988; Bidard et al., 1989; Coleman et al., 1992), and damage to the neurons can occur if injected in high doses (Bagetta et al., 1997). Riluzole blocks the convulsant action of dendrotoxin I to some extent (Stutzmann et al., 1991), but it is not blocked by lemakalim, which is a potassium channel opener (Heurteaux and Lazdunski, 1991). In mice the activity of α-dendrotoxins are blocked by "phenyoin" and "vaproate", but not by "diazepam" (Coleman et al., 1992). The dendrotoxins labelled as 125I have been used to study the distribution of binding sites in the brain (Bidard et al., 1989; Pelchen-Matthews and Dolly, 1989; Awan and Dolly, 1991). The areas that are synapses-rich mostly have dense labelling. The thalamus, midbrain, and the neocortex are the high-density binding sites in the brains of rats to which "$^{125}$I-tøxin I" binds (Bidard et al., 1989). δ-dendrotoxin does not block all the $^{125}$I-α-dendrotoxin binding (Awan and Dolly, 1991), and indicates the various subtypes of binding sites for dendrotoxins, probably showing various "hetero-oligomeric combinations" of potassium channel subunits. It has also been found that, for "$^{125}$I-α-dendrotoxin", binding sites are present in the brain sections of monkeys (Barrezueta et al., 1994).

Responses of isolated "skeletal-muscle preparations" are elevated by dendrotoxins to indirect stimulation. The small change in the responses to "cholinoceptor stimulation" happens when there is utmost increase of responses to the stimulation of nerves (Harvey and Karlsson, 1980). The effects of dendrotoxins slowly develop, and it seems that they are irreversible with the nerve-muscle preparation of chick biventer cervicis. By increasing the toxin concentration, the time taken to reach utmost twitch growth is reduced, but this utmost increase in the height of twitch clearly does not depend on the concentration which is above the threshold value (Harvey and Karlsson, 1980; Harvey and Karlsson, 1982). It was reported that dendrotoxins only take 15 minutes to bind with their receptors; however, they do not show any effect for many hours (Harvey et al., 1984b). Ca ions, nerve-terminal activity, or the release of transmitter are not required for dendrotoxins for their binding (Harvey et al., 1984b). Thus, there is a free access of binding site to the toxin and during the nerve-terminal depolarization by action potentials or during the influx of Ca and release of acetylcholine, the binding sites are not exposed to the toxin.

## 20.6 ISOLATION OF TARGET SITES

The labelling of dendrotoxin can be done with a "$^{125}$1 to a specific activity of 300–400 Ci/mmol" without losing its biological activity. From the brains of rats and chicks, particular binding of "$^{125}$I-dendrotoxin" to membranes can be detected (Harvey and Karlsson, 1984; Harvey et al., 1984b;

Dolly et al., 1984, 1986; Black and Dolly, 1986). The binding of dendrotoxin, particularly to a class of non-interacting sites present in the synaptic membranes or synaptosomes from the brains of rats. It has been found that o.3 nM was the $K_D$ and 1.2–1.7 pmol/mg protein was the binding site concentration. Black et al. (1986) found comparable results from cerebral cortex and membranes of hippocampus area.

There is no requirement of the presence of Ca ions for the dendrotoxin binding to the brain of rats. The proteins appear to be the binding site for the toxins, because when membranes were pre-treated with typsin or chymotrypsin, or treatment was given by heat or acid, the binding of toxin was greatly decreased (Black et al., 1986). The presence of apamin, or presence of K+ channel blocker like "tetraethyl ammonium", "4 aminopyridine", etc., at high concentration or Ca channel blocker like "nifedipine", or "nimodipine", etc., does not decrease the binding of toxin. There was partial reduction in the binding of toxin when there was presence of "the presynaptic phospholipase $A_2$ toxins", "taipoxin and flbungarotoxin" and by phospholipase $A_2$, which is present in the venom of honey bee. A similar type of "phospholipase $A_2$" was found in the cobra venom (*Naja melanoleuca*) which shows zero inhibition, but it depends upon the activity of enzyme it means that there may be an interaction between the protein binding sites of dendrotoxins and particular types of lipids present in the surrounding membrane. The related experiments regarding the binding of dendrotoxin have been carried out by the use of membranes which are isolated from the cerebral cortices of chick (Black and Dolly, 1986). Again, a site for protein binding was specified by the loss in the particular binding of dendrotoxin after treatment with proteases, heat, or acid. There was no effect on the binding of dendrotoxin when treatment was given with "neuraminidase" and "deoxyribonuclease". Contrary to the finding with the brain of rat, dendrotoxin binding was not standardized. A "Scatchard plot" was nonlinear but two components which are having different affinities for dendrotoxin can resolve it. The sites with higher affinity "$K_D$ = 0.5 nM" was there in low amount "Bmax = 90 fmol/mg", protein as compared to the sites having lower affinity "$K_D$ approx 15 nM; Bmax = 400 fmol/mg protein". It has been indicated in the kinetic experiments that dendrotoxin association is similar in these two sites but dissociation of dendrotoxin from the sites having low affinity is faster. It has been found in the competition studies that no discrimination is done by facilitatory toxins between the two sites, and inactive homologs such as B-protein, bovine pancreatic trypsin inhibitor, crotoxin, apamin, and trypsin inhibitor of soyabean do not affect that binding. Nevertheless, the binding of dendrotoxin is particularly blocked by the β-bungarotoxin to the high affinity site. The protein found in the rat's brain bound to dendrotoxin has a molecular weight of 65,000 daltons. However, this is certainly part of a large molecule. Experiments regarding radiation inactivation of binding site in situ showed that it has a molecular weight of "240,000 to 265,000 daltons" (Dolly et al., 1984), and it has been estimated that the centrifugation of the solubilized binding site has 390,000 to 450,000 daltons (Dolly et al., 1986). In the brain of chicks, the labelling of two components was done by $^{125}$I-dendrotoxin, the main components have molecular weight of 75,000 daltons and minor component has molecular weight of 68,000 daltons. β-bungarotoxin partially reduces the labelling to both the proteins and both of these seem like a part of binding sites having high and low affinity. Black and Dolly (1986) separated two forms of dendrotoxin binding sites of rats. From the "cerebral cortical membranes" of rats, binding sites for dendrotoxins have been isolated successfully without any loss of dendrotoxin binding affinity (Mehraban et al., 1985).

## 20.7 CONCLUSION

It has been concluded that dendrotoxins are the homologous group of proteins, but these are dissimilar from "Kunitz-type protease inhibitors" (Dufton, 1985). The pharmacological action that they show is to facilitate the release of neurotransmitters. There are many studies available which show that dendrotoxins block some types of $K^+$ channels in the neuromuscular junction. There are various important characteristics about dendrotoxins which have yet to be clarified. The nature of the binding site is one of them.

## REFERENCES

Akins, P.T. and McCleskey, E.W. 1993. Characterization of potassium currents in adult rat sensory neurons and modulation by opioids and cyclic AMP. *Neuroscience*, 56(3), 759–769.

Alessandri-Haber, N., Lecoq, A., Gasparini, S., Grangier-Macmath, G., Jacquet, G., Harvey, A.L., de Medeiros, C., Rowan, E.G., Gola, M., Ménez, A. and Crest, M. 1999. Mapping the functional anatomy of BgK on Kvl. 1, Kvl. 2, and Kvl. 3: Clues to design analogs with enhanced selectivity. *Journal of Biological Chemistry*, 274(50), 35653–35661.

Anderson, A.J. 1985. The effects of protease inhibitor homologues from mamba snake venoms on autonomic neurotransmission. Toxicon, 23(6), 947–954.

Anderson, A.J. and Harvey, A.L. 1988. Effects of the potassium channel blocking dendrotoxins on acetylcholine release and motor nerve terminal activity. *British Journal of Pharmacology*, 93(1), 215–221.

Arseniev, A.S., Wider, G., Joubert, F.J. and Wüthrich, K. 1982. Assignment of the 1H nuclear magnetic resonance spectrum of the trypsin inhibitor E from Dendroaspis polylepis polylepis: Two-dimensional nuclear magnetic resonance at 500 MHz. *Journal of Molecular Biology*, 159(2), 323–351.

Awan, K.A. and Dolly, J.O. 1991. K+ channel sub-types in rat brain: Characteristic locations revealed using β-bungarotoxin, α-and δ-dendrotoxins. *Neuroscience*, 40(1), 29–39.

Bagetta, G., Palma, E., Piccirilli, S., Nisticò, G. and Dolly, J.O. 1997. Seizures and hippocampal damage produced by dendrotoxin-K in rats is prevented by the 21-aminosteroid U-74389G. *Experimental Neurology*, 147(1), 204–210.

Baker, M., Howe, J.R. and Ritchie, J.M. 1993. Two types of 4-aminopyridine-sensitive potassium current in rabbit Schwann cells. *The Journal of Physiology*, 464(1), 321–342.

Baker, M.D. and Ritchie, J.M. 1996. Characteristics of type I and type II K+ channels in rabbit cultured Schwann cells. *The Journal of physiology*, 490(1), 79–95.

Barrett, J.C. and Harvey, A.L. 1979. Effects of the venom of the green mamba, Dendroaspis angusticeps on skeletal muscle and neuromuscular transmission. *British Journal of Pharmacology*, 67(2), 199.

Barrezueta, N.X., Pearsall, D.M., Schechter, L.E. and Rhodes, K.J. 1994. Distribution of (125I) α-dendrotoxin binding sites in the amygdala, hippocampus, and entorhinal cortex of the monkey. *Society for Neuroscience*, 20, 1524.

Benishin, C.G., Sorensen, R.G., Brown, W.E., Krueger, B.K. and Blaustein, M.P. 1988. Four polypeptide components of green mamba venom selectively block certain potassium channels in rat brain synaptosomes. *Molecular Pharmacology*, 34(2), 152–159.

Benoit, E. and Dubois, J.M. 1986. Toxin I from the snake Dendroaspis polylepis polylepis: A highly specific blocker of one type of potassium channel in myelinated nerve fiber. *Brain Research*, 377(2), 374–377.

Bidard, J.N., Mourre, C., Gandolfo, G., Schweitz, H., Widmann, C., Gottesmann, C. and Lazdunski, M. 1989. Analogies and differences in the mode of action and properties of binding sites (localization and mutual interactions) of two K+ channel toxins, MCD peptide and dendrotoxin I. *Brain Research*, 495(1), 45–57.

Black, A.R., Breeze, A.L., Othman, I.B. and Dolly, J.O. 1986. Involvement of neuronal acceptors for dendrotoxin in its convulsive action in rat brain. *Biochemical Journal*, 237(2), 397–404.

Black, A.R. and Dolly, J.O. 1986. Two acceptor sub-types for dendrotoxin in chick synaptic membranes distinguishable by β-bungarotoxin. *European Journal of Biochemistry*, 156(3), 609–617.

Black, A.R., Donegan, C.M., Denny, B.J. and Dolly, J.O. 1988. Solubilization and physical characterization of acceptors for dendrotoxin and beta-bungarotoxin from synaptic membranes of rat brain. *Biochemistry*, 27(18), 6814–6820.

Bräu, M., Dreyer, F., Jonas, P., Repp, H. and Vogel, W. 1990. A K+ channel in Xenopus nerve fibres selectively blocked by bee and snake toxins: Binding and voltage-clamp experiments. *The Journal of Physiology*, 420(1), 365–385.

Cochran, S.M. and Pratt, J.A. 1997. Regionally selective changes in the displacement of a-dendrotoxin binding by charybdotoxin and toxin K in the rat septohippocampal pathway during aging. *British Journal of Pharmacology-Proceedings Supplement*, 256P.

Coleman, M.H., Yamaguchi, S.I. and Rogawski, M.A. 1992. Protection against dendrotoxin-induced clonic seizures in mice by anticonvulsant drugs. *Brain Research*, 575(1), 138–142.

Corrette, B.J., Repp, H., Dreyer, F. and Schwarz, J.R. 1991. Two types of fast K+ channels in rat myelinated nerve fibres and their sensitivity to dendrotoxin. *Pflügers Archiv*, 418(4), 408–416.

Danse, J.M., Rowan, E.G., Gasparini, S., Ducancel, F., Vatanpour, H., Young, L.C., Poorheidari, G., Lajeunesse, E., Drevet, P., Ménez, R. and Pinkasfeld, S. 1994. On the site by which α-dendrotoxin binds to voltage-dependent potassium channels: Site-directed mutagenesis reveals that the lysine triplet 28–30 is not essential for binding. *Federation of European Biochemical Societies Letters*, 356(2–3), 153–158.

Dauplais, M., Lecoq, A., Song, J., Cotton, J., Jamin, N., Gilquin, B., Roumestand, C., Vita, C., de Medeiros, C.C., Rowan, E.G. and Harvey, A.L. 1997. On the convergent evolution of animal toxins: Conservation of a diad of functional residues in potassium channel-blocking toxins with unrelated structures. *Journal of Biological Chemistry*, 272(7), 4302–4309.

Deisenhofer, J. and Steigemann, W. 1975. Crystallographic refinement of the structure of bovine pancreatic trypsin inhibitor at l. 5 Å resolution. *Acta Crystallographica Section B: Structural Crystallography and Crystal Chemistry*, 31(1), 238–250.

Dolly, J.O., Black, J.D., Black, A.R., Pelchen-Matthews, A. and Halliwell, J.V. 1986. Novel roles of neural acceptors for inhibitory and facilitatory toxins. *Natural Toxins: Animal, Plant and Microbial*, 1, 237–264.

Dolly, J.O., Halliwell, J.V., Black, J.D., Williams, R.S., Pelchen-Matthews, A., Breeze, A.L., Mehraban, F., Othman, I.B. and Black, A.R. 1984. Botulinum neurotoxin and dendrotoxin as probes for studies on transmitter release. *Journal de Physiologie*, 79(4), 280–303.

Dolly, J.O. and Parcej, D.N. 1996. Molecular properties of voltage-gated K+ channels. *Journal of Bioenergetics and Biomembranes*, 28(3), 231–253.

Dreyer, F. 1990. Peptide toxins and potassium channels. *Special Issue on Ionic Channels II*, 115, 93–136.

Dreyer, F. and Penner, R. 1987. The actions of presynaptic snake toxins on membrane currents of mouse motor nerve terminals. *The Journal of Physiology*, 386(1), 455–463.

Dufton, M.J. 1985. Proteinase inhibitors and dendrotoxins: Sequence classification, structural prediction and structure/activity. *European Journal of Biochemistry*, 153(3), 647–654.

Dufton, M.J. and Harvey, A.L. 1998. Dendrotoxins: How does structure determine function?. *Journal of Toxicology: Toxin Reviews*, 17(2), 161–182.

Eder, C., Fischer, H.G., Hadding, U. and Heinemann, U. 1995. Properties of voltage-gated potassium currents of microglia differentiated with granulocyte/macrophage colony-stimulating factor. *The Journal of Membrane Biology*, 147(2), 137–146.

Foehring, R.C. and Surmeier, D.J. 1993. Voltage-gated potassium currents in acutely dissociated rat cortical neurons. *Journal of Neurophysiology*, 70(1), 51–63.

Gasparini, S., Danse, J.M., Lecoq, A., Pinkasfeld, S., Zinn-Justin, S., Young, L.C., de Medeiros, C.C., Rowan, E.G., Harvey, A.L. and Ménez, A. 1998. Delineation of the functional site of α-dendrotoxin: The functional topographies of dendrotoxins are different but share a conserved core with those of other Kvl potassium channel-blocking toxins. *Journal of Biological Chemistry*, 273(39), 25393–25403.

Grissmer, S., Nguyen, A.N., Aiyar, J., Hanson, D.C., Mather, R.J., Gutman, G.A., Karmilowicz, M.J., Auperin, D.D. and Chandy, K.G. 1994. Pharmacological characterization of five cloned voltage-gated K+ channels, types Kvl. 1, 1.2, 1.3, 1.5, and 3.1, stably expressed in mammalian cell lines. *Molecular Pharmacology*, 45(6), 1227–1234.

Guillemare, E., Honore, E., Pradier, L., Lesage, F., Schweitz, H., Attali, B., Barhanin, J. and Lazdunski, M., 1992. Effects of the level of mRNA expression on biophysical properties, sensitivity to neurotoxins, and regulation of the brain delayed-rectifier K+ channel Kvl. 2. *Biochemistry*, 31(49), 12463–12468.

Hall, A., Stow, J., Sorensen, R., Dolly, J.O. and Owen, D. 1994. Blockade by dendrotoxin homologues of voltage-dependent K+ currents in cultured sensory neurones from neonatal rats. *British Journal of Pharmacology*, 113(3), 959–967.

Halliwell, J.V., Othman, I.B., Pelchen-Matthews, A. and Dolly, J.O. 1986. Central action of dendrotoxin: Selective reduction of a transient K conductance in hippocampus and binding to localized acceptors. *Proceedings of the National Academy of Sciences*, 83(2), 493–497.

Harvey, A. and Karlsson, E. 1980. Dendrotoxin from the venom of the green mamba, Dendroaspis angusticeps. *Naunyn-Schmiedeberg's Archives of Pharmacology*, 312(1), 1–6.

Harvey, A.L. and Anderson, A.J. 1985. Dendrotoxins: Snake toxins that block potassium channels and facilitate neurotransmitter release. *Pharmacology and Therapeutics*, 31(1–2), 33–55.

Harvey, A.L. and Anderson, A.J. 1987. Pharmacological actions of facilitatory neurotoxins on peripheral synapses. In *Neurotoxins and Their Pharmacological Implications* (pp. 97–114).

Harvey, A.L., Anderson, A.J. and Karlsson, E. 1984b. Facilitation of transmitter release by neurotoxins from snake venoms. *Journal de Physiologie*, 79(4), 222–227.

Harvey, A.L., Anderson, A.J., Mbugua, P.M. and Karlsson, E. 1984a. Toxins from mamba venoms that facilitate neuroiluscular transmission. *Journal of Toxicology: Toxin Reviews*, 3(2–3), 91–137.

Harvey, A.L. and Karlsson, E. 1982. Protease inhibitor homologues from mamba venoms: Facilitation of acetylcholine release and interactions with prejunctional blocking toxins. *British Journal of Pharmacology*, 77(1), 153–161.

Harvey, A.L. and Karlsson, E. 1984. Polypeptide neurotoxins from mamba venoms that facilitate transmitter release. *Trends in Pharmacological Sciences*, 5, 71–72.

Harvey, A.L., Rowan, E.G., Vatanpour, H., EngstrÖM, Å., Westerlund, B. and Karlsson, E. 1997. Changes to biological activity following acetylation of dendrotoxin I from Dendroaspis polylepis (black mamba). *Toxicon*, 35(8), 1263–1273.

Heurteaux, C. and Lazdunski, M. 1991. MCD peptide and dendrotoxin I activatec-fos andc-jun expression by acting on two different types of K+ channels. A discrimination using the K+ channel opener lemakalim. *Brain Research*, 554(1–2), 22–29.

Hollecker, M. and Creighton, T.E. 1983. Evolutionary conservation and variation of protein folding pathways: Two protease inhibitor homologues from black mamba venom. *Journal of Molecular Biology*, 168(2), 409–437.

Hollecker, M., Creighton, T.E. and Gabriel, M. 1982. Preliminary circular dichroism study of the conformations of intermediates trapped during protein folding. *Biochimie*, 63(11–12), 835–839.

Hopkins, W.F. 1998. Toxin and subunit specificity of blocking affinity of three peptide toxins for heteromultimeric, voltage-gated potassium channels expressed in Xenopus oocytes. *Journal of Pharmacology and Experimental Therapeutics*, 285(3), 1051–1060.

Huber, R., Kukla, D., Rühlmann, A. and Steigemann, W. 1972, January. Pancreatic trypsin inhibitor (kunitz) part I: Structure and function. In *Cold Spring Harbor Symposia on Quantitative Biology* (Vol. 36, pp. 141–150). Cold Spring Harbor Laboratory Press.

Hurst, R.S., Busch, A.E., Kavanaugh, M.P., Osborne, P.B., North, R.A. and Adelman, J.P. 1991. Identification of amino acid residues involved in dendrotoxin block of rat voltage-dependent potassium channels. *Molecular Pharmacology*, 40(4), 572–576.

Imredy, J.P., Chen, C. and MacKinnon, R. 1998. A snake toxin inhibitor of inward rectifier potassium channel ROMK1. *Biochemistry*, 37(42), 14867–14874.

Imredy, J.P. and MacKinnon, R. 2000. Energetic and structural interactions between δ-dendrotoxin and a voltage-gated potassium channel. *Journal of Molecular Biology*, 296(5), 1283–1294.

Jonas, P., Bräu, M.E., Hermsteiner, M. and Vogel, W. 1989. Single-channel recording in myelinated nerve fibers reveals one type of Na channel but different K channels. *Proceedings of the National Academy of Sciences*, 86(18), 7238–7242.

Joubert, F.J. and Taljaard, N. 1980. The amino acid sequence of two proteinase inhibitor homologues from Dendroaspis angusticeps venom. *Zeitschrift für Physiologische Chemie*, 361, 661–674.

Keighley, W.W., Newcombe, J., Templeton, D. and Treherne, J.M. 1994. Binding of I-125 labeled dendrotoxin to demyelinated human multiple-sclerosis lesions. *Journal of Physiology*, 480, 68–69.

Keller, R.M., Baumann, R., Hunziker-Kwik, E.H., Joubert, F.J. and Wüthrich, K. 1983. Assignment of the 1H nuclear magnetic resonance spectrum of the trypsin inhibitor homologue K from Dendroaspis polylepis polylepis: Two-dimensional nuclear magnetic resonance at 360 and 500 MHz. *Journal of Molecular Biology*, 163(4), 623–646.

Koh, D.S. and Vogel, W. 1996. Single-channel analysis of a delayed rectifier K+ channel in Xenopus myelinated nerve. *The Journal of Membrane Biology*, 149(3), 221–232.

Kondo, T., Ikenaka, K., Fujimoto, I., Aimoto, S., Kato, H., Ito, K.I., Taguchi, T., Morita, T., Kasai, M. and Mikoshiba, K. 1992. K+ channel involvement in induction of synaptic enhancement by mast cell degranulating (MCD) peptide. *Neuroscience Research*, 13(3), 207–216.

Kumar, A. and Gupta, V. 2018. Neurological Implications of Dendrotoxin: A Review. *Pharmacology and Toxicology*, 6.6, 469–476.

Lauridsen, L.P., Laustsen, A.H., Lomonte, B. and Gutiérrez, J.M. 2016. Toxicovenomics and antivenom profiling of the Eastern green mamba snake (Dendroaspis angusticeps). *Journal of Proteomics*, 136, 248–261.

Laustsen, A.H., Lomonte, B., Lohse, B., Fernández, J. and Gutiérrez, J.M. 2015. Unveiling the nature of black mamba (Dendroaspis polylepis) venom through venomics and antivenom immunoprofiling: Identification of key toxin targets for antivenom development. *Journal of Proteomics*, 119, 126–142.

MacKinnon, R. 1991. Determination of the subunit stoichiometry of a voltage-activated potassium channel. *Nature*, 350(6315), 232–235.

Majumder, K., De Biasi, M., Wang, Z. and Wible, B.A. 1995. Molecular cloning and functional expression of a novel potassium channel β-subunit from human atrium. *Federation of European Biochemical Societies Letters*, 361(1), 13–16.

Marshall, d.l. and Harvey, A.L. 1992. Protease inhibitor homologues of dendrotoxin do not bind to dendrotoxin acceptors on synaptosomal membranes or facilitate neuromuscular transmission. *Biological Chemistry Hoppe-Seyler*, 373, 707–714.

McAlexander, M.A. and Undem, B.J. 2000. Potassium channel blockade induces action potential generation in guinea-pig airway vagal afferent neurones. *Journal of the Autonomic Nervous System*, 78(2–3), 158–164.

McGivern, J., Scholfield, C.N. and Dolly, J.O. 1993. Action of α-dendrotoxin on K+ currents in nerve terminal regions of axons in rat olfactory cortex. *British Journal of Pharmacology*, 109(2), 535–538.

Mehraban, F., Black, A.R., Breeze, A.L., Green, D.G. and Dolly, J.O. 1985. A functional membranous acceptor for dendrotoxin in rat brain: Solubilization of the binding component. *Biochemical Society Translation*, 13(2), 507–508.

Mehraban, F., Haines, A. and Dolly, J.O. 1986. Monoclonal and polyclonal antibodies against dendrotoxin: Their effects on its convulsive activity and interaction with neuronal acceptors. *Neurochemistry International*, 9(1), 11–22.

Morales, M.J., Castellino, R.C., Crews, A.L., Rasmusson, R.L. and Strauss, H.C. 1995. A novel β subunit increases rate of inactivation of specific voltage-gated potassium channel α subunits. *Journal of Biological Chemistry*, 270(11), 6272–6277.

Newitt, R.A., Houamed, K.M., Rehm, H. and Tempel, B.L. 1991. Potassium channels and epilepsy: Evidence that the epileptogenic toxin, dendrotoxin, binds to potassium channel proteins. *Epilepsy Research*, 4, 263–273.

Nishio, H., Katoh, E., Yamazaki, T., Inui, T., Nishiuchi, Y. and Kimura, T. 1999. Structure-activity relationships of calcicludine and dendrotoxin-I, homologous peptides acting on different targets, calcium and potassium channels. *Biochemical and Biophysical Research Communications*, 262(2), 319–321.

Owen, D.G., Hall, A., Stephens, G., Stow, J. and Robertson, B. 1997. The relative potencies of dendrotoxins as blockers of the cloned voltage-gated K+ channel, mKvl. 1 (MK-1), when stably expressed in Chinese hamster ovary cells. *British Journal of Pharmacology*, 120(6), 1029–1034.

Parcej, D.N. and Dolly, J.O. 1989. Dendrotoxin acceptor from bovine synaptic plasma membranes. Binding properties, purification and subunit composition of a putative constituent of certain voltage-activated K+ channels. *Biochemical Journal*, 257(3), 899–903.

Parcej, D.N., Scott, V.E. and Dolly, J.O. 1992. Oligomeric properties of. alpha.-dendrotoxin-sensitive potassium ion channels purified from bovine brain. *Biochemistry*, 31(45), 11084–11088.

Pardi, A., Wagner, G. And Wüthrich, K. 1983. Protein conformation and proton nuclear-magnetic-resonance chemical shifts. *European Journal of Biochemistry*, 137(3), 445–454.

Pelchen-Matthews, A. and Dolly, J.O. 1989. Distribution in the rat central nervous system of acceptor subtypes for dendrotoxin, a K+ channel probe. *Neuroscience*, 29(2), 347–361.

Penner, R., Petersen, M., Pierau, F.K. and Dreyer, F. 1986. Dendrotoxin: A selective blocker of a non-inactivating potassium current in guinea-pig dorsal root ganglion neurones. *Pflügers Archiv*, 407(4), 365–369.

Poulter, M.O., Hashiguchi, T. and Padjen, A.L. 1989. Dendrotoxin blocks accommodation in frog myelinated axons. *Journal of Neurophysiology*, 62(1), 174–184.

Rehm, H. and Lazdunski, M. 1988. Purification and subunit structure of a putative K+-channel protein identified by its binding properties for dendrotoxin I. *Proceedings of the National Academy of Sciences*, 85(13), 4919–4923.

Rehm, H., Pelzer, S., Cochet, C., Chambaz, E., Tempel, B.L., Trautwein, W., Pelzer, D. and Lazdunski, M. 1989. Dendrotoxin-binding brain membrane protein displays a potassium channel activity that is stimulated by both cAMP-dependent and endogenous phosphorylations. *Biochemistry*, 28(15), 6455–6460.

Reid, G., Scholz, A., Bostock, H. and Vogel, W. 1999. Human axons contain at least five types of voltage-dependent potassium channel. *The Journal of Physiology*, 518(3), 681–696.

Rettig, J., Heinemann, S.H., Wunder, F., Lorra, C., Parcej, D.N., Dolly, J.O. and Pongs, O. 1994. Inactivation properties of voltage-gated K+ channels altered by presence of β-subunit. *Nature*, 369(6478), 289–294.

Robertson, B., Owen, D., Stow, J., Butler, C. and Newland, C. 1996. Novel effects of dendrotoxin homologues on subtypes of mammalian Kvl potassium channels expressed in Xenopus oocytes. *Federation of European Biochemical Societies Letters*, 383(1–2), 26–30.

Safronov, B.V., Kampe, K. and Vogel, W. 1993. Single voltage-dependent potassium channels in rat peripheral nerve membrane. *The Journal of Physiology*, 460(1), 675–691.

Schechter, L.E., Pearsall, D.M., Nawoschik, S.P., Barrezueta, N.X. and Rhodes, K.J. 1994. A comparative profile of 125I-α-dendrotoxin binding to voltage-dependent potassium channels in rodent nonhuman primate and human brain. *Society for Neuroscience Abstract*, 20, 1524.

Schweitz, H., Bruhn, T., Guillemare, E., Moinier, D., Lancelin, J.M., Béress, L. and Lazdunski, M. 1995. Kalicludines and Kaliseptine: Two different classes of sea anemone toxins for voltage-sensitive K+ channels. *Journal of Biological Chemistry*, 270(42), 25121–25126.

Scott, V.E., Muniz, Z.M., Sewing, S., Lichtinghagen, R., Parcej, D.N., Pongs, O. and Dolly, J.O. 1994. Antibodies specific for distinct Kv subunits unveil a heterooligomeric basis for subtypes of. alpha.-dendrotoxin-sensitive potassium channels in bovine brain. *Biochemistry*, 33(7), 1617–1623.

Scott, V.E., Parcej, D.N., Keen, J.N., Findlay, J.B. and Dolly, J.O. 1990. Alpha-dendrotoxin acceptor from bovine brain is a K+ channel protein. Evidence from the N-terminal sequence of its larger subunit. *Journal of Biological Chemistry*, 265(33), 20094–20097.

Silveira, R., Barbeito, L. and Dajas, F. 1988. Behavioral and neurochemical effects of intraperitoneally injected dendrotoxin. *Toxicon*, 26(3), 287–292.

Smith, L.A., Olson, M.A., Lafaye, P.J. and Dolly, J.O. 1995. Cloning and expression of mamba toxins. *Toxicon*, 33(4), 459–474.

Smith, L.A., Reid, P.F., Wang, F.C., Parcej, D.N., Schmidt, J.J., Olson, M.A. and Dolly, J.O. 1997. Site-directed mutagenesis of dendrotoxin K reveals amino acids critical for its interaction with neuronal K+ channels. *Biochemistry*, 36(25), 7690–7696.

Sorensen, R.G. and Blaustein, M.P. 1989. Rat brain dendrotoxin receptors associated with voltage-gated potassium channels: Dendrotoxin binding and receptor solubilization. *Molecular Pharmacology*, 36(5), 689–698.

Southan, A.P. and Robertson, B. 1998. Patch-clamp recordings from cerebellar basket cell bodies and their presynaptic terminals reveal an asymmetric distribution of voltage-gated potassium channels. *Journal of Neuroscience*, 18(3), 948–955.

Southan, A.P. and Robertson, B. 2000. Electrophysiological characterization of voltage-gated K+ currents in cerebellar basket and Purkinje cells: Kvl and Kv3 channel subfamilies are present in basket cell nerve terminals. *Journal of Neuroscience*, 20(1), 114–122.

Stansfeld, C.E., Fagni, L., Marsh, S.J., Brown, D.A. and Feltz, A. 1991. Kinetics of the dendrotoxin-sensitive k current in dissociated dorsal rootganglion (drg) neurones of the rat. *Journal of Physiology*, 434.

Stansfeld, C.E., Marsh, S.J., Halliwell, J.V. and Brown, D.A. 1986. 4-Aminopyridine and dendrotoxin induce repetitive firing in rat visceral sensory neurones by blocking a slowly inactivating outward current. *Neuroscience Letters*, 64(3), 299–304.

Stansfeld, C.E., Marsh, S.J., Parcej, D.N., Dolly, J.O. and Brown, D.A. 1987. Mast cell degranulating peptide and dendrotoxin selectively inhibit a fast-activating potassium current and bind to common neuronal proteins. *Neuroscience*, 23(3), 893–902.

Storm, J.F. 1988. Temporal integration by a slowly inactivating K+ current in hippocampal neurons. *Nature*, 336(6197), 379–381.

Strydom, D.J.S. 1973. Protease inhibitors as snake venom toxins. *Nature Chemical Biology* 243(124), 88–90.

Strydom, D.J. 1976. Snake venom toxins: Purification and properties of low-molecular-weight polypeptides of dendroaspis polylepis polylepis (Black Mamba) venom. *European Journal of Biochemistry*, 69(1), 169–176.

Stutzmann, J.M., Böhme, G.A., Gandolfo, G., Gottesmann, C., Lafforgue, J., Blanchard, J.C., Laduron, P.M. and Lazdunski, M. 1991. Riluzole prevents hyperexcitability produced by the mast cell degranulating peptide and dendrotoxin I in the rat. *European Journal of Pharmacology*, 193(2), 223–229.

Swaminathan, P., Hariharan, M., Murali, R. and Singh, C.U. 1996. Molecular structure, conformational analysis, and structure: Activity studies of dendrotoxin and its homologues using molecular mechanics and molecular dynamics techniques. *Journal of Medicinal Chemistry*, 39(11), 2141–2155.

Tytgat, J., Debont, T., Carmeliet, E. and Daenens, P. 1995. The α-dendrotoxin footprint on a mammalian potassium channel. *Journal of Biological Chemistry*, 270(42), 24776–24781.

Velluti, J.C., Caputi, A. and Macadar, O. 1987. Limbic epilepsy induced in the rat by dendrotoxin, a polypeptide isolated from the green mamba (Dendroaspis angusticeps) venom. *Toxicon*, 25(6), 649–657.

Wagner, G. and Wüthrich, K. 1982. Sequential resonance assignments in protein 1H nuclear magnetic resonance spectra: Basic pancreatic trypsin inhibitor. *Journal of Molecular Biology*, 155(3), 347–366.

Wang, F.C., Bell, N., Reid, P., Smith, L.A., McIntosh, P., Robertson, B. and Dolly, J.O. 1999a. Identification of residues in dendrotoxin K responsible for its discrimination between neuronal K+ channels containing Kv1. 1 and 1.2 α subunits. *European Journal of Biochemistry*, 263(1), 222–229.

Wang, F.C., Parcej, D.N. and Dolly, J.O. 1999b. α Subunit compositions of Kv1. 1-containing K+ channel subtypes fractionated from rat brain using dendrotoxins. *European Journal of Biochemistry*, 263(1), 230–237.

Wang, S.Y., Castle, N.A. and Wang, G.K. 1992. Identification of RBK1 potassium channels in C6 astrocytoma cells. *Glia*, 5(2), 146–153.

Weller, U., Bernhardt, U., Siemen, D., Dreyer, F., Vogel, W. and Habermann, E. 1985. Electrophysiological and neurobiochemical evidence for the blockade of a potassium channel by dendrotoxin. *Naunyn-Schmiedeberg's Archives of Pharmacology*, 330(2), 77–83.

Wlodawer, A., Walter, J., Huber, R. and Sjölin, L. 1984. Structure of bovine pancreatic trypsin inhibitor: Results of joint neutron and X-ray refinement of crystal form II. *Journal of Molecular Biology*, 180(2), 301–329.

Wu, R.L. and Barish, M.E. 1992. Two pharmacologically and kinetically distinct transient potassium currents in cultured embryonic mouse hippocampal neurons. *Journal of Neuroscience*, 12(6), 2235–2246.

CHAPTER **21**

# Batrachotoxin

**Arashdeep Singh and Reshu Rajput**

## CONTENTS



## 21.1 INTRODUCTION

Batrachotoxins, classified as steroidal alkaloid neurotoxins, were discovered in the mid-1960s in the skin extracts of poison-dart frogs of Colombia belonging to the *Phyllobates* genus. These frogs belong to the *Dendrobatidae* family and have particular skin glands which store and release poison toxins, and these glands are believed to be jam-packed densely on the frog's back. Several studies revealed that the frog acquires this toxin from the nutritional resource, yet the exact foundation of these poisons found in frog skin has not been acknowledged so far. Most toxic frogs of genus *Phyllobates* are bright in colour as compared to other congeners. These frogs were directly profited not only due to the poisonous nature of batrachotoxin (active principle) that helps them to defend themselves from predation, but also to a great degree due to their effects on mucous and buccal membranes causing irritation, numbness, and sneezing in the predator arising from only minute amounts of the poison (Daly and Witkop, 1971). These effects were often noticed during handling of these frogs and also during purification of extracts of skin. Batrachotoxin finds a route into the bloodstream with a small scratch or ulceration resulting in the manifestation of the toxic properties of batrachotoxins (Daly and Witkop, 1971). Among all the known frogs used for poisoning darts, merely three species of genus *Phyllobates* were in reality utilized by Native Americans for dart-tip poisoning and the key noxious substance accountable for inducing poisoning was batrachotoxin.

DOI: 10.1201/9781003178446-21

The term batrachotoxin was coined by the American chemist Bernhard Witcop, who organized the National Institute of Health's (NIH) search for the toxic frogs in Colombia. Batrachotoxin derives its name was from '*batrachos*', which is a Greek word meaning frog. Batrachotoxin is a multifaceted alkaloid steroidal that leads to depolarization and persistent activation of voltage-gated sodium ion channels. Batrachotoxins bind to voltage-gated sodium channels (Nav) in nerve and muscle membranes with high affinity and lock them open, allowing sodium to freely flow across the membrane with a massive influx of sodium, resulting in depolarization of muscle and nerve membranes (Albuquerque et al., 1971). Batrachotoxins have been extensively used to study the functioning of sodium channels due to their potency and specificity (Dumbacher et al., 2004; Strichartz et al., 1987). Although researchers and scientists have not elucidated the structure of this small toxin molecule until the mid-1960s, the native folks of the Choco area of North Western Colombia and the Eastern and Central Highlands provinces in Papua New Guinea had knowledge about the potential properties of the toxin for centuries. Frogs of the Colombian rainforest used to produce secretions which were milky white on their backs that contained the toxin. Native peoples have always utilised the batrachotoxin, which they name 'kokoi,' to poison their arrows and blow-darts (Marki and Witkop, 1963). In earlier times, the locals of Papua New Guinea used to avoid certain species of beetles also including *Pitohui* and Blue-capped *Ifrita* birds as their skin shows burning and numbing sensation when contacted with the skin of these groups (Dumbacher et al., 2004) without knowing the presence of toxin in these species.

Batrachotoxin, which is a hydrophobic alkaloid, when penetrates into the cell membranes of nerve, muscle, and heart, triggers the voltage-gated sodium channels of the system. A number of naturally found batrachatoxins have been identified in frogs and birds and the main widespread toxins are batrachotoxin and homobatrachotoxin, which consist of a pyrrole ring. The presence of a pyrrole ring was already confirmed by the observations of Ehrlich colour reactions that were found to be positive for both batrachotoxin and homobatrachotoxin (Daly et al., 1965), followed by detailed analysis by NMR spectra and NMR comparisons with ethyl dimethylpyrrole-3-carboxylates, which show the way to the establishment of the structures of the very lethal batrachotoxin and homobatrachotoxin (Tokuyama et al., 1969). These are found in almost equal proportions in frogs and have a lethal effect ($LD_{50}$) in mice. The pyrrole ring can be altered naturally and also in lab conditions to produce a non-pyrrole form known as batrachotoxin-A, which is about 500 times less toxic than batrachotoxin. Several experiments revealed that this toxin in both birds and frogs was acquired from dietary sources. It has previously been reported that frogs who are raised in cages lose their toxicity; frogs that are fed normal, toxic-free diets in cages do not produce batrachotoxins. When a batrachotoxin-containing diet is given to frogs, they accumulate the toxins readily in their skin.

## 21.2 OCCURRENCE

The batrachotoxin alkaloids differ in various features pertaining to structures, particularly 3,9 hemiketal function, 2,4-dialkylpyrrole-3-carboxylate moiety, and the homomorpholine bridge. Batrachotoxins were only known to be obtained from the frogs of the genus *Phyllobates* which belong to the neotropical family *Dendrobatidae*. Among the five Colombian species only three species, namely *P. terribilis*, *P. aurotaenia*, and *P. bicolor* contain high a level of toxin that is employed to poison tips of blow-darts. Because of this, all three classes deserve to be designated as poison-dart frogs. Maimum levels of toxin occurs in skin of *P. terribilis*containing batrachotoxin, homobatrachotoxin and batrachotoxin A in the amount of about 500 µg, 300 and 200 µg respectively (Myers et al., 1978). About 20 µg batrachotoxin, 10 µg homobatrachotoxin and 50 µg batrachotoxin A was found to be present in the skins of the less toxic *P. bicolor* and *P. aurotaenia*. Costa Rican species *P. Vittatus* skin has been reported to contain about 0.2 µg batrachotin, 0.2 µg homobatrachotoxin and 2 µg batrachotoxin A. Daly et al. (1980) reported that the content of batrachotoxin gradually declined in the skin of wild-caught *P. terribilis* fed on fruit flies and crickets for years and also no detectable levels of batrachotoxins was found in the progeny of feral -caught *P. terribilis*. The most likely explanation of these observations is that these *Phyllobates* species were dependent upon their dietary sources for batrachotoxins and with time they might have developed a proficient uptake routine for batrachotoxins storage and related alkaloids in the skins secretory glands. According to Daly et al. (1980), muscle sodium channels of *P. terribilis* were insensitive to batrachotoxin and the basis for this conclusion was that BTX unsuccessful in depolarization of membrane capability of muscle cells at 5 μM concentration. Some procreation trial established that BTX auto-resistance was heritable in *P. Terribilis* (Wang and Wang, 2017). The species *P. bicolor* having no batrachotoxin in skin when kept captive and provided with alkaloid sprinkle fruit flies were capable to build up batrachotoxin A into their skin (Daly et al., 1994).

Dumbacher et al. (1992) discovered one of the batrachotoxin in feathers and skin parts of New Guinean birds from genus *Pitohui* belonging to the family Muscicapidae and in the initial study only homobatrachotoxin was detected. The hooded pitohui bird (*Pitohui dichrous*) has the greatest levels of homobatrachotoxin in its skin and feathers i.e. about 20 μg, about ten times lower found in the erratic pitohui (*Pitohui kirhocephalus*) and yet below than these in corroded pitohui (*Pitohui ferrugineus*) (Dumbacher et al., 1992). Homobatrachotoxin content of in feathers and skin part of black pitohui (*Pitohui nigrescens*) were reported to be comparable with rusty pitohui (Dumbacher et al., 1992).

Dumbacher et al. (2004), investigated the occurrence of batrachotoxins in melyrid beetles which belongs to genus *Choresine* which was potential source of the alkaloids batrachotoxin reported in toxic-dart frogs and poisonous passerine birds. They have carried out a research on a not much examined beetles group which belongs to genus *Choresine*and family Melyridae to describe the presence of high levels of batrachotoxins. The tiny insect and presence of higher levels of poison suggested that they could be the toxin source for birds of New Guinea. The analysis of stomach contents of *Pitohui* exposed the presence of beetles of genus *Choresine* along many tiny other beetles and arthropods in their diets.

## 21.3 ISOLATION AND CHARACTERIZATION OF BATRACHOTOXIN

In the year 1962, two biologists Marte Latham and Fritz Marki travelled to Western Colombia particularly Choco region, a densely jungled area located between the Pacific Ocean and the Andes mountains. Both Latham and Markiwere part of an NIH program led by the Bernhard Witcop and John Daly for the isolation and characterization of poison from Colombian dart frog (Saporito et al., 2009). Due to the collaborative and constant efforts over a period of 15 years by John Daly and his fellow scientists in that region, more than 10,000 frogs were collected and tested (Saporito et al., 2009). It was necessary to use thousands of frogs for the isolation of toxin as skin of each frog contains only 1–2 μg of *kokoi* venom (Daly et al., 1980). There were numerous challenges associated with collecting such a large number of frogs. Morphologically all frogs of family *Dendrobatidae* possess similar poison glands (Neuwirth et al., 1979), but only three species in this family found to contain the toxin those are *Phyllo batesbicolor*, *Phyllo batesaurotaenia* and *Phyllo batesterribilis*. The largest species of *P. Terribilis* measure only about 50 mm in adulthood therefore locating these frogs was another significant logistical problem (Myers et al., 1978). The preferred habitat of these frogs was near the ground in dense jungle undergrowth which further complicated the process. With the help from the native people only, the researchers were able to locate and collect the frogs as these people were able to imitate the peeping sound of frogs.

For the isolation of toxin, the frogs were killed with ether and immediately skinned. The skins were extracted numerous times with aqueous methanol, once cut into small squares (Marki and Witkop, 1963). Concentration was done under reduced pressure, followed by the removal of concomitant azeotropic water. The extract was stored at low temperature to avoid degradation of toxin. The neutral aqueous solution of the residue then undergoes further purification involving chloroform extractions, chromatography on silicic acid, countercurrent distribution, and finally at least three rounds of thin-layer chromatography (Marki and Witkop, 1963).

After the first TLC separation, sections of the plate were assayed for toxicity in order to determine which portion contained the active venom. In this standard assay, samples were dissolved in 100 μL of 0.9% v/v aqueous NaCl and injected subcutaneously into male white mice. The time difference between injection and animal death was then calculated, and the TLC section corresponding to the sample that elicited the shortest time of death was selected for further purification. Once the toxin-containing section was identified, subsequent rounds of TLC ultimately resolved the active material into one homogeneous spot that was visible upon exposure of the plate to iodine vapour. In this fashion, a few 100 μg of pure toxin was extracted from 330 frogs (Marki and Witkop, 1963). The initial report indicates that this material was a solid, but because so little material was available, no attempts at crystallization were performed (Marki and Witkop, 1963). Although future reports would indicate that the toxin was actually a mixture of components that were separable under the TLC conditions utilized during the initial isolation (Daly et al., 1965, Tokuyama et al., 1968), this first record makes no mention of additional toxic substances purified. It is possible that, as a result of the assay method employed (time to death), these substances were overlooked in an effort to purify the most toxic material.

Despite the small amount of toxin purified, preliminary chemical analyses were performed, and the information gleaned from these studies would later facilitate a more streamlined purification procedure that would ultimately lead to the complete chemical characterization of the *kokoi* venom (Marki and Witkop, 1963). In particular, the behaviour of the compound on different ion exchange resins was studied, and based on a strong adsorption to an ammonium ion column, it was ascertained that the substance contained a basic moiety. The pKa of this basic group was determined by measuring the percent of total activity extracted into the organic layer of either a water/chloroform or water/10% benzene-cyclohexane mixture at varying pH values of the aqueous phase. Using this method, the pKa of the venom was determined to be 7.1 and 8.0 in the two systems, respectively. Further, sharp absorption bands in the IR spectrum at approximately 3,000 $cm^{-1}$ and 1,700 $cm^{-1}$ suggested the presence of both amine and carbonyl functional groups.

## 21.4 STRUCTURE OF BATRACHOTOXIN (BTX)

The elucidation of structural components of *kokoi* venom was very complicated due to the highly unstable nature of the toxin. For the structure of the most active principle compound batrachotoxin, the first high-resolution mass spectrometry incorrectly determined the empirical formula as $C_{31}H_{42}N_2O_6$ (Daly et al., 1965). Batrachotoxinin A, which is the most abundant among minor components, was correctly assigned the molecular formula of $C_{24}H_{35}NO_5$. The element map revealed that a contiguous skeleton of at least 17 carbon atoms was present in both these compounds suggesting steroidal framework (Figure 21.1). Batrachotoxins' structure consists of a steroid skeleton and oxazapane ring.

Despite the presence of similar carbon atoms, both these compounds exhibited remarkable differences in various chemical and analytical tests performed. For instance, the IR spectrum of BTX showed a concentrated band absorption at 1,690 $cm^{-1}$ which was not present in batrachotoxin A (Tokuyama et al., 1968). Batrachotoxin gives an immediate strong red colour when treated with Ehrlich reagent and colour upon treatment with *p*-dimethylaminocinnamaldehyde (Daly et al., 1965). These chemical tests suggested that BTX contained a pyrrole moiety. Contradictory results were obtained when other chemical tests were performed, suggesting the presence of nitrogen in BTX as carbinolamine ether. Upon reduction of BTX with lithium aluminium hydride ($LiAlH_4$),

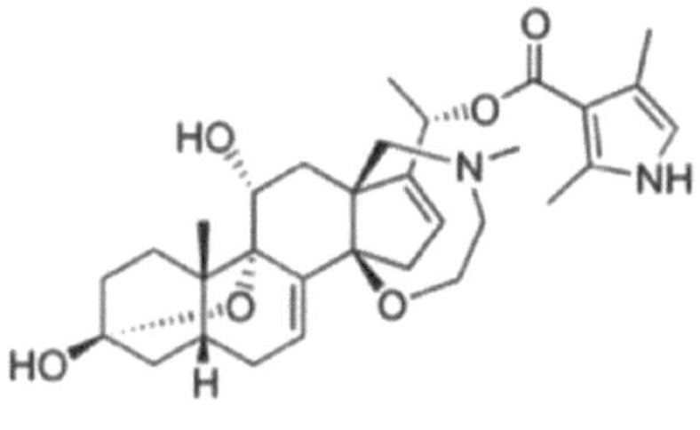

**Figure 21.1** Structure of batrachotoxins

the Ehrlich test came to be negative, whereas, on the other hand, MeI resulted in an Ehrlich-positive quaternary salt. The results from these studies were observed to be inconsistent with the occurrence of a pyrrole moiety as the source of nitrogen, because under former conditions BTX should have been Ehrlich-positive and should be Ehrlich-negative under latter conditions. As a final result it was established that batrachotoxin and batrachotoxin A were structurally distinct and also the $LD_{50}$ of BTX on white mice was determined to be 2 µg/kg, while the $LD_{50}$ of batrachotoxin A was found to be significantly higher at 1 mg/kg (Tokuyama et al., 1969).

When O-p-bromobenzoate derivatives were discovered in the crystal structure of batrachotoxin A, many of the structural and chemical conflicts were resolved. It was observed that batrachotoxin A acylation with *p*-bromobenzic anhydride under Schotten-Baumann conditions gave a crystalline solid. After that, purification on silica gel was carried out and the obtained product was recrystallized for fine needles production from acetone. The batrachotoxin is a steroidal alkaloid, of a single crystal of purified compound was revealed by the X-ray diffraction technique (XRD). Batrachotoxin A had several structural features that were never seen before in any natural product. Furthermore, 9α-hydroxy 3β-hemiketal were also observed in batrachotoxin A, and these structural elements were not observed in any other known natural steroidal product (Tokuyama et al., 1969). Partial synthesis confirmed the final molecular structure of batrachotoxin. Under basic conditions, hydrolysis of sterically hindered ester of BTX was carried out to batrachotoxin A with difficulty at 60°C with 2.0 N aqueous NaOH for a period of 16 hours. The conversion of batrachotoxin A to batrachotoxin was done by treating with 9.2 equivalents of 2,4-dimethylpyrrole-3-carboxylic acid anhydride and 0.2 N aqueous KOH in chloroform for 5 h. Even though the esterification was not completed, batrachotoxin purified on silica gel and 35% yield was isolated and the identity of BTX was confirmed through TLC, NMR, Mass spectrometry, and toxicity analysis. The NIH team of Daly and Witkop had identified 4β-hydroxybatrachotoxin and 4β-hydroxyhomobatrachotoxin and successful elucidation of the structures of five novel compounds forming a small batrachotoxin alkaloid family.

## 21.5 MECHANISM OF ACTION

Being extremely toxic, batrachotoxin having a lethal dosage of homobatrachotoxin as < 100 µg for mice (Daly and Spande, 1986). The batrachotoxins tend to attach purposely to voltage-gated sodium channels in nerve and muscle membranes (Albuquerque et al., 1971) and significantly affect the functioning of the channel in four ways. Firstly, the activation gating 30–50 mV is significantly shifted towards the hyperpolarization. Therefore, a batrachotoxin-adjoined ion channel is more eagerly triggered, steady at resting potential of membrane. Secondly, both rapid and decelerated inactivation gating that keeps the active channels open for hours or more are eliminated or reduced by batrachotoxin. Thirdly, single-channel conductance can be reduced by up to 50% by batrachotoxin. And fourthly, ion-based selectivity of voltage-gated sodium channel can be altered by batrachotoxin. In brief, batrachotoxins bind to a sodium channel that is open and also stabilize the channel in its open conformation, thus the closing of the channel is prevented (Daly et al., 1999). This causes sodium ions to readily flow across the membrane, with a massive influx of sodium and depolarization of muscle and nerve membrane occurs. This results in the blockage of membrane functioning which leads to irritation, tingling, and numbness in peripheral nervous tissue. It has been reported that, at higher concentrations, batrachotoxins will lead to paralysis, convulsions, and failure of the heart or lungs, because the membrane can be depolarized even with considerably small proportion of activated channels. As these batrachotoxins have a high affinity for binding with proteins that act as sodium channels, this type of binding is frequently referred to as irreversible.

Due to the important influence on voltage-sensitive sodium channels, batrachotoxin and its derivatives have been employed as important tools for researching membrane excitability. Brown and Bradley (1985) carried out batrachotoxin A 20-α-N-methylanthranilate production. The new fluorescent compound had the same receptor site for binding with the sodium channels which are voltage-sensitive, such as batrachotoxin having a symmetrical dissociation constant $K_d$= 180 nM in scorpion poison presence, which is found to be highly toxic. The binding and fluorescence properties of the newly synthesized compound have been explored for achieving successful visualization of sodium channels at Ranvier's mammalian nodes. With the development of a batrachotoxin A 20-α-N-methylanthranilate, the study of sodium channel distribution was facilitated (Brown and Bradley, 1985). Kongsamut et al. (1985) reported partial inhibition of calcium channel activity by batrachotoxin with the help of dihydropyridine. Daly and Spande (1986) reviewed the detailed biological activity of batrachotoxin. Creveling and Daly (1992) discussed the use of batrachotoxinin A 20β-[$^3$H]benzoate as a radio-ligand for studying the consequence of local anti-convulsants, sedative, and erstwhile pills on sodium channels which are voltage-dependent. Casebolt and Brown (1993) reported that a photosensitive derivative of batrachotoxinnamely 20β-[$^3$H]*o*-azidobenzoate binds precisely to the cerebral cortical synaptoneurosome site of rats batrachotoxin sodium channel upon irradiation with a covalent bond. Following that, one transmembrane region of the sodium channel was mentioned as the main location of photoaffinity labelling with batrachotoxinin. A 20β-[$^3$H]*o*-azidobenzoate (Trainer et al., 1996). The batrachotoxin congener's interaction, [$^3$H]batrachotoxin-A 20-α-benzoate, increased by compounds such as α-polypeptide scorpion toxins and α-cyano-pyrethroid poison (Brown, 1988). Poisonous effects of batrachotoxin might be suppressed with the help of tetrodotoxin (Warnick et al., 1971), a chemical compound responsible for sodium ion transport obstruction via excited membrane. The first constriction of muscle induced by batrachotoxin resulted from hyperpolarization of the muscles is recognized by permeability enhancement of sodium in membranes, whereas the appearance of a secondary persistent contraction which includes intracellular calcium discharge via an osmotically disturbed sarcotubular network (Warnick et al., 1971).

It is indeed worth noting that BTX has little impact on the membrane permeability and action potential of lobster and crayfish muscles (Albuquerque et al., 1973), which are believed to generate action potentials via increasing transmembrane resistance to calcium rather than sodium (Werman and Grundfest, 1961). Preliminary data suggests that perhaps the sulfhydryl moieties of protein complexes are required for BTX to have its action (Albuquerque et al., 1971). The impact of BTX is prevented by pre-treatment of lobsters gigantic axons using p-chloromercuribenzenesulfonate (PCMBS), dithiothreitol (DTT), or N-ethylmaleimide (NEM), but not through TTX. TTX and BTX appear to operate on distinct locations or biomolecules of the membranes. An additional piece of substantial evidence of distinct BTX and TTX receptor is acquired using the rodent's abdominal and pelvic muscle tissue (Albuquerque et al., 1973).

## 21.6 TOXICITY OF BATRACHOTOXINS

For the toxicity of batrachotoxins in humans only very little information is available. If mouse and human toxicity are nearly similar at 2.5 μg/kg through percutaneous injection, a low fatal dose for a 68 kg person is around 170 μg of batrachotoxin. Some researchers have found that rats are much less sensitive to neurotoxins than humans, thus another calculation could be relied mostly on lethality correlations of batrachotoxin to aconitine, digitoxin, and strychnine, and also its neurotoxicity. On the basis of these relationships it can be assumed that a smaller dose of around 2–10 μg pure batrachotoxin is administered intravenously; it has the potential to be fatal to humans. Likewise, even small amounts of 120–500 μg are predicted to be deadly to humans if consumed. So far, only the direct negative consequences on voltage-gated ion channels were examined, whereas additional toxicology pathways such as acute exposure, hepatotoxicity, cytotoxicity, and carcinogenic effects have not been investigated.

Dumbacher et al. (2000) investigated and isolated batrachotoxin alkaloids from passerine birds. In this study they extracted batrachotoxins in five New Guinean bird species which belong to the genus *Pitohui*, as well as a species of a second poisonous bird genus, *Ifrita kowaldi*, and evaluated the relative quantities of poisons using high-performance liquid chromatography spectrometry. The alkaloids identified were batrachotoxin-A cis-crotonate, batrachotoxin-A and a derivative, batrachotoxin, homobatrachotoxin, batrachotoxin-A 3'-hydroxylated derivatives of homo-batrachotoxin and mono- and di-hydroxylated isomers of homo-batrachotoxin. They discovered that the greatest concentrations of batrachotoxins were found within contouring feathers of the abdomen, legs, and breast in *Pitohuikirhocephalus*, *Pitohuidichrous*, and *Ifritakowaldi*. They have reported that the quantities and ratios among those batrachotoxins found to be variedly different among various *Pitohui* and *Ifrita* tribes of birds. As a result of the research, it was shown that these birds do not generate these toxins and instead get batrachotoxin alkaloids from the environment through their diet.

Marquez et al. (2018), investigated whether auto-resistance of batrachotoxin *Phyllobates* poison-dart amphibians co-evolve with toxicity. According to them, toxin tolerance evolution might include physiological constraints, thus auto-resistance is frequently predicted to develop gradually following toxicity, manifesting in a connection in between levels of toxicity and auto-resilience amongst poisonous species. They have investigated correlation between toxicity and auto-resistance in poison frogs of genus *Phyllobates*, known for the secretion of deadly batrachotoxin (BTX), a potent neurotoxin that affects the function of ion channels by using ancient sequencing restorations of BTX-sensing regions of the muscular voltage-gated ion channel. According to restorations, batrachotoxin resistance develops mostly in base of *Phyllobates*, corresponding with the emergence of batrachotoxin production. Although significant increases in poison across these amphibians' evolutionary history, hardly any further development of auto-tolerance appears to have happened after this occurrence. Hence, the study of Marquez et al. (2018) does not provide any further evidence in the support of an evolutionary correlation between toxicity and auto-resistance, which contradicted with the earlier findings reported by Dobler et al. (2011). Deeper analysis mostly on physiological risks and advantages of BTX resistant strains, and also their occurrence in wild populations, could offer insight on the conceptual frameworks behind the link between cytotoxicity and bio tolerance among *Phyllobates* amphibians.

Finol-Urdaneta et al. (2019) investigated the encounter of Batrachotoxin on the homo-tetrameric prokaryotic voltage-gated sodium channels such as NaChBac and NavSp1. They have shown that BTX performs activation in a use-dependent manner and this may be accomplished by combining mutagenesis research, full sequence number clamping, and kinetics and structural simulation. Their molecular model represented the horse-shoe shaped BTX particle bided inside the open hole and formed hydrophobic H-bonds with the helices of pore-lining. This paradigm doesn't really enable slightly desiccated sodium ions to reach the hydrophilic horseshoe's inner layer. From this, they came to the conclusion that the hefty BTX component bided at the unlocking residues region inhibited the S6 alterations that were required to close the activating gate. Their research found significant commonalities among prokaryotic and eukaryotic amperage ion channels (Nav) and focused upon tractability of bacterial Nav channels as analogues of voltage-dependent sodium ion channels gating.

### 21.6.1 Exposure Routes and Pathways

The exposure of toxin in humans occurs thorough ingesting skin and flesh of the frogs. The handling of these frogs is very dangerous due to the high quantity of toxin present in them and also some of the absorption in the body may happen via the skin. The toxins contact arises due to subcutaneous injection, which is a puncture caused by a toxic-dart point. Exposure through birds could also occur by ingesting meat; also, even touching the birds might result in mild discomfort and allergic responses such as a runny nose, tingling around the buccal membrane, itchy eyes, and sneezing. Batrachotoxins are fat-soluble steroidal alkaloids, which are soluble in various organic solvents such as ethanol, chloroform, ether, and methanol. Batrachotoxins may be soaked up via skin and even through gastrointestinal tract (GI). The impacts of certain poisons are felt in 10 minutes and might persist for many hours to a day.

### 21.6.2 Pharmacology

Batrachotoxin is believed to irrevocably inhibit neuromuscular signalling and to cause muscle contraction in an isolated neuronal formulation. Batrachotoxin is the most potent naturally occurring non-peptidic toxin known, with an $LD_{50}$ of 2 μg/kg in mice. Homobatrachotoxin is also potent, with an $LD_{50}$ of 3 μg/kg.12 Daly noted that subcutaneous injection of a mouse with 2 μg of purified batrachotoxin induces short hopping movements, followed by full-body spasms, convulsions, and gasping for breath in the animal. The mouse was dead within one minute of injection (Marki and Witkop, 1963). Early studies performed on rat diaphragm muscle fibers revealed that batrachotoxin irreversibly blocked the ability of muscle cells to respond to electrical stimulation. Even in these preliminary studies, it was clear that batrachotoxin interfered with nervous system function, and it was speculated that the toxin might interfere with the function of proteins involved in sodium trafficking across membranes (Marki and Witkop, 1963). The pharmacological effects of batrachotoxins on Purkinje fibers, nerve axons, and papillary muscle of the heart, brain, and both pre- and post-synaptic aspects of the neuromuscular junction were described by Albuquerque et al. (1971). The detailed review of these studies has been carried out (Albuquerque and Daly, 1976). Based on a review of the biological studies performed thus far, Albuquerque et al. (1971) concluded with the increase in permeability of membrane towards the sodium ions, batrachotoxin leads to a dose-dependent and irreversible depolarization of electrically excitable membranes. In normal bathing medium, the squid large axon is deprotonated by batrachotoxin, but no effect was observed when mutually intra- and extra-cellular section were filled with solution devoid of sodium (Narahashi et al. 1971). Tedrodoxin is responsible for completely blocking the depolarized excitable membranes by batrachotoxin (Catterall, 1975; Albuquerque, Daly and Witkop, 1971). In several excitable tissues, measurement of the concentration-dependence of batrachotoxin depolarization has been carried out. However, this research does not provide any information of the relationship between accumulation and outcome, due to the highly nonlinear relationship between sodium permeability and membrane potential. The ability of cells to return to resting potential reduces upon treatment with batrachotoxin and to respond to electrical stimuli results in secondary effects such as spontaneous neurotransmitter release and muscle contracture. Ultimately, the inability of the muscle and nerve cells to generate and respond to electrical signals as a result of toxin binding results in death through heart failure and/or asphyxiation (Narahashi, 1974).

Further studies revealed that batrachotoxin causes membrane depolarization by modifying the function of voltage-gated sodium ion channels (Nav) (Catterall, 1980). These channels were large proteins with disulfide bridges that were accountable for quick initiation of movement capabilities in all electrically impulsive cells (Catterall, 1992). Electrophysiological experiments have revealed that BTX causes a complex array of responses when applied to Nav (Wang and Wang, 2003), as can be seen from a comparison of the traces recorded from recombinant Nav1.3-expressing oocytes in either the absence (control) or presence of BTX (Li et al., 2002). First, BTX ties to the channel's free state and hyperpolarizes the threshold of activation. In the control cell, Navs are mostly closed at -50 mV and -35 mV. As a result, little current is observed. However, in the presence of BTX, a portion of the channel population opens at -50 mV. A significant number of channels have opened once a potential of -35 mV has been reached, resulting in current flow. Second, BTX blocks channel inactivation. In untreated cells, membrane depolarization causes Navs to open to allow sodium ion influx. The protein then enters a non-conductive inactive state and then finally returns to the closed state. However, treatment with BTX causes channels to remain open at voltages that normally affect channel inactivation. The synergy of these two aspects is that a portion of Nav is persistently activated at stationary action potentials in the company of BTX. In other words, in the company of BTX, a net depolarization of the membrane takes place. Third, BTX reduces single-channel conductance. As can be seen in the current traces at 0 mV, the peak current in the presence of BTX is smaller in magnitude than in the control. Finally, BTX alters the ion selectivity of Nav, boosting the channel's porosity to bigger ionic species (e.g., $K^+$, $Ca^{2+}$). Despite the limited amount of batrachotoxin available from natural sources, preliminary structure–activity relationship and mutagenesis studies have been performed in an attempt to deconvolute these different biological responses as well as to obtain a better physical understanding of the BTX binding site in these channels. As expected, there is a strong correlation between drug toxicity and its ability to move the threshold of commencement to additional hyperpolarized prospective. Most remarkably, batrachotoxinin A, having an $LD_{50}$ that is approximately 100 times higher than BTX, depolarized diaphragm muscle of rat by less than 10% (Warnick et al., 1975). Furthermore, the C20 esters of 7,8-dihydrobatrachotoxinin A with 2,4,5-trimethylpyrrole-3-carboxylic acid and benzoic acid resulted in modification of Navs that was substantially comparable to the response persuaded by BTX at 10-50M (Khodorov et al., 1992). Supporting these results was the earlier finding that the analogue of batrachotoxin containing a 2,4,5-trimethylpyrrole-3-carboxylic acid C20 side chain is quite potent, with an $LD_{50}$ that is lower than BTX itself (1 μg/kg) (Tokuyama et al., 1969). From this data it has been concluded that an aromatic C20 ester group is critical for activity.

Li et al. (2002) carried out research wherein they protected the batrachotoxin receptors onto voltage-gated ion channel by the channel's activation region. Batrachotoxin (BTX), extracted from South American amphibians of the genera *Phyllobates*, caused the irreversible activation of voltage-gated ion channels. The 260-kDa subunit is the most important structural component of sodium channel, which consist of four areas (I–IV), in each of the four fields, the regions between S5 and S6 form aperture loops that descend in to trans-membrane to form a small selective screen just at ion-conducting pore's outer ends. Some studies based site-directed mutation experiments had indicated that particular amino acids residues in each of the four S6 regions were critical. On site-directed mutagenesis has revealed that specific amino acid residues within each of the four S6 segments are vital factors for determining action of batrachotoxin (Linford et al., 1998; Li et al., 2002). A few of these acids have also been involved in the action of localized anaesthetics and sodium channel blockers. In this work, scientists induced a variety of mutations at this location inside the Nav sodium channel, produced ferocious and mutation circuits in Xenopus laevis oocytes, and used voltage clamp monitoring to assess their susceptibility to BTX. It was discovered that substituting alanine or isoleucine significantly lowered poison susceptibility, but cysteine, tyrosine, or tryptophan had just a little effect. These findings point to an electromagnetic ligand-receptor interaction at this location, which might include a chargeable tertiary amine on BTX. They examined the characteristics of the toxin-receptor response in further depth using a mutation channel (mutant F1710C) with moderate toxin sensitivities. Unlike ferocious channels, that engage BTX virtually permanently, toxin separation from mutation channels is fast, but only if the streams are opened, not shut. These findings point to a blocked activation barrier trapping coupled toxin. Even though BTX separation requires channel stimulation, it was curiously delayed by significant depolarisation, indicating that the poison-adsorption process is impacted by further state-dependent and/or electrical effects. They hypothesise that BTX travels in and out of its receptors via the cytoplasmic ends of the wide ion-conducting pores, much as quaternary local anaesthetics like QX314.

## 21.7 SYNTHETIC APPROACHES TO BATRACHOTOXIN ALKALOIDS

The batrachotoxins exhibit several distinct structural features, comprising a steroid-based pentacyclic core skeleton, a seven-membered oxazapane ring and an intramolecular 3β-hemiketal. These chemical compounds are potential neurotoxins having toxicity, $LD_{50}$ in mice is 2 μg/kg and acting as irrevocable activators of sodium channel (Albuquerque et al., 1971). Since its first isolation in the last 50 years, few important reports have been published elaborating total synthesis of batrachotoxin. Batrachotoxin A fractional production from progesterone was completed by Imhof et al. (1972), whereas numerous other artificial attempts towards ABA ring system have been documented (Keana et al., 1976). The following section focuses on arguably the two most fruitful endeavours, the syntheses of 20*S*-batrachotoxinin A and (±)-batrachotoxinin A by Wehrli and associated scientists and Kishi and associated scientists (Kurosu et al., 1998), respectively. Both these pathways have significant difference in their approach. In the Wehrli synthesis, 11-acetoxyprogesterone was manipulated into 20*S*-batrachotoxinin A, whereas in the Kishi synthesis, (±)-batrachotoxinin A was formed from simple starting materials. Although each pathway was ultimately successful, both syntheses were lengthy procedures involving sequence of reactions. A closer examination of these pathways reveals the challenges associated with the efficient construction of such a highly oxidized steroidal natural product.

### 21.7.1 Wehrli Synthesis of 20S-Batrachotoxinin A

Wehrli and associated scientists reported the first effort towards the total synthesis of batrachotoxin in a study published in the year 1972 about the synthesis of 20*S*-batrachotoxinin A (Kurosu et al., 1998). This strategy featured manipulation of an available steroid through a sequence of transformation involving oxidation and reduction reactions in order to achieve the required functionality found in the natural product. The formation of the final homomorpholine ring occurred at the later stage. The steroid chosen as the starting material was 11α-acetoxy progesterone, which already contains the necessary C11α- oxygenation as well as a two-carbon units at C17. To accomplish the synthesis, five oxidative and two reductive transformations were necessary on the steroidal backbone. At the outset, the most challenging of these manipulations would appear to be the introduction of the C14 tertiary alcohol with concomitant inversion of the C/D ring fusion geometry from *transto cis*.

The first reactant in the Wehrli synthesis was 11α-acetoxyprogesterone. A typical sequence of ten steps was required for the conversion of steroid into intermediate an oxidized C18 derivative of ester. After the oxidation of C18, the 3α,9α-hemiketal as well as a C7 hydroxy group were installed by a sequence of 11 steps. For the synthesis of 20*S*-batrachotoxin, several sequences of reactions took place involving a number of chemical compounds required for the synthesis, followed by formation of various intermediate compounds, resulting in the final synthesis of 20*S*-batrachotoxinin A.

### 21.7.2 Kishi Synthesis of (±)-Batrachotoxin A

Twenty-five years on from Wehrli et al.'s published work, Kishi and associates accomplished the first complete synthesis of (±)-batrachotoxin A. They tried to construct the batrachotoxin core in a convergent manner that enabled them to install various required functional groups at an early stage in the synthesis (Grinsteiner and Kishi, 1994). In this method, batrachotoxinin A would be achieved from tetracycle, formed through an intra-molecular Diels-Alder reaction of furan-annulated A/B ring system attached to an electron-withdrawn alkene. One of the key questions posed by Kishi retrosynthetic analysis of BTX was the feasibility of the proposed Diels-Alder process. While it may be argued that the Kishi route is more convergent than the Wehrli synthesis, both preparations require more than 40 linear steps. Among the highlights of the Kishi work is the intra-molecular furan Diels-Alder reaction that forms both the A or B or C or D ring system and the C13 quaternary centre in a single step. However, as in the Wehrli synthesis, successive functional group transformations quickly add to the overall length of the synthesis. Nevertheless, for its time, the Kishi synthesis stands as a notable achievement in natural products research.

## 21.8 BATRACHOTOXIN USES

Batrachotoxin inhibits sodium channel function in nerve and muscle cells as it tends to bind specifically to voltage-gated channels of sodium in nerves and membranes of muscle and thus obstruct the conveying of electrical impulses throughout the body. Because of its ability to keep voltage-gated sodium channels open as well as its actions at other ligand-binding sites, it is an essential research tool in pharmacology and clinical medical studies. It has been regularly used in research of ion channel and ligand. It is currently not used in medical clinical trials for two main reasons: its high toxicity and the risk of using it for clinical purposes. If it is to be used, then synthetic forms should be produced with alterations in properties for clinical trials. Secondly, no commercial sources are available for batrachotoxins and no commercially viable synthetic pathways.

## 21.9 CONCLUSION

Batrachotoxins are steroidal alkaloid neurotoxins extracted from Colombian poison-dart frogs skins which belong to *Phyllobates* genus. Several researchers have proved the hypothesis stating that *Phyllobates* frogs acquire these batrachotoxins from the dietary sources and not produced inside their body. Batrachotoxin diffuses inside cell membranes and stimulates voltage-gated sodium ion channels of nerve, muscle, and heart. A number of naturally found batrachatoxins have been identified in frogs and birds and the prime most toxins are batrachotoxin and homobatrachotoxin that consist of a pyrrole ring. Gradually, the structures of these batrachotoxins were elucidated by the scientists. Batrachotoxin has proved to be an important research tool due to its strong binding towards voltage-gated sodium channels. Several studies have been published confirming the action of batrachotoxin on the voltage-gated sodium channel and this has further helped to widely study the mechanism of action with different alterations. However, due to its highly toxic nature, batrachotoxin has no clinical usage but it is extensively used to study batrachotoxin receptor sites in the sodium channel.

## REFERENCES

Albuquerque, E. X. and Daly, J. W. 1976. Batrachotoxin, a selective probe for channels modulating sodium conductances in electrogenic membranes. In *Receptors and Recognition*, ed. P. Cuatrecasas, London: Chapman and Hall Press, pp. 299–336.

Albuquerque, E. X., Daly, J. W. and Witkop, B. 1971. Batrachotoxin: Chemistry and pharmacology. *Science*, 172: 995–1002.

Albuquerque, E. X., Seyama, I. and Narahashi, T. 1973. Characterization of batrachotoxin induced depolarization of the squid giant axons. *Journal of Pharmacology and Experimental Therapeutics*, 184: 308–314.

Brown, G. B. 1988. Batrachotoxin: A window on the allosteric nature of the voltage-sensitive sodium channel. *International Review of Neurobiology*, 29: 7–116.

Brown, G. B. and Bradley, R. J. 1985. Batrachotoxinin-A N-methylanthranilate, a new fluorescent ligand for voltage-sensitive sodium channels. *Journal of Neuroscience Methods*, 13: 119–129.

Casebolt, T. L. and Brown, G. B. 1993. Batrachotoxinin-A-ortho-azidobenzoate: A photoaffinity probe of the batrachotoxin binding site of voltage-sensitive sodium channels. *Toxicon*, 31: 1113–1122.

Catterall, W. A. 1975. Activation of the action potential sodium ionophore of cultured neuroblastoma cells by veratridine and batrachotoxin. *Journal of Biological Chemistry*, 250: 4053–4059.

Catterall, W. A. 1980. Neurotoxins that act on voltage-sensitive sodium channels in excitable membranes. *Annual Review of Pharmacology and Toxicology*, 20: 15–43.

Catterall, W. A. 1992. Cellular and molecular biology of voltage-gated sodium channels. *Physiological Reviews*, 72 (Supplement): S15–S48.

Creveling, C. R. and Daly, J. W. 1992. Batrachotoxin A [$^3$H] benzoate binding to sodium channels. *Methods in Neuroscience*, 8: 25–37.

Daly, J. and Witkop, B. 1971. Batrachotoxin, an extremely active cardio- and neurotoxin from the Colombian arrow poison frog *Phyllobates aurotaenia*. *Clinical Toxicology*, 4: 331–342.

Daly, J., Myers, C., Warnick, J. and Albuquerque, E. 1980. Levels of batrachotoxin and lack of sensitivity to its action in poison-dart frogs (*Phyllobates*). *Science*, 208: 1383–1385.

Daly, J. W. and Spande, T. F. 1986. *Alkaloids: Chemical and Biological Perspectives*, ed. S. W. Pelletier, New York, Wiley, Vol. 4, pp. 1–254.

Daly, J. W., Witkop, B., Bommer, P. and Biemann, K. 1965. Batrachotoxin-The active principle of the Colombian arrow ppoison frog, *phyllobates bicolor*. *Journal of the American Chemical Society*, 87: 124–126.

Daly, J. W., Myers, C. W., Warnick, J. E. and Albuquerque, E. X. 1980. Levels of batrachotoxin and lack of sensitivity to its action in poison-dart frogs (*Phyllobates*). *Science*, 208: 1383–1385.

Daly, J. W., Secunda, S. I., Garraffo, H. M., Spande, T. F., Wisnieski, A. and Cover, J. F. 1994. An uptake system for dietary alkaloids in poison frogs (*Dendrobatidae*). *Toxicon*, 32: 657–663.

Daly, J. W., Garraffo, H. M. and Spande, T. F. 1999. Alkaloids from amphibian skins. In *Alkaloids: Chemical and Biological Perspectives*, ed. S. W. Pelletier, New York, Wiley, Vol. 13, pp. 1–161.

Dobler, S., Petschenka, G. and Pankoke, H. 2011. Coping with toxic plant compounds: The insect's perspective on iridoid glycosides and cardenolides. *Phytochemistry*, 72: 1593–1604.

Dumbacher, J. P., Beehler, B. M., Spande, T. F., Garraffo, H. M. and Daly, J. W. 1992. Homobatrachotoxin in the genus Pitohui: chemical defense in birds? *Science*, 258: 799–801.

Dumbacher, J. P., Spande, T. F. and Daly, J. W. 2000. Batrachotoxin alkaloids from passerine birds: A second toxic bird genus (*Ifritakowaldi*) from New Guinea. *Proceedings of the National Academy of Sciences of the United States of America*, 97: 12970–12975.

Dumbacher, J. P., Wako, A., Derrickson, S. R., Samuelson, A., Spande, T. F. and Daly, J. W. 2004. Melyrid, beetles (Choresine): A putative source for the batrachotoxin alkaloids found in poison-dart frogs and toxic passerine birds. *Proceedings of the National Academy of Sciences of the United States of America*, 101: 15857–15860.

Finol-Urdaneta, R. K., McArthur J. R., Goldschen, M. P., Gaudet, R., Tikhonov, D. B., Zhorov, B. S. and French, R. J. 2019. Batrachotoxin acts as a stent to hold open homotetrameric prokaryotic voltage-gated sodiumchannels. *Journal of General Physiology*, 151: 186–199.

Grinsteiner, T. J. and Kishi, Y. 1994. Synthetic studies towards batrachotoxin 2. Formation of the oxazepane ring system via a Michael reaction. *Tetrahedron Letters*, 35: 8337–8340.

Imhof, R., Gossinger, M. E., Graf, W., Berner, H., Berner-Fenz, M. L. and Wehrli, H. 1972. Steroids and sex hormones. Part 245. Partial synthesis of batrachotoxinin A. Preliminary communication. *Helvetica ChimicaActa,* 55(4): 1151–1153.

Khodorov, B. I., Yelin, E. A., Zaborovskaya, L. D., Maksudov, M. Z., Tikhomirova, O. B. and Leonov, V. N. 1992. Comparative analysis of the effects of synthetic derivatives of batrachotoxin on sodium currents in frog node of Ranvier. *Cellular and Molecular Neurobiology*, 12: 59–81.

Kongsamut, S., Freedman, S. B., Simon, B. E. and Miller, R. J. 1985. Interaction of steroidal alkaloid toxins with calcium channels in neuronal cell lines. *Life Sciences,* 36(15): 1493–1501.

Kurosu, M., Marcin, L. R., Grinsteiner, T. J. and Kishi, Y. 1998. Total synthesis of (±)-batrachotoxinin A. *Journal of the American Chemical Society*, 120: 6627–6628.

Li, H. L., Hadid, D. and Ragsdale, D. S. 2002. The batrachotoxin receptor on the voltage-gated sodium channel is guarded by the channel activation gate. *Molecular Pharmacology*, 61: 905–912.

Linford, N. J., Cantrell, A. R., Qu, Y., Scheuer, T. and Catterall, W. A. 1998. Interaction of batrachotoxin with the local anesthetic receptor site in transmembrane segment IVS6 of the voltage-gated sodium channel. *Proceedings of the National Academy of Sciences USA*, 95: 13947–13952.

Marki, F. and Witkop, B. 1963. The venom of the Colombian arrow poison frog *Phyllobates* bicolor. *Experientia*, 19: 329–376.

Marquez, R., Ramirez-Castaneda, V. and Amezquita, A. 2018. Does batrachotoxinautoresistance coevolve with toxicity in *Phyllobates* poison-dart frogs? *The Society for the Study of Evolution*, 73: 390–400.

Myers, C. W., Daly, J. W. and Malkin, B. 1978. A dangerously toxic new frog (*Phyllobates*) used by Embera Indians of Western Colombia with discussion of blowgun fabrication and dart poisoning. *Bulletin of the American Museum of Natural History*, 161.

Narahashi, T. 1974. Chemicals as tools in the study of excitable membranes. *Physiological Reviews*, 54: 813–889.

Narahashi, T., Albuquerque, E. X. and Deguchi, T. 1971. Effects of batrachotoxin on membrane potential and conductance of squid giant axons. *Journal of General Physiology*, 58: 54–70.

Neuwirth, M., Daly, J. W., Myers, C. W. and Tice, L. W. 1979. Morphology of the granular secretory glands in skin of poison-dart frogs (*Dendrobatidae*). *Tissue and Cell*, 11: 755–771.

Saporito, R. A., Spande, T. F., Garraffo, H. M. and Donnelly, M. A. 2009. Arthropod alkaloids in poison frogs: A review of the dietary hypothesis. *Heterocycles*, 79: 277–297.

Strichartz, G., Rando, T. and Wang, G. K. 1987. An integrated view of the molecular toxinology of sodium channel gating in excitable cells. *Annual Review of Neuroscience*, 10: 237–267.

Tokuyama, T., Daly, J., Witkop, B., Karle, I. L. and Karle, J. 1968. The structure of batrachotoxin A, a novel steroidal alkaloid from the Colombian arrow poison frog, *Phyllobates aurotaenia*. *Journal of the American Chemical Society*, 90: 1917–1918.

Tokuyama, T., Daly, J. and Witkop, B. 1969. The structure of batrachotoxin, a steroidal alkaloid from the Colombian arrow poison frog, *Phyllobates aurotaenia*, and partial synthesis of batrachotoxin and its analogs and homologs. *Journal of the American Chemical Society*, 91: 3931–3938.

Trainer, V. L., Brown, G. B. and Catterall, W. A. 1996. Site of covalent labeling by a photoreactive batrachotoxin derivative near trans membrane segment IS6 of the sodium channel subunit. *Journal of Biological Chemistry*, 271: 11261–11267.

Wang, S. Y. and Wang, G. K. 2003. Voltage-gated sodium channels as primary targets of diverse lipid-soluble neurotoxins. *Cell Signal*, 15: 151–159.

Wang, S. Y. and Wang, G. K. 2017. Single rat muscle $Na^+$ channel mutation confers batrachotoxin auto resistance found in poison-dart frog *Phyllobates terribilis*. *Proceedings of the National Academy of Sciences*, 114: 10491–10496.

Warnick, J. E., Albuquerque, E. X. and Sansone, F. M. 1971. The pharmacology of batrachotoxin. I. Effects on the contractile mechanism and on neuromuscular transmission of mammalian skeletal muscle. *Journal of Pharmacology and Experimental Therapeutics*, 176: 497–510.

Warnick, J. E., Albuquerque, E. X., Onur, R., Jansson, S. E., Daly, J. W., Tokuyama, T. and Witkop, B. 1975. The pharmacology of batrachotoxin. VII. Structure-activity relationships and the effects of pH. *The Journal of Pharmacology and Experimental Therapeutics*, 193: 232–245.

Werman, R. and Grundfest, H. 1961. Graded and all-or-none electrogenesis in arthropod muscle. II. The effects of alkali-earth and onium ions on lobster muscle fibers. *Journal of General Physiology*, 44: 997–1027.

CHAPTER 22

# Conotoxin

**Avinash Kumar Jha, Muzamil Ahmad Rather, Mukesh S. Sikarwar, Subhamoy Dhua, Panchi Rani Neog, Rajeev Ranjan, Somya Singhal, Abhinay Shashank, and Arun Kumar Gupta**

## CONTENTS



DOI: 10.1201/9781003178446-22

## 22.1 INTRODUCTION

Conotoxins are invaluable, disulfide-rich neuroactive peptides targeting neuronal receptors, most of the G protein-coupled receptors (GPCRs), several ion channels, and enzymes. They are obtained from the venom produced by the epithelial secretory cells of more than 750 marine snails of the genus *Conus* (Dao et al. 2017). Although the terms conopeptide and conotoxin are nowadays interchangeable, there are two categories of conopeptides on the bases of disulfide-bonds, *viz.*, a) disulfide-poor peptides, which include contulakins, conolysins, conophans, contryphans, conomap, conantokins, conorfamides, conomarphins, and conopressins; and b) disulfide-rich (containing multiple disulfide bonds) peptides referred as conotoxins (Akondi et al. 2014). Each species of genus *Conus* can secrete about 1,000 conotoxins and it has been reported that over 1,000,000 conopeptides are being secreted by cone snails (Davis et al. 2009). The conotoxins are structurally stable, small in size, and possess high target specificity that makes them an ideal candidate for validation of target and discovery of peptide drugs. Generally, conotoxins consist of 2–4 or more disulfide bonds and a sequence of 10–40 amino acid residues. In the Endoplasmic reticulum (ER) and Golgi apparatus, their RNA-encoded precursor proteins are transported and processed into mature peptides. The conopeptide precursor contains three important regions a) highly conserved ER signal region, b) variable mature peptide region, and c) pro-region (Yang and Zhou 2020; Fu et al. 2018). Post-transcriptional modifications (PTMs), bromylation of tryptophan, hypermutation, C-terminal α-carboxamidation, mutation-induced premature termination, γ-carboxylation of glutamate, stereochemical inversion of specific L-amino acids to D-amino acids and fragment insertion/deletion of conotoxin-encoding transcripts are collectively responsible for the stability, potency, efficacy, and diversity of conotoxins (Lu et al. 2014; Craik and Adams 2007). On the bases of disulfide connectivity and N-terminal precursor sequence, conotoxins have been classified into 16 superfamilies *viz.*, A, D, I1, I2, I3, J, L, M, O1, O2, O3, P, S, T, V, and on the basis of cysteine organization, Y has been further categorised into multiple families (Dao et al. 2017). On the basis of their affinity for ion channels, they have been classified as calcium channel-targeted conotoxins (Ca-conotoxins), potassium channel-targeted conotoxins (K-conotoxins), and sodium channel-targeted conotoxins (Na-conotoxins) (Ramirez et al. 2017).

Conotoxins as voltage-gated calcium channel (VGCC) modulators may be used in the development of potent drugs to treat neuropathic pain (Adams and Berecki 2013). Similarly, conotoxins could be used to inhibit voltage-gated sodium channels (VGSCs, $Na_vS$) to act as local anaesthetic. μ–, δ–, ι–, μO–, and μO§– conotoxins are five pharmacologically different conotoxins targeting VGSCs and could be promising agents for the development of next-generation analgesics (Morales Duque et al. 2019; Abraham et al. 2017). It has been reported that μ–conotoxins act as channel or pore blockers as they bind to site 1 on VGSCs, thus showing promising analgesic potential in different animal models of acute, inflammatory, and neuropathic pain (Durek and Craik 2015). Likewise, μO– conotoxins bind at or near neurotoxin site II and inactive voltage sensor in domain II, and thus act as long-lasting analgesic in neuropathic and inflammatory pain (Munasinghe and Christie 2015). Conotoxins bind to nicotinic acetylcholine receptors (nAChRs), which are ligand-gated synaptic transmitters in the central and peripheral nervous systems (Lebbe et al. 2014). By attaching efficiently to the acetylcholine ligand-binding site, α-conotoxins display antagonistic competition. As these receptors mediate wide range of biological processes, α-conotoxins have been proposed for usage as plant insecticides and muscle relaxants., diagnostic agents, as well as therapeutic targets for curing cardiovascular disorders, drug addiction, cancer, and pain (Durek and Craik 2015). The structural variety, distribution, biochemistry, and toxicity of conotoxins are discussed in this chapter. The chapter also discusses the mechanism of action, safety, and preventive measures, as well as their extensive therapeutic uses.

## 22.2 CHEMISTRY

Conopeptides, initially translated as prepropeptide precursors are genetically encoded small proteins consists of a signal sequence (i.e., "pre" region) followed by a "pro" region, and at mature toxin region is represented by the C-terminal part. An enzymatic cleavage generates the pharmacologically active peptide in the C-terminal part of the prepropeptide (Terlau and Olivera 2004).

The precursors synthesized from conotoxins are composed of a typical structure having three domains which includes: 1) hydrophobic N-terminal signal region which is highly conserved (towards the cellular secretory pathway and the endoplasmic reticulum conotoxin precursor is guided); 2) an intervening propeptide region which is moderately conserved (for some conotoxins participates in post-translational modification, folding and secretion) (Buczek et al. 2004); and 3) a C-terminal region, (comprising mature functional peptide) (Kaas et al. 2010). The signal region's conserved sequence profiles are used to classify the conotoxin precursors into 40–50 protein superfamilies (with alphabet letters they are named originally) (Puillandre et al. 2012; Lavergne et al. 2013; Robinson et al. 2014; Li et al. 2017). Furthermore, despite the fact that the majority of these protein superfamilies contain more than one cysteine framework, sequence comparison of mature peptides reveals conotoxin precursor superfamilies connected with 26 conserved cysteine frameworks identified by Roman numerals (Lavergne et al. 2015; Robinson et al. 2014; Lavergne et al. 2015). However, certain mature peptides are cysteine-deficient or entirely lacking in cysteines (Abalde et al. 2018).

The connections between organisms mediated by well-known conotoxin hyperdiversity, which is characteristic of gene families (Barghi et al. 2015a), can be explained by a combination of various (evolutionary) processes: 1) duplication of gene in an extensive manner (Puillandre et al. 2010; Chang and Duda 2012); 2) rate of mutation is high and mature domain selection is diversifying (Conticello et al. 2001,3); 3) events of recombination (Espiritu et al. 2001; Wu et al. 2013); and 4) peptide processing is variable (Dutertre et al. 2013) and post-translational modifications (Lu et al. 2014; Abalde et al. 2018).

To date, the majority of identified conotoxins contain disulfide bonds between cysteine residues, which confer resistance against proteolytic degradation and structural stability (Safavi-Hemami et al. 2018). However, cysteines are not contained in all conotoxins and therefore, it has been suggested to be classified into two groups: (1) rich-cysteine (more than one disulfide bond is contained) and (2) poor-cysteine (no or only one disulfide bond is contained). The latter group was named by the term "conopeptide". Conotoxins are broadly classified into distinct groups based on three biochemical and pharmacological features: their gene superfamily (Latin letters are used to designate them), their cysteine framework (Roman numerals are used to designate them) and their pharmacological target and activity (Greek letters are used to designate them). Five pharmacological types of conotoxins with all target ion channels have been explored in the neurological and locomotor systems: μ (inhibits voltage-gated sodium channels, VGSC), κ (inhibits voltage-gated potassium channels, VGKC), ω (inhibits voltage-gated calcium channels, VGCC), α (inhibits nAChR), and δ (delays the activation of voltage-gated sodium channels, VGSC) (Table 22.1). Greek letter designation is not given to all pharmacological classes of conotoxins. As a result, their phenotypic impact in mice (e.g., sleep-like condition in mice produced by toxin termed Conantokins, Filipino word for sleep, "antok" is used to name it) or similarities to other peptides are utilised to name them or sequence homology (Bjørn-Yoshimoto et al. 2020).

Conotoxin sequence diversity has been discovered by liquid chromatography, fractionation, second-generation sequencing, Edman degradation, and mass spectroscopy. It has been reported that conotoxins depict several post-transcriptional modifications (PTMs) as well. The PTMs imparts structural and functional variability to conotoxins (Buczek et al. 2005). Between cysteine residues, the cross-linked disulfide-bond formation is one such PTM that influences protein structure.

**Table 22.1 Pharmacological Families of Conotoxins**

| Sl. No. | Pharmacological Family | Molecular Target | Molecular Mechanism | Reference Conotoxin | Reference |
|---|---|---|---|---|---|
| 1. | α (alpha) | Nicotinic acetylcholine receptors (nAChR) | Receptor antagonists | GI | Cruz et al. (1978) |
| 2. | γ (gamma) | Neuronal pacemaker cation Channels | Channel activator, potentially indirect effect | PnVIIA | Fainzilber et al. (1998) |
| 3. | δ (delta) | Voltage-gated Na channel | Delay channel inactivation | PVIA | Shon et al. (1995) |
| 4. | ι (iota) | Voltage-gated Na channels | Channel activators | RXIA | Jimenez et al. (2003) |
| 5. | κ (kappa) | Voltage-gated K channels | Channel blockers | PVIIA | Terlau et al. (1996) |
| 6. | σ (sigma) | 5-hydroxytryptamine 3 receptor (HTR3A) | Receptor antagonist | GVIIIA | England et al. (1998) |
| 7. | τ (tao) | Somatostatin receptor (SSTR) | Receptor antagonist | CnVA | Petrel et al. (2013) |
| 8. | χ (chi) | Norepinephrine Transporter | Inhibitor | MrIA | Sharpe et al. (2001) |
| 9. | Φ (phi) | Promotes cell proliferation | Not determined | MiXXVIIA | Jin et al. (2017) |
| 10. | Conantokins | N-methyl-D-aspartate receptor (NMDAR) | Receptor antagonists | Conantokin-G | Olivera et al. (1985) |
| 11. | Coninsulins | Insulin receptor | Receptor agonists | Con-Insulin G1 | Safavi-Hemami, et al. (2015) |

Adapted from Olivera et al. 2015; Bjørn-Yoshimoto et al. 2020

Conotoxins' chemical diversity is due to a variety of changes, including glutamate-carboxylation, proline hydroxylation, and C-terminal amidation, in addition to disulfide bond formation (Akondi et al. 2014). Thus, the diversity of conotoxins at the protein level could be attributed to many factors including PTMs, conservative bioactive propeptide regions (Dutertre et al. 2013), transcriptomics at the gene level (Jin et al. 2013) and differential processing of conotoxins (Dutertre et al. 2013).

The NMR spectroscopy is performed to determine the structural diversity of conotoxins. On the bases of disulfide cross-links spatial position and shapes four different groups commonly referred to 'fold classes' (A-D) have been reported. Folds with four cysteine residues includes a) "fold A" having globular disulfide connectivity [1–3, 2–4] and cysteine Framework I (CC-C-C) (Muttenthaler et al. 2011) and b) "fold D" with ribbon like structures with four cysteine and connectivity [1–4, 2–3] (Dutton et al. 2002). Whereas folds having six residues includes a) "fold B" having cysteine Framework III and similar in shape to fold A however, disulfide bonds spatial arrangement is different (Poppe et al. 2012) and b) "fold C" is like fold B having same disulfide-bond connectivity (1–4, 2–5, 3–6) but exhibit cysteine knots due to the knotted arrangement of disulfide bonds (Gracy et al. 2007; Akondi et al. 2014).

## 22.3 DISTRIBUTION AND ECOLOGY OF CONOTOXIN

In the environments of tropical Indo-Pacific reef, *Conus* (marine invertebrate's most diverse genus) substantially contribute to the massive biodiversity (Kohn 1978). The toxicology and morphology of genus *Conus* is evidence of speciation and rich endemism (Rockel et al. 1995). Throughout all tropical oceans *Conus* is widely distributed and it comprises one quarter of earth's ocean area (Hubbss 1974), however, specifically in the Indo-Pacific region, their 60% (approx.) habitation occurs. More than 20 species have been seen on reef platforms, but just 27 species have been seen in Indonesia (Kohn and Nybakken 1975; Kohn 1990). In recent investigations, Kohn has found 36 species on the reef platform that surrounds Laing Island and 32 species of *Conus* on four small reefs in Northeast Papua Guinea's Near Madang (Kohn 2001). In Dampier Archipelago's inner region, the dominant species in intertidal habitats are *Conus anemone* and *Conus victoriae*. Their recorded densities (estimated) were 0.2–2.6 and 0.1–0.3 individuals/10 $m^2$, respectively in favourable habitats. Predominantly, on limestone substrate or sand (specifically under rocks) both the species occurred (Kohn 2003; Kumar et al. 2015).

There are around 100 species found in the intertidal and subtidal sections of Indian beaches; however, sixteen of these species have yet to be validated due to a lack of sufficient information (Kohn 1978). *Conus generalis* and *Conus litoglyphus* were not considered as verified species however, being a native species of Indian Coastal waters, it is confirmed (Kohn 2003; Kohn 2001; Rockel et al. 1995). Based on IUCN study in 1996, *Conus nobrei*, *Conus africanus*, *Conus cepasi*, and *Conus zebroides* are vincible and *Conus kohni* remains data insufficient (Hammond et al. 2008; Kumar et al. 2015). Cone snails are divided into three families based on the prey they pursue: molluscivorous species (which hunt other gastropods), piscivorous species (which quickly paralyze and swallow fish), and vermivorous species (which hunt other vertebrates) (feed on polychaetes and other worms). About 75% of all cone snails are accounted by the vermivorous species, are predominant among those three groups of cone snails (Kohn and Perron 1994). However, close relationship between human beings and those cone snails drives people to be long focused on mollusc- and fish-hunting cone snails. In contrast, few studies have been performed on vermivorous species (Figure 22.1). According to recent research, a number of new conotoxin families found only in worm-hunting cone snails have substantial neuropharmaceutical activity (Kauferstein et al. 2004; Jiang et al. 2006). Vermivorous species might be logically claimed to have equal promising pharmaceutical treasuries (Pi et al. 2006).

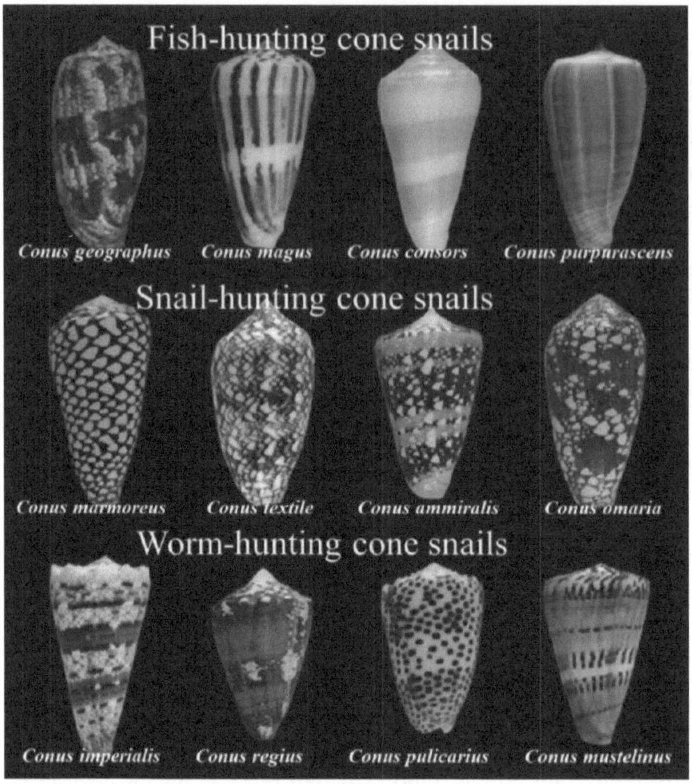


**Figure 22.1** Shells of nine subgenera of cone snail species. Shells not to scale. (Adapted from Bjørn-Yoshimoto et al. 2020.)

## 22.4 BIOLOGY OF *CONUS*

The importance of cone snail venom in foraging and defence strategies has ensured its survival (McDougal et al. 2008). The use of paralyzing neuronic peptide toxin's deadly combination makes Cone snail effective venomous predators of small fish, worms, and other molluscs. The gut content and faecal analyses have discovered the singular preferential prey choice (Kohn and Nybakken 1975; Kohn 1986) among all species, however, to categorize the numerous species into three important groups only a few have become the way, which generally provide their venom's projected threat level toward humans. The piscivorous class is considered as deadly to humans however, it contains the smallest number of species. Molluscivorous class is considered as dangerous due to their aggressive behaviour (although confirmed fatalities have not been implicated by some members) and it has a greater diversity of species. The main vermivorous class (which accounts for roughly 80% of the genus) is determined to be nonthreatening and timorous. Individual species have a tendency to specialise in areas where large numbers of congeners co-occur; nonetheless, diet variety is a genus level issue (Kohn 1978; Kohn 1986), and most *Conus* species hunt only one of the three types of prey indicated above (Kumar et al. 2015).

However, the diet of one prey category is less than a few species span. Among all *Conus* species *Conus californicus* exhibits a noticeable exception with the broadest diet which includes molluscs, fish (gastropods and bivalves included), crustaceans, and polychaetes (Kohn 1966). It has been observed that *Conus bullatus* (*C. bullatus*) feed on both molluscs and fish (Kohn 2001) as reported by Rockel et al. (1995). Also, prey on hemichordates, sedentary polychaetes, and errant polychaetes have been reported for various vermivorous species, including *Conus eburneus* (*C. eburneus*),

*C. arenatus*, *C. lividus*, *C. miliaris*, and *C. sponsalis* in several geographic locations. Moreover, *C. eburneus* and *C. tessulatus* occasionally prey on fishes as well (Kumar et al. 2015).

Geometric morphometric techniques have been used in systematic biology study and this technique allows direct quantification and variation analysis in biological shape. Geometric morphometric examination of shell shape variation in *Conus spp.* reveals the efficacy of geometric morphometric methods in capturing interspecific changes in shell form (Cruz et al. 2012). Around 30 recorded fatalities have caused by human envenomation [majorly by piscivorous *Conus geographus* (*C. geographus*)]. The first recorded death due to envenomation was attributed to molluscivorous *Conus* textile in 1705 (Rumphine 1999), but additional envenomations (including fatalities) are believed to have gone unreported due to the growing popularity of ornamental cone shells around the world. As a result, it must be underlined that collecting live cone snails from the wild is a risky endeavour that necessitates prior experience, meticulous attention to species ethology, and accurate identification (Bingham et al. 2014; Kumar et al. 2015).

## 22.5 MECHANISM OF ACTION OF CONOTOXIN

The different mechanism action of conotoxin is shown in Figure 22.2.

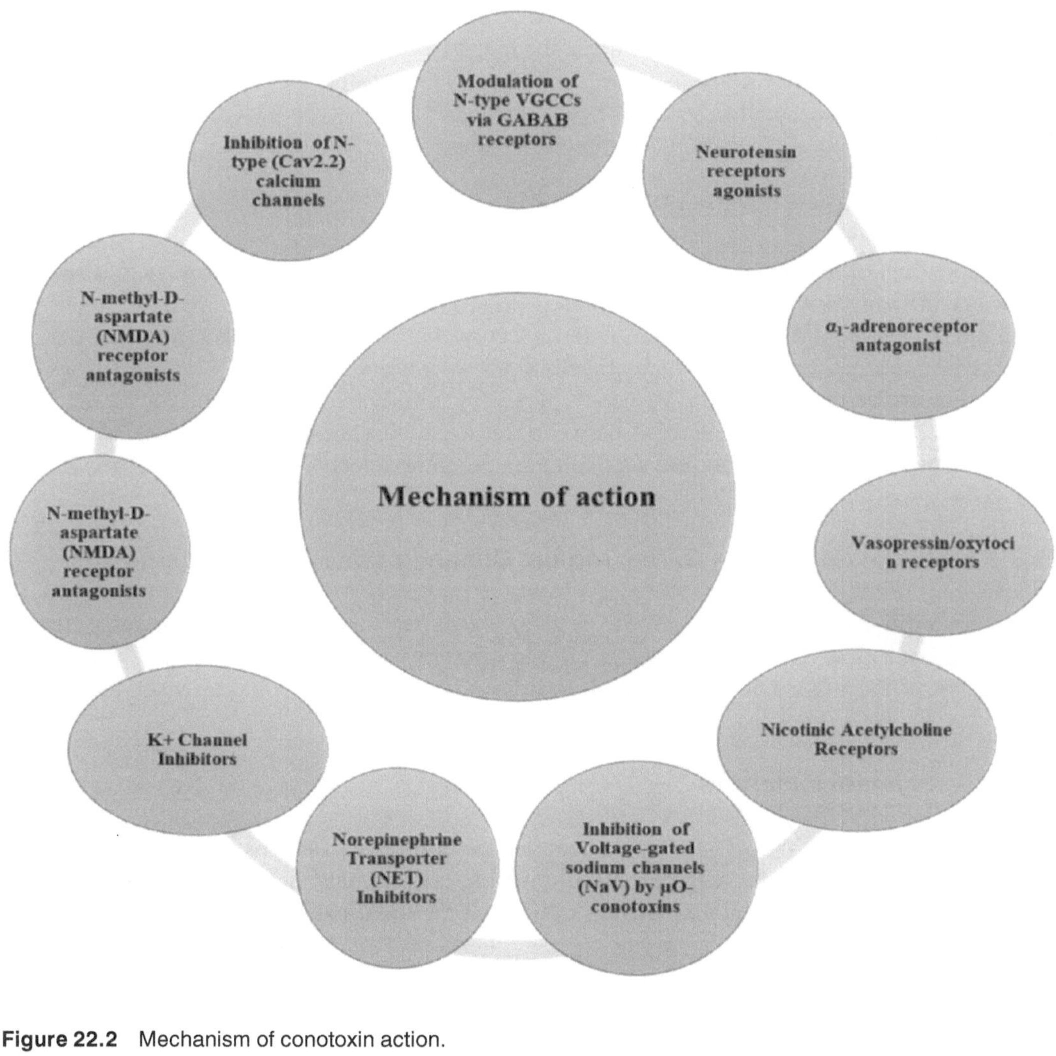


**Figure 22.2** Mechanism of conotoxin action.

### 22.5.1 Inhibition of N-Type (Cav2.2) Calcium Channels

This pathway helps to regulate calcium homeostasis and consequently plays a crucial role in pain processing by transferring electrical activity into other cellular processes. It may be possible to treat neuropathic pain with N-type VGCC modulators or inhibitors. N-type VGCCs are selectively inhibited by conotoxins. VGCCs targeted by the ω-conotoxins are exclusively of the N type, while the α-conotoxins also block VGCCs that are activated by G protein-coupled GABAB receptors. Important voltage-dependent and $Ca^{2+}$-dependent inactivation mechanisms are found in N-type calcium channels. A growing body of research involving recombinant N-type calcium channels has demonstrated that N-, P/Q-, and R-type channels differ in terms of how they shut off and what subunits do within the cell. The "ultra-slow" kinetics are partially regulated by the auxiliary β3 subunit, even when the cell is in the closed state (Adams and Berecki 2013).

### 22.5.2 Modulation of N-Type VGCCs via GABAB Receptors

The μ-conotoxins have amino acid chains coupled to a disulfide-bonded cysteine structure with two connected side chains, such as a C-1 to C-3 and C-2 to C-4. Vc1.1, RgIA, and PeIA are -conotoxins, which are powerful antagonists of 910 nAChRs found in both neuronal and non-neuronal cells. The Vc1.1 and RgIA do not interact with N-type VGCCs directly or through unique G protein-coupled GABABR-mediated pathway (Cav2.2). GPCR-mediated modulation of N-type VGCCs, which are regulated by the src tyrosine kinase activity, is principally responsible for controlling these voltage-independent intracellular pathways. It has been established that N-type VGCC modulators can be used as pain medications for neuropathic disorders (Adams and Berecki 2013).

### 22.5.3 Nicotinic Acetylcholine Receptors

The composition of nAChRs is variable in the pathophysiology of many neurological disorders. While crystallizing with acetylcholine binding protein in a co-crystallization experiment, the conotoxins displayed a distinct orientation in the acetylcholine binding pocket. Many of the participants in this study made significant contributions to conserved hydrophobic interactions and to a protein involved in the biotransformation of Acetylcholine. Because of the electrostatic interactions and hydrogen bonds generated between the α-conotoxin and the Nicotinic cholinergic receptor subunits, different nicotinic acetylcholine receptor selectivity profiles emerged (Lebbe et al. 2014).

### 22.5.4 Inhibition of Voltage-Gated Sodium Channels (NaV) by μO-Conotoxins

Both scorpion β-toxins and μO-conotoxin lead to "blocking" of NaV channels to some degree. However, μO-conotoxins are only capable of "resting state voltage sensor trapping. The voltage dependency of the μO-conotoxin action shows that the toxin has a voltage sensor mechanism (Leipold et al. 2007).

### 22.5.5 $K^+$ Channel Inhibitors

Both scorpion β-toxins and μO-conotoxin lead to "blocking" of NaV channels to some degree. However, μO-conotoxins are only capable of "resting state voltage sensor trapping". The voltage dependency of the μO-conotoxin action shows that the toxin has a voltage sensor mechanism (Leipold et al. 2007).

### 22.5.6 N-Methyl-D-Aspartate (NMDA) Receptor Antagonists

Conantokin G (Con G) is a substance discovered in the venom of the marine cone snail that blocks the NMDA receptor's activity. Con G selectively blocks NMDA receptors that contain the NR2B subunit. Con G was discovered to be an NMDA receptor subunit-specific competitive antagonist. Because Con G shows subunit selectivity, it may describe its favourable *in vivo* profile. The NMDA receptor specific inhibitors have therapeutic applications in managing pain (Donevan and McCabe 2000).

### 22.5.7 Neurotensin Receptors Agonists

Contulakin-G has a C-terminus that is very similar to glycosylated neurotensin, which is required for neurotensin receptor activation. While Contulakin-G has a lesser affinity and activity as an agonist for neurotensin receptors than glycosylated neurotensin, it shares a comparable sequence with glycosylated neurotensin. Contulakin-G is a weak agonist and has a longer half-life in the circulation and produces significantly less cell-surface receptor desensitization than other agonists (Lee et al. 2015).

### 22.5.8 Norepinephrine Transporter (NET) Inhibitors

An analogue of chi-MrIA interacts with NET predominantly through amino acids in the first loop, such as Tyr7, Lys8, and Leu9, which are present in an orientation that favours high affinity NET contact. Within the transporter, a huge hydrophobic pocket interacts with a second, smaller loop (Brust et al. 2009).

### 22.5.9 $\alpha_1$-Adrenoreceptor Antagonist

In addition to this, the predatory marine snail secretes a peptide called r-TIA into its venom. Tissue and cellular α1-adrenoreceptor antagonism to norepinephrine-evoked increases in cytosolic free $Ca^{2+}$ concentration and contractility is exhibited by ρ-TIA. Because of its antagonistic impact on the α1-adrenoreceptor-mediated contractile response, the peptide acts as a non-competitive antagonist, lowering the amount of norepinephrine required to fully activate the contractile response (Sharpe et al. 2003).

### 22.5.10 Vasopressin/Oxytocin Receptors

Conopressin-T is a V1a receptor antagonist, with selectivity that favours humans. Leu7 and Val9 replace Exocyclic tripeptide (Pro7 and Gly9) in conopressin-T. Despite conopressin-oxytocin-binding T's properties, a L7P counterpart had a higher affinity for the V1a receptor and a lower affinity for the V2. Dutertre et al. (2008) changed Gly9 with Val9 in oxytocin and vasopressin to see if the V1a receptor activation position would serve as an agonist/antagonist switch, and this position was found to be an agonist/antagonist switch at the V1a receptor.

## 22.6 TOXICOLOGY

This is currently considered to be the most famous conotoxin yet discovered (or ziconotide). It was first discovered at the University of Utah in 1982 after the venom of the magician cone

(*C. magus*) was extracted (McIntosh et al. 1982). Fish-hunting cone snail venom is believed to have paralytic properties, and ω-MVIIA was discovered in the course of that research (Figure 22.1). Neuromuscular transmission was blocked at the presynaptic terminus in fish thanks to the inhibition of ω-MVIIA, a specific voltage-gated calcium channel (Kerr and Yoshikami 1984; McCleskey et al. 1987). However, until the early 1980s, no one knew how many different voltage-gated calcium channels existed in the vertebrate nervous system. Understanding the operations of voltage-gated calcium channels was helped by isolating the ω-MVIIA and a related peptide from *C. geographus*, which provided pharmacological tools to distinguish between different types of voltage-gated calcium channels.

The peptides were especially selective for a previously identified calcium channel subtype (initially known as the N-type calcium channel, and later as Cav2.2). Specific binding to layers of the dorsal horn of the spinal cord, which has been demonstrated to be important for pain perception in the past (Todd 2010). Researchers were able to develop ω-MVIIA as an analgesic as a result of this discovery (Miljanich 2004; Bjorn-Yoshimoto et al. 2020).

Several conotoxins have been studied as potential treatments for pain, epilepsy, heart disease, and diabetes, but only -MVIIA is now in clinical trials (Safavi-Hemami et al. 2019; Pennington et al. 2018; Robinson and Safavi-Hemami 2017). None of these conotoxins have obtained clinical approval, despite their fascinating medicinal potential (yet). It is difficult to assess the underlying reasons for development when information on commercial developments of a drug is not made public (e.g., lack of efficacy in clinical trials, safety concerns, a change in a company's development programme) (Bjørn-Yoshimoto et al. 2020).

Most of these toxins have evolved into tools of modern pharmacology and biomedical science, regardless of their pharmaceutical development status (Bjørn-Yoshimoto et al. 2020).

Selective for a particular receptor subtype or subunit composition, depending on the conotoxin molecule. A beneficial feature had been presented for the use of conotoxins in various pharmacological, neuroscience, biochemistry, and structural biology research areas (Bjørn-Yoshimoto et al. 2020).

Also, the *vermivorous conus imperialis* (including the later discovered α-conotoxin, ImII) produced another example of α-conotoxin, ImI. (Ellison et al. 2003). The neuronal α7 subtype of the nAChRs is inhibited by ImI and ImII (Broxton et al. 1999). This form of conotoxin has been employed in a variety of studies, including disease and physiology, to emphasise the relevance of receptor subunits (Terlau and Olivera 2004; Giribaldi and Dutertre 2018). In addition, they have also seen other more specialised uses for these. Heghinian and colleagues studied *D. melanogaster* α7 nAChRs and used a variety of α-conotoxins to facilitate structural-guided mutations in this receptor to make it selective for certain conotoxins. The primary result of this was the creation of D. melanogaster cholinergic synapses that mimic vertebrate synapses, making the mutant flies better suited for the *in vivo* drug discovery process (Heghinian et al. 2015; Bjørn-Yoshimoto et al. 2020).

In a study conducted in 2015, Mei et al. (2015) used the specificity of α-ImI for targeting the chemotherapy drug, paclitaxel, to examine cellular components. According to the authors, when the micelles used to encapsulate paclitaxel were linked to α-ImI rather than unlinked paclitaxel-filled micelles or free paclitaxel, the tumour mass in mice was considerably reduced. The toxicity of the α-ImI-linked micelles in the body was found to be lower than expected.

Conotoxins have also been used to investigate the various methods of receptor activation and particular receptor binding sites in structural biology. The molecular mechanism behind receptor activation was also disclosed by the GluR2 AMPA receptor subunit complex and the X-ray crystal structure of the conotoxin con-ikot-ikot from *C. striatus* (Walker et al. 2009; Chen et al. 2014). Con-Insulin G1 is a conotoxin from *C. geographus* that has a minimal insulin binding motif in the human insulin receptor (Menting et al. 2016).

Conotoxins go through post-translational processing (folding and modification) in the ER and Golgi before being packaged and secreted into the venom gland.

Because of their small size, chemical variety, and high degree of post-translational modifications, conotoxins are good candidates for investigations on peptide folding, folding techniques, and secretion. Substrates including α-GI (Buczek et al. 2004), μ-SmIIIA (Safavi-Hemami et al. 2016), and conantokin-G (Safavi-Hemami et al. 2010; 2016) were used to investigate enzyme-assisted peptide production and folding (Bandyopadhyay et al. 1998; Bulaj et al. 2003).

To summarise, conotoxins have been used in a variety of studies looking at how dietary factors, prey taxa, age, and geographic diversity influence the evolution of venom genes, as well as studies looking at the effects of duplication and diversification, as well as positive selection on venom gene expression (Chang and Duda 2012; Puillandre et al. 2010; Safavi-Hemami et al. 2016; Phuong et al. 2016). To date, human fatalities from cone snail stings have been reported for more than 350 years. Over the past 141 years, at least 36 fatalities have been recorded (Kohn 2019). Hovering over 20 years, there have been no reported human casualties. Of the total number of 36 human fatalities resulting from cone snail stings, nearly all (97%) can be attributed to just one species, *C. geographus* (Kohn 2019). There have also been no reports of cone snail poison being utilised as a murder weapon. This was all accidental.

The symptoms that result from cone snail envenomation in humans vary depending on a number of factors, including the species of cone snail. Oedema, fatigue, faintness, loss of reflexes, vision impairment, dyspnoea, and nausea are reported to frequently occur, but symptoms can include pain, numbness, oedema, and swelling. Some victims of the sting report feeling a burning sensation near the site of the sting. However, the sting itself goes unnoticed to some of the victims. The following are additional common symptoms that occur in more severe cases: reports of light-headedness, dysphagia, ptosis of the eyelids, and poor vision and speech. Furthermore, there are no signs prior to the beginning of muscle paralysis, which, in the worst-case scenario, might result in death within a few hours owing to respiratory or cardiac arrest (Kizer 1983; Halford et al. 2015). No effective anti-venom is currently available for cone snail venom.

While only a small portion of cone snail venom is toxic to humans, the other venomous animals' venom may cause thousands of human envenomations. Snake bite is clearly the most important cause of human envenomation. Estimation places the number of annual snakebites at 2,700,000, which leads to 400,000 permanent disabilities, including amputations, and 81,000–138,000 deaths annually (Bjørn-Yoshimoto et al. 2020). Aside from the significant rise in human-snake encounters, there are a significant number of snakebite deaths. Contrary to cone snails, which do not pose a significant threat to human health and life, snake envenomation has clear and obvious dangers.

There are estimated to be more than 3,250 deaths from human envenomation each year due to scorpions, and scorpions are a significant contributor to human envenomation (Chippaux and Goyffon 2008). The eastern red scorpion, *Hottentotta tamulus*, is one of the deadliest stingers, with a death rate of 30% when left untreated. By adding an anti-hypertension drug, such as prazosin, the fatality rate can be lowered to between 2% and 4%. (Kularatne et al. 2015; Rodrigo and Gnanathasan 2017). Among the many beneficial applications of the poisonous cone snail are biomedical and biological research, research instruments, as well as medications and drug leads. Snake venom has produced a number of pharmaceuticals, including blood pressure medicines, clotting factors, and anti-coagulants, all of which have had a major impact on public health (Slagboom et al. 2017; Serrano 2013). Additionally, there has been extensive research on multiple scorpion venom components, such as novel peptide anti-microbial drugs, to investigate their possible biomedical applications (Ortiz et al. 2015).

## 22.7 CONOTOXIN TOXICITY

Cone snails, their venom, or toxin components have never been used for malicious purposes in real life, despite their portrayal as formidable murder weapons in fiction. This section contains studies on the toxicity of conotoxins used as weapons in fiction, as well as regulatory efforts aimed at limiting conotoxin research. The median $LD_{50}$ of several poisons and hazardous compounds is compared in Table 22.2.

**Table 22.2 Toxic Substance Comparison Based on $LD_{50}$**

| Sl. No. | Toxin | $LD_{50}$ in Mice (µg/kg) | Route of Administration | Type of Toxin | Source | Known Anti-Venom/ Antidote | Reference |
|---|---|---|---|---|---|---|---|
| 1. | α-conotoxin GI | 12 | IP | Peptide | *Conus geographus* | No | Cruz et al. (1978) |
| 2. | ω-conotoxin GVIA | ≈60 | IP | Peptide | *Conus geographus* | No | Suszkiw et al. (1989) |
| 3. | Volkensin | 1.38–1.73 | IP | Protein | *Adenia volkensii* | No | Stirpe et al. (1985) |
| 4. | Ciguatoxin-1 | 0.25 | IP and oral | Polycyclic poylethers | *Various dinoflagellates* | No | Lewis et al. (1991) |
| 5. | Maitotoxin | 0.13 | IP | Polycyclic poylethers | *Various dinoflagellates* | No | Yokoyama et al. (1988) |
| 6. | Palytoxin | 0.15 | IV | Polycyclic poylethers | Palythoa corals and dinoflagellates (or bacteria living on these) | No | Moore and Scheuer (1971) |
| 7. | Batrachotoxin | 2 | SC | Alkaloid | Various beetles, birds, and frogs | No | Tokuyama et al. (1968) |
| 8. | Saxitoxin | 10 | IP | Alkaloid | Various marine dinoflagellates | In guinea pigs # | Halstead and Schantz (1984) |
| 9. | Tetrodotoxin | 8 | IV | Alkaloid | Various marine bacteria (e.g., *Pseudoalteromonas tetraodonis*) symbiotically living with numerous marine animals, e.g., Tetraodontidae fish, Hapalochlaena octopodes, and Naticidae snails | No | Stonik and Stonik (2010) |

Because mice are the traditional testing method for conotoxins, the most potent toxins need to be found first (McIntosh et al. 1982; Gray et al. 1981). A toxin derived from *C. geographus* is an inhibitor of nicotinic acetylcholine receptors of the neuromuscular junction (McManus et al. 1981; Groebe et al. 1997). α-conotoxin GI of *C. geographus* envenomation results in the paralysis of muscle and the ultimate paralysis of the diaphragm, which results in respiratory arrest (Almquist et al. 1989). This toxin was originally written about over 40 years ago, and we know of no reports of its misuse thus far. The anti-convulsant α-conotoxin GII, contrary to popular assumption, has proved a useful study tool in neurology and biochemistry. The majority of Cone Snail toxins (which aren't harmful to humans) are found in the venom. The advantages of α-conotoxin GI and other *C. geographus* toxins include several pharmacological leads and biomedical tools, as well as one diagnostic agent. In addition to the large variety of biochemical targets in various species, a wide range of orders of magnitude has been covered by mammalian toxicity of a variety of conotoxins. A 12 µg/kg intraperitoneal (IP) injection of α-conotoxin GI yields a median Lethal Dose ($LD_{50}$, Lethal Dose 50%) of 12 µg/kg in mice (Cruz et al., 1978). On the neuromuscular junction, muscle-type nicotinic acetylcholine receptors are particularly vulnerable to α-conotoxins, which operate on muscle-type nicotinic acetylcholine receptors. Nonetheless, this category of -conotoxins (targeting nAChR subtypes in the nervous system and generating little to no toxicity in mammals) makes up a tiny subset of -conotoxins and a vanishingly small portion of all conotoxins. Due to their low toxicity, the $LD_{50}$ for practically all other conotoxins has never been measured. This includes not just many poisons from fish-hunting animals that have little to no effect on vertebrates, but also countless poisons from animals that hunt and consume them, such as snails and worms.

For instance, in the *C. geographus* snake's venom, the vasopressin-like toxin (conopressin-G) elicits a mouse-like grooming behaviour when injected into the brain and lowers blood sugar in fish by activating the fish's insulin-like toxins (coninsulins) (Ahorukomeye et al. 2019). For those who may have missed it, above it was stated that most of the α-conotoxins toxins are devoid of toxicity in mammals. α-conotoxin GIC, found in the species *C. geographus*, specifically targets neuronal nAChRs, and mice injected with doses of 5 nmol IP were unaffected (McIntosh et al. 2002).

Many conotoxins are harmful to humans, while others are generated in other species and are far less hazardous. Textilotoxin, a protein toxin found in the eastern brown snake *Pseudonaja textilis*, outperforms ciguatoxins and maitotoxins generated by dinoflagellate species by more than a factor of ten.

Furthermore, only when conotoxins are administered do they appear to be toxic. It has been attempted to increase the oral activity of conotoxin drug leads, although this has only been done using experimental delivery methods. To improve the oral bioactivity of -conotoxin Vc1.1, various modifications were explored. The analogue constructed illustrated that, regardless of route of administration, the most bioactive oral dosage was 1000-fold (approximately) less effective than injection dosage (Satkunanathan et al. 2005; Clark et al. 2010; Bjørn-Yoshimoto et al. 2020).

## 22.8 IDENTIFICATION AND QUANTIFICATION

Identification and quantification of various conotoxins is shown in Table 22.3.

### 22.8.1 Safety and Precautions

#### *22.8.1.1 Minimum Personal Protective Equipment (PPE)*

At the very least, personal protective equipment should include eye protection, a face shield, nitrile gloves, a respirator, and protective clothing.

**Table 22.3 Identification and Quantification of Various Conotoxins**

| Sr. No. | Conotoxin | Marine Drug Source | Identification/Quantification | References |
|---|---|---|---|---|
| 1. | T1-conotoxin | *C. bandanus* | Bn5a conotoxin possesses unique $C_1$-$C_4$/$C_2$-$C_3$ disulfide connectivity, unlike other T1-conotoxins ($C_1$-$C_3$/$C_2$-$C_4$) | Bao et al. (2020) |
| 2. | Conotoxins | *C. leopardus* | Novel Odd Number of Cysteine Residues | Rajesh and Franklin (2018) |
| 3. | kM-conotoxin RIIIK | *C. radiatus* | kM-conotoxin RIIIK, the first conotoxin to block human Kv1.2 potassium channels | Ferber et al. (2004) |
| 4. | Conotoxins | *C. betulinus* | 215 unique putative conopeptide transcripts from the combination of five transcriptomes and one EST sequencing dataset | Peng et al. (2016) |
| 5. | α-Conotoxin EI | *Conus spp.* | Identify crucial residues that are significantly affecting potency of E1 for mouse α1β1δε nAChR | Ning et al. (2019) |
| 6. | α-conotoxins | Cone snails | 16 α-conotoxins, as well as a pseudogene and three kappa A conotoxins, were identified from their genomic DNAs. | Yuan et al. (2007) |
| 7. | Conotoxins | *C. victoriae* | Discovered 100 unique conotoxin sequences from 20 gene superfamilies, two of the conotoxins identified showed cysteine frameworks not previously associated with their specific superfamily | Robinson et al. (2014) |
| 8. | Conotoxin GS | *C. geographus* | The established distribution of amino acid sidechains in the structure creates several polar and charged patches, and comparisons with -conotoxins provide a foundation for determining conotoxin GS polypeptide binding surface | Hill et al. (1997) |
| 9. | Conopeptides | *C. inscriptus* | Venom peptides showed 6 distinct molecular weight bands over 30 kDa following in-gel enzymatic digestion (37, 51, 60, 70, 80, and 90 kDa). The results showed that 29 proteins with disulfide connections of various molecular masses were scattered in the range of 387–1536 m/z. T-superfamily of conotoxins with 78 kDa heat shock proteins were the proteins that were noticed | Kumari et al. (2019) |
| 10. | V-superfamily conotoxins | *C. virgo* | Vi15a has a unique cysteine residue arrangement (C-C-CC-C-C-C-C), defining the new V-superfamily conotoxins | Peng et al. (2008) |

#### 22.8.1.2 Hazardous Warning Signs

"Caution" should be posted in the room where conotoxins/conopeptides are used.

#### 22.8.1.3 Safety while delivery of Conotoxins and Conopeptides

During shipment of conotoxins/conopeptides, it is mandatory to include the enclosed shipment specification sheet which contains quantity and date information. Any shipping damage should be noted and notified so that it can be decontaminated.

#### 22.8.1.4 Handling

A chemical that must be kept below the glove box/Class III biosafety cabinet temperature should be handled in a glove box or biosafety cabinet.

#### 22.8.1.5 *Storage*

In a secondary sealed container, upright, within a lockable freezer, a vial of conotoxins and conopeptides is placed.

### 22.8.2 Regulations Regarding Conotoxin Usage

Regulations of the federal government: The Federal Select Agent Program is a collaborative endeavour of the CDC's Division of Select Agents and the APHIS' Agricultural Select Agents Program, which is part of the Animal and Plant Health Inspection Service (APHIS). According to the CDC, of the conotoxins that have been discovered, only a minority are sufficiently toxic to pose a significant threat to human health. This subclass of conotoxin, which we call "short paralytic alpha conotoxins", have all of these characteristics, according to available data.

The CDC defines an entity as "any government agency (federal, state, or local), academic institution, corporation, company, partnership, society, association, firm, sole proprietorship, or other legal entity" that can store any of the short, paralytic α-conotoxins that are allowed by the select agent registry.

For disulfide-reduced conotoxin sequences lacking oxidised cysteines, or resin-bound synthetic peptides, there is no restriction on the amount of disulfide reduced conotoxin sequences that may be employed. No doubt, bioengineering of conotoxins has offered a whole new series of regulatory challenges. It is time to introduce a new regulatory approach for conotoxins.

Conotoxins are select agents, and are under federal regulation at part 73 of the Code of Federal Regulations. Informal Possession of select agent toxins above the maximum amount, as determined by the CDC, is a criminal offence.

The stingray *C. geographus* is believed to have a fatality rate of 65%, prompting biosecurity experts to speculate on possible weaponization and legislation that sets restrictions on research into specific conopeptide classes by the U.S. federal government. It is possible, however, that other conopeptides will turn out to be bioterrorism threats, as there is a vast space of chemicals and many of them have not been suspected of posing threats. Conopeptides have proven to be excellent templates for rational medication design in pain management, allowing researchers to better understand the physiological roles of their target proteins (Mansbach et al. 2019). More recently, the Danish Center of Biosecurity and Bio-preparedness has adopted the narrower definition of α-Conotoxins.

Conotoxins are short, paralysis inducing amino acid sequences that have the following chemical formula: X1CCX2PACGX3X4X5X6CX7, where C denotes cysteine residues with the 1st and 3rd cysteine linked via disulfide bridges; An amino acid can be any of the following: Asparagine, Histidine, Alanine, Glycine, Arginine, Lysine, Tyrosine, Phenylalanine, or Tryptophan. Some examples are Proline, Asparagine, Histidine, Lysine, Arginine, Tyrosine, Phenylalanine, or Tryptophan.

One such example would be until 2012, the United States' select agent list included "conotoxins". The prior assertion still applies, even though this version now eliminates paralytic α-conotoxins with a different sequence pattern that is connected to the sequence patterns seen in muscle-type nicotinic acetylcholine receptor blocking conotoxins.

An informal arrangement known as the "Australia Group" was established in 1985 to harmonise exports while minimizing the risk of these exports being used to assist in the proliferation of chemical and biological weapons. It's worth noting that even the most venomous cone snail species have never been subjected to legislation. Even when the term "conotoxins" is used to encompass all venom components, only the "conotoxin" components are regulated (Bjørn-Yoshimoto et al. 2020).

## 22.9 CONCLUSIONS AND FUTURE PERSPECTIVES

As discussed, conotoxins are peptides obtained from predatory cone snails that modulate numerous molecular receptors with high potency and selectivity. Due to decrease in translation of small molecules into drugs, scientists have shifted their paradigm of drug discovery towards natural products. In this regard conotoxins are becoming potent natural products for drug discovery due to their high diversity, potency, selectivity, specificity, lower cost and enhanced pharmacokinetics. Since conotoxins selectively inhibit and modulate different channels (sodium, calcium, potassium), and receptors (nicotinic acetylcholine, N-methyl-D-aspartate, neurotensin, and noradrenaline transporters), therefore, they could be used in the development of potent drugs to treat neuropathic pain, chronic pain, spasticity, neurodegenerative diseases, cancer, and cardiovascular diseases. As a result, more research, including spectroscopic structure elucidation of conotoxins, is urgently needed to better understand the function and therapeutic potential of conotoxins.

Although a huge number of cone snails and conopeptides provide an efficient field for drug discovery, their translation from research into application is still lagging. In this context, transcriptomics, proteomics, high-throughput omic and multi-omic techniques need to be prioritized to enhance conotoxin discovery, purification, and efficiency. Furthermore, machine learning approaches should be advanced for predicting peptide cleavage sites, position of disulfide bonds and target prediction. Over 8,000 peptide sequences of conotoxins have been already reported but most of the sequences (98%) lack 3-D structural and functional information that could be addressed by advancement in bioinformatics and genomics. From a clinical standpoint, conotoxins' inability to penetrate the blood–brain barrier necessitates intrathecal delivery, which has become a major roadblock to conotoxins' broad therapeutic use. Last but not the least the futuristic approach for enhancing their pharmacological properties lies in the development of re-engineered conotoxin analogues, and improving their *in vivo* stability and efficacy.

## REFERENCES

Abalde, S., Tenorio, M.J., Afonso, C.M. and Zardoya, R. 2018. Conotoxin diversity in *Chelyconus ermineus* (Born, 1778) and the convergent origin of piscivory in the Atlantic and Indo-Pacific cones. *Genome Biology and Evolution*, 10(10): 2643–2662.

Abraham, N., Healy, M., Ragnarsson, L., Brust, A., Alewood, P.F. and Lewis, R.J. 2017. Structural mechanisms for α-conotoxin activity at the human α3β4 nicotinic acetylcholine receptor. *Scientific Reports*, 7(1): 1–12.

Adams, D.J. and Berecki, G. 2013. Mechanisms of conotoxin inhibition of N-type (Cav2. 2) calcium channels. *Biochimica et Biophysica Acta (BBA)-Biomembranes*, 1828(7): 1619–1628.

Ahorukomeye, P., Disotuar, M.M., Gajewiak, J., Karanth, S., Watkins, M., Robinson, S.D., Salcedo, P.F., Smith, N.A., Smith, B.J., Schlegel, A. and Forbes, B.E. 2019. Fish-hunting cone snail venoms are a rich source of minimized ligands of the vertebrate insulin receptor. *Elife*, 8: 41574.

Akondi, K.B., Muttenthaler, M., Dutertre, S., Kaas, Q., Craik, D.J., Lewis, R.J. and Alewood, P.F. 2014. Discovery, synthesis, and structure–activity relationships of conotoxins. *Chemical Reviews*, 114(11): 5815–5847.

Almquist, R.G., Kadambi, S.R., Yasuda, D.M., Weitl, F.L., Polgar, W.E. and Toll, L.R. 1989. Paralytic activity of (des-Glu1) conotoxin GI analogs in the mouse diaphragm. *International Journal of Peptide and Protein Research*, 34(6): 455–462.

Bandyopadhyay, P.K., Colledge, C.J., Walker, C.S., Zhou, L.M., Hillyard, D.R. and Olivera, B.M. 1998. Conantokin-G precursor and its role in γ-carboxylation by a vitamin K-dependent carboxylase from a conussnail. *Journal of Biological Chemistry*, 273(10): 5447–5450.

Bao, N., Lecaer, J.P., Nghia, N.D. and Vinh, P.T.K., 2020. Isolation and structural identification of a new T1-conotoxin with unique disulfide connectivities derived from *Conus bandanus. Journal of Venomous Animals and Toxins Including Tropical Diseases*, 26: 1–9.

Barghi, N., Concepcion, G.P., Olivera, B.M. and Lluisma, A.O. 2015. Comparison of the venom peptides and their expression in closely related Conus species: Insights into adaptive post-speciation evolution of *Conus exogenomes. Genome Biology and Evolution*, 7(6): 1797–1814.

Bingham, J. P., Likeman, R. K., Hawley, J. S., Yu, P. Y. C., Halford, Z. A. 2014. Conotoxins. In: Liu, D., editor. *Manual of security sensitive microbes and toxins*. CRC Press.

Bjørn-Yoshimoto, W.E., Ramiro, I.B.L., Yandell, M., McIntosh, J.M., Olivera, B.M., Ellgaard, L. and Safavi-Hemami, H. 2020. Curses or cures: A review of the numerous benefits versus the biosecurity concerns of conotoxin research. *Biomedicines*, 235(8):1–22.

Broxton, N.M., Down, J.G., Gehrmann, J., Alewood, P.F., Satchell, D.G. and Livett, B.G. 1999. α-Conotoxin ImI inhibits the α-bungarotoxin-resistant nicotinic response in bovine adrenal chromaffin cells. *Journal of Neurochemistry*, 72(4): 1656–1662.

Brust, A., Palant, E., Croker, D.E., Colless, B., Drinkwater, R., Patterson, B., Schroeder, C.I., Wilson, D., Nielsen, C.K., Smith, M.T. and Alewood, D. 2009. χ-Conopeptide pharmacophore development: Toward a novel class of norepinephrine transporter inhibitor (Xen2174) for pain. *Journal of Medicinal Chemistry*, 52(22): 6991–7002.

Buczek, O., Bulaj, G. and Olivera, B.M. 2005. Conotoxins and the posttranslational modification of secreted gene products. *Cellular and Molecular Life Sciences CMLS*, 62(24): 3067–3079.

Buczek, O., Olivera, B.M. and Bulaj, G. 2004. Propeptide does not act as an intramolecular chaperone but facilitates protein disulfide isomerase-assisted folding of a conotoxin precursor. *Biochemistry*, 43(4): 1093–1101.

Bulaj, G., Buczek, O., Goodsell, I., Jimenez, E.C., Kranski, J., Nielsen, J.S., Garrett, J.E. and Olivera, B.M. 2003. Efficient oxidative folding of conotoxins and the radiation of venomous cone snails. *Proceedings of the National Academy of Sciences*, 100(suppl 2): 14562–14568.

Chang, D. and Duda Jr, T.F. 2012. Extensive and continuous duplication facilitates rapid evolution and diversification of gene families. *Molecular Biology and Evolution*, 29(8): 2019–2029.

Chen, L., Dürr, K.L. and Gouaux, E. 2014. X-ray structures of AMPA receptor–cone snail toxin complexes illuminate activation mechanism. *Science*, 345(6200): 1021–1026.

Chippaux, J.P. and Goyffon, M., 2008. Epidemiology of scorpionism: A global appraisal. *Acta Tropica*, 107(2): 71–79.

Clark, R.J., Jensen, J., Nevin, S.T., Callaghan, B.P., Adams, D.J. and Craik, D.J. 2010. Inside cover: The engineering of an orally active conotoxin for the treatment of neuropathic pain. *Angewandte Chemie*, 122 (37): 6606–6606.

Conticello, S.G., Gilad, Y., Avidan, N., Ben-Asher, E., Levy, Z. and Fainzilber, M. 2001. Mechanisms for evolving hypervariability: The case of conopeptides. *Molecular Biology and Evolution*, 18(2): 120–131.

Craik, D.J. and Adams, D.J. 2007. Chemical modification of conotoxins to improve stability and activity. *ACS Chemical Biology*, 2(7): 457–468.

Cruz, L.J., De Santos, V., Zafaralla, G.C., Ramilo, C.A., Zeikus, R., Gray, W.R. and Olivera, B.M. 1987. Invertebrate vasopressin/oxytocin homologs. Characterization of peptides from *Conus geographus* and *Conus straitus* venoms. *Journal of Biological Chemistry*, 262(33): 15821–15824.

Cruz, L.J., Gray, W.R. and Olivera, B.M. 1978. Purification and properties of a myotoxin from *Conus geographus* venom. *Archives of Biochemistry and Biophysics*, 190(2): 539–548.

Cruz, R.A.L., Pante, M.J.R. and Rohlf, F.J. 2012. Geometric morphometric analysis of shell shape variation in Conus (Gastropoda: Conidae). *Zoological Journal of the Linnean Society*, 165(2): 296–310.

Dao, F.Y., Yang, H., Su, Z.D., Yang, W., Wu, Y., Hui, D., Chen, W., Tang, H. and Lin, H. 2017. Recent advances in conotoxin classification by using machine learning methods. *Molecules*, 22(7): 1057.

Davis, J., Jones, A. and Lewis, R.J. 2009. Remarkable inter-and intra-species complexity of conotoxins revealed by LC/MS. *Peptides*, 30(7): 1222–1227.

Donevan, S.D. and McCabe, R.T. 2000. Conantokin G is an NR2B-selective competitive antagonist of N-methyl-d-aspartate receptors. *Molecular Pharmacology*, 58(3): 614–623.

Durek, T. and Craik, D.J. 2015. Therapeutic conotoxins: A US patent literature survey. *Expert Opinion on Therapeutic Patents*, 25(10): 1159–1173.

Dutertre, S., Croker, D., Daly, N.L., Andersson, Å., Muttenthaler, M., Lumsden, N.G., Craik, D.J., Alewood, P.F., Guillon, G. and Lewis, R.J. 2008. Conopressin-T from *Conus tulipa* reveals an antagonist switch in vasopressin-like peptides. *Journal of Biological Chemistry*, 283(11): 7100–7108.

Dutertre, S., Jin, A.H., Kaas, Q., Jones, A., Alewood, P.F. and Lewis, R.J. 2013. Deep venomics reveals the mechanism for expanded peptide diversity in cone snail venom. *Molecular & Cellular Proteomics*, 12(2): 312–329.

Dutton, J.L., Bansal, P.S., Hogg, R.C., Adams, D.J., Alewood, P.F. and Craik, D.J. 2002. A new level of conotoxin diversity, a non-native disulfide bond connectivity in α-conotoxin AuIB reduces structural definition but increases biological activity. *Journal of Biological Chemistry*, 277(50): 48849–48857.

Ellison, M., McIntosh, J.M. and Olivera, B.M. 2003. α-Conotoxins ImI and ImII: Similar α7 nicotinic receptor antagonists act at different sites. *Journal of Biological Chemistry*, 278(2): 757–764.

England, L.J., Imperial, J., Jacobsen, R., Craig, A.G., Gulyas, J., Akhtar, M., Rivier, J., Julius, D. and Olivera, B.M. 1998. Inactivation of a serotonin-gated ion channel by a polypeptide toxin from marine snails. *Science*, 281(5376): 575–578.

Espiritu, D.J.D., Watkins, M., Dia-Monje, V., Cartier, G.E., Cruz, L.J. and Olivera, B.M. 2001. Venomous cone snails: Molecular phylogeny and the generation of toxin diversity. *Toxicon*, 39(12): 1899–1916.

Fainzilber, M., Nakamura, T., Lodder, J.C., Zlotkin, E., Kits, K.S. and Burlingame, A.L. 1998. γ-Conotoxin-PnVIIA, a γ-carboxyglutamate-containing peptide agonist of neuronal pacemaker cation currents. *Biochemistry*, 37(6): 1470–1477.

Ferber, M., Al-Sabi, A., Stocker, M., Olivera, B.M. and Terlau, H. 2004. Identification of a mammalian target of κM-conotoxin RIIIK. *Toxicon*, 43(8): 915–921.

Fu, Y., Li, C., Dong, S., Wu, Y., Zhangsun, D. and Luo, S. 2018. Discovery methodology of novel conotoxins from Conus species. *Marine Drugs*, 16(11): 417.

Giribaldi, J. and Dutertre, S. 2018. α-Conotoxins to explore the molecular, physiological and pathophysiological functions of neuronal nicotinic acetylcholine receptors. *Neuroscience Letters*, 679: 24–34.

Gracy, J., Le-Nguyen, D., Gelly, J.C., Kaas, Q., Heitz, A. and Chiche, L. 2007. KNOTTIN: The knottin or inhibitor cystine knot scaffold in 2007. *Nucleic Acids Research*, 36(suppl_1): 314–D319.

Gray, W.R., Luque, A., Olivera, B.M., Barrett, J. and Cruz, L.J. 1981. Peptide toxins from *Conus geographus* venom. *Journal of Biological Chemistry*, 256(10): 4734–4740.

Groebe, D.R., Gray, W.R. and Abramson, S.N. 1997. Determinants involved in the affinity of α-conotoxins GI and SI for the muscle subtype of nicotinic acetylcholine receptors. *Biochemistry*, 36(21): 6469–6474.

Halford, Z.A., Yu, P.Y., Likeman, R.K., Hawley-Molloy, J.S., Thomas, C. and Bingham, J.P. 2015. Cone shell envenomation: Epidemiology, pharmacology and medical care. *Diving and Hyperbaric Medicine*, 45: 200–207.

Halstead, B.W., Schantz, E.J. and World Health Organization. 1984. *Paralytic Shellfish Poisoning*. World Health Organization.

Hammond, P.S., Bearzi, G., Bjørge, A., Forney, K., Karczmarski, L., Kasuya, T., Perrin, W.F., Scott, M.D., Wang, J.Y., Wells, R.S. and Wilson, B. 2008. Lagenorhynchus obscurus. *The IUCN Red List of Threatened Species*, 2008: e. T11146A3257285.

Heghinian, M.D., Mejia, M., Adams, D.J., Godenschwege, T.A. and Marí, F. 2015. Inhibition of cholinergic pathways in *Drosophila melanogaster* by α-conotoxins. *The Federation of American Societies for Experimental Biology Journal*, 29(3): 1011–1018.

Hill, J.M., Alewood, P.F. and Craik, D.J. 1997. Solution structure of the sodium channel antagonist conotoxin GS: A new molecular caliper for probing sodium channel geometry. *Structure*, 5(4): 571–583.

Hubbs, C.L. 1974. *Review*, Marine zoogeography, by John C. Briggs. Copeia. 1002–1005.

Jiang, H., Wang, C.Z., Xu, C.Q., Fan, C.X., Dai, X.D., Chen, J.S. and Chi, C.W. 2006. A novel M-superfamily conotoxin with a unique motif from *Conus vexillum*. *Peptides*, 27(4): 682–689.

Jimenez, E.C., Shetty, R.P., Lirazan, M., Rivier, J., Walker, C., Abogadie, F.C., Yoshikami, D., Cruz, L.J. and Olivera, B.M. 2003. Novel excitatory Conus peptides define a new conotoxin superfamily. *Journal of Neurochemistry*, 85(3): 610–621.

Jin, A.H., Dekan, Z., Smout, M.J., Wilson, D., Dutertre, S., Vetter, I., Lewis, R.J., Loukas, A., Daly, N.L. and Alewood, P.F. 2017. Conotoxin Φ-MiXXVIIA from the superfamily G2 employs a novel cysteine framework that mimics granulin and displays anti-apoptotic activity. *Angewandte Chemie International Edition*, 56(47): 14973–14976.

Jin, A.H., Dutertre, S., Kaas, Q., Lavergne, V., Kubala, P., Lewis, R.J. and Alewood, P.F. 2013. Transcriptomic messiness in the venom duct of Conus miles contributes to conotoxin diversity. *Molecular & Cellular Proteomics*, 12(12): 3824–3833.

Kaas, Q., Westermann, J.C. and Craik, D.J. 2010. Conopeptide characterization and classifications: An analysis using ConoServer. *Toxicon*, 55(8): 1491–1509.

Kauferstein, S., Huys, I., Kuch, U., Melaun, C., Tytgat, J. and Mebs, D. 2004. Novel conopeptides of the I-superfamily occur in several clades of cone snails. *Toxicon*, 44(5): 539–548.

Kerr, L.M. and Yoshikami, D. 1984. A venom peptide with a novel presynaptic blocking action. *Nature*, 308(5956): 282–284.

Kizer, K.W., 1983. Marine envenomations. *Journal of Toxicology: Clinical Toxicology*, 21(4–5): 527–555.

Kohn, A. 2001. Maximal species richness in Conus: Diversity, diet and habitat on reefs of northeast Papua New Guinea. *Coral Reefs*, 20(1): 25–38.

Kohn, A.J. 1966. Food specialization in Conus in Hawaii and California. *Ecology*, 47(6): 1041–1043.

Kohn, A.J. 1978. The Conidae (Mollusca: Gastropoda) of India. *Journal of Natural History*, 12(3): 295–335.

Kohn, A.J. 1986 Type specimens and identity of the described species of Conus IV. The species described by Hwass, Brugiére and Olivi in 1792. *Journal of The Linnean Society of London*, 47: 431–503.

Kohn, A.J. 1990. Tempo and mode of evolution in Conidae. *Malacologia*, 32(1): 55–67.

Kohn, A.J., 2001. The conidae of India revisited. *Phuket Marine Biological Center Special Publication*, 25(2): 357–362.

Kohn, A.J. 2019. Conus envenomation of humans: In fact and fiction. *Toxins*, 11(1): 10.

Kohn, A.J. and Nybakken, J.W. 1975. Ecology of Conus on eastern Indian Ocean fringing reefs: Diversity of species and resource utilization. *Marine Biology*, 29(3): 211–234.

Kohn, A.J. and Perron, F.E., 1994. *Life History and Biogeography: Patterns in Conus* (Vol. 9). Oxford University Press on Demand.

Kularatne, S.A., Dinamithra, N.P., Sivansuthan, S., Weerakoon, K.G., Thillaimpalam, B., Kalyanasundram, V. and Ranawana, K.B. 2015. Clinico-epidemiology of stings and envenoming of *Hottentotta tamulus* (Scorpiones: Buthidae), the Indian red scorpion from Jaffna Peninsula in northern Sri Lanka. *Toxicon*, 93: 85–89.

Kumar, P.S., Kumar, D.S. and Umamaheswari, S. 2015. A perspective on toxicology of Conus venom peptides. *Asian Pacific Journal of Tropical Medicine*, 8(5): 337–351.

Kumari, A., Ameri, S., Ravikrishna, P., Dhayalan, A., Kamala-Kannan, S., Selvankumar, T. and Govarthanan, M. 2019. Isolation and characterization of conotoxin protein from *Conus inscriptus* and its potential anticancer activity against cervical cancer (HeLa-HPV 16 associated) cell lines. *International Journal of Peptide Research and Therapeutics*, 26, 1051–1059.

Lavergne, V., Dutertre, S., Jin, A.H., Lewis, R.J., Taft, R.J. and Alewood, P.F. 2013. Systematic interrogation of the *Conus marmoreus* venom duct transcriptome with ConoSorter reveals 158 novel conotoxins and 13 new gene superfamilies. *BMC Genomics*, 14(1): 1–12.

Lavergne, V., Harliwong, I., Jones, A., Miller, D., Taft, R.J. and Alewood, P.F. 2015. Optimized deep-targeted proteotranscriptomic profiling reveals unexplored Conus toxin diversity and novel cysteine frameworks. *Proceedings of the National Academy of Sciences*, 112(29): E3782–E3791.

Lebbe, E.K., Peigneur, S., Wijesekara, I. and Tytgat, J. 2014. Conotoxins targeting nicotinic acetylcholine receptors: An overview. *Marine Drugs*, 12(5): 2970–3004.

Lee, H.K., Zhang, L., Smith, M.D., Walewska, A., Vellore, N.A., Baron, R., McIntosh, J.M., White, H.S., Olivera, B.M. and Bulaj, G. 2015. A marine analgesic peptide, Contulakin-G, and neurotensin are distinct agonists for neurotensin receptors: Uncovering structural determinants of desensitization properties. *Frontiers in Pharmacology*, 6: 11.

Leipold, E., DeBie, H., Zorn, S., Adolfo, B., Olivera, B.M., Terlau, H. and Heinemann, S.H. 2007. μO-conotoxins inhibit Nav channels by interfering with their voltage sensors in domain-2. *Channels*, 1(4): 253–262.

Lewis, R.J., Sellin, M., Poli, M.A., Norton, R.S., MacLeod, J.K. and Sheil, M.M. 1991. Purification and characterization of ciguatoxins from moray eel (*Lycodontis javanicus*, Muraenidae). *Toxicon*, 29(9): 1115–1127.

Li, Q., Barghi, N., Lu, A., Fedosov, A.E., Bandyopadhyay, P.K., Lluisma, A.O., Concepcion, G.P., Yandell, M., Olivera, B.M. and Safavi-Hemami, H. 2017. Divergence of the venom exogene repertoire in two sister species of Turriconus. *Genome Biology and Evolution*, 9(9): 2211–2225.

Lu, A., Yang, L., Xu, S. and Wang, C. 2014. Various conotoxin diversifications revealed by a venomic study of *Conus flavidus. Molecular & Cellular Proteomics*, 13(1): 105–118.

Mansbach, R.A., Travers, T., McMahon, B.H., Fair, J.M. and Gnanakaran, S. 2019. Snails in silico: A review of computational studies on the conopeptides. *Marine Drugs*, 17(3): 145.

McCleskey, E.W., Fox, A.P., Feldman, D.H., Cruz, L.J., Olivera, B.M., Tsien, R.W. and Yoshikami, D. 1987. Omega-conotoxin: Direct and persistent blockade of specific types of calcium channels in neurons but not muscle. *Proceedings of the National Academy of Sciences*, 84(12): 4327–4331.

McDougal, O.M., Turner, M.W., Ormond, A.J. and Poulter, C.D. 2008. Three-dimensional structure of conotoxin tx3a: An m-1 branch peptide of the M-superfamily. *Biochemistry*, 47(9): 2826–2832.

McIntosh, J.M., Dowell, C., Watkins, M., Garrett, J.E., Yoshikami, D. and Olivera, B.M. 2002. α-Conotoxin GIC from *Conus geographus*, a novel peptide antagonist of nicotinic acetylcholine receptors. *Journal of Biological Chemistry*, 277(37): 33610–33615.

McIntosh, M., Cruz, L.J., Hunkapiller, M.W., Gray, W.R. and Olivera, B.M. 1982. Isolation and structure of a peptide toxin from the marine snail *Conus magus*. *Archives of Biochemistry and Biophysics*, 218(1): 329–334.

McManus, O.B., Musick, J.R. and Gonzalez, C. 1981. Peptides isolated from the venom of *Conus geographus* block neuromuscular transmission. *Neuroscience Letters*, 25(1): 57–62.

Mei, D., Lin, Z., Fu, J., He, B., Gao, W., Ma, L., Dai, W., Zhang, H., Wang, X., Wang, J. and Zhang, X. 2015. The use of α-conotoxin ImI to actualize the targeted delivery of paclitaxel micelles to α7 nAChR-overexpressing breast cancer. *Biomaterials*, 42: 52–65.

Menting, J.G., Gajewiak, J., MacRaild, C.A., Chou, D.H.C., Disotuar, M.M., Smith, N.A., Miller, C., Erchegyi, J., Rivier, J.E., Olivera, B.M. and Forbes, B.E. 2016. A minimized human insulin-receptor-binding motif revealed in a *Conus geographus* venom insulin. *Nature Structural & Molecular Biology*, 23(10): 916–920.

Miljanich, G.P. 2004. Ziconotide: Neuronal calcium channel blocker for treating severe chronic pain. *Current Medicinal Chemistry*, 11(23): 3029–3040.

Moore, R.E. and Scheuer, P.J. 1971. Palytoxin: A new marine toxin from a coelenterate. *Science*, 172(3982): 495–498.

Morales Duque, H., Campos Dias, S. and Franco, O.L. 2019. Structural and functional analyses of cone snail toxins. *Marine Drugs*, 17(6): 370.

Munasinghe, N.R. and Christie, M.J. 2015. Conotoxins that could provide analgesia through voltage gated sodium channel inhibition. *Toxins*, 7(12): 5386–5407.

Muttenthaler, M., B Akondi, K. and F Alewood, P. 2011. Structure-activity studies on alpha-conotoxins. *Current Pharmaceutical Design*, 17(38): 4226–4241.

Ning, J., Ren, J., Xiong, Y., Wu, Y., Zhangsun, M., Zhangsun, D., Zhu, X. and Luo, S. 2019. Identification of crucial residues in α-Conotoxin EI inhibiting muscle nicotinic acetylcholine receptor. *Toxins*, 11(10): 603.

Olivera, B.M., McIntosh, J.M., Clark, C., Middlemas, D., Gray, W.R. and Cruz, L.J. 1985. A sleep-inducing peptide from *Conus geographus* venom. *Toxicon*, 23(2): 277–282.

Olivera, B.M., Safavi-Hemami, H., Horvarth, M.P. and Teichert, R.W. 2015. Conopeptides, marine natural products from venoms: Biomedical applications and future research applications. *Marine Biomedicine: From Beach to Bedside*; Baker, B.J., Ed. CRC Press.

Ortiz, E., Gurrola, G.B., Schwartz, E.F. and Possani, L.D. 2015. Scorpion venom components as potential candidates for drug development. *Toxicon*, 93: 125–135.

Peng, C., Liu, L., Shao, X., Chi, C. and Wang, C. 2008. Identification of a novel class of conotoxins defined as V-conotoxins with a unique cysteine pattern and signal peptide sequence. *Peptides*, 29(6): 985–991.

Peng, C., Yao, G., Gao, B.M., Fan, C.X., Bian, C., Wang, J., Cao, Y., Wen, B., Zhu, Y., Ruan, Z. and Zhao, X. 2016. High-throughput identification of novel conotoxins from the Chinese tubular cone snail (*Conus betulinus*) by multi-transcriptome sequencing. *GigaScience*, 5(1): 1–14.

Pennington, M.W., Czerwinski, A. and Norton, R.S. 2018. Peptide therapeutics from venom: Current status and potential. *Bioorganic & Medicinal Chemistry*, 26(10): 2738–2758.

Petrel, C., Hocking, H.G., Reynaud, M., Upert, G., Favreau, P., Biass, D., Paolini-Bertrand, M., Peigneur, S., Tytgat, J., Gilles, N. and Hartley, O. 2013. Identification, structural and pharmacological characterization of τ-CnVA, a conopeptide that selectively interacts with somatostatin sst3 receptor. *Biochemical Pharmacology*, 85(11): 1663–1671.

Phuong, M.A., Mahardika, G.N. and Alfaro, M.E. 2016. Dietary breadth is positively correlated with venom complexity in cone snails. *BMC Genomics*, 17(1): 1–15.

Pi, C., Liu, J., Peng, C., Liu, Y., Jiang, X., Zhao, Y., Tang, S., Wang, L., Dong, M., Chen, S. and Xu, A. 2006. Diversity and evolution of conotoxins based on gene expression profiling of *Conus litteratus*. *Genomics*, 88(6): 809–819.

Poppe, L., Hui, J.O., Ligutti, J., Murray, J.K. and Schnier, P.D. 2012. PADLOC: A powerful tool to assign disulfide bond connectivities in peptides and proteins by NMR spectroscopy. *Analytical Chemistry*, 84(1): 262–266.

Puillandre, N., Koua, D., Favreau, P., Olivera, B.M. and Stöcklin, R. 2012. Molecular phylogeny, classification and evolution of conopeptides. *Journal of Molecular Evolution*, 74(5): 297–309.

Puillandre, N., Watkins, M. and Olivera, B.M. 2010. Evolution of Conus peptide genes: Duplication and positive selection in the A-superfamily. *Journal of Molecular Evolution*, 70(2): 190–202.

Rajesh, R.P. and Franklin, J.B. 2018. Identification of conotoxins with novel odd number of cysteine residues from the venom of a marine predatory gastropod *Conus leopardus* found in Andaman Sea. *Protein and Peptide Letters*, 25(11): 1035–1040.

Ramírez, D., Gonzalez, W., Fissore, R.A. and Carvacho, I. 2017. Conotoxins as tools to understand the physiological function of voltage-gated calcium (CaV) channels. *Marine Drugs*, 15(10): 313.

Robinson, S.D. and Safavi-Hemami, H. 2017. Venom peptides as pharmacological tools and therapeutics for diabetes. *Neuropharmacology*, 127: 79–86.

Robinson, S.D., Safavi-Hemami, H., McIntosh, L.D., Purcell, A.W., Norton, R.S. and Papenfuss, A.T. 2014. Diversity of conotoxin gene superfamilies in the venomous snail, *Conus victoriae. PloS one*, 9(2): e87648.

Röckel, D., Korn, W. and Kohn, A.J. 1995. Manual of the living Conidae. Vol. I, indo-pacific. *Verlag Christa Hemmen, DM*, 1: 5–13.

Rodrigo, C. and Gnanathasan, A. 2017. Management of scorpion envenoming: A systematic review and meta-analysis of controlled clinical trials. *Systematic Reviews*, 6(1): 1–12.

Rumphine, G. E. 1999. *The Ambonese curiosity cabinet.* Yale University Press, 148.

Safavi-Hemami, H., Brogan, S.E. and Olivera, B.M. 2019. Pain therapeutics from cone snail venoms: From Ziconotide to novel non-opioid pathways. *Journal of Proteomics*, 190: 12–20.

Safavi-Hemami, H., Bulaj, G., Olivera, B.M., Williamson, N.A. and Purcell, A.W. 2010. Identification of Conus peptidylprolyl cis-trans isomerases (PPIases) and assessment of their role in the oxidative folding of conotoxins. *Journal of Biological Chemistry*, 285(17): 12735–12746.

Safavi-Hemami, H., Foged, M.M. and Ellgaard, L. 2018. Evolutionary adaptations to cysteine-rich peptide folding. *Oxidative Folding of Proteins*, 9:99–128.

Safavi-Hemami, H., Gajewiak, J., Karanth, S., Robinson, S.D., Ueberheide, B., Douglass, A.D., Schlegel, A., Imperial, J.S., Watkins, M., Bandyopadhyay, P.K. and Yandell, M. 2015. Specialized insulin is used for chemical warfare by fish-hunting cone snails. *Proceedings of the National Academy of Sciences*, 112(6): 1743–1748.

Safavi-Hemami, H., Li, Q., Jackson, R.L., Song, A.S., Boomsma, W., Bandyopadhyay, P.K., Gruber, C.W., Purcell, A.W., Yandell, M., Olivera, B.M. and Ellgaard, L. 2016. Rapid expansion of the protein disulfide isomerase gene family facilitates the folding of venom peptides. *Proceedings of the National Academy of Sciences*, 113(12): 3227–3232.

Safavi-Hemami, H., Lu, A., Li, Q., Fedosov, A.E., Biggs, J., Showers Corneli, P., Seger, J., Yandell, M. and Olivera, B.M. 2016. Venom insulins of cone snails diversify rapidly and track prey taxa. *Molecular Biology and Evolution*, 33(11): 2924–2934.

Satkunanathan, N., Livett, B., Gayler, K., Sandall, D., Down, J. and Khalil, Z. 2005. Alpha-conotoxin Vc1. 1 alleviates neuropathic pain and accelerates functional recovery of injured neurones. *Brain Research*, 1059(2): 149–158.

Serrano, S.M. 2013. The long road of research on snake venom serine proteinases. *Toxicon*, 62: 19–26.

Sharpe, I.A., Gehrmann, J., Loughnan, M.L., Thomas, L., Adams, D.A., Atkins, A., Palant, E., Craik, D.J., Adams, D.J., Alewood, P.F. and Lewis, R.J. 2001. Two new classes of conopeptides inhibit the α1-adrenoceptor and noradrenaline transporter. *Nature Neuroscience*, 4(9): 902–907.

Sharpe, I.A., Thomas, L., Loughnan, M., Motin, L., Palant, E., Croker, D.E., Alewood, D., Chen, S., Graham, R.M., Alewood, P.F. and Adams, D.J. 2003. Allosteric α1-adrenoreceptor antagonism by the conopeptide ρ-TIA. *Journal of Biological Chemistry*, 278(36): 34451–34457.

Shon, K.J., Grilley, M.M., Marsh, M., Yoshikami, D., Hall, A.R., Kurz, B., Gray, W.R., Imperial, J.S., Hillyard, D.R. and Olivera, B.M. 1995. Purification, characterization, synthesis, and cloning of the lockjaw peptide from *Conus purpurascens* venom. *Biochemistry*, 34(15): 4913–4918.

Slagboom, J., Kool, J., Harrison, R.A. and Casewell, N.R. 2017. Haemotoxic snake venoms: Their functional activity, impact on snakebite victims and pharmaceutical promise. *British Journal of Haematology*, 177(6): 947–959.

Stirpe, F., Barbieri, L., Abbondanza, A., Falasca, A.I., Brown, A.N., Sandvig, K., Olsnes, S. and Pihl, A. 1985. Properties of volkensin, a toxic lectin from *Adenia volkensii. Journal of Biological Chemistry*, 260(27): 14589–14595.

Stonik, V.A. and Stonik, I.V. 2010. Studies on marine toxins: Chemical and biological aspects. *Russian Chemical Reviews*, 79(5): 397.

Suszkiw, J.B., Murawsky, M.M. and Shi, M. 1989. Further characterization of phasic calcium influx in rat cerebrocortical synaptosomes: Inferences regarding calcium channel type (s) in nerve endings. *Journal of Neurochemistry*, 52(4): 1260–1269.

Terlau, H. and Olivera, B.M. 2004. Conus venoms: A rich source of novel ion channel-targeted peptides. *Physiological Reviews*, 41–68.

Terlau, H., Shon, K.J., Grilley, M., Stocker, M., Stühmer, W. and Olivera, B.M. 1996. Strategy for rapid immobilization of prey by a fish-hunting marine snail. *Nature*, *381*(6578): 148–151.

Todd, A.J. 2010. Neuronal circuitry for pain processing in the dorsal horn. *Nature Reviews Neuroscience*, 11(12): 823–836.

Tokuyama, T., Daly, J., Witkop, B., Karle, I.L. and Karle, J. 1968. The structure of batrachotoxinin A, a novel steroidal alkaloid from the Colombian arrow poison frog, *Phyllobates aurotaenia*. *Journal of the American Chemical Society*, 90(7): 1917–1918.

Walker, C.S., Jensen, S., Ellison, M., Matta, J.A., Lee, W.Y., Imperial, J.S., Duclos, N., Brockie, P.J., Madsen, D.M., Isaac, J.T. and Olivera, B. 2009. A novel Conus snail polypeptide causes excitotoxicity by blocking desensitization of AMPA receptors. *Current Biology*, 19(11): 900–908.

Wu, Y., Wang, L., Zhou, M., You, Y., Zhu, X., Qiang, Y., Qin, M., Luo, S., Ren, Z. and Xu, A. 2013. Molecular evolution and diversity of Conus peptide toxins, as revealed by gene structure and intron sequence analyses. *PloS One*, 8(12): e82495.

Yang, M. and Zhou, M. 2020. Insertions and deletions play an important role in the diversity of conotoxins. *The Protein Journal*, 1–6.

Yokoyama, A., Murata, M., Oshima, Y., Iwashita, T. and Yasumoto, T. 1988. Some chemical properties of maitotoxin, a putative calcium channel agonist isolated from a marinedinoflagellate. *The Journal of Biochemistry*, 104(2): 184–187.

Yuan, D.D., Han, Y.H., Wang, C.G. and Chi, C.W. 2007. From the identification of gene organization of α conotoxins to the cloning of novel toxins. *Toxicon*, 49(8): 1135–1149.

## CHAPTER 23

# Toxins in Sea Anemone

**Sunanda Biswas**

### CONTENTS



## 23.1 INTRODUCTION

Sea anemones are invertebrate marine animals and belong to the phylum *Cnidaria*. They are simple, predatory animals and are referred to as the flower of the sea. *Cnidaria* comes from the Latin *cnidae*, which means 'nettle', and all Cnidarians have radial symmetry. Cnidarians have two body plans: polyp (tubular body, sessile) and medusa (bell-shaped body, motile). A small digestive cavity surrounded by three layers (endodermis, ectodermis, and an intermediate noncellular matrix, mesoglea) is found, also known as coelenteron, which has a single opening called a mouth. This mouth is surrounded by tentacles, which are capable of capturing prey (Arai, 1997). Phylum *Cnidaria* includes corals, sea pens, sea anemones, jellyfish and hydras, having five classes: Hydrozoa, Scyphozoa, Cubozoa, Staurozoa, and Anthozoa (D'Ambra & Lauritano, 2020). According to phylogenetic methods based on DNA sequencing, Anthozoa is the basal group of Cnidarians because it has circular mitochondrial DNA, whereas others have a linear molecule. Class Anthozoa sea anemones differ from all other Cnidarians. Anthozoa is also evolutionary separated from others because it has only the polyp stage (embryo > larva > polyp) life cycle, whereas Hydrozoa, Scyphozoa, and

DOI: 10.1201/9781003178446-23

**Table 23.1 Life Stages of Different Classes of the Phylum *Cnidaria***

| Types of Life Stages | Different Classes of Phylum Cnidaria |
|---|---|
| Alternance polyp/medusa | Hydrozoa |
| | Scyphozoa |
| | Cubozoa |
| | Staurozoa |
| Polyp only | Anthozoa |

Cubozoa have metagenic (embryo > larva > polyp > medusa) life cycle (Technau & Steele, 2012) (Table 23.1). Nearly 1,200 species of sea anemones are found, organised in 46 families, creating a great diversity within Anthozoa.

Sea anemones are considered as poisonous animals for their capability of producing venom, a complex mixture of small molecules, proteins, and peptides (Prentis et al., 2018). Anemone venom is delivered from specialised stinging capsules called nematocysts. Sea anemones have specialised subcellular organelles having different structures and function called cnidae. Cnidae can be classified into three types; nematocysts (deliver the venom through the skin), spirocysts (acts as adhesive), and ptychocysts (involved in protection) (Nevalainen et al., 2004). The nematocyst having tiny threads pushed by the osmotic pressure outside the cell is started up by chemical and physical stimulation, which stimulates the cnidocil and supplies substances combined with mixed toxic substances. The venom is presented on the inner side of the inverted tubule, which is then exhibited and injected into the prey at the time of discharge everts outside.

Research into anemone toxin to date already focused much attention on the molecular structure and protein function of venom. In humans, generally, most sea anemones are harmless, whereas some of them cause severe symptoms. Anemone toxins cause swelling, itching, dermatitis, pain, cardiotoxicity, erythema, paralysis, and necrosis. In vivo, it causes neurotoxicity and cardiotoxicity (Martins et al., 2009). From sea anemones, several metabolites, anticancer, and antioxidant substances have been already isolated. In research, it has been observed that these compounds show their activity at the cellular level and can be considered a potential source of new drugs for therapeutic use against neurologic, hematologic, infectivologic, and oncologic diseases (Mariottini & Pane, 2013). This chapter will explore composition, mechanism of action, toxicology, and state of the art techniques used for extraction of sea anemone venom, and determine how this venom can be most beneficial in evidence-based clinical practice in the future.

## 23.2 COMPOSITION

Most sea anemones are harmless, but some species are toxic and may cause severe harm. Several research studies have been conducted on them to identify venomous lineage, and the characteristics of sea anemone venom, but detailed information on the toxin is still not known. It has been determined that toxins released by sea anemone are cytolytic toxin, neuropeptide, and protease inhibitor type. According to research, sea anemone toxins are contained with proteinaceous and non-proteinaceous compounds. Proteinaceous include peptides, proteins, enzymes, and proteinase inhibitors, whereas non-proteinceous includes purine, biogenic amines, and quaternary ammonium compounds and betains (Martins et al., 2009). Maximum molecular mass identified to date in sea anemone 220 kDa. The functional components which are observed in sea anemone venom can be grouped into four types: (1) phospholipase $A_{2,}$ which is very common to all *Cnidaria*, degrades neuronal and muscle cell membrane phospholipid and causes muscle inflammation and nerve damage; (2) neurotoxins which may act as receptor or inhibitor of voltage-gated channels which may obstruct regular neuromuscular transmission activity; (3) cytolysins which mostly do their function on cell membranes and causes cell lysis; (4) non-proteinaceous compounds responsible for pain during envenomation (Madio et al., 2019).

Sea anemone venom includes voltage-gated sodium ($Na_v$) channels and voltage-gated potassium ($K_v$) channels (Mariottini et al., 2015). To date, no existence of systematic nomenclature of sea anemone toxin is present. Recently, the researcher Norton (2013) suggested avoiding confusion and overlapping naming of the same sea anemone toxin; the nomenclature could be organised according to toxin type, such as $K_v$1, $K_v$2. Different kinds of anemone toxins have been discussed below.

### 23.2.1 Voltage-Gated Sodium ($Na_v$) Channel Toxins

A significant portion of sea anemone venom is included in this type of toxin. Three receptor sites have been identified to bind at the time of depolarisation. Type I and II $Na_v$ toxin have 46-51 amino acids and anti-parallel β- sheet (with four β-strands), whereas type III $Na_v$ toxins include 27-32 amino acids and β and γ turns. Type I and II $Na_v$ toxins are available in sea anemone venom, but type III is limited to few species.

Table 23.2 indicates $Na_v$ toxin with mentioning their toxin family type and name of species of sea anemone from which they derived.

### 23.2.2 Voltage-Gated Potassium ($K_v$) Channel Toxins

Voltage-gated potassium ($K_v$) channel toxin can be typed into four classes. Type I, Type II, and Type III all have three disulphide bridges, except Type IV, with two disulphide bridges. Amino acid residues vary in these types of $K_v$ channel toxin. Type I, Type II, Type III, and Type IV contain amino acid residues35–37, 58-59, 41-42, and 28. Some examples of $K_v$ toxin mentioned with their toxin family type and name of species of sea anemone from which they derived have been listed in Table 23.3.

Among $K_v$ toxin, type I interfere between radiolabelled dendrotoxin and synaptosomal membranes and block the K(Ca) channels (Frazão et al., 2012). Type II $K_v$ toxins are similar to Kunitz-type

**Table 23.2 Voltage-Gated Sodium ($Na_v$) Channel Toxin of Sea Anemones Including Toxin Family Type and Species Name**

| Toxin Family Type | Name of the Toxin | Species of Sea Anemone |
|---|---|---|
| Type I | Ae I | *A. equina* |
| | AETX-I | *A. erythraea* |
| | ATX-I, II, III,V | *A. viridis* |
| | ATX Ia, Ib, II, V, | *A. sulcata* |
| | ApC Norton, APE 1–1, 1–2, and 2–2 | *Anthopleura elegantissima* |
| | AFT I and II | *Anthopleura fuscoviridis* |
| | Hk2a, 7a, 8a, and 16a | *Anthopleura sp* |
| | Cangitoxin, Cangitoxin-2, 3 | *Bunodosoma cangicum* |
| | Bc III | *Bunodosoma caissarum* |
| | Am III | *Antheopsis maculata* |
| | Rc I | *Radianthus (Heteractis) crispus* |
| | Gigantoxin II | *S. gigantea* |
| Type II | RTX I, II, III, IV, and V | *Radianthus (Heteractis) macrodactylus* |
| | Rp II, III | *Radianthus (Heteractis) paumotensis* |
| | Sh I | *S. helianthus* |
| | Gigantoxin III | *S. gigantea* |

(Frazão et al., 2012)

**Table 23.3 Voltage-Gated Potassium ($K_v$) Channel Toxin of Sea Anemones Including Toxin Family Type and Species Name**

| Toxin Family Type | Name of the Toxin | Species of Sea Anemone |
|---|---|---|
| Type I | AeK | *A. equina* |
| | Kaliseptin | *A. viridis* |
| | Bgk | *B. granulifera* |
| | ShK | *S. helianthus* |
| Type II/ Kunitz-type proteinase inhibitor | SA5 II, kalicludin-1, 2, 3, BDS-I | *A. viridis* |
| | Analgesic Polypeptide HC1, Kunitz-type Trypsin inhibitor IV | *H. crispa* |
| | SHPI-1, 2 | *S. helianthus* |
| | SHTX-3 | *S. haddoni* |
| Type III | BDS-II | *A. viridis* |
| | APET x1, APET x2 | *Anthopleura elegantissima* |
| | Am-2 | *Antheopsis maculata* |
| | BcIV, V | *Bunodosoma caissarum* |
| Type IV | SHTX-1, 2 | *S. haddoni* |

(Frazão et al., 2012)

protease inhibitors. They inhibit venom from rapid degradation by endogenous proteases in animals themselves or of the prey. Type III $K_v$ toxins block currents involving $K_V3$ subunits or ERG (ether-a-go-go, KV11.1) channels, an important component of human cardiac cells, whereas Type IV shifts dendrotoxin binding synaptosomal membranes, but channel-blocking specificity of them is still unknown (Messerli & Greenberg, 2006).

### 23.2.3 Cytolysin Toxin

Several sea anemones produce cytolytic peptides with cytolysins amino acids. Cytolysins are essential for their cardio-stimulating and dermatonecrotic properties, act as a model protein for studying protein–lipid interaction and eradicate tumour cells and parasites (Klyshko et al., 2004). Four polypeptide groups have been identified in cytolysins. Polypeptides are present in type I 5–8 kDa, type II 20 kDa, type III 30–40 kDa, and type IV 80 kDa. Another group of cytolysins are also found known as membrane-attack complex/perforin (MACPF). In the immune system, the MACPF is best studied. Among these cytolysins, type I have antihistamine activity and type II are inhibited by sphingomyelin. Cytolysins toxin with mentioning their toxin family type and name of species of sea anemone from which they derived have been listed in Table 23.4.

### 23.2.4 PhospholipaseA$_2$ Toxin

PhospholipaseA$_2$ ($PLA_2$) produces fatty acid and lysophospholipid through cleaving the *sn*-2 acyl ester bond of glycerophospholipids. Generally, $PLA_2$ plays a dual role, like one secreted from the pancreas, which acts as a digestive enzyme, and another is active components of the venom. The secreted $PLA_2$s characterised by low molecular weight (13–15 kDa) are disulphide linked proteins. For enzymatic activity $PLA_2$ depends on $Ca^{2+}$-ion. Except for secreted $PLA^2$s, there are also other types of $PLA_2$s; cytosolic $Ca^{2+}$-dependent and $Ca^{2+}$ independent. According to molecular structure, $PLA_2$s have been grouped into several classes numbered from I to XIV and numerous subgroups (Nevalainen et al., 2004). Several Cnidarians comprise presynaptic neurotoxin, albeit $PLA_2$, that blocks nerve terminals through nerve membrane binding and membrane lipids hydrolysis. In Table 23.5, we described $PLA_2$ toxins mentioning the species that have an amino acid sequence.

**Table 23.4 Cytolysins Toxin of Sea Anemoness Including Toxin Family Type and Species Name**

| Toxin Family Type | Name of the Toxin | Species of Sea Anemone |
|---|---|---|
| Type I | Cytolysin RTX-A, RTX-S-II | *Heteractis crispa* |
| Type II | Avt-I, Avt-II | *A. villosa* |
| | Equinatoxin-I, Ia, II, III, IV, V | *A. equina* |
| | Fragaceatoxin C | *A. fragacea* |
| | Tenebrosin-A, B, C | *A. tenebrosa* |
| | Bandaporin | *A. asiatica* |
| | Pstx-20A | *P. semoni* |
| | HMgI, HMgII, HMgIII, Hemolytic toxin | *Radianthus magnifica* |
| | Sticholysin-I, II | *S. helianthus* |
| Type III | Uc-I, Urticinatoxin | *U. crassicornis* |
| Membrane-attack complex/ perforin (MACPF) | PsTX-60A, PsTX-60B | *Phyllodiscus semoni* |

(Frazão et al., 2012)

**Table 23.5 Sea Anemones with Phospholipase$A_2$ Toxins Having Amino Acid Sequence with Their Species Name**

| Name of the Toxin | Species of Sea Anemone |
|---|---|
| $PLA_2$ | *Condylactis gigantea* |
| $AcPLA_2$ | *Adamsia palliata* |
| $UcPLA_2$ | *U. crassicornis* |
| Cationic protein $C_1$ | *Bunodosoma caissarum* |

(Frazão et al., 2012)

### 23.2.5 Other Toxins

Apart from the described toxins, some other toxins are not fully characterised, so classifications of those toxins are yet unknown. Examples of such toxins are the toxins isolated from acrorhagin of a sea anemone. This type of toxins have not any sequence similarity with other sea anemones toxin and a low similarity with venom toxins, so it is not still incorporated in any earlier described groups (Bartosz et al., 2008). In Table 23.6, we have detailed such types of sea anemone toxins that are not still incorporated in the earlier classification, including features that differentiate them from the others.

## 23.3 DISTRIBUTION

Sea anemone is a colourful inhabitant of coastal waters. They are found all over the world but are primarily available in tropical oceans. Anemones are available in various ocean depths, intertidal to deep oceans (more than 10,000 metres). They are radially symmetric, have a columnar body with a mouth surrounded by tentacles, and live attached with rocks, seafloor, shells, mud, and sand. Several cultures that report having consumed sea anemone suggest they may contain enzymes, pore-forming toxins, neurotoxins, and enzyme inhibitors which show their toxic effects on humans. Different coloured and different species of sea anemone can be gathered year-round for consumption by some groups of coastal areas. Several groups also consume the giant green anemone, a large and common species (Ellis & Swan, 1981). Sea anemones are a famous delicacy. Generally, people living in the coastal regions consume sea anemone to cope with their feeding needs. Anemones are eaten like deep-fried fish chips and are also diced in soup.

**Table 23.6 Sea Anemone Toxins That Are Not Still Incorporated in Earlier Classifications Type with Their Species Name and Their Special Distinguishing Features**

| Species | Toxin | Special Distinguishing Features |
|---|---|---|
| *A. equina* | Acrorhagin 1, 1a, 2a | Produced by acrorhagi |
| *A. villosa* | Avt120 | May<br>inhibit nerve cells/possible nephrotoxin |
| *erythraea* | AETX-II, III | Toxin type unknown/possible neurtoxin |
| *A. maculata* | Peptide toxin Am-1 | Inhibits ion channels |
| *B. granulifera* | Granulitoxin | Neurotoxin |
| *P semoni* | Nephrotoxin PsTX-115 | Nephrotoxin |
| *S. haddoni* | EGF-like peptide SHTX-5 | Has both toxicity and EGF activity |
| *S. gigantea* | Gigantoxin-1 | |

(Frazão et al., 2012)

## 23.4 MECHANISM OF ACTION

Sea anemone toxins may comprise enzymes, neurotoxins, pore-forming toxins, and enzyme inhibitors. A large scale of bioactive peptides is also available from the sea anemones. Sea anemone toxins act its different toxic action to humans, which may also consider as a potential source for drug development due to its pharmacological actions. Sea anemone's neurotoxins help them to paralyse their prey quickly and to protect against predators. These neurotoxins affect the $Na_v$ channel gating or $K_v$ channel gating and carry on the action potential of both the excitable and non-excitable membranes in cardiac cells, sensory neurons, and skeletal muscle cells. For this reason, the cell becomes hyperactive and secretes many neurotransmitters at the synapse and neuromuscular junctions, which causes an early spastic stage followed by descending flaccid paralysis. Voltage-gated ion channel toxins of sea anemones show their affinity with sodium and potassium channels, showing how to treat ion channel dysfunctions related to neurological diseases with new compounds (Liao et al., 2019). Sticholysine I and II toxins derived from *Stichodactyla helianthus* and equinatoxin II derived from *Actinia equina*, all are proved to kill *Giardia duodenalis* specifically, whereas anti-Giardia antibodies can do better (Tejuca et al., 1999; Jayathilake & Gunathilake, 2020). Another sea anemone toxin derived from *Aiptasia mutabilis* shows its haemolytic effects against human erythrocytes via pore-forming mechanism (Marino et al., 2009). $PLA_2$ fraction from *Aiptasia pallida* nematocytes shows its hemolytic activity (Hessinger & Lenhoff, 1976). Actinoporis present in sea anemones responsible for different types of toxicity and bioactivity through its interaction exclusively with sphingomyelin containing membranes. Kunitz peptides made up with cross-linked three disulphide bridges, usually function against chymotrypsin and trypsin proteinases and inhibit the quick venom degradation by endogenous enzymes. Kalicludin 1-3 from *A. sulcate* is this type of toxin. Compound ShK derived from *Stoichactis helianthus* is a effective Kv1.3 channel blocker toxin. This Kv1.3 channel is vital in the proliferation and cytokine production of human effector memory T cells ($T_{EM}$)( Chi et al., 2012). Table 23.7 described the biological activity of some sea anemone toxins with the species name from which they have been derived.

## 23.5 TOXICOLOGY

The crude venom derived from sea anemones has different cytotoxic, cytolytic, haemolytic, and neurotoxic effects on human. Some studies have been conducted in vitro, some studies in vivo, yet lack of data regarding toxicity detail is still unrevealed. Envenomation by sea anemones in the

**Table 23.7 Sea Anemone Toxins Including Their Species Name and Biological Activity**

| Species of Sea Anemone | Name of the Toxin | Biological Activity |
|---|---|---|
| *A. equina* | Acrorhagin I and II, AeI | Lethal activity to crabs |
| *A. erythraea* | AETX-I, II and III | |
| *Radianthus (Heteractis) crispus)* | Rc I | |
| *S. haddoni* | SHTX IV | |
| *A. villosa* | Avt120 | Lethal activity to mice, cytotoxic |
| *A. equina* | Equinatoxin-IV | Hemolytic |
| *A. villosa* | Avt-I | |
| *Radianthus (Heteractis) crispus)* | Actinoporin RTX-A, RTX-S II | |
| *Anthopleura asiatica* | Bandaporin | |
| *S. helianthus* | Sticholysin-I and II | |
| *Heteractis magnifica* | Magnificalysins I and II | |
| *Urticina piscivora* | Up-I | |
| *A. villosa* | Avt-II | Cytolysis |
| *Urticina crassicornis* | Uc-I | |
| *Heteractis magnifica* | HMgIII | Cytolytic and hemolytic |
| *A. equina* | Equinatoxin-I, II, and III | |
| | AEPI-I, II, III, and IV | Kunitz-type toxins |
| *S. helianthus* | SHPI-1 | Kunitz-type proteinase inhibitor |
| *A. sulcata* | Kalicludin 1, 2, 3 | |
| *S. haddoni* | SHTX-III | |
| *A. sulcata* | SA5 II | Kunitz-type proteinase toxin |
| *Radianthus (Heteractis) crispus)* | HCRG1, HCRG2 | Kunitz-type inhibitor |
| | HCIQ2c1 | |
| | HGRC21 | |
| | InhVJ | |
| *Heteractis magnifica* | HMIQ3c1 | |
| | HMGS1 | |
| *Anthopleura xanthogrammica* | AXPI-I and II | |
| *Anthopleura elegantissima* | Anthopleurin-C | Cardiotoxic to rats |
| *A. sulcata* | ATX-II | |
| *Anthopleura xanthogrammica* | Anthopleurin-A and B | |
| *Radianthus (Heteractis) crispus* | APHC1, APHC2, APHC3 | Analgesic (TRPV1 modulation) |
| | Hcr 1b-1 | ASIC3 channel inhibitor |
| | Hcr1b-2, 3, 4 | Neurotoxic (ASIC1 channel inhibitors) |
| | HCGS 1.20 | Anti-inflammatory |
| *Heteractis magnifica* | HmK | $K_v$ channel inhibitor |
| *S. helianthus* | ShK | |
| *Bunodosoma caissarum* | BcsTx3 | |
| *S. gigantea* | Gigantoxins I–III | $Na_v$ channel inhibitor, Crab toxicity |
| *S. haddoni* | SHTX I–III | Crab-paralysing activity |
| *Anthopleura spp* | Hk2a, Hk7a, Hk8a, Hk16a | Rat heart stimulation |
| *A. villosa* | AvTX-60A | Toxic to mice |
| *Stoichactis sp* | Phospholipase A2 | PLA2 catalytic activity |
| *S. helianthus* | Sh1 | Neurotoxic on crabs |
| *Bunodosoma cangicum* | Bcg 21.75, 23.41, 21.00, Bcg 31.16, 28.78, 25.52, 29.21 | |
| *Heteractis magnifica* | RpI, RpII, RpIII, and RpIV | Toxic in mice and crabs |
| | Magnificamide | Alpha-amylase inhibitor |
| *S. helianthus* | Helianthamide | |

(D'Ambra & Lauritano, 2020)

human body can cause several effects like tissue damage, pain, cardiovascular collapse, and even death. The sea anemone venom targets the tissues, e.g., epidermis, vasculature, lymphatic system, dermis, and subcutaneous or muscular structures, to initiate an prompt and delayed toxicological and immunological response. Venom content, injected volume, duration of tentacle-skin contacts, and conditions of patient's health differs the envenomation symptoms (D'Ambra & Lauritano, 2020; Jouiaei et al., 2015). It has been observed from cellular and vivo effects of anemone toxins that Kv1 blockers and other toxins have immunosuppressive action, whereas equinatoxin from *Actinia equina* functioned as a reversible block of potassium current toxin (Suput, 2009). APETx2 from *Anthopleura elegantissima* is an acid-sensing ion channel blocker and permeates several cations. Injection of the lethal neurotoxin GRX isolated from *Bunodosoma granulifera* in mice effects circular movements and may cause aggressive behaviour, convulsions, and even death (Santana et al., 1998).

Many sea anemone toxins like cytolysins and neurotoxins are found to have notable cardiotonic actions. In five toxins (APE 1–APE 5) of *A. elegantissima*, all are neurotoxins, but APE 1-1, APE 2-1 and APE 5-3 show their positive inotropic effect on the mammalian heart muscle. On the other hand, a crude extract of *Bunodosoma cavernata* dose-dependent intervention causes rat blood pressure changes.

We need updated knowledge on vitro cytotoxicity of sea anemone toxins to utilise cultured cells for therapeutic use. It was observed that Src I extracted from *Sagartia rosea* showed its cytotoxic effects on cultured NIH/3T3 (Swiss mouse embryo), U251 (glioblastoma), BEL-7402 (liver carcinoma), NSCLC (non-small cell lung carcinoma), and BGC-823 (stomach adenocarcinoma) cells (Santana et al., 1998). Then Bc2 derived from *Bunodosoma caissarum* also showed its cytotoxic effect against human glioblastoma. Table 23.8 shows a summary of data regarding cytotoxicity of compounds produced by sea anemones (Mariottini & Pane, 2013).

## 23.6 EXTRACTION AND PURIFICATION

In recent years, anemone toxins have been extensively investigated for their notable biological activity. Venom, consisting of peptides and proteins, is available from sea anemones nematocysts.

**Table 23.8 Cytotoxicity of Different Compounds Derived from Sea Anemones**

| Species of Sea Anemone | Compound | Tissue/Organ/Histology | Organism |
|---|---|---|---|
| *A. equina* | Equinatoxin II, Crude venom | Normal lung fibroblasts | Chinese hamster |
| *A. sulcata* | Crude venom | | |
| *Heteractis crispa* | Actinoporin RTX-A | Promyelocytic leukemia, monocytic leukemia, cervix carcinoma, colon cancer, breast cancer | Human |
| *Sagartia rosea* | Acidic actinoporin Src I | Non-small cell lung carcinoma, glioblastoma, stomach adenocarcinoma, liver carcinoma | |
| *U. piscivora* | Crude extract, UpI (protein) | Embryonic lung, epidermoid carcinoma | |
| *Aiptasia mutabilis* | Crude venom | Epithelial carcinoma | |
| *Bunodosoma caissarum* | Bc2 | Glioblastoma | |
| *A. equina* | Equinatoxin II-I18C mutant | Breast carcinoma | |
| | EqTx-II | Glioblastoma | |

(Martins et al., 2009)

Autolysis of venom-containing nematocysts can be proceeded by several extraction methods, different from each other. For extraction and purification, first cnidocysts from both fresh and frozen specimens are thoroughly noticed to compare these organelles' physical condition. These sea anemone cnidocysts can be extracted using either seawater (fresh/artificial/filtered) or through .reverse osmosis of purified water to different concentrations of saline solutions (Jayathilake & Gunathilake, 2020; Frazão & Antunes, 2016). Then, mechanical techniques like centrifugation can be used to remove insoluble material from the mass (Kem et al., 1989). For purification of protein and identification of venom components, liquid chromatography or gel electrophoresis (SDS-PAGE and 2DE) are most commonly utilized due to their efficacy and short duration. Western blot analysis is best used to perform for the detection of known compounds in a venom (Frazão & Antunes, 2016).

## 23.7 SAFETY, PRECAUTIONS, AND REGULATION

Sea anemone toxins are considered as marine biotoxins. Marine biotoxin consumption can cause severe illness and even death to humans, and as such is now part of a public health concern. In humans, envenomation may cause muscle spasms and cramps, nausea, vomiting, diarrhea, diaphoresis, and cardiorespiratory failure. Envenomation symptoms depend on the venom content, injected volume, patient's health, and tentacle–skin contact duration (Burnett, 2009). For treatment of human envenomation, first physical attempts to detach remaining tentacles from the victim's skin is necessary because it may cause a massive discharge of venom. Then the use of specific fluids is vital to prevent further nematocyst discharge. Urea, seawater, vinegar, methylated spirits, etc., are used as traditional remedies for inactivating the undischarged nematocysts on the adhered tentacles and/or alleviating pain. The action of these chemicals may differ on different sea anemones (Jouiaei et al., 2015).

With the consumption of increasing seafood plates, emerging biotoxins are being reported, and new guidelines are now needed mentioning their management. In 2006, The European Food Safety Authority (EFSA), at the European Commission's (EC) request, has developed a series of scientific opinions related to marine biotoxins. Emerging toxins such as palytoxins (PTXs), ciguatoxins (CTXs), and tetrodotoxins (TTXs) have been included in it based on the report of the prevalence of health risk in some geographical areas and to raise awareness in others (Estevez et al., 2019). Few countries set their regulations regarding marine biotoxins based on the mouse bioassay. Sea anemones are primarily harmless, where few show harmful activity. Lethality and neurotoxicity were assessed only in a few species. Very few systemic reviews and meta-analyses were found related to sea anemone toxicity. Risk assessment was not still done with this sea anemone venom. Scientific opinions on sea anemone toxin need to be more developed and standardised for safety.

## 23.8 EFFECT OF PROCESSING

For food and nutritional security, peoples of several coastal areas consume sea anemone as food. Before cooking sea anemone food, tentacles from the sea anemone need to be detached, though it may consist of nematocytes from where the toxin is secreted. Vinegar helps to inactivate the discharged nematocysts wholly and rapidly (Hartwick et al., 1980). So, before cooking, bathing in vinegar or baking soda is essential to prevent nematocyst secretions. No other information regarding other processing of sea anemone is available.

## 23.9 FUTURE SCOPE

Compounds isolated from sea anemones affect human health due to their neurotoxic, cytotoxic action. However, different findings .from different researchers have suggested that sea anemone toxins may be essential pharmacological active agents in the therapy of several human diseases.

Researchers found that a number of cytolysins and protease inhibitors were isolated from *Actinia equina*. Among them, Equinatoxin II (EqT II), a pore-forming protein, .showed its toxic effect against Ehrlich ascites tumour and cell line of L1210 leukaemia as well as. Chinese hamster's diploid lung fibroblasts (Giraldi et al., 1976). Equistatin is also a potent inhibitor of papain-like cysteine proteases that are involved with central nervous system-related diseases (Brömme & Petanceska, 2002), and aspartic proteinase cathepsin D, related to breast carcinoma (Liaudet-Coopman et al., 2006).

ShK isolated from *Stoichactis helianthus* is a effective Kv1.3 channel-blocker toxin, responsible for proliferation and cytokine production effector memory T cells (TEM) of humans. For this function, ShK can be used as a important immunosuppressant for the treatment of T cell-mediated autoimmune diseases. It is also effective against obesity and insulin resistance (Upadhyay et al., 2013).

So, researchers have considered sea anemones for a decade as an important source of peptide and protein toxins. Recent research developments related to multiple 'omic' technologies like genomics, transcriptomics, proteomics, and advanced bioinformatics, have opened diverse dimensions in wide-ranging discovery of novel sea anemone toxins; among those toxins, many will be helpful as pharmacological tools and valuable therapeutic leads.

## 23.10 CONCLUSION

Sea anemones are sources of under-explored peptide toxins, and different habitats, including various species, have been investigated. To date, there is more to explore. Transcriptomes and genomes of several anemones have already analysed. Sea anemone venoms are considered as a substantial source of peptides for their pharmacological importance. Most research on sea anemone toxins have pointed their focus on functions of sea anemone toxins with its .toxicity of medical significance as well as therapeutic capacity, and consequent fundamental studies. related to venom composition and its ecological role, compositional changes in different temperature and pH are scarce. The growing interest in sea anemone toxin is indeed for therapeutic application, but in several coastal regions, the sea anemone is accepted as food; necessary research needs to focus on consumption patterns, behaviour, processing, and toxic effects of sea anemone as food.

## REFERENCES

Arai, M.N. 1997. *A Functional Biology of Scyphozoa*; 315. London: Chapman & Hall.

Bartosz, G., Finkelshtein, A., Przygodzki, T., Bsor, T., Nesher, N., Sher, D., Zlotkin, E.A 2008. Pharmacological solution for a conspecific conflict: ROS-mediated territorial aggression in sea anemones. *Toxicon* 5:1038–1050.

Brömme, D., and Petanceska, S. 2002. Papain-like cysteine proteases and their implications in neurodegenerative diseases. In *Role of Proteases in the Pathophysiology of Neurodegenerative Diseases*; 47–61. New York: Springer.

Burnett, J.W. 2009. Treatment of Atlantic cnidarian envenomations. *Toxicon* 54:1201–1205.

Chi, V., Pennington, M.W., Norton, R.S., Tarcha, E.J., Londono, L.M., Sims-Fahey, B., Upadhyay, S.K., Lakey, J.T., Iadonato, S., Wulff, H. 2012. Development of a sea anemone toxin as an immunomodulator for therapy of autoimmune diseases. *Toxicon* 59:529–546.

D'Ambra, I., and Lauritano, C. 2020. A review of toxins from Cnidaria. *Mar. Drugs* 18(10):507.

Ellis, D.W., and Swan, L. 1981. *Teachings of the Tides: Uses of Marine Invertebrates by the Manhousat People*, 1st edition. Nanaimo, BC: Theytus Books Ltd.

Estevez, P., Castro, D., Pequeño-Valtierra, A., Giraldez, J., Gago-Martinez, A. 2019. Emerging marine biotoxins in seafood from European Coasts: incidence and analytical challenges. *Foods* 8(5):49.

Frazão, B., and Antunes, A. 2016. Jellyfish bioactive compounds: methods for wet-lab work. *Mar. Drugs* 14(4):75.

Frazão, B., Vasconcelos, V., Antunes, A. 2012. Sea anemone (Cnidaria, Anthozoa, Actiniaria) toxins: an overview. *Mar. Drugs* 10(8):1812–1851.

Giraldi, T., Ferlan, I., Romeo, D.1976.Antitumour Activity of Equinatoxin. *Chem.-Biol. Interact.* 13:199–203.

Hartwick R., Callanan V., Williamson J. 1980. Disarming the box-jellyfish: nematocyst inhibition in *Chironex fleckeri*. *Med. J. Aust.* 1:15–20.

Hessinger, D.A., and Lenhoff, H.M. 1976. Mechanism of hemolysis induced by nematocyst venom: roles of phospholipase A and direct lytic factor. *Arch. Biochem. Biophys.* 173:603–613.

Jayathilake, J.M.N.J., and Gunathilake, K.V.K. 2020. Cnidarian toxins: recent evidences for potential therapeutic uses. *Eur. Zool. J.* 87(1):708–713.

Jouiaei, M.,Yanagihara, A.A., Madio, B., Nevalainen, T.J., Alewood, P.F., Fry, B.G. 2015. Ancient venom systems: a review on Cnidaria toxins. *Toxins* 7(6):2251–71.

Kem, W.R., Parten, B., Pennington, M.W., Dunn, B.M., Price, D. 1989. Isolation and characterisation, and amino acid sequence of a polypeptide neurotoxin occurring in the sea anemone Stichodactyla helianthus. *Biochem. J.* 28:3483–3489.

Klyshko, E.V., Issaeva, M.P., Monastyrnaya, M.M., Il'yna, A.P., Guzev, K.V., Vakorina, T.I., Dmitrenok, P.S., Zykova, T.A., Kozlovskaya, E.P. 2004. Isolation, properties and partial amino acid sequence of a new actinoporin from the sea anemone Radianthus macrodactylus. *Toxicon* 44:315–324.

Liao, Q., Feng, Y., Yang, B., Lee, S.M.-Y. 2019. Cnidarian peptide neurotoxins: a new source of various ion channel modulators or blockers against central nervous systems disease. *Drug Discov. Today* 24:189–197.

Liaudet-Coopman, E., Beaujouin, M., Derocq, D., Garcia, M., Glondu-Lassis, M., Laurent-Matha, V., Prébois, C., Rochefort, H.,Vignon, F. 2006. Cathepsin D: newly discovered functions of a long-standing aspartic protease in cancer and apoptosis. *Cancer Lett.* 237:167–179.

Madio, B., King, G.F., Undheim, E.A.B. 2019. Sea anemone toxins: a structural overview. *Mar. Drugs* 17:325.

Marino, A., Morabito, R., La Spada, G. 2009. Factors altering the haemolytic power of crude venom from *Aiptasia. mutabilis* (Anthozoa) nematocysts. *Comp. Biochem. Physiol. A* 152:418–422.

Mariottini, G., and Pane, L. 2013.Cytotoxic and cytolytic cnidarian venoms. A review on health implications and possible therapeutic applications. *Toxins* 6(1):108–151.

Mariottini, G.L., Bonello, G., Giacco, E., Pane, L. 2015.Neurotoxic and neuroactive compounds from Cnidaria: five decades of research….and more. *Cent. Nerv. Syst. Agents Med. Chem.* 15(2):74–80.

Martins, R.D., Alves, R.S., Martins, A.M., Barbosa, P.S., Evangelista, J.J., Evangelista, J.S., Ximenes, R.M., Toyama, M.H., Toyama, D.O., Souza, A.J., Orts, D.J., Marangoni, S., Menezes, D.B., Fonteles, M.C., Monteiro, H.S. 2009. Purification and characterization of the biological effects of phospholipase A2 from sea anemone *Bunodosoma caissarum*. *Toxicon* 54:413–420.

Messerli, S.M., and Greenberg, R.M. 2006. Cnidarian toxins acting on voltage-gated ion channels. *Mar. Drugs* 4:70–81.

Nevalainen, T.J., Peuravuori, H.J., Quinn, R.J., Llewellyn, L.E., Benzie, J.A., Fenner, P.J., Winkel, K.D. 2004. Phospholipase A2 in cnidaria. *Comp. Biochem. Physiol.* 139:731–735.

Norton, R.S. 2013. *Sea anemone peptides*. In *Handbook of Biologically Active Peptides*, 2nd edition; Ribeiro, S.M., Porto, W.F., Silva, O.N., Santos, M.d.O., Dias, S.C., Franco, O.L., Eds.; 430–436, Berkeley, CA: Elsevier.

Prentis, P.J., Pavasovic, A., Norton, R.S. 2018. Sea anemones: quiet achievers in the field of peptide toxins. *Toxins* 10(1):36.

Santana, A.N., Leite, A.B., Franca, M.S., Franca, L., Vale, O.C., Cunha, R.B., Ricart, C.A., Sousa, M.V., Carvalho, K.M. 1998. Partial sequence and toxic effects of granulitoxin, a neurotoxic peptide from the sea anemone Bundosoma granulifera. *Braz. J. Med. Biol.* 31(10):1335–1338.

Suput, D. 2009. In vivo effects of cnidarian toxins and venoms. *Toxicon* 54(8):1190–200.

Technau, U., and Steele, R.E. 2012. Evolutionary crossroads in developmental biology: *Cnidaria. Development* 138:1447.

Tejuca, M., Anderluh,G., Maček, P., Marcet, R., Torres, D., Sarracent, J., Alvarez, C., Lanio, M.E., Dalla Serra, M., Menestrina, G. 1999. Antiparasite activity of sea-anemone cytolysins on Giardia duodenalis and specific targeting with anti-Giardia antibodies. *Int. J. Parasitol.* 29(3):489–498.

Upadhyay, S.K., Eckel-Mahan, K.L., Mirbolooki, M.R., Tjong, I., Griffey, S.M., Schmunk, G., Koehne, A., Halbout, B., Iadonato, S., Pedersen, B. et al. 2013. Selective Kv1.3 channel blocker as therapeutic for obesity and insulin resistance. *Proc. Natl. Acad. Sci. USA*.110(24):E2239-48.

## CHAPTER 24

# Biogenic Amines

**Ghulam Mustafa Kamal, Waliya Zubairi, Jalal Uddin, Makhdoom Ibad Ullah Hashmi, Muhammad Khalid, and Asma Sabir**

## CONTENTS



DOI: 10.1201/9781003178446-24

## 24.1 INTRODUCTION

The Biogenic amines (BAs) are essential nitrogen-based compounds which are produced naturally by decarboxylation of amino acid or by aldehyde and ketone amination and transamination. These are organic bases with low molecular weight which may beheterocyclic, aromatic, or aliphatic (Table 24.1) (Özogul and Özogul, 2007).

BAs are formed through different metabolism of microorganisms, plants, and animals (Bermúdez et al., 2012, Shalaby, 1996). Their presence in food products is mostly due to the occurrence of decarboxylase-active microorganisms; the elimination of the alpha carboxyl group from the amino acid forms the respective biogenic amine. Generally, the name of a biogenic amine is based on amino acid that derives specific BA (Figure 24.1), like histamine is derived from histidine amino acid. Likewise, tyramine formed by tyramine, etc.

BAs have a vital role in the performance of the human brain, body-temperature regulation, and pH regulation, secretion of gastric acid, cell growth, and differentiation and immune response system, etc. Biogenic amines are nitrogen-containing compounds and are precursors for synthesis of alkaloids, nucleic acids, proteins, and different hormones.

Excessive oral intake of BAs, however, can stimulate adverse effects such as headaches, nausea, rashes, and blood pressure changes. This is particularly true for people having low immunity and those in whom detoxification of BA is impaired. Biogenic amines are formed in food and beverages by raw material enzymes and generated by microbial amino acid decarboxylation (Ruiz-Capillas and Jiménez-Colmenero, 2005, Linares et al., 2011). The total amount and type of amines therefore mainly depends on the nature of the microorganisms present and the food. By spoilage and fermentation of food the presence of biogenic amines is noticed. Other amines intensify the effects; hence they are considered as a food hazard (Linares et al., 2016, Mohammed et al., 2016). Other BAs like histamine and tyramine show toxic characteristics as these poison the food (Taylor and Eitenmiller, 1986).

They cause water pollution as their formation results in the production of amino acids and microorganisms. Consumption of a high amount causes intoxication.

**Table 24.1 Classification of Biogenic Amines**

| | | Biogenic Amine | | |
|---|---|---|---|---|
| | **Precursor-Aminoacid** | **Aliphatic** | **Aromatic** | **Hetrocyclic** |
| *Biogenic Amines* | Ornithine | Putrescine<br>Butane-1,4-diamine | | |
| | Lysine | Cadaverine<br>1,5-pentanediamine | | |
| | | Spermine<br>N,N'-bis(3-aminopropyl)butane-1,4-diamine | | |
| | | Spermidine<br>N'-(3-aminopropyl) butane-1,4-diamine | | |
| | Arginine | Agmatine<br>2-(4-aminobutyl)guanidine | | |
| | Tyrosine | | Tyramine | |
| | Phenylalanine | | Phenylethylamine | |
| | Histidine | | | Histamine<br>2-(1h-imidazol-4-yl) ethanamine |
| | Tryptophan | | | Tryptamine |

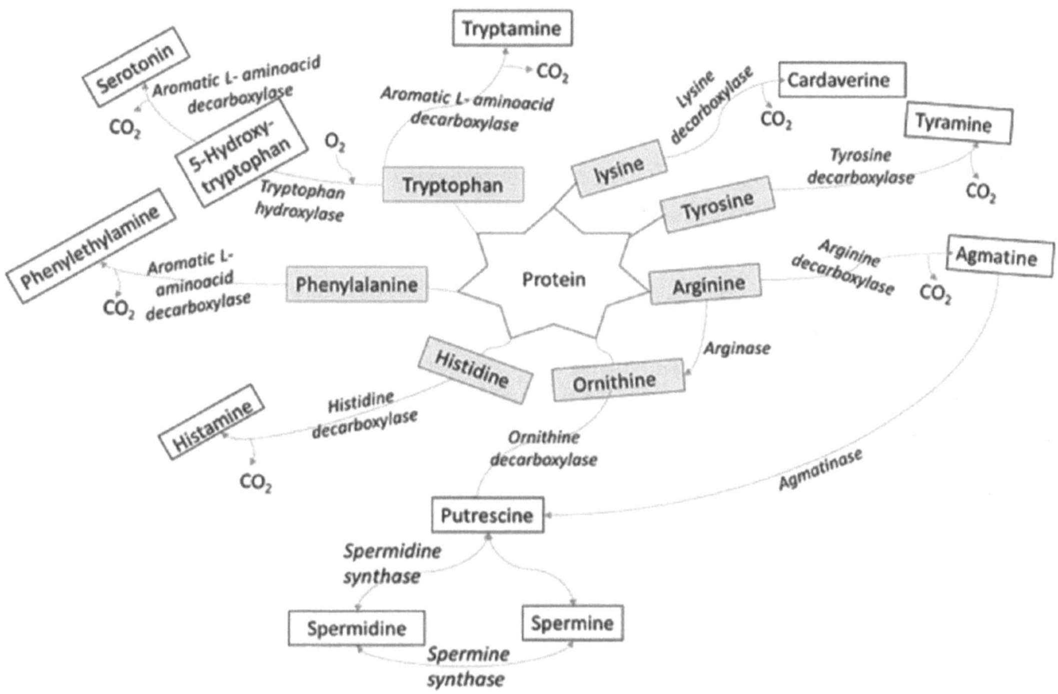


**Figure 24.1** Synthesis of biogenic amines from precursor amino acids.

## 24.2 CHEMISTRY

Amino acid decarboxylation:

Biogenic amines are derivatives of amino acids. The enzymatic reaction catalyzed by pyridoxal phosphate to decarboxylate the amino acid results in the formation of $CO_2$ and biogenic amine (Sebastian et al., 2011).

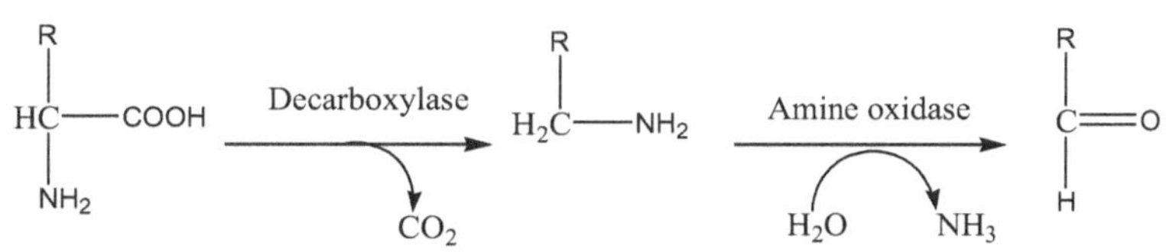


Aminoacid Biogenic amine Aldehyde

Biogenic amines are bioactive molecules as they are produced during normal metabolic processes by amino acid decarboxylation or amination and transamination of aldehydes and ketones. Biogenic amines promote the differentiation and proliferation of cells. They stimulate the metabolism of body cells by entering in the structure of vitamins, hormones, and coenzyme A.

### 24.2.1 Histamine

Histidine amino acid undergoes decarboxylation resulting in formation of histamine biogenic amine.

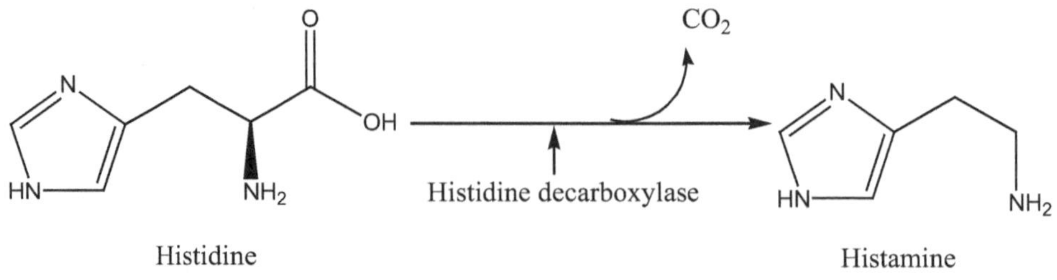


The distribution and accumulation of histamine varies in all vertebrate tissues. It is found in hypothalamus of brain and plays role in learning and memory. Histamine plays several roles and functions in several processes. It is involved in regulation of gastric acid secretion, vasodilation, regulating the stomach pH and volume and balancing the body temperature. It performs cerebral activities, e.g., functions as neurotransmission and vascular permeability. It also causes stimulation in allergic reactions (Feng et al., 2016).

### 24.2.2 Tryptamine

Tryptamine is derived from tryptophan amino acid. It is produced as a result of decarboxylase activity of aromatic L-amino acid.

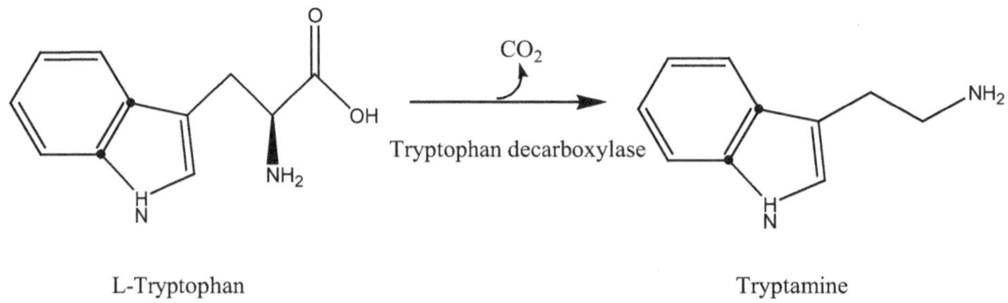


It is the type of monoamine alkaloids present in animals, plants, and fungi. Its presence is also found in trace amount in brain which acts as neurotransmitter and increases blood pressure.

### 24.2.3 Phenylethylamine

Phenylalanine amino acid undergoes enzymatic activity of L-amino acid decarboxylase forming phenylethylamine BA.

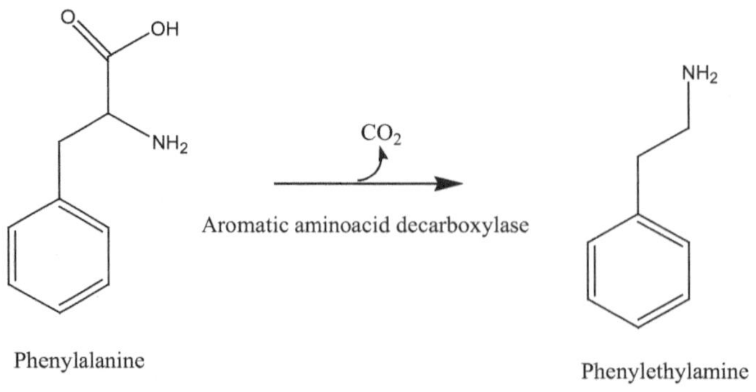


Phenylethylamine is the neurotransmitter present in human CNS.

### 24.2.4 Tyramine

Tyrosine amino acid undergoes enzymatic activity of tyrosine decarboxylase forming tyramine BA.

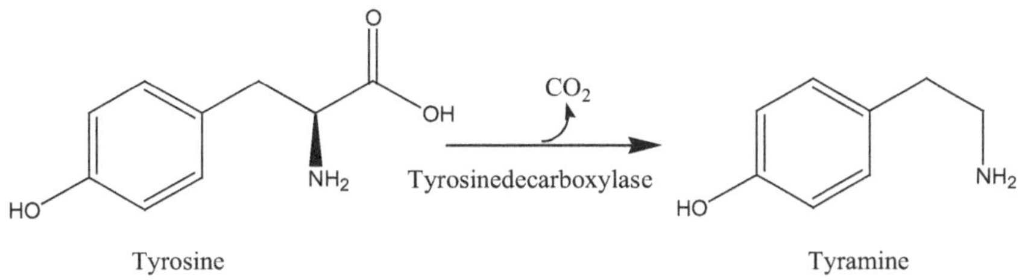


It regulates many physiological reactions like vasoconstriction, regulates the blood pressure, noradrenalin secretion, and controls several functions of body. It is present in neurons. Tyramine causes increase in salvation, production of tears. It has a significant antioxidant activity, which rises with its concentration (Doeun et al., 2017).

### 24.2.5 Serotonin

It is derived from tryptophan by action of L-amino acid decarboxylase and tryptophan hydroxylase enzyme.

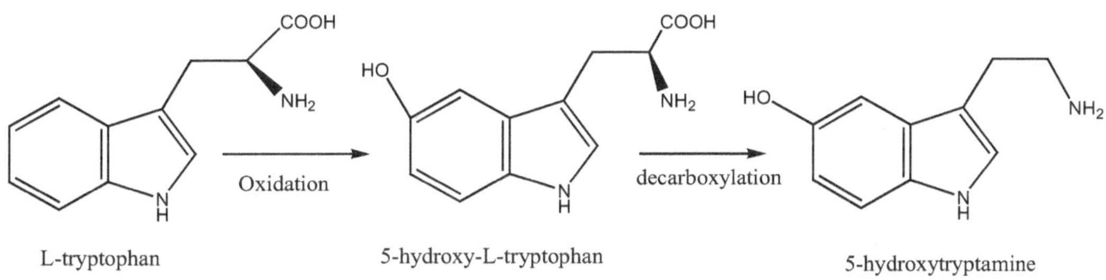


It is essential neurotransmitter of CNS and has control over physiological mechanisms, mood disorders, appetite regulation, sleep, cerebral blood flow regulation, and sexual behaviour. Its activity is blocked by lysergic acid diethylamide (LSD) and used to treat depression. It is a mood elevator.

### 24.2.6 Putrescine

Putrescine is the diamine. Ornithine amino acid undergoes ornithine decarboxylase enzyme activity forming putrescine biogenic amine.

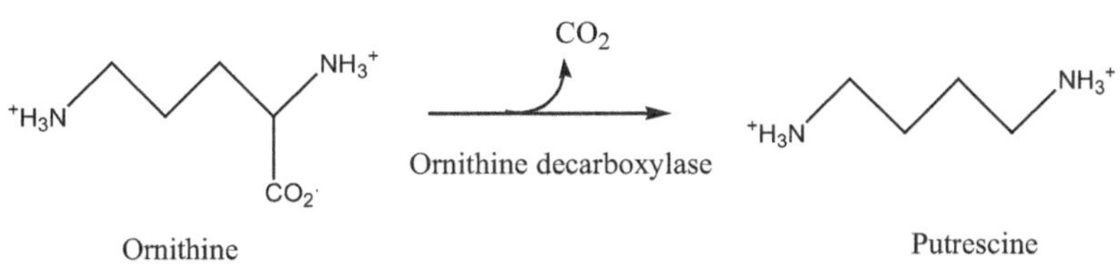


It can also be formed by arginine via agmatine and carbamoyl putrescine. Putrescine is also produced by fungi and bacteria which promote angiogenesis, cell growth and cell division.

### 24.2.7 Cadaverine

Amino acid lysine undergoes lysine decarboxylase enzyme activity synthesizing cadaverine biogenic amine. It acts as free radical scavenger (Lu et al., 2015).

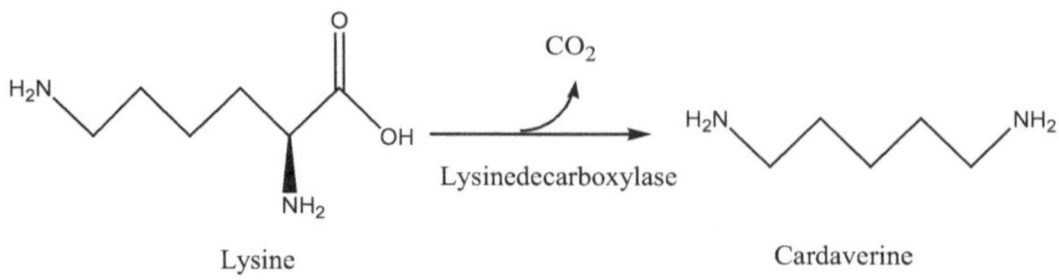


### 24.2.8 Spermidine

Putrescine amino acid results in formation of spermidine. It is a precursor of many other biogenic amines like spermine and thermospermine isomer (Igarashi and Kashiwagi, 2000).

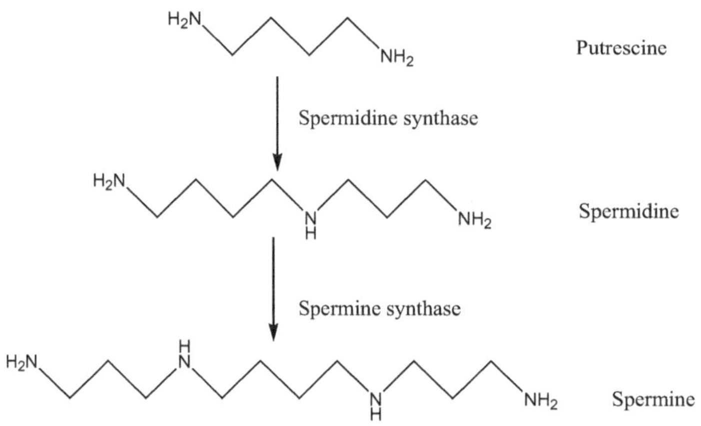


Spermidine plays role in regulating many biological processes, controls pH and volume of cell and protects membrane potential. It is involved in cellular metabolism, intestinal tissue development, synthesis of nitric oxide (Lim and Lee, 2016).

### 24.2.9 Spermine

It is derived from ornithine, which under goes enzymatic action forming spermidine leading to formation of spermine biogenic amine. Spermine is present in all eukaryotic cells performing cellular metabolism. It maintains the helical structure in virus and also plays role in development of intestinal tissue. It is involved in physiological processes like flowering, fruit growth, cell division, response to senescence and stress (Jansen et al., 2003).

### 24.2.10 Agmatine

Arginine amino acid undergoes the arginine decarboxylase enzyme activity, forming the agmatine biogenic amine.

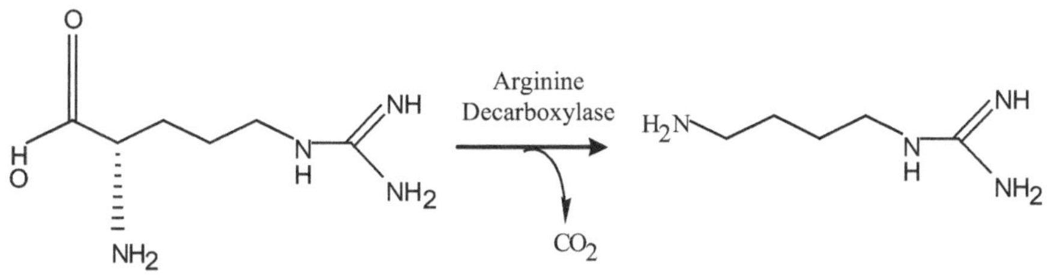


L-Arginine Agmatine

Agmatine enzyme is used in synthesis of nitric oxide, production of hydrogen peroxide, polyamine metabolism, and matrix metalloproteinase.

## 24.3 DISTRIBUTION

Biogenic amines are most commonly present in food products like fish, vegetables, meat, cheese fermented vegetables, sausages, and wines. Histamine is the most important biogenic amine present in foods whereas, other BAs include tyramine, cadaverine, β-phenylethylamine, serotonin, spermidine, putrescine, agmatine, tryptamine, and spermine.

These amines are named as dietary amines which may be aromatic and aliphatic polyamines according to their structural chemistry. The level of biogenic amines present in food depends upon the type of food product, nature, and availability of bacteria. Biogenic amines are formed naturally by plants, animals and microorganisms performing many physiological functions like neurotransmission, vasoactivity, cell differentiation and growth, immune response, gastric secretions, psychoactive, regulating gene expression, inflammatory processes, etc. (Maijala et al., 1993). Biogenic amines are the polyamines chemically formed by decarboxylation of amino acids followed by respective enzyme action. The formation of biogenic amines is influenced by several factors including raw materials, microorganisms and their processing and storage conditions. Distribution of biogenic amines in different food products is discussed below.

### 24.3.1 Sea Food

Histamine, putrescine, cadaverine, and tyramine are the most common biogenic amines found in fish and other sea foods. Histidine free amino acid is present in *Scombridae* family of fish species. Histidine by the action of histidine decarboxylase bacteria results in formation of histamine BA. Occurrence of BAs in fish and fish products is related with the storage duration and temperature. Fish products including fish sauce, fish paste, shrimp paste, dried fish, and fermented anchovies contain abundant amount of histamine BAs. FDA proposed maximum level of 50 ppm of histamine in fish products (Prester, 2011).

### 24.3.2 Sausages

Putrescine and tyramine are the abundant biogenic amines found in sausages. The production of tyramine is facilitated by bacteria like coagulase negative *staphylococci* and lactic acid bacteria. Other than that yeast and mould have ability of formation of biogenic amines in sausages. 13% *staphylococci* and 48% lactic acid bacteria are found in sausages and are responsible for the decarboxylation of amino acids. The sausage thickness, ripening technique, ingredients, additives, and raw materials are the factors which influence the presence and production of biogenic amines.

### 24.3.3 Cheese

Cheese is formed by activity of decarboxylase bacteria on raw material, which provides an ideal environment for the production of biogenic amines. The factors stimulating the BAs formation in cheese includes water activity, presence of oxygen, use of starter culture or enzymes, pH, temperature, amount of proteolysis, relative humidity, availability of microorganisms, and period of ripening. FDA concludes that, in cheese, level of biogenic amines could exceed from 2,000 ppm (Ščavničar et al., 2018, Mayer and Fiechter, 2018).

### 24.3.4 Fermented Vegetables

Tyramine and histamine are the biogenic amines found in fermented soybean. Fermented soyabean products also contain putrecine, cadaverine, spermine, spermidine, agmatine, tryptamine, and phenylethylamine. Soybean products include soy sauce, which is formed by hydrolysis of soybean protein. Fermentation of cabbage also results in formation of biogenic amines like histamine, tyramine, putrescine, and cadaverine (Spano et al., 2010, Pircher et al., 2007).

### 24.3.5 Wine

The biogenic amines found in wine are histamine, tyramine, phenylethylamine, spermine, agamatine, spermidine, putrescine, and tryptamine. The most abundant BA in wine is putrescine. Grapes are the source of wine and must possess spermidine and putrescine biogenic amines. During the alcoholic fermentation and malolactic fermentation, metabolism of yeast and lactic acid bacteria produce biogenic amines. The production of biogenic amine can be controlled by optimizing the growth of lactic acid bacteria. It is observed that white wine is formed without malolactic formation which results in less production of biogenic amine than that of produced in red wine (Özogul and Özogul, 2019, Almeida et al., 2012).

## 24.4 MECHANISM OF ACTION

Biogenic amines are produced by decarboxylation of amino acid. Microorganisms acting on precursor amino acid are discussed in Table 24.2. The removal of α-carboxyl group of the amino acid results in decarboxylation. By process of proteolysis (bacterial or autolytic) free amino acid is formed from tissue proteins. Amino acid acts as substrate for the decarboxylase bacteria. Amino acid decarboxylation can occur by following two mechanisms of action.

### 24.4.1 Pyridoxal Phosphate Dependent Reaction

The formation of active site of enzyme occurs while pyridoxal phosphate binds in Schiff base linkage with amino group of lysyl residue. Pyridoxal phosphate itself catalyzes many free amino acid reactions which are dependent on pyridoxal phosphate enzyme. Amino acid reacts with carbonyl group of pyridoxal phosphate to form Schiff base intermediates which then eliminates water on decarboxylation and yield corresponding amino acid and original pyridoxal phosphate (Özogul and Özogul, 2019).

### 24.4.2 Non-Pyridoxal Phosphate Dependent Reaction

The decarboxylation in non-pyridoxal phosphate reaction occurs with the help of pyruvoyl residue rather than of pyridoxal 5-phosphate.

**Table 24.2 Classification of BAs on the Basis of Precursors, Decarboxylase Enzyme and Their Producers' Microorganisms**

| Biogenic Amine | Precursor | Classification | Decarboxylase enzyme | Lactic Acid Bacteria-Producing Species |
|---|---|---|---|---|
| *Histamine* | Histidine | Hetrocyclic | Histidine decarboxylase (HDC) | *E. faecium, E. faecalis, L. sakei, L. curvatus, L. parabuchneri, L. buchneri, L. plantarum, L. brevis, L. casei, L. paracasei, L. vaginalis, L. reuteri, L. hilgardii, L. mali, L. rhamnosus, L. paracollinoides, L. rossiae, L. helveticus, S. thermophilus, O. oeni, P. parvulus, Leuc. mesenteroides, W. cibaria, W. confusa, W. paramesenteroides, T. muriaticus, T. halophilus* |
| *Phenylethyl amine* | Phenylalanine | Aromatic | Tyrosine decarboxylase (TDC) | *E. faecium, E. faecalis, E. durans, E. hirae, E. casseliflavus, E. mundtii, L. brevis, Lc. lactis, Leuc. mesenteroides, C. divergens* |
| *Tyramine* | Tyrosine | Aromatic | Tyrosine decarboxylase (TDC) | *E. faecium, E. faecalis, E. durans, E. hirae, E. casseliflavus, E. mundtii, L. sakei, L. curvatus, L. plantarum, L. brevis, L: buchneri, L. casei, L. paracasei, L. reuteri, L. hilgardii, L. homohiochii, L. delbrueckii subsp. bulgaricus, S. thermophilus, S. macedonicus, Lc. lactis, Leuc. mesenteroides, W. cibaria, W. confusa, W. paramesenteroides, W. viridescens, C. divergens, C. maltaromaticum, C. galliranum, T. halophilus, Sporolactobacillus sp* |
| *Cadaverine* | Lysine | Aliphatic | Lysine decarboxylase (LDC) | *E. faecium, E. faecalis, L. curvatus, L. brevis, L. casei, L. paracasei, S. thermophilus, Pediococcus spp., Leuc. mesenteroides, T. halophilus* |
| *Putrescine* | Agmatine | Aliphatic | Agmatine deiminase (AgDI) | *E. faecalis, E. faecium, E. durans, E. hirae, E. mundtii, L. curvatus, L. plantarum, L. brevis, S. thermophilus, S. mutans, Lc. lactis, O. oeni, P. parvulus, P. pentosaceus, Leuc. mesenteroides, W. halotolerans, C. divergens, C. maltaromaticum, C. gallinarum* |
| | Arginine | Aliphatic | Ornithine decarboxylase (ODC) | *E. faecium, E. faecalis, E. durans, E. hirae, E. casseliflavus, L. sakei, L. curvatus, L. buchneri, L. plantarum, L. brevis, L. paracasei, L. mali, L. rhamnosus, L. rossiae, L. homohiochii, Lc. lactis, S. thermophilus, S. mutans, P. parvolus, O. oeni, T. halophilus* |

## 24.5 TOXICOLOGY

Biogenic amines have their significance in cellular physiology. Optimized concentration is needed to control the biosynthesis, absorption, and catabolism in cells and tissues of the body. Excess of intake of food abundant in biogenic amines results in accumulation of BAs in body which can disturb the proper activity of BAs in various metabolic processes. Studies have highlighted the toxicological reactions of some biogenic amines present even in small amounts. Improper intake of these biological compounds results in digestive, respiratory, and circulatory disorders (Table 24.3).

In human body diamine oxidase (DAO), histamine-N-methyl transferase (HNMT), monoamine oxidase (MAO) and polyamine oxidase (PAO) are the enzymes which play role in detoxification

**Table 24.3 Toxicological and Physiological Aspects of Various BAs in Human Health**

| Biogenic Amine | Toxic Effects | Physiological Effects |
|---|---|---|
| *Histamine* | Oedema, headache, rashes, sweating, extrasystoles, blood pressure disorders, dizziness, diarrhoea, blood pressure imbalance, respiratory problem, urticaria | Hormone, neurotransmitter, cell growth and differentiation, food intake, regulation of body temperature, allergic reactions, gastric acid secretion, immune response, learning, and memory |
| *Putrescine* | Carcinogenic effects, increase cardiac activity, hypotension | Cell growth and differentiation, regulation of gene expression, intestine maturation |
| *Tyramine* | Migraine, nausea, hypertension, respiratory disorders, neurological disorders | Neurotransmitter, support respiration, release norepinephrine from CNS, increase cardiac activity, vasoconstriction, increase blood glucose |

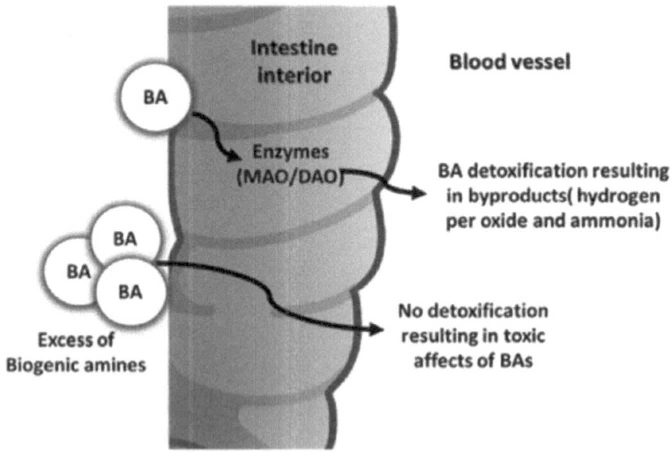


**Figure 24.2** Role of biogenic amines in human intestine.

of biogenic amines (Figure 24.2). Figure 24.3 show the role of biogenic amines in human intestine when it is accumulated in optimum and excessive amount.

### 24.5.1 Histamine Toxicity

By intake of large amount of food having histamine biogenic amine, histamine poisoning is caused. Due to excessive accumulation of amines, the oxidases are unable to detoxify the BAs resulting in a serious adverse effect. Histamine fish poisoning is commonly observed worldwide also referred to as "Scombroid Poisoning". The first cases were first observed in 1799 in Britain and then the disease again out broke in 1950s in Japan (Feng et al., 2016). Besides fish, excessive utilization of cheese also results in histamine poisoning.

Fish from *Scombridae* family like mackerel and tuna have high level of free histidine amino acid in their muscles which lead to Scombroid Poisoning (Ruiz-Capillas and Moral, 2004). Other than that, anchovies, yellowtail steak, herring, blue fish, tuna, and fish products like different sauces and roasted fish also result in histamine toxicity (Šimat and Dalgaard, 2011, Alfonzo et al., 2018). In tuna fish, the level of histidine is 15 g/kg, in herring it is 1 g/kg while fresh fish has minimum amount of histamine usually less than 0.1 mg/100 g (Burt et al., 1992, Frank et al., 1981). Scombroid poisoning is a foodborne toxicity which happens when a high amount of histamine is ingested. In raw fish, different enzymes and bacteria act on histidine amino acid converting it into histamine BA.

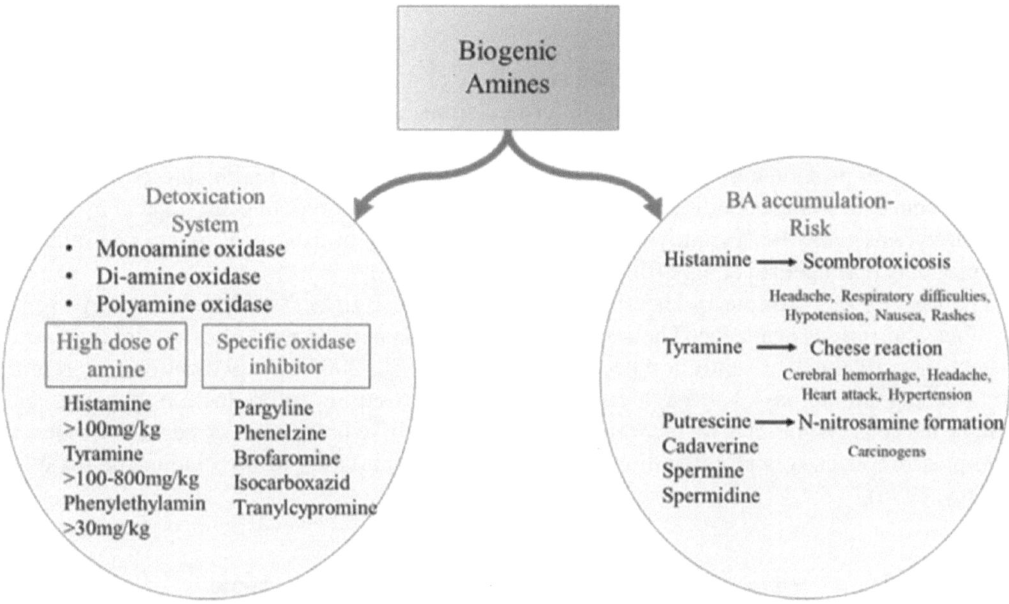


**Figure 24.3** Toxicity and mechanism of detoxification of biogenic amines.

Histidine metabolism has two mechanisms of action. First histidine is degraded to urocanic acid by the action of histidase enzyme and converting it into glutamic acid. Glutamic acid is further converted into α-ketoglutarate which is an intermediate product formed in Kreb's cycle (Tortorella et al., 2014).

In second mechanism the removal of carboxyl group occurs by the action of histidine decarboxylase enzyme forming histamine. Enzymes for decarboxylation are produced by gram negative bacteria like *E. coli*, *Pseudomonas aeruginosa*, *Morganella morganii*, and *Klebsiella* specie. These microorganisms are found in skin, gills, and intestine of fish (Taylor et al., 1989). Other bacteria-producing biogenic amines include *Salmonella*, *Escherichia*, *Lactobacillus*, *Shigella*, *Enterobacter*, and *Streptococcus* (Pinho et al., 2004). To control the production of BAs and their toxicity, the storage conditions are to be optimized, which includes a cold temperature environment. If the food is not properly processed, then it is the most likely to cause the conversion of histidine into histamine biogenic amine above the safety levels. Other parameters affecting BAs production include pH, addition of additives, drying, water activity, and sodium chloride concentration (Chong et al., 2011, Suzzi and Gardini, 2003). High levels of histamine are observed in fermented foods like cheese, wine, soy sauce, sausage, and miso. In intestine DAO is the enzyme which detoxifies histamine by catabolism. Due to drug usage (DAO inhibitors DAOI), e.g., verapamil, metoclopramide, clavulanic acid, and acetylcysteine or deficiency of DAO histamine accumulation could be occurring. Sensitive persons should avoid the intake of fermented foods.

The histamine poisoning symptoms are just like allergy symptoms which could be misled by food allergy. Histamine poisoning causes the following symptoms (Ohnuma et al., 2001);

- **Circulatory Disorders:** Hypertension or hypotension, palpitations, conjunctival injection, and tachycardia.
- **Gastric Disorders:** Vomiting, diarrhoea, cramping, nausea, and epigastric pain.
- **Skin:** Swelling, urticarial, rash and erythema on trunk, neck, face.
- **CNS Disorder:** Cramps, palpitations, loss of sight, cramps, headache, and warmth around mouth.
- **Respiratory Problems:** Bronchoconstriction.

### 24.5.2 Tyramine Toxicity

Cheese is a fermented dairy product which is a source of many biogenic amines like tyramine, histamine, cadaverine, and putrescine. During fermentation, activity of microorganisms enhances the production of BAs by decarboxylation of free amino acids. The production of biogenic amines in cheese is further promoted by presence of free amino acids, temperature, Ph, and presence of salts. It also depends on storage conditions. Tyramine is produced from tyrosine amino acid by the action of decarboxylase enzyme. Tyramine is also found abundantly in fish, meat, wine, and other dairy food products (Evangelista et al., 2016).

The toxicity of tyramine in cheese leads to the "Cheese Effect" which causes hypertension, migraine, and serious headache. The toxicity of tyramine is noticed more than that of histamine as it affects intestinal cells resulting in necrosis (Gennaro et al., 2003). Detoxification of tyramine is not simple, tyramine passes through circulatory system, resulting in production of noradrenaline from the nervous system. It is further reported that diseases like brain haemorrhage, diarrhoea, high blood pressure, nausea, and palpitations also result in accumulation of tyrosine to the toxic levels (Shalaby, 1996).

## 24.6 IDENTIFICATION AND QUANTIFICATION

Analytical techniques have played a great role in determining the biogenic amines in food and providing information about their toxicity levels. Variety of modern analytical methods are reported to detect and isolate the biogenic amines to their estimation but no single method is enough for the detection of all the biogenic amines in all foods. Figure 24.4 highlights the food source of biogenic amines and the analytical techniques for their estimation.

As indicated above, according to the perspective of food handling and to evaluate the possible poisonous impact of biogenic amine, it is essential to inhibit and figure out which BAs ought to be tended to. Various quick and precise insightful techniques have been developed to detect BA levels in various food products. These methods vary from the common colorimetric and fluorometric techniques most often used for the determination of histamine separately, to the ELISA catalyst

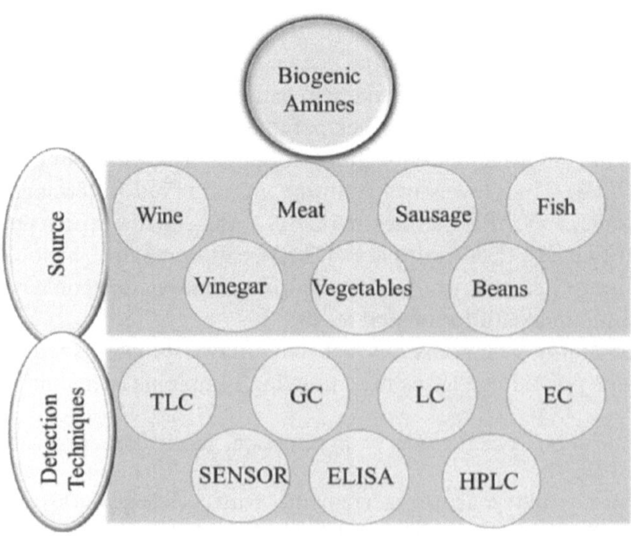


**Figure 24.4** Biogenic amines: food source and detection techniques.

immunoassay to identify histamine in fish. Other techniques for the analysis of biogenic amines include high-performance liquid chromatography, gas chromatography and gas chromatographic-mass spectrometry, HPLC-mass spectrometry, capillary electrophoresis, etc. Of these techniques, HPLC is the most sensitive and accurate for detection and measurement of biogenic amines. This technique provides accuracy and flexibility. In addition, it helps in analysis of all BAs in one go. The HPLC technique provides separation and detection of BAs from the food products. The extraction of BAs is accomplished by utilizing various solvents, for example, hydrochloric acid, trichloroacetic acid, per-chloric acid, methanol, etc. (Danchuk et al., 2020).

High-performance liquid chromatography is the advanced technique in which the separation column could be modified according to the nature of analyte to be separated. The column could be modified as reversed phase polarity, i.e., non-polar stationary phase or by using ion exchange chromatographic column. By adding functionalities to the column and using the selective mobile phase, the sensitivity of determining the biogenic amines is enhanced, especially those BAs which lack chromophores and have low volatility. The commonly used reagents to modify the column are benzoyl chloride, 3-(4-fluorobenzoyl)-2-quinolinecarboxylaldehyde, dansyl chloride, methane-sulfonic acid, p-phenyldiazonium sulfonate, and ortho-ophtaldehyde (OPA). Dansyl chloride and ortho-ophtaldehyde are mostly used in determination (Omanovic-Miklicanin and Valzacchi, 2017).

To determine the biogenic amines, more advancements are also made in analytical routine methods like flow injection analysis. This method provides rapid reaction system and control on chemical reaction along with all the steps being automatically controlled in online system. The detectors used are UV-visible spectrophotometer, fluorescent detector, and diode array detector. Flow injection analysis is coupled with mass spectroscopy or electrodes/reactors using enzymes like peroxidase, amine oxidase, and histaminase for BA analysis by using chemiluminescence or amperometry.

Analysis of biogenic amines in food is challenging work due to complex nature of sample matrix and presence of interfering compounds in the same aliquot. Chemical reagents like hydrochloric acid, trichloroacitic acid, perchloric acid, and other solvents are used for BAs extraction from food. Chromatographic techniques including paper chromatography, thin layer chromatography, gas chromatography, and high-performance liquid chromatography are used for separation and identification of BAs or their derivatives. For individual analysis of biogenic amines flourometric methods are also used.

Staruszkiewicz et al. devised the method to determine the amount of histamine present in the fish. The biogenic amines were extracted using methanol followed by the ion exchange chromatography for separation and detection by using flourometric method.

Lerke and Bell introduce the similar extraction procedure with modification of using 10%TCA and cation/anion exchange resin instead of methanol.

Further modifications in procedure were done by Taylor et al. by using sequential extraction. This method is used to determine tyramine amino acid in food (Taylor et al., 1978). Gas liquid chromatography and ultra-performance liquid chromatography are used to analyze the biogenic amines. The analytical techniques provide separation, identification, and quantification of most of the biogenic amines (Santos-Buelga et al., 1981).

Karmas and Mietz introduced the high-performance liquid chromatography method for analysis of spermine, cadaverine, histamine, putrescine, and spermidine in fish. The BAs were first reacted with dansyl chloride before estimation (Eerola et al., 1993).

Hui and Taylor proposed the process of derivatization of HPLC column for determination of cadaverine, tyramine, phenylethylamine, histamine, and putrescine in fish, sausage, and cheese. To determine histamine, putrescine, tyramine, and phenylethylamine in meat post-column derivatization is done using 3-mercaptopropionic acid ando-phthalaldehyde reagent (Joosten and Olieman, 1986).

Further modifications are being made in analytical techniques like gas liquid chromatographic techniques and amino acid analyzer for separation and determination of biogenic amines in food.

HPLC is the advanced technique with high sensitivity and resolution but problems may occur while analyzing BAs due to mobile phase either solvent or carrier gas. Mobile phase carries analyte with itself, which on reaching the detector may dilute the results, whereas thin layer chromatography is more sensitive as the mobile phase does not interfere with detection. Procedures for identification and estimation of biogenic amines should not be time-consuming as toxicity and amount of Bas increases if source (food) is not stored under optimum conditions. Improvement and novelty should be bought in current analytical methods to obtain rapid and precise results. Improvements should be bought in selection of extracting solvents, derivative formation, elution procedure in selection of appropriate stationary/mobile phase and detection technique. Development could not be possible without cooperation of government and industry. For such purpose international agencies and more laboratories should be made. Such programs will be helpful in registering the worldwide data on biogenic amines, in addition to establish a standard analytical method (Önal, 2007).

## 24.7 SAFETY, PRECAUTION, AND REGULATION

Biogenic amines are the cause of food intoxication especially histamine and tyramine. Putrescine and cadaverine also show toxic effects. People who lack the natural mechanisms triggered by genetic factors to detoxify BAs and take antidepressant drugs indicate that they are more vulnerable to poisoning with BAs. The toxicity level of BAs depends on individual characteristics. However, level of 750–900 mg/kg is proposed to be toxic (Ordóñez et al., 2016).

Histamine is a heat-stable biogenic amine due to which cooking, freezing or canning of food cannot eliminate it, and hence it has significant issues regarding public health. Therefore, one must know the amount of histamine in fish products before consumption (Ruiz-Capillas and Herrero, 2019).

It is not easy to determine the level of toxicity produced by biogenic amine as it depends on several factors including detoxification ability of individual intestine (Stadler and Lineback, 2008). The level of toxicity of BAs is extremely hard to determine since it is dependent on intestinal detoxification ability of person as well as the involvement of other factors. Table 24.4 describes the toxic level of histamine in fish. Legally, 100 mg of histamine/kg of food and 2 mg/L of alcoholic drinks are proposed to be safe. According to a report by European Food Safety Authority, despite the fact that an amount of 50 mg histamine is considered to fall under the No Observed Adverse Effect Level (NOAEL), a healthy person should not feel symptoms until he/she consumes more histamine than the NOAEL. Food toxic doses were stated to be 100 to 800 mg/kg of tyramine and 30 mg/kg of phenylethylamine.

Foodstuffs having 30 mg/kg of phenylethylamine is considered to be at toxic level, which is considered dangerous in food products. To certain sensitive individuals, 5–10 mg of histamine is considered normal, while 10 mg is almost normal, 100 mg has an average poisonous capacity and 1,000 mg is fatal and considered hazardous to one's well-being. For fish species belonging to *Clupeidae* and *Scombridae* family, the European Union has proposed guidelines for histamine accumulation levels. According to those guidelines, histamine levels should be less than 100 mg/kg in raw fish, and in salted fish it should be less than 200 mg/kg. The Slovak Republic's Nutritional Codex determined

**Table 24.4 Toxicity of Histamine in Fish**

| | Histamine (mg) | |
|---|---|---|
| *Amount of Fish (100g)* | <5 mg | Safe |
| | 5–10 mg | May be toxic |
| | 20–100 mg | Maybe toxic |
| | >100 mg | Toxic |

the maximum tolerated level of tyramine to be 200 mg/kg and histamine (20 mg/kg in lager and 200 mg/kg in fish and fish products) (Linares et al., 2016).

FDA has proposed 50 mg histamine/100g of fish as risk activity fixation. In the Turkish Food Codex, histamine at 200 mg/kg for fish and 10 mg/kg for wines is recognized as an abnormal indicator. The histamine accumulation for mackerel and herring angles is considered safe by German Fish Order at 200 mg/kg. To prevent unintended adverse effects, it would be beneficial to manufacture foods with low levels of BAs from a toxicological point of view (Küçük and Torul, 2018).

FDA proposed the Threat Analysis and Hazard Analysis Critical Control Point (HACCP) software in 1996 to avoid foodborne illnesses caused by seafood production hazards. At the harbour, a limit of 50 mg/kg was set for scombroid or scombroid-like fish (Feng et al., 2016). The toxic level of histamine was identified in many fish verities, such as the *Scombridae*, *Coryfenidae*, *Clupeidae*, *Pomatomide*, *Scombresosidae*, and *Engraulidae* families. The amount of mercury in fish products is 200 mg/kg. For fresh fish European law sets regulatory limits of 200 mg/kg and 400 mg/kg for fish products treated with different enzymes. The histamine biogenic amine is classified as a food additive by Codex Alimentarius. Levels of histamine in fish and fish products in Brazil and Mercosur are limited to 100 mg/kg, while in Europe its levels in fish and fish products are limited to 100 and 200 mg/kg (Magro et al., 2020, Rai et al., 2013).

The FDA89 guideline's key goal is to stop bacteria from producing histamine during the handling and preservation of fish products. The amount of time it takes to reduce the heat of fish after capturing depends on a variety of factors, which includes the harvesting and cooling techniques used, as well as the fish size. The scombrotoxin-producing fish should be frosted as possible before it is eaten (Lehane and Olley, 2000).

Tao et al. measured histamine levels in fresh scombroid (tuna, mackerel, etc.) and non-scombroid fish as well as fish products (sauce, dried fish) from China, Thailand, Philippines, Fiji, Netherlands, Cambodia, Japan, and Norway. Fiji's fish analyses had a low amount of histamine (12–31 ppm). Histamine was used in two of the 12 analyses from Germany (68 ppm in herring while 184 ppm in sardine). These levels were found to be higher than the FDA's limit of 50 ppm of histamine. In two of nine specimens from the Netherlands, histamine was found (1,439 ppm in Tuna while 39 ppm in horse mackerel). Even though tuna products seemed to be very new at that time, the histamine amount in the tuna (1,439 ppm) increased according to the EC control of histamine (100–200 ppm) from Netherlands. Histamine levels between 56 and 1,964 ppm was present in 4 4 of 11 Thai fish samples. In 3 processed freshwater fish tests from Cambodia, histamine levels ranged from 25 to 148 ppm. Histamine was found in 60% of preserved bonito extracts from the Philippines, with levels ranging from 19 to 1,530 ppm. In the Japanese specimens, no histamine or microbial amines were found. One study from China reported 15 ppm of histamine. In tested substances like (horse mackerel and saury), putrescence (13–25 ppm) as well as cadaverine (6 ppm) were found to be in one horse mackerel analysis. To certify the quality of imported fish and fish products globally, histamine levels must be monitored (Tao et al., 2011).

Users' alimentary susceptibility to single biogenic amines as well as the bioactive amines was assessed and overall, the highest tolerable levels of tyramine were found in Austrian foods. They found that people who aren't sensitive to tyramine have a higher risk of developing sugar disease. The NOAEL of 200 mg tyramine per meal is considered appropriate. In cheese, fermented sausage, fish/fishery goods, and sauerkraut, recommended maximum tyramine amounts may be 1,000 mg/kg, 2,000 mg/kg, 950 mg/kg, and 800 mg/kg, etc. It has been stated that typical tyramine intake is between 100 and 800 mg/kg, with amounts greater than 1,080 mg/kg considered to be hazardous. People who take MAOIs, on the other hand, are more vulnerable to tyramine intake, with 60 mg/kg in the food causing a moderate problem and 100–250 mg/kg causing extreme headache with intracranial haemorrhage and squeal (Doeun et al., 2017, Stadnik and Dolatowski, 2010).

Acute symptoms after oral ingestion are a major concern due to tryptamine's high metabolism. Foods have tryptamine levels of a 100 mg/kg or less. In the EFSA's scientific opinion, the highest recorded tryptamine content in fish and fish products was 362 mg/kg, whereas fermented fish meat had a value of 10.1 mg/kg. In the EFSA's scientific opinion, which summarized evidence from over 2,000 cheese tests from across Europe, the highest recorded tryptamine amount in cheese was 312 mg/kg in an Austrian semi-hard cheese. However, tryptamine levels above the sensitivity and specificity limit were found in 4% of the overall EFSA cheese samples. Allowable maximum values were found to be 1,650, 3,200, 2,840, 4,800, 14, 120, 1,740, and 2,400 mg/kg, collectively, for fresh/cooked seafood, frozen fish, cheese, raw sausage, seasonings, sauerkraut, and fermented tofu. Tryptamine levels in raw sausages and beer are well below the suggested allowable maximum tryptamine dose (Wüst et al., 2017).

The physicochemical regulation of six Italian-style salami products available in Niteroi area. Just half of the salami products met the Brazilian law's criteria for humidity and protein-rich, implying that quality management is critical. Two products had histamine levels that were higher than the permissible limit (100 mg/kg). It has been suggested that the bioactive amine amounts would have a huge impact in susceptible users, depending on the volume and duration of these goods consumed. Based on data and eating patterns in Austria, Rauscher-Gabernig et al. proposed acceptable amounts for putrescine and cadaverine in sausages, pork, cheese, sauerkraut, and flavourings. Allowable maximum ranges for putrescine in pork, sausage, sauerkraut, cheese and flavourings are suggested to be 140, 170, 180, 360, and 510 mg/kg, respectively, while maximum ranges allowed for cadaverine in sauerkraut, fish, cheese, preserved sausages and flavourings are 430, 510, 540, 1,080, and 1,540 mg/kg, respectively. Furthermore, experiments have shown that tyramine and histamine have unique and powerful inhibitory effects on intestinal cell cultures. It was also found that histamine, at levels below the recommended level, would increase the cytotoxicity of tyramine at levels commonly found in dietary fiber (Rauscher-Gabernig et al., 2012).

## 24.8 EFFECT OF PROCESSING

To ensure the safety of food it is important to monitor the presence of biogenic amines as they are toxic in nature and cause serious health issues. Managing the quality of food implements to the food safety and health guarantee. The quality of food refers to the nutrition, freshness, integrity, convenience, and its availability. There are different impacts of processing of food on biogenic amines concentration. It depends on raw material, storage temperature, addition of additives, presence of microorganisms, and packaging conditions.

The storage temperature of final products is also one of the critical factors in the formation of BAs (Tapingkae et al., 2010). By optimizing all these conditions, the shelf-life of food can be improved. We have to look for new strategies to preserve the food as a massive amount of food is needed globally. For this, deeper knowledge is required to develop new conservation systems to supply the food with optimum quality.

Drying of biogenic amine includes the freeze-drying method and fluidized bed-drying method. Freeze-drying method shows significant decrease in formation of biogenic amines (Topuz et al., 2021).

The process of fermentation allows the action of bacteria and other microorganisms action on substrate which is the step co-relating the production of biogenic amine (Bover-Cid et al., 2001). Hence process of fermentation promotes the growth of biogenic amines like putrescine, cadaverine, and tyramine. Using the optimized level of bacterial action can control the growth of BAs. The fermented food includes sausage, wine, cheese, cabbage, and other vegetables (Nout et al., 1993, Suzzi and Gardini, 2003).

Boiling at certain temperature decreases the formation of BAs in processed foods. The thermal processing of milk before cheese formation shows significant decrease in biogenic amines production (Bozkurt and Erkmen, 2004). By cooking or using additives, the formation of biogenic amines can be controlled. By addition of malic acid, succinic acid, and ascorbic acid in food prevents the histamine formation (Jairath et al., 2015, Lorenzo et al., 2007). Freezing up to low temperature inhibits the growth of microorganisms (*Proteus vulgaris*, *Morganella morganii*) by which the rate of formation of biogenic amines is also decreased. By maintaining the low temperature, the level of BAs can be stabilized in foods, e.g., yellowfin tuna can be stored at freezing temperature for nine days with low level of histamine production (Maijala et al., 1995). Roasting successfully reduces the quantity of histamine, cadaverine, spermine, tyramine, and putrescine biogenic amines. It leads to products having aseptic characteristics which decrease the biogenic amines formation by inhibiting the growth of decarboxylating bacteria. Roasted sausage has fewer BAs compared to the fermented sausage (Ekici and Omer, 2020).

## 24.9 FUTURE SCOPE

Biogenic amines are abundantly found in food products and are need to be investigated further. This is the subject of research for providing innovation to different food product storage procedures in the view of microbiological and toxicological actions. Further research should be conducted to overcome the toxicity of biogenic amines. To guarantee the human health and food safety, different factors should be studied which promote the production of biogenic amines. Histamine and tyramine are the leading biogenic amines causing toxicity in foods. Their accumulation in food should be controlled by modifying and improving the food preservation methods, thus controlling the growth of microorganisms. Biosensors sensing the production of BAs at toxic levels should be devised. Today's market is advancing to developing new materials and technologies to save human health and to increase shelf-life of foods. The activity of decarboxylase enzyme could be controlled to inhibit the production of biogenic amines. It could be done by optimizing pH, temperature, and other external conditions. Many analytical methods have been developed for quantifying the biogenic amines as a whole. Further research is still required to introduce simple, accurate, and precise methods to determine the concentration of individual biogenic amines. These developed methods and technologies should be accessible to public laboratories and regulatory authorities in order to ensure the food safety and quality.

It is challenging to monitor the concentration of biogenic amines in fish as it requires longer time duration as well as trained analysts. The first step of pre-concentration is hard and time-consuming. It is highly desired to develop automated techniques in order to run the samples in online mode. The chromatographic columns are first to be derivitized according to the polarity of biogenic amines. Immune-linked enzymatic assays like ELISA, biosensors, and several colorimetric techniques are used to determine the histamine level in raw fish and fish products but only semi quantitative results are provided by ELISA kits. Capillary electrophoresis is also a not very sensitive technique for BAs analysis but provides results in a short time period. Electrodes made of amine oxidase are used to catalyze deamination of biogenic amines to produce hydrogen per oxide and ammonia.

Electrochemical detectors are rapid and sensitive towards the detection of analyte qualitatively and quantitatively. In today's research, certain nano-materials like graphene, dendrimer, and carbon nanotubes have resulted in improved detection speed (as less amount of sample is required for analysis) and decreased cost.

## 24.10 CONCLUSIONS

Biogenic amines are considered to be the essential elements of human body as they play vital role in metabolism, normal development, and other physiological functions. They may cause toxic affects if are taken in excess amounts. The elevated concentration of biogenic amines is also proved to be carcinogenic.

Biogenic amines play great role in regulating the metabolic pathways, their source being the food which we ingest. The present chapter describes the occurrence, chemistry, biosynthesis, measuring techniques, toxicity, safety regulations of biogenic amines in foods. Such studies will provide the information about appropriate intake of biogenic amines up to the safe level for ensuring human health and well-being. Biogenic amines also show synergic effects, their activity pathways, and potential should also be noted. The progress and research in this regard provides food companies with new analytical techniques and methods to understand the factors which lead to the accumulation of biogenic amines. Thus, they may monitor and optimize them to keep the concentration of biogenic amines below toxic limits. The food industry should also progress to make food products free of biogenic amines for sensitive people.

## REFERENCES

Alfonzo, A., Gaglio, R., Francesca, N., Barbera, M., Saiano, F., Santulli, A., Matraxia, M., Rallo, F. and Moschetti, G. 2018. Influence of salt of different origin on the microbiological characteristics, histamine generation and volatile profile of salted anchovies (Engraulis encrasicolus L.). *Food Control*, 92: 301–311.

Almeida, C., Fernandes, J. and Cunha, S. 2012. A novel dispersive liquid–liquid microextraction (DLLME) gas chromatography-mass spectrometry (GC–MS) method for the determination of eighteen biogenic amines in beer. *Food Control*, 25(1): 380–388.

Bermúdez, R., Lorenzo, J., Fonseca, S., Franco, I. and Carballo, J. 2012. Strains of Staphylococcus and Bacillus Isolated from Traditional Sausages as Producers of Biogenic Amines. *Frontiers in Microbiology,* 3(151) https://doi.org/10.3389/fmicb.2012.00151

Bover-Cid, S., Hugas, M., Izquierdo-Pulido, M. and Vidal-Carou, M. C. 2001. Amino acid-decarboxylase activity of bacteria isolated from fermented pork sausages. *International Journal of Food Microbiology*, 66(3): 185–189.

Bozkurt, H. and Erkmen, O. 2004. Effects of temperature, humidity and additives on the formation of biogenic amines in sucuk during ripening and storage periods. *Food Science and Technology International*, 10(1): 21–28.

Burt, J. R., Hardy, R. and Whittle, K. J. 1992. *Pelagic Fish: The Resource and Its Exploitation*. Fishing News Books.

Chong, C., Abu Bakar, F., Russly, A., Jamilah, B. and Mahyudin, N. 2011. The effects of food processing on biogenic amines formation. *International Food Research Journal*, 18(3): 867-876.

Danchuk, A. I., Komova, N. S., Mobarez, S. N., Doronin, S. Y., Burmistrova, N. A., Markin, A. V. and Duerkop, A. 2020. Optical sensors for determination of biogenic amines in food. *Analytical and Bioanalytical Chemistry*, 412: 4023–4036.

Doeun, D., Davaatseren, M. and Chung, M.-S. 2017. Biogenic amines in foods. *Food Science and Biotechnology*, 26(6): 1463–1474.

Eerola, S., Hinkkanen, R., Lindfors, E. and Hirvi, T. 1993. Liquid chromatographic determination of biogenic amines in dry sausages. *Journal of AOAC International*, 76(3): 575–577.

Ekici, K. and Omer, A. K. 2020. Biogenic amines formation and their importance in fermented foods. BIO Web of Conferences: EDP Sciences, 00232.

Evangelista, W. P., Silva, T. M., Guidi, L. R., Tette, P. A., Byrro, R. M., Santiago-Silva, P., Fernandes, C. and Gloria, M. B. A. 2016. Quality assurance of histamine analysis in fresh and canned fish. *Food Chemistry*, 211: 100–106.

Feng, C., Teuber, S. and Gershwin, M. E. 2016. Histamine (scombroid) fish poisoning: a comprehensive review. *Clinical Reviews in Allergy & Immunology*, 50(1): 64–69.

Frank, H. A., Yoshinaga, D. H. and Nip, W. 1981. Histamine formation and honeycombing during decomposition of skipjack tuna, Katsuwonus pelamis, at elevated temperatures. *Marine Fisheries Review*, 43(10): 9–14.

Gennaro, M., Gianotti, V., Marengo, E., Pattono, D. and Turi, R. 2003. A chemometric investigation of the effect of the cheese-making process on contents of biogenic amines in a semi-hard Italian cheese (Toma). *Food Chemistry*, 82(4): 545–551.

Igarashi, K. and Kashiwagi, K. 2000. Polyamines: mysterious modulators of cellular functions. *Biochemical and Biophysical Research Communications*, 271(3): 559–564.

Jairath, G., Singh, P. K., Dabur, R. S., Rani, M. and Chaudhari, M. 2015. Biogenic amines in meat and meat products and its public health significance: a review. *Journal of Food Science and Technology*, 52(11): 6835–6846.

Jansen, S. C., van Dusseldorp, M., Bottema, K. C. and Dubois, A. E. 2003. Intolerance to dietary biogenic amines: a review. *Annals of Allergy, Asthma & Immunology*, 91(3): 233–241.

Joosten, H. and Olieman, C. 1986. Determination of biogenic amines in cheese and some other food products by high-performance liquid chromatography in combination with thermo-sensitized reaction detection. *Journal of Chromatography A*, 356: 311–319.

Küçük, A. and Torul, O. 2018. Voltammetric sensor based on poly (3-methylthiophene) synthesized in dichloromethane for tyramine determination in moldy cheese. *Synthetic Metals*, 237: 23–28.

Lehane, L. and Olley, J. 2000. Histamine fish poisoning revisited. *International Journal of Food Microbiology*, 58(1–2): 1–37.

Lim, E.-S. and Lee, N.-G. 2016. Control of histamine-forming bacteria by probiotic lactic acid bacteria isolated from fish intestine. *Korean Journal of Microbiology*, 52(3): 352–364.

Linares, D. M., Martín, M., Ladero, V., Alvarez, M. A. and Fernández, M. 2011. Biogenic amines in dairy products. *Critical Reviews in Food Science and Nutrition*, 51(7): 691–703.

Linares, D. M., del Rio, B., Redruello, B., Ladero, V., Martin, M. C., Fernandez, M., Ruas-Madiedo, P. and Alvarez, M. A. 2016. Comparative analysis of the in vitro cytotoxicity of the dietary biogenic amines tyramine and histamine. *Food Chemistry*, 197: 658–663.

Lorenzo, J. M., Martínez, S., Franco, I. and Carballo, J. 2007. Biogenic amine content during the manufacture of dry-cured lacón, a Spanish traditional meat product: effect of some additives. *Meat Science*, 77(2): 287–293.

Lu, S., Ji, H., Wang, Q., Li, B., Li, K., Xu, C. and Jiang, C. 2015. The effects of starter cultures and plant extracts on the biogenic amine accumulation in traditional Chinese smoked horsemeat sausages. *Food Control*, 50: 869–875.

Magro, S. L., Summa, S., Iammarino, M., D'Antini, P., Marchesani, G., Chiaravalle, A. E. and Muscarella, M. 2020. A 5-years (2015–2019) control activity of an EU laboratory: contamination of histamine in fish products and exposure assessment. *Applied Sciences*, 10(23): 8693.

Maijala, R., Nurmi, E. and Fischer, A. 1995. Influence of processing temperature on the formation of biogenic amines in dry sausages. *Meat Science*, 39(1): 9–22.

Maijala, R. L., Eerola, S. H., Aho, M. A. and Hirn, J. A. 1993. The effect of GDL-induced pH decrease on the formation of biogenic amines in meat. *Journal of Food Protection*, 56(2): 125–129.

Mayer, H. K. and Fiechter, G. 2018. UHPLC analysis of biogenic amines in different cheese varieties. *Food Control*, 93: 9–16.

Mohammed, G., Bashammakh, A., Alsibaai, A., Alwael, H. and El-Shahawi, M. 2016. A critical overview on the chemistry, clean-up and recent advances in analysis of biogenic amines in foodstuffs. *TrAC Trends in Analytical Chemistry*, 78: 84–94.

Nout, M., Ruikes, M., Bouwmeester, H. and Beljaars, P. 1993. Effect of processing conditions on the formation of biogenic amines and ethyl carbamate in soybean tempe. *Journal of Food Safety*, 13(4): 293–303.

Ohnuma, S., Higa, M., Hamanaka, S., Matsushima, K. and Yamamuro, W. 2001. An outbreak of allergy-like food poisoning. *Internal Medicine*, 40(8): 833–835.

Omanovic-Miklicanin, E. and Valzacchi, S. 2017. Development of new chemiluminescence biosensors for determination of biogenic amines in meat. *Food Chemistry*, 235: 98–103.

Önal, A. 2007. A review: current analytical methods for the determination of biogenic amines in foods. *Food Chemistry*, 103(4): 1475–1486.

Ordóñez, J. L., Troncoso, A. M., García-Parrilla, M. D. C. and Callejón, R. M. 2016. Recent trends in the determination of biogenic amines in fermented beverages: a review. *Analytica Chimica Acta*, 939: 10–25.

Özogul, F. and Özogul, Y. 2007. The ability of biogenic amines and ammonia production by single bacterial cultures. *European Food Research and Technology*, 225(3): 385–394.

Özogul, Y. and Özogul, F. 2019. *Biogenic Amines Formation, Toxicity, Regulations in Food, pp 1-7; Royal Society of Chemistry London, UK.*

Pinho, O., Pintado, A. I., Gomes, A. M., Pintado, M. M. E., Malcata, F. X. and Ferreira, I. M. 2004. Interrelationships among microbiological, physicochemical, and biochemical properties of Terrincho cheese, with emphasis on biogenic amines. *Journal of Food Protection*, 67(12): 2779–2785.

Pircher, A., Bauer, F. and Paulsen, P. 2007. Formation of cadaverine, histamine, putrescine and tyramine by bacteria isolated from meat, fermented sausages and cheeses. *European Food Research and Technology*, 226(1): 225–231.

Prester, L. 2011. Biogenic amines in fish, fish products and shellfish: a review. *Food Additives & Contaminants: Part A*, 28(11): 1547–1560.

Rai, K. P., Pradhan, H. R., Sharma, B. K. and Rijal, S. K. 2013. Histamine in foods: its safety and human health implications. *Journal of Food Science and Technology Nepal*, 8: 1–11.

Rauscher-Gabernig, E., Gabernig, R., Brueller, W., Grossgut, R., Bauer, F. and Paulsen, P. 2012. Dietary exposure assessment of putrescine and cadaverine and derivation of tolerable levels in selected foods consumed in Austria. *European Food Research and Technology*, 235(2): 209–220.

Ruiz-Capillas, C. and Herrero, A. M. 2019. Impact of biogenic amines on food quality and safety. *Foods*, 8(2): 62.

Ruiz-Capillas, C. and JimÉNez-Colmenero, F. 2005. Biogenic amines in meat and meat products. *Critical Reviews in Food Science and Nutrition*, 44(7–8): 489–599.

Ruiz-Capillas, C. and Moral, A. 2004. Free amino acids and biogenic amines in red and white muscle of tuna stored in controlled atmospheres. *Amino Acids*, 26(2): 125–132.

Santos-Buelga, C., Nogales-Alarcon, A. and Marine-Font, A. 1981. A method for the analysis of tyramine in meat products: its content in some Spanish samples. *Journal of Food Science*, 46(6): 1794–1795.

Ščavničar, A., Rogelj, I., Kočar, D., Köse, S. and Pompe, M. 2018. Determination of biogenic amines in cheese by ion chromatography with tandem mass spectrometry detection. *Journal of AOAC International*, 101(5): 1542–1547.

Sebastian, P., Herr, P. and Fischer, U. 2011. Molecular identification of lactic acid bacteria occurring in must and wine. *South African Journal of Enology and Viticulture*, 32(2): 300–309.

Shalaby, A. R. 1996. Significance of biogenic amines to food safety and human health. *Food Research International*, 29(7): 675–690.

Šimat, V. and Dalgaard, P. 2011. Use of small diameter column particles to enhance HPLC determination of histamine and other biogenic amines in seafood. *LWT-Food Science and Technology*, 44(2): 399–406.

Spano, G., Russo, P., Lonvaud-Funel, A., Lucas, P., Alexandre, H., Grandvalet, C., Coton, E., Coton, M., Barnavon, L. and Bach, B. 2010. Biogenic amines in fermented foods. *European Journal of Clinical Nutrition*, 64(3, Supplement 3): S95–S100.

Stadler, R. H. and Lineback, D. R. 2008. *Process-induced Food Toxicants: Occurrence, Formation, Mitigation, and Health Risks.* Wiley.

Stadnik, J. and Dolatowski, Z. J. 2010. Biogenic amines in meat and fermented meat products. *ACTA Scientiarum Polonorum Technologia Alimentaria*, 9(3): 251–263.

Suzzi, G. and Gardini, F. 2003. Biogenic amines in dry fermented sausages: a review. *International Journal of Food Microbiology*, 88(1): 41–54.

Tao, Z., Sato, M., Zhang, H., Yamaguchi, T. and Nakano, T. 2011. A survey of histamine content in seafood sold in markets of nine countries. *Food Control*, 22(3–4): 430–432.

Tapingkae, W., Tanasupawat, S., Parkin, K. L., Benjakul, S. and Visessanguan, W. 2010. Degradation of histamine by extremely halophilic archaea isolated from high salt-fermented fishery products. *Enzyme and Microbial Technology*, 46(2): 92–99.

Taylor, S. L. and Eitenmiller, R. R. 1986. Histamine food poisoning: toxicology and clinical aspects. *CRC Critical Reviews in Toxicology*, 17(2): 91–128.

Taylor, S. L., Leatherwood, M. and Lieber, E. R. 1978. Histamine in sauerkraut. *Journal of Food Science*, 43(3): 1030–1030.

Taylor, S. L., Stratton, J. E. and Nordlee, J. A. 1989. Histamine poisoning (scombroid fish poisoning): an allergy-like intoxication. *Journal of Toxicology: Clinical Toxicology*, 27(4–5): 225–240.

Topuz, O. K., Yatmaz, H. A., Alp, A. C., Kaya, A. and Yerlikaya, P. 2021. Biogenic amine formation in fish roe in under the effect of drying methods and coating materials. *Journal of Food Processing and Preservation*, 45(1): e15052.

Tortorella, V., Masciari, P., Pezzi, M., Mola, A., Tiburzi, S. P., Zinzi, M. C., Scozzafava, A. and Verre, M. 2014. Histamine poisoning from ingestion of fish or scombroid syndrome. *Case Reports in Emergency Medicine*, 4825311(04 pages).

Wüst, N., Rauscher-Gabernig, E., Steinwider, J., Bauer, F. and Paulsen, P. 2017. Risk assessment of dietary exposure to tryptamine for the Austrian population. *Food Additives & Contaminants: Part A*, 34(3): 404–420.

CHAPTER 25

# Emerging Food Toxins and Contaminants

**Sheikh Firdous Ahmad, Snehasmita Panda, Triveni Dutt, Manjit Panigrahi, and Bharat Bhushan**

## CONTENTS



## 25.1 INTRODUCTION

The world population is ever-increasing while food resources are limited. According to Malthusian theory, the human population increases in geometric fashion while food resources increase following an arithmetic progression. The world civilization has experienced many high-impact developments that have long-lasting effects on future generations and their sustainability. These mainly include developments such as industrialization, advanced transportation, mechanization, urbanization, and others. Along with positive impact, these processes have negative effects too on overall human races and the environmental patterns. These negatives have the potential to create havoc within the shortest possible time that many populations of flora and fauna can get destroyed with their effects. The modern human perception says that everything is toxic; it is only the dose that decides the toxicity. Even clean water and food, if taken in excess amounts may prove to be toxic, given that scientific reasons play their role in generating the toxicity (Dolan, Matulka, and Burdock 2010). Excessive water intake within short periods may case hyponatremia (less sodium in body) and cerebral edema while too much of food may lead to stagnation and hamper the sojourn of gastro-intestinal tract (GIT) and eventually cause enterotoxaemia. Similarly, too much intake of Vitamin A may lead to liver damage/hepatotoxicity (Sy et al. 2020). Emerging toxins are produced due to food processing and/or interaction with different integral parts of food items, demographic, and environmental factors. Emerging toxins are generally recently discovered, whose toxic potential has not been studied/identified yet, unregulated, or not strictly regulated by existing legislation with a potential to cause disorders in human/animal populations at present or in future.

DOI: 10.1201/9781003178446-25

Nature has bestowed humankind with many things without which its existence within the universe would have been very difficult and nearly impossible. Emerging toxins are produced due to food processing and/or interaction with different integral parts of food items, demographic, and environmental factors. Emerging toxins are generally recently discovered, whose toxic potential has not been studied/identified yet, unregulated, or not strictly regulated by existing legislation with a potential to cause disorders in human/animal populations at present or in future, not only for humans but for all non-human species. However, for one or other reasons, all food items contain ingredients that may prove to be toxic in their natural forms or after handling, storage, processing, or other similar procedures. From growth of plants/animals and journey of food items to the platter, every step is potentially toxic if proper precautions are not undertaken.

Initially during evolution, the plant- and animal-derived foods contained many toxic metabolites that hindered their consumption by humans and other higher hierarchical members of the food chain, thereby rendering them inedible. However, natural selection and efforts from artificial selection coupled with domestication events have led to the decrease of these harmful ingredients in foods of plant and animal origin. The human civilization has made much progress and chemical substances continuously gain entry into the living routines of humans. These include preservatives, sweeteners, drugs and residues, veterinary drugs, heavy metals, and others (Campo and Picó 2020). Sometimes, different environmental contaminants are also included in this group of toxins. In the current era, the list of environmental toxins and contaminants is continuously growing (Kantiani et al. 2010). There may be multiple reasons responsible for occurrence of emerging toxins in food products that include food processing steps, transportation under unhygienic/poor sanitary conditions and addition of chemicals as preservatives, chemicals for shelf-life improvement and others (Rather et al. 2017).

Basically, the food toxins may broadly be divided into two classes, i.e., conventional toxins and emerging toxins. Conventional toxins refer to those which occur naturally in the food ingredients, are majorly known to humankind and processes for their removal or management exists since long periods of time. Whereas, emerging toxins are produced due to food processing and/or interaction with different integral parts of food items, demographic, and environmental factors. Emerging toxins are generally recently discovered, whose toxic potential has not been studied/identified yet, unregulated, or not strictly regulated by existing legislation with a potential to cause disorders in human/animal populations at present or at futuristic times (Thapa, Shrestha, and Anal 2020; Campo and Picó 2020). Emerging toxins may be generated from an unknown or known source and perceived via a naive exposure to human population or identified through application of novel and advanced scientific methodologies in their detection (Gavrilescu et al. 2015; Murnyak et al. 2011). The food habits of previous generations were so different from those of the present generation that susceptibility to some toxins has vanished while tolerance to other toxins has decreased. Waste materials are continuously generated from different industrial and domestic processes which include the production of chemicals, hormones, fertilizers, pharmaceuticals, etc., and their subsequent release into the environment. These wastes, under certain environmental conditions, can potentially lead to the generation of various types of emerging toxins. Through this way, the concept of emerging toxins is ever-evolving. Emerging toxins and contaminants are often reported to be associated with many health hazards that vary from simple allergic reaction to many systemic syndromes including cancerous states. Therefore, it is important to review and study the emerging toxins so that food safety of masses is ensured in a sustainable way. In the recent decades, many emerging toxins and contaminants have been reported to exist, courtesy mainly to the advancement in analysis and detection principles/ methodology (Lei et al. 2015). Recently, attempts to classify different emerging toxins into broad groups have been made. In this chapter, an attempt is made to initially introduce the concept of emerging toxins followed by detailed analysis about the emerging toxins and contaminants in food.

Emerging toxins are an intricate part of modern human civilization with increased use of modern technology and chemicals such as pesticides, fertilizers, deep seepage of chemicals, pollution of water with chemical effluents from various industries, aerosols, cosmetics, etc. The human civilization as well as science have taken many leaps and has made these processes indispensable with modern life (Thomaidis & Asimakopoulos 2012). Consequently, the production of anthropogenically produced chemicals has increased by many-folds in the modern world (Gavrilescu et al. 2015). The emerging toxins can be classified based on source at which they are generated viz. plant- and animal-generated toxins. In plant-derived foods, several toxicants are usually present that vary from alkenyl Benzenes to Xanthin alkaloids. Hajšlová et al. (2018) have reviewed the occurrence of these plant toxicants in members of different plant families. The emerging toxins from animal foods include mycotoxicosis and several other pathogenic agents that were previously commensals or non-pathogenic to normal individuals but have emerged as pathogens under modern era due to changes in environment and other aspects.

## 25.2 EMERGING CHEMICAL AND BIOLOGICAL TOXINS

The nature of emerging toxins in terms of their chemistry, distribution, toxicology and other important aspects is so varied which hampers elaborate discussion on them in traditional ways. Newell et al. (2010) reported more than 200 chemical and biological toxins to be existent in food and food products. In the environment, micropollutants get converted to emerging toxins after chemical degradation of conventional organic toxins and/ or subsequent persistence of metabolites thereby (Sørensen et al. 2007). At many instances, pharmaceutical wastes are continuously accumulated at a single place that leads to maintenance of conducive environment needed for the production of emerging toxins. With increased mechanization and changes in farming practices coupled with intensive production approaches, chances of leaching of surface and groundwater resources are increased. This leads to generation of chemical metabolites and emerging toxins and subsequently increased incidence of health hazards in humans and animals. Currently, research studies are targeted towards studying the interaction of these chemical metabolites with internal hormonal and other chemical-messenger based organ systems of human body (Gavrilescu et al. 2015).

Anthropogenic activities have resulted in contamination of majority of natural resources including water and air. This has given rise to new pathogenic biological organisms including bacteria, viruses, and fungi that are capable of causing diseases in humans and animals, especially under immunocompromised states. At other instances, human activities generate the conducive environment for the development of microbial pathogens. Environmental interactions change, thereby posing new challenges due to varying trends in the growth of emerging and re-emerging pathogenic organisms. The spectrum of toxins from emerging and re-emerging pathogens is widening and is one of the biggest threats to human civilization via increased incidence of antibiotic resistant strains of pathogens. Mycotoxins are one of the important emerging toxins that have the potential to cause food poisoning and allergic reactions in mammalian species consuming it.

Under the current era, different chemicals are routinely being poured out into the environment due to various anthropogenic activities. These mainly include disinfectants, detergents, chemical insecticides and pesticides, sanitizers, etc. These chemicals sooner or later gain access to the food chain and pose serious threat to human life. Different classes of emerging toxins and contaminants of chemical nature have been identified to date that include polyhalogenated compounds (including perfluorinated, perchlorinated, and polybrominated compounds), organophosphorus compounds (like organophosphorus flame retardants), pharmaceutical compounds, and compounds formed during processing and storage of food products (like perfluoroalkyl substances and microplastics), biotoxins of alkaloid nature (like amygdaline or pyrrolizidine), and other compounds (like cyanogen glucosides and pyrrolizidine alkaloids, gasoline additives, cosmetic wastes) (Lei et al. 2015; Campo and Picó 2020; Sharma and Ghoshal 2018).

### 25.2.1 Perfluorinated Compounds as Emerging Toxins

Perfluorinated compounds are special substances that are produced when all alkyl groups attached to hydrophobic part of a hydrocarbon chain are fully fluorinated. The perfluorinated compounds mainly include Perfluorooctanesulfonate (PFOS) and Perfluorooctanoic acid (PFOA) along with their salts. These compounds are both water as well as oil repellents and thus find applications in many products, especially for surface treatments (Kantiani et al. 2010). They have emerged as an indispensable part of modern life and are part of major industrial processes leading to production of various consumer goods (Stahl, Mattern, and Brunn 2011). They form important ingredients in paint and paint accessories, inks, various wall coating formulations, detergent products, non-stick coatings in cooking utensils and even textile industry (Lei et al. 2015). These compounds are resistant to microbial metabolism and degradation and are thus considered bio-accumulative. Ahrens (2011) reported the presence of perfluorinated compounds (PFOA and PFOS) on land surface, water (both drinking and sea water sources) and even in different body fluids (serum, milk, etc.). Mostly, the perfluorinated compounds are termed as persistent organic pollutants with high thermo-chemical stability mainly due to the presence of peculiar Carbon-Fluorine bonds (Stahl, Mattern, and Brunn 2011).

Perfluorinated compounds reach food chain of humans through various paths that include ingestion of contaminated foods, contact with contaminated non-food items, aerosol route, and others. In other words, ingestion, inhalation, and skin contact cum penetration are three important ways for perfluorinated compounds to reach the human body. Some studies have reported the crossing of perfluorinated compounds even through the placental barrier during prenatal life (Hinderliter et al. 2005; Midasch et al. 2007; Stahl, Mattern, and Brunn 2011) and its transfer to newborn babies through milk of lactating mothers (Stahl, Mattern, and Brunn 2011; Hinderliter et al. 2005; So et al. 2006; Kärrman et al. 2007). Various perfluorinated compounds have been reported to be associated with incidences of different diseases in humans and animals, including cancer, thyroid and reproductive dysfunction, hormonal and endocrine disruption, and other metabolic diseases, etc. (Lei et al. 2015).

### 25.2.2 Disinfection By-Products in Water

The usage of drinking water is indispensable for human civilizations. Concurrently, water is an optimum carrier for many pathogens and can cause numerous diseases. Disinfection products are routinely used to purify water resources and make it fit for human consumption. When disinfection products are used in drinking water tanks, swimming pools, and other water resources, purification is based on the oxidizing power of these chemicals. However, the oxidation process is coupled with reduction reactions, too, wherein these interactions lead to generations of different emerging toxins which may prove hazardous to human and animal health (Richardson 2009). Emergence of disinfection by-products along with their interaction with different pollutants in water is an untoward and unintentional consequence of the water purification processes (Li and Mitch 2018). Similar to perfluorinated compounds, the disinfection products reach human body through different ways that include ingestion, inhalation, and absorption/penetration via skin. Disinfection by-products have also been reported to be associated with cancer, other reproductive disorders, foetal anomalies, and other malformations (Lei et al. 2015; Richardson 2003; Li and Mitch 2018).

### 25.2.3 Pharmaceutical Products

With scientific advancement in therapeutics, pharmaceuticals and pharmaceutical products are routinely used for maintaining physiological functions and addressing different pathological conditions both in humans and animals/poultry. Many pharmaceutical compounds are used for growth promotion and prevention of different diseases in animals, especially in poultry. Some of the pharmaceutical compounds persist in the meat and other food products of these animals and thus gain entry into the food chain and gain access to the human body. Improper disposal of hospital waste and other pharmaceutical products also results in their accumulation and generation of metabolic substances when conducive environmental conditions are met. Many pharmaceutical substances are routinely used in the current era for personal care. These have long-lasting physiological effects, even at small doses (Ebele, Abou-Elwafa Abdallah, and Harrad 2017). Bioactivity of these pharmacological by-products leads to toxicological and hazardous effects in humans and animals (Chopra and Kumar 2018). Different classes of pharmaceutical substances and by-products vary in their level of persistency in different environments. This way they also get entry into the ground water and other food products and ultimately reach the food chain. These pharmaceutical by-products are not easily filtered via sewage treatments too and thus pose risk of health hazard to humans and animals (Ebele, Abdallah, and Harrad 2017). The entry of pharmaceutical by-products into the human body is mainly through drinking water and other aquatic environments. Moreover, the metabolites formed after interaction of primary pharmacological products in aquatic and other environments also threaten human civilizations with possibility of many adversities.

In the current era, nutritional supplements, anabolic steroids, diagnostic kits, hormonal preparations, and antibiotics are routinely used and leave long-lasting traces on the environment. These compounds are continuously discarded in aquatic and ecological niches and possess bioactivity even at smaller amounts. Similarly, coccidiostatic and coccidiocidal drugs are continuously used in poultry. The drug residues persist in different food products originating from these species (food and eggs) or are voided via faeces and thereby gain entry into the food chain of humans.

### 25.2.4 Microplastics

The use of plastics has seen a rapid rise in the twentieth century, especially in developing countries. Microplastics are small sized particles of plastic nature which are less than 5 mm in size (Peng et al. 2018). They are generated originally at this size range or are result of fragmentation process of plastic products due to varied reasons. Microplastics are generally classified into primary and secondary types. On one hand, primary microplastics are inherently less than 5 mm in size and are not generally the degradation products before entering the environment. These mostly generate from clothing, plastic pellets, and beads. Whereas secondary microplastics are generated due to the degradation process from different sources that include plastic bottles, nets, bags, and containers. Microplastics mainly include low-weight polymeric compounds like low-density polyethylene (LDPE), polyethylene terephthalate (PET), polystyrene (PS), poly vinyl chloride (PVC), polyurethane (PUR), and others (Pandey et al. 2020). Microplastics are increasingly being generated under different environmental conditions, especially aquatic ecosystems. They are considered as emerging toxins and their entry into the food chain through aquatic food and food products has been reported in many studies (Rainieri and Barranco 2019). Microplastics adsorb, along with themselves, several heavy and toxic metals that can easily reach the food chain and can cause nephrotoxic and hepatotoxic effects in the human body. The microplastics are also eaten away by fishes and other aquatic species. Microplastics, through this way, reach the stomach of fishes and other aquatic species. However, stomach parts of fish are inedible and generally not eaten by humans. The microplastics in stomach are eaten by animals when fish GIT is used as non-conventional food resources for them. Through animal food, microplastics reach the food chain and ultimately pose a threat to humans.

An additional threat posed by microplastics is through adsorption sites that are made available for various toxic contaminants, especially in aquatic resources. This has also been reported to be associated with adsorption of carcinogens and chemical substances that are inherently endocrine disruptors and can prove really lethal for human and animal life in the long run. Moreover, pesticides and organic pollutants also get adsorbed on to the surface of microplastics. This generates major problems for drinking water as natural and artificial processes to sequestrate pollution are affected, especially in developing nations (Peng et al. 2018). Furthermore, the disintegration/degradation of microplastics is associated with the release of more toxic compounds including phthalates and ethers (Pandey et al. 2020). Drinking water is considered a sink for microplastics due to its peculiarity to resist the phenomenon of biodegradability. It provides longevity to microplastics and helps its aggregation.

### 25.2.5 Emerging Biological Food Toxins

Several microorganisms exist as commensals inside the human and animal body and play important roles in maintaining optimal physiological states. However, at some instances, these commensal organisms become pathogenic when the individual is under stress or immunocompromised. At other instances, different kinds of chemical substances (metabolites and co-metabolites) are produced by microorganisms, especially by fungal organisms which contaminate food and food products. The chemical metabolites produced by fungal species are termed as mycotoxins. Mycotoxins are basically the toxic secondary metabolites of fungal activity, mainly produced during food storage. These possess abundant health hazard and health risk to the consumers (Karlovsky et al. 2016). Aflatoxins, Ochratoxins, Zearalenone, trichothecenes, zearalenone, fumonisins, etc., are some of the important mycotoxins that produce hepatotoxic and nephrotoxic effects in consuming species. Aspergillus, Pencillium, and Fusarium species of fungi mainly produce these toxins (Hajšlová et al. 2018). Unlike the enterotoxins produced by *Staphylococcus* and *Bacillus* species in food items, mycotoxins are heat-labile and are not easy to be removed via thermal processing of food stuffs. Some of the mycotoxins are able to penetrate the body barriers and are secreted via milk and can reach food chain via this route too. Similarly, phytotoxins are produced by unicellular algae and microalgal species. These toxins are present mainly in and around aquatic or semi-aquatic environments and gain entry to food chain via drinking water. The emerging biological toxins mainly lead to diarrhoeal states, hepatotoxicity, typhoid symptoms, fever, gastritis, vomition, rashes, and sometimes neurological symptoms (Newell et al. 2010).

## 25.3 ANALYTICAL TECHNIQUES TO DETECT EMERGING TOXINS AND CONTAMINANTS

Advanced scientific technologies are needed to deal with such emerging toxins so that they are meticulously identified and the natural resources polluted with these toxins are purified for immediate human use. Perfluorinated compounds (PFCs) are polar and need processing to be analysed through conventional gas chromatography techniques. Therefore, the method of choice for analysis of PFCs is liquid chromatography coupled with mass spectrometry (LC-MS) (Dorman and Reiner 2012). However, for less polar PFCs, gas chromatography technique may be employed for analytical procedures. For analysis of microplastics in food and food products, visual sorting using microscopy followed by spectroscopy are usually used (Shim, Hong, and Eo 2017; Hanvey et al. 2017). Similarly, a combination of liquid chromatography and mass spectrometry is advocated for analysis of disinfection by-products and pharmaceutical products in food and food products (Zwiener and Richardson 2005). The emerging analytical methods for disinfection by-products in water include high-resolution mass spectrometry, total organic halogen analysis, and total ion current-toxic potency testing (Yang, Liberatore, and Zhang 2019). Application of nanomaterials and nanotechnology are some of the emerging aspects that may help in purification of food stuffs affected with emerging toxins and ensuring food safety. In the near future, it will be really important to develop semi-automatic or automatic techniques in order to improve the accuracy regarding identification cum quantification of emerging toxins and pollutants in food and food products. However, cost implications, field application, and other relevant aspects need to be taken into account.

## 25.4 CONCLUSION

The world population is ever-evolving while the food resources are limited. Safe, nutritious, and affordable food is needed for every living being. However, food toxicity is a big challenge that hinders the availability of quality, nutritious food to all human beings across the world. Though some scientific advances have helped in the understanding and removal of a few conventional toxins, food toxicity is still a huge issue. An additional challenge is posed by continuously emerging chemical and biological toxins. Emerging toxins are generally recently discovered, whose toxic potential has not been studied/identified yet, unregulated, or not strictly regulated by existing legislation with a potential to cause disorders in human/animal populations at present or at futuristic times. Emerging toxins are sometimes produced due to food processing and/or interaction with different integral parts of food items, demographic, and environmental factors. Environmental contaminants are routinely classed with emerging toxins. With increased developments including mechanization, industrialization, advanced transportation, and others, chemical substances are routinely voided out into the environment which are potential sources of several types of emerging toxins. Some biological agents that were previously non-toxic or remained commensals facilitating optimal physiological states in humans and animals have gained the pathogenic capacity and lead to the production of emerging toxins in food and food products. Though many routine techniques are available for analysis of emerging toxins and contaminants, advanced analytical techniques, including the use of nanomaterials and nanotechnology, can be of immense help in controlling the issue of toxicity in food and food products with regard to emerging toxins and contaminants.

## REFERENCES

Ahrens, L. 2011. Polyfluoroalkyl compounds in the aquatic environment: a review of their occurrence and fate. *Article in Journal of Environmental Monitoring*, 13(1): 20–31.

Campo, J. and Picó, Y. 2020. Emerging contaminants and toxins. In Elsevier and Y. Picó (Ed.), *Chemical Analysis of Food*, pp. 729–758. Academic Press.

Chopra, S. and Kumar, D., 2018. Pharmaceuticals and personal care products (PPCPs) as emerging environmental pollutants: toxicity and risk assessment. In *Advances in Animal Biotechnology and Its Applications*, pp. 337–353. Springer.

Dolan, L.C., Matulka, R.A. and Burdock, G.A. 2010. Naturally occurring food toxins. *Toxins*, 2(9): 2289–2332.

Dorman Jr, F.L. and Reiner, E.J. 2012. Emerging and persistent environmental compound analysis. In *Gas Chromatography*, pp. 647–677. Elsevier Inc.

Ebele, A.J., Abdallah, M.A.E. and Harrad, S. 2017. Pharmaceuticals and personal care products (PPCPs) in the freshwater aquatic environment. *Emerging Contaminants*, 3(1): 1–16.

Gavrilescu, M., Demnerová, K., Aamand, J., Agathos, S. and Fava, F. 2015. Emerging pollutants in the environment: present and future challenges in biomonitoring, ecological risks and bioremediation. *New Biotechnology*, 32(1): 147–156.

Hajšlová, J., Schulzová, V., Botek, P. and Lojza, J. 2018. Natural toxins in food crops and their changes during processing. *Czech Journal of Food Science*, 22: S29–S34.

Hanvey, J.S., Lewis, P.J., Lavers, J.L., Crosbie, N.D., Pozo, K. and Clarke, B.O. 2017. A review of analytical techniques for quantifying microplastics in sediments. *Analytical Methods*, 9(9):1369–1383.

Hinderliter, P.M., Mylchreest, E., Gannon, S.A., Butenhoff, J.L. and Kennedy Jr, G.L. 2005. Perfluorooctanoate: placental and lactational transport pharmacokinetics in rats. *Toxicology*, 211(1–2): 139–148.

Kantiani, L., Llorca, M., Sanchís, J., Farré, M. and Barceló, D. 2010. Emerging food contaminants: a review. *Analytical and Bioanalytical Chemistry*, 398(6): 2413–2427.

Karlovsky, P., Suman, M., Berthiller, F., De Meester, J., Eisenbrand, G., Perrin, I., Oswald, I.P., Speijers, G., Chiodini, A., Recker, T. and Dussort, P. 2016. Impact of food processing and detoxification treatments on mycotoxin contamination. *Mycotoxin Research*, 32(4): 179–205.

Kärrman, A., Ericson, I., van Bavel, B., Darnerud, P.O., Aune, M., Glynn, A., Lignell, S. and Lindström, G. 2007. Exposure of perfluorinated chemicals through lactation: levels of matched human milk and serum and a temporal trend, 1996–2004, in Sweden. *Environmental Health Perspectives*, 115(2): 226–230.

Lei, M., Zhang, L., Lei, J., Zong, L., Li, J., Wu, Z. and Wang, Z. 2015. Overview of emerging contaminants and associated human health effects. *BioMed Research International*, 2015. https://doi.org/10.1155/2015/404796

Li, X.F. and Mitch, W.A. 2018. Drinking water disinfection byproducts (DBPs) and human health effects: multidisciplinary challenges and opportunities. *Environmental Science and Technology*, 52(4): 1681–89.

Midasch, O., Drexler, H., Hart, N., Beckmann, M.W. and Angerer, J. 2007. Transplacental exposure of neonates to perfluorooctanesulfonate and perfluorooctanoate: a pilot study. *International Archives of Occupational and Environmental Health*, 80(7): 643–648.

Murnyak, G., Vandenberg, J., Yaroschak, P.J., Williams, L., Prabhakaran, K. and Hinz, J. 2011. Emerging contaminants: presentations at the 2009 Toxicology and Risk Assessment Conference. *Toxicology and Applied Pharmacology*, 254(2): 167–169.

Newell, D.G., Koopmans, M., Verhoef, L., Duizer, E., Aidara-Kane, A., Sprong, H., Opsteegh, M., Langelaar, M., Threfall, J., Scheutz, F. and van der Giessen, J. 2010. Food-borne diseases: the challenges of 20 years ago still persist while new ones continue to emerge. *International Journal of Food Microbiology*, 139(Supplement 1): S3–S15.

Pandey, D., Singh, A., Ramanathan, A. and Kumar, M. 2020. The combined exposure of microplastics and toxic contaminants in the floodplains of north India: a review. *Journal of Environmental Management*, 279(1): 111557. https://doi.org/10.1016/j.jenvman.2020.111557.

Peng, G., Xu, P., Zhu, B., Bai, M. and Li, D. 2018. Microplastics in freshwater river sediments in Shanghai, China: a case study of risk assessment in mega-cities. *Environmental Pollution*, 234: 448–456.

Rainieri, S. and Barranco, A., 2019. Microplastics, a food safety issue? *Trends in Food Science & Technology*, 84: 55–57.

Rather, I.A., Koh, W.Y., Paek, W.K. and Lim, J. 2017. The sources of chemical contaminants in food and their health implications. *Frontiers in Pharmacology*, 8: 830.

Richardson, S.D. 2003. Disinfection by-products and other emerging contaminants in drinking water." *TrAC: Trends in Analytical Chemistry*, 22(10): 666–84.

Richardson, S. D. 2009. Water analysis: emerging contaminants and current issues. *Analytical Chemistry*, 81(12): 4645–77.

Sharma, Rajan and Gargi Ghoshal. 2018. Emerging trends in food packaging. In *Nutrition and Food Science*. Emerald Group Publishing Ltd. https://doi.org/10.1108/NFS-02-2018-0051

Shim, W.J., Hong, S.H. and Eo, S.E. 2017. Identification methods in microplastic analysis: a review. *Analytical Methods*, 9(9): 1384–1391.

So, M.K., Yamashita, N., Taniyasu, S., Jiang, Q., Giesy, J.P., Chen, K. and Lam, P.K.S. 2006. Health risks in infants associated with exposure to perfluorinated compounds in human breast milk from Zhoushan, China. *Environmental Science & Technology*, 40(9): 2924–2929.

Sørensen, S.R., Holtze, M.S., Simonsen, A. and Aamand, J. 2007. Degradation and mineralization of nanomolar concentrations of the herbicide dichlobenil and its persistent metabolite 2, 6-dichlorobenzamide by Aminobacter spp. isolated from dichlobenil-treated soils. *Applied and Environmental Microbiology*, 73(2): 399–406.

Stahl, T., Mattern, D. and Brunn, H. 2011. Toxicology of perfluorinated compounds. *Environmental Sciences Europe*, 23(1): 1–52.

Sy, A.M., Kumar, S.R., Steinberg, J., Garcia-Buitrago, M.T. and Benitez, L.R.A. 2020. Liver damage due to hypervitaminosis. *ACG Case Reports Journal*, 7(7): e00431.

Thapa, S.P., Shrestha, S. and Anal, A.K. 2020. Addressing the antibiotic resistance and improving the food safety in food supply chain (farm-to-fork) in Southeast Asia. *Food Control*, 108: 106809.

Thomaidis, N.S. and Asimakopoulos, A.G. 2012. Emerging contaminants: a tutorial mini review. *Global NEST Journal*, 14(1): 72–79.

Yang, M., Liberatore, H.K. and Zhang, X. 2019. Current methods for analyzing drinking water disinfection byproducts. *Current Opinion in Environmental Science & Health*, 7: 98–107.

Zwiener, C. and Richardson, S.D., 2005. Analysis of disinfection by-products in drinking water by LC–MS and related MS techniques. *TrAC: Trends in Analytical Chemistry*, 24(7): 613–621.

# Index